IARC Handbooks of Cancer Prevention

Volume 8

Fruit and Vegetables

IARC Handbooks of Cancer Prevention
Programme Head: Harri Vainio

Volume 8:

Editors: Harri Vainio, M.D., Ph.D.
Franca Bianchini, Ph.D

Technical editor: John Cheney, Ph.D

Bibliographic assistance: Annick Rivoire

Photographic assistance: Georges Mollon

Layout: Josephine Thévenoux

Printed by: LIPS, Lyon, France

Publisher: IARC*Press*
International Agency for Research on Cancer
150 cours Albert Thomas, 69372, Lyon, France
Tel. +33 4 72 73 84 85
Fax. +33 4 72 73 83 19

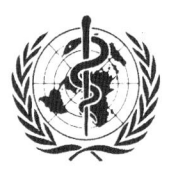

WORLD HEALTH ORGANIZATION

INTERNATIONAL AGENCY FOR RESEARCH ON CANCER

IARC Handbooks of Cancer Prevention

Volume 8

Fruit and Vegetables

IARC*Press*

Lyon, 2003

Published by the International Agency for Research on Cancer,
150 cours Albert Thomas, F-69372 Lyon cedex 08, France

© International Agency for Research on Cancer, 2003

Distributed by Oxford University Press, Walton Street, Oxford, OX2 6DP, UK (Fax: +44 1865 267782) and in the USA by Oxford University Press, 2001 Evans Road, Carey, NC 27513, USA (Fax: +1 919 677 1303).
All IARC publications can also be ordered directly from IARC*Press*
(Fax: +33 4 72 73 83 02; E-mail: press@iarc.fr)
and in the USA from IARC*Press*, WHO Office, Suite 480, 1775 K Street, Washington DC, 20006

Publications of the World Health Organization enjoy copyright protection in
accordance with the provisions of Protocol 2 of the Universal Copyright Convention.
All rights reserved.

The designations used and the presentation of the material in this publication do not imply the
expression of any opinion whatsoever on the part of the Secretariat of the World Health Organization
concerning the legal status of any country, territory, city, or area or of its authorities,
or concerning the delimitation of its frontiers or boundaries.

The mention of specific companies or of certain manufacturers' products does not imply
that they are endorsed or recommended by the World Health Organization in preference to others
of a similar nature that are not mentioned. Errors and omissions excepted,
the names of proprietary products are distinguished by initial capital letters.

The authors alone are responsible for the views expressed in this publication.

The International Agency for Research on Cancer welcomes requests for permission to
reproduce or translate its publications, in part or in full. Applications and enquiries should be addressed
to the Communications Unit, International Agency for Research on Cancer,
which will be glad to provide the latest information on any changes made to the text, plans for new
editions, and reprints and translations already available.

IARC Library Cataloguing in Publication Data

Fruit and vegetables/
   IARC Working Group on the Evaluation of
   Cancer-Preventive Strategies (2003 : Lyon, France)

(IARC handbooks of cancer prevention ; 8)

1. Neoplasms – prevention & control 2. Fruit 3. Vegetables   I. IARC Working Group on the Evaluation of Cancer Preventive Strategies. II. Series

ISBN 92 832 3008 6   (NLM Classification: W1)
ISSN 1027-5622

Printed in France

International Agency For Research On Cancer

The International Agency for Research on Cancer (IARC) was established in 1965 by the World Health Assembly, as an independently financed organization within the framework of the World Health Organization. The headquarters of the Agency are in Lyon, France.

The Agency conducts a programme of research concentrating particularly on the epidemiology of cancer and the study of potential carcinogens in the human environment. Its field studies are supplemented by biological and chemical research carried out in the Agency's laboratories in Lyon and, through collaborative research agreements, in national research institutions in many countries. The Agency also conducts a programme for the education and training of personnel for cancer research.

The publications of the Agency contribute to the dissemination of authoritative information on different aspects of cancer research. Information about IARC publications, and how to order them, is available via the Internet at: http://www.iarc.fr/

> This publication represents the views and opinions of an IARC Working Group on the Evaluation of Cancer-Preventive Strategies which met in Lyon, France, March 4–11, 2003

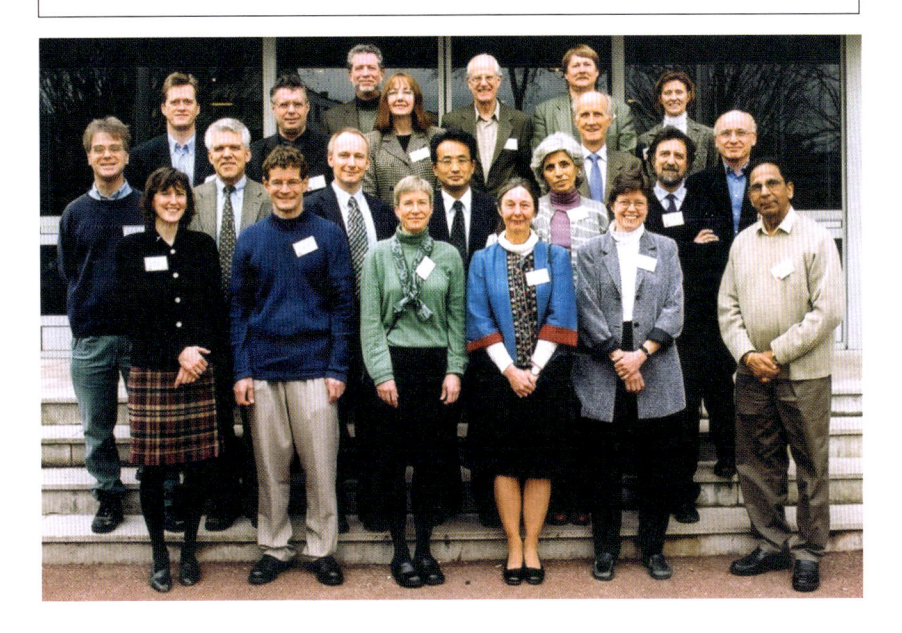

From left to right:
Front: S. Smith-Warner; J. Little; J.W. Lampe; J. Pennington; J. Freudenheim; B. Reddy
Middle: T. Key; T. Byers; L. Dragsted; S. Tsugane; A. Ferro-Luzzi; P. Vineis; F. Levi
Back: P.A. van den Brandt; G. Alink; A. Schatzkin; A. Wolk; A.B. Miller; H. Boeing; P. Elmer

Note to the Reader

Anyone who is aware of published data that may influence any consideration in these *Handbooks* is encouraged to make the information available to the Unit of Chemoprevention, International Agency for Research on Cancer, 150 Cours Albert Thomas, 69372 Lyon Cedex 08, France

Although all efforts are made to prepare the *Handbooks* as accurately as possible, mistakes may occur. Readers are requested to communicate any errors to the Unit of Chemoprevention, so that corrections can be reported in future volumes.

Acknowledgements

We would like to acknowledge generous support from the Foundation for Promotion of Cancer Research, Japan (the 2nd Term Comprehensive 10-Year Strategy for Cancer Control), and from the World Cancer Research Fund, London, United Kingdom (WCRF Grant 2001/45).

Contents

List of participants ix
Preface xi

1. **Definitions and classifications for fruit and vegetables**
   Botanical and culinary definitions 1
      Botanical definitions 1
      Culinary definitions 2
      Cultural differences in culinary definitions ... 3
      Summary of definition issues 3
   Subgroup classifications for plants, fruit and vegetables 4
      Botanical families 5
      Growing conditions 9
      Fruit development from flowers 9
      Food supply and consumption data 13
      Edible parts of plants 13
      Colour 14
      Processing and preparation 14
   Considerations for epidemiological studies 18
      Fruit and vegetable groupings used in dietary assessment tools 18
      Fruit and vegetable groupings familiar to survey participants 19

2. **Measuring intake of fruit and vegetables**
   Household measures of food availability 23
      Household dietary surveys 23
      Household budget surveys 23
      Food balance sheets 23
   Methods to measure dietary intake at the individual level 24
      Questionnaire methods 24
         Diet history 25
         Food frequency questionnaire 25
         Brief food frequency questionnaires 27
      Recording-based measures of actual intake .. 27
         The 24-hour dietary recall 27
         Food records 28
   Quantification of fruit and vegetable portions ... 28
   Measurement error and validity 29
      Sources of error 29
      Validity 29
   Effects of dietary measurement error 30
      Approaches to evaluating impact of dietary assessment error 32
      Estimated validity of measured fruit and vegetable consumption 32

3. **Consumption, availability and food policies**
   Fruit and vegetable consumption 35
      Categories of fruit and of vegetables 35
      Age and sex groupings 36
      National surveys 36
      Selected multi-centre studies 37
      Developing countries 40
      Availability and time trends in large regions .. 40
      Variations within countries 41
   Nutrition and food policies and special campaigns 45
      Historical perspective 45
      Current policy and dietary guidelines 46
      Programmes to implement dietary guidelines and nutrition policy 47
      Recommended amounts of fruit and vegetables 47
      Campaigns to increase fruit and vegetable intake 48
         5 A Day Program—USA 49
         Australia 51
         Europe 51

4. **Cancer-preventive effects**
   Human studies 53
      General issues 53
         Study design 53
         Statistical analysis 60
         Study context 61
         Integration of evidence 61
      Effects by site 62
         Grouped sites of the upper gastrointestinal tract 62
         Oral cavity and pharynx 62
         Oesophagus 63
         Stomach 66
         Colon and rectum 72
         Liver 76
         Biliary tract 78
         Pancreas 78
         Larynx 79
         Lung 81
         Breast 84

Table of contents

    Cervix 89
    Endometrium 92
    Ovary 92
    Prostate 94
    Testis 95
    Bladder 95
    Kidney 98
    Brain 101
    Thyroid 101
    Non-Hodgkin lymphoma 103
    Leukaemia 103
  Preventable fraction 246
  Ecological studies 246
    Cross-sectional studies between countries 248
    Cross-sectional studies between regions within countries 248
    Time trend studies 252
    Migrant studies 252
    Summary 252
  Intermediate markers of cancer 252
    Intervention studies 254
    Observational studies 272
  Experimental studies 272
    Animal studies 272
      Effects on spontaneous tumours 272
      Effects on carcinogen-induced tumours . 280
    Biomarkers 286
      Effects on phase I and II enzymes 286
      Inhibition of damage to macromolecules 289
      Oxidative damage and defence 290
      Effects on mutation and DNA strand breaks 292
      Effects on DNA repair 292
      Intermediary markers related to the cell cycle 292
  Mechanisms of cancer prevention 293
    Inhibition of endogenous carcinogen formation 293
      Inhibition of radical formation 293
      Inhibition of nitrosation 294
    Modulation of carcinogen bioavailability ... 294
    Modulation of enzyme systems 294
      Phase I and II enzymes 294
      Antioxidant enzymes 296
    Inhibition of damage to macromolecules ... 297
      Decreased oxidative damage to lipids, proteins and DNA 297

      Decreased carcinogen–DNA binding or increased DNA repair 297
      Decreased mutation or cytogenetic damage 298
    Post-initiation effects 299
      Modulation of cell proliferation or apoptosis 299
      Immune function 299

5. Associations with diseases other than cancer
  Cardiovascular diseases 301
  Other diseases 302

6. Carcinogenic effects
  Human studies 311
  Animal studies 311

7. Toxic effects
  Human studies 313
  Animal studies 313

8. Summary of data
  Definitions and classifications for fruit and vegetables 315
  Measuring intake of fruit and vegetables 315
  Consumption of fruit and vegetables and relevant policies 316
  Cancer-preventive effects 316
    Human studies 316
    Experimental studies 320
    Mechanisms of cancer prevention 321
  Associations with diseases other than cancer . 321
  Carcinogenic effects 321
  Toxic effects 321

9. Evaluation
  Cancer-preventive activity 323
    Humans 323
    Experimental animals 323
  Overall evaluation 323

10. Recommendations
  Research recommendations 325
  Public health recommendations 326

References 327

Working procedures 369

List of participants

G. Alink
Division of Toxicology
Wageningen University
Tuinlaan 5
6703 HE Wageningen
The Netherlands

H. Boeing
German Institute of Human Nutrition
Department of Epidemiology
Arthur Scheunert Allee 114–116
14558 Potsdam-Rehbruecke
Germany

T. Byers
Department Preventive Medicine & Biometrics
University of Colorado School of Medicine
Box C245
4200 East Ninth Avenue
Denver CO 80262
USA

L.O. Dragsted
Institute of Food Safety and Nutrition
Danish Veterinary & Food Administration
19 Morkjoj Bygade
2860 Soborg
Denmark

P.J. Elmer
Center for Health Research
Division of Epidemiology & Disease Prevention
3800 N. Interstate Avenue
Portland OR 97227
USA

A. Ferro-Luzzi
WHO Collaborating Centre
National Institute of Research for Food & Nutrition
INRAN
Via Ardeatina 546
00178 Rome
Italy

J.L. Freudenheim
Department of Social & Preventive Medicine
University at Buffalo
3434 Main Street
Buffalo NY 14214–0001
USA

T. Key
Cancer Research UK
Epidemiology Unit
University of Oxford
Gibson Building
Radcliffe Infirmary
Oxford OX2 6HE
UK

J.W. Lampe
Cancer Prevention Research Program
Fred Hutchinson Cancer Research Center
1100 Fairview Avenue North
MP-900
Seattle WA 98109
USA

F. Levi
Registre Vaudois
Unité d'Epidémiologie du Cancer
Univ. de Médecine Sociale & Préventive
CHUV-Falaises 1
1011 Lausanne
Switzerland

J. Little *(Vice-Chairman)*
Epidemiology Group
Department of Medicine & Therapeutics
University of Aberdeen
Foresterhill
Aberdeen AB25 2ZD
UK

A.J. McMichael *(Chairman)*
The Australian National University
National Centre for Epidemiology and Population Health
Canberra ACT 0200
Australia

A.B. Miller
Deutches Krebsforschungszentrum
Division of Clinical Epidemiology
Im Neuenheimer Feld 280
69120 Heidelberg
Germany

J. Pennington
National Institutes of Health
Division of Nutrition Research Coordination
6707 Democracy Boulevard,
Room 629,
Bethesda, MD 20892-5461
USA

B.S. Reddy
Division of Nutritional Carcinogenesis
Institute for Cancer Prevention
1 Dana Road
Valhalla NY 10595
USA

IARC Handbooks of Cancer Prevention Volume 8: Fruit and Vegetables

R. Saracci
IFC-National Research Council
Division of Epidemiology
Via Trieste 41
56100 Pisa
Italy

A. Schatzkin
National Cancer Institute/NIH
Nutritional Epidemiological Branch
EPS 3040
6120 Executive Boulevard
Bethesda, MD 20852-7232
USA

S. Smith-Warner
Harvard School of Public Health
Department of Nutrition
665 Huntington Avenue
Boston MA 02115
USA

G. Stoner*
School of Public Health
Ohio State University
1148 CHRI
300 W. 10th Avenue
Colombus OH 43210-1240
USA

S. Tsugane
National Cancer Center Research
Institute East
Epidemiology and Biostatistics
Division
6-5-1 Kashiwanoha
Kashiwa
Chiba 277-8577
Japan

P.A. van den Brandt
Maastricht University
Department of Epidemiology
P.O. Box 616
6200 MD Maastricht
The Netherlands

P. Vineis
University of Turin
Department of Biomedical Science &
Human Oncology
Unit of Cancer Epidemiology
Via Santena 7
10126 Turin
Italy

A. Wolk
Karolinska Institutet
National Institute of Environmental
Medicine
Division of Nutritional Epidemiology
Box 210
171 77 Stockholm
Sweden

Observers

World Cancer Research Fund International

L. Miles
Scientific Officer
19 Harley Street
London
WIG 9QJ
UK

M. Wiseman
19 Harley Street
London
WIG 9QJ
UK

WHO

I. Keller
Noncommunicable Diseases and
Mental Health
Nutrition and NCD Prevention
World Health Organization
CH-1211 Geneva 27
Switzerland

A. Ullrich
Cancer Control Programme
World Health Organization
CH-1211 Geneva 27
Switzerland

European Cancer League

M. Rautalahti
Chief Medical Officer
Liisankatu 21 B
FIN-00170
Helsinki
Finland

Secretariat

W. Al-Delaimy
F. Bianchini
J. Cheney
P. Ferrari
S. Franceschi
M. Friesen
Y. Grosse
R. Kaaks
T. Norat
E. Riboli
T. Sawa
B. Secretan
N. Slimani
K. Soldan
K. Straif
H. Vainio
E. Weiderpass-Vainio

Technical assistance

S. Egraz
B. Kajo
J. Mitchell
A. Rivoire
J. Thévenoux

*Unable to attend

Preface
Why a Handbook on fruit and vegetables ?

Nutritional research and food policy have shifted focus during the last hundred years. In the early 1900s the focus was on identifying and preventing nutrient deficiency diseases; in the latter part of the last century the attention was on identifying nutrient requirements. More recently, investigations have turned to the role of diet in maintaining health and reducing the risk of non-communicable diseases, such as heart diseases and osteoporosis.

All types of diet have potential health risks as well as benefits associated with their consumption, both at the individual and collective level. During the past 30 years, while meat intake has been associated with increased risk for a variety of chronic diseases such as ischaemic heart disease and some cancers, abundant consumption of fruit and vegetables, legumes, unrefined cereals have been associated with a lower risk for many chronic degenerative diseases and total mortality (see WHO, 2003).

The low consumption of fruit and vegetables in many regions of the world, especially in the developing part, is a persistent phenomenon. Only a small or negligible minority of the world's population at present consumes the generally recommended high average intakes of fruit and vegetables. In 1998, only six of the 14 WHO regions had an availability of fruit and vegetables equal to or greater than the recommended intakes of 400 g/d (WHO, 2003).

Nutritional epidemiology provides the only direct approach to the assessment of health effects from diet in humans. There are special problems associated with the measurement of diet, including fruit and vegetable intake, particularly in case–control studies. However, in prospective studies within single populations, where there is little dietary variation between individuals, large measurement error can be associated with each assessment.

In 1997, scientists assembled by the World Cancer Research Fund (WCRF) and the American Institute for Cancer Research (AICR) concluded that diets rich in fruits and vegetables 'decreased the risk of many cancers', and perhaps cancer in general and they endorsed fruit and vegetables as parts of a diet that would reduce risk of various cancers (WCRF/AICR, 1997).

This evaluation originated mainly from the results of case–control studies. Since then, the messages have been clouded by more recent prospective cohort studies that found that such diets may not be protective against cancer. As these newer findings have introduced doubt about the role of fruit and vegetables in cancer prevention, the IARC has considered it important to make a new evidence-based evaluation of the current state of the evidence of a diet rich in fruit and vegetables.

The purpose of this *IARC Handbook* is to provide an up-to-date review of knowledge about fruit and vegetables collectively. Since various types of fruit and vegetables, such as cruciferous vegetables, allium vegetables and citrus fruits, have also been investigated separately, specialist panels will be convened later to look into the evidence concerning these specific categories separately, including the evidence on their main individual chemical components. The first such *Handbook* will consider cruciferous vegetables, isothiocyanates and indoles, and will be published in 2004.

Chapter 1
Definitions and classifications for fruit and vegetables

Botanical and culinary definitions

Botanical definitions
Broadly, the botanical term *fruit* refers to the mature ovary of a plant, including its seeds, covering and any closely connected tissue, without any consideration of whether these are edible. As related to food, the botanical term *fruit* refers to the edible part of a plant that consists of the seeds and surrounding tissues. This includes fleshy fruits (such as blueberries, cantaloupe, peach, pumpkin, tomato) and dry fruits, where the ripened ovary wall becomes papery, leathery, or woody as with cereal grains, pulses (mature beans and peas) and nuts.

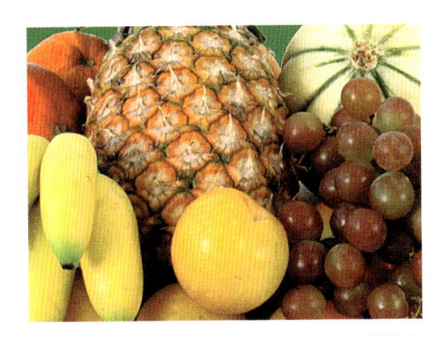

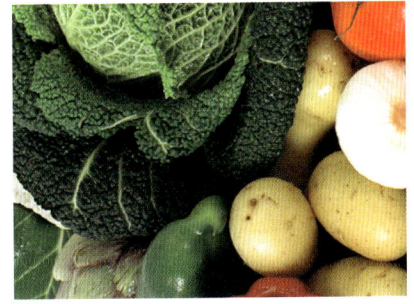

In the broadest sense, the botanical term *vegetable* refers to any plant, edible or not, including trees, bushes, vines and vascular plants, and distinguishes plant material from animal material and from inorganic matter. There are two slightly different botanical definitions for the term *vegetable* as it relates to food. According to one, a vegetable is a *plant* cultivated for its edible part(s); according to the other, a vegetable is the *edible part(s) of a plant,* such as the stems and stalk (celery), root (carrot), tuber (potato), bulb (onion), leaves (spinach, lettuce), flower (globe artichoke), fruit (apple, cucumber, pumpkin, strawberries, tomato) or seeds (beans, peas). The latter definition includes fruits as a subset of vegetables.

Definition of fruit and vegetables applicable in epidemiological studies

Fruit and vegetables

Edible plant foods excluding cereal grains, nuts, seeds, tea leaves, coffee beans, cacao beans, herbs and spices

Fruit

Edible parts of plants that contain the seeds and pulpy surrounding tissue; have a sweet or tart taste; generally consumed as breakfast beverages, breakfast and lunch side-dishes, snacks or desserts

Vegetables

Edible plant parts including stems and stalks, roots, tubers, bulbs, leaves, flowers and fruits; usually includes seaweed and sweet corn; may or may not include pulses or mushrooms; generally consumed raw or cooked with a main dish, in a mixed dish, as an appetizer or in a salad

Whether mushrooms and seaweed (foods commonly used as vegetables) are regarded as part of the plant kingdom depends on the choice of one out of four schemes used to classify living organisms into kingdoms. The traditional scheme of two kingdoms (plant and animal) places fungi and algae (sources of food mushrooms and seaweed, respectively) in the plant kingdom. In the other three schemes, the fungi and algae are placed either together in the Protista kingdom or separately in the Protista and fungi kingdoms (Stern, 1988).

Culinary definitions

The main culinary groupings for edible plant materials are fruit, vegetables, cereal grains, nuts, and seeds. (Minor groupings include herbs or spices and plant parts used to make coffee, tea and chocolate). Populations are accustomed to these culinary groupings and use them to communicate about plant foods and to distinguish the types of plant food used in meals. These culinary groupings are used in households for meal planning and preparation, in educational settings where nutrition professionals communicate cooking skills and dietary advice to consumers, in the market place, where people purchase plant foods for home use, and in restaurants, where people order and consume prepared foods.

The culinary term *fruit and vegetables* may be defined as edible plant foods excluding cereal grains, nuts, seeds, coffee, tea, cacao and herbs and spices. Domel *et al.* (1993b) provided a similar but more detailed definition for fruit and vegetables, noting the exclusion of nuts, seeds, peanuts, peanut butter, grains and vegetables when used as grains and the inclusion of olives, avocados, pickles, coconut and products and mixed dishes that contain any amount of fruit and vegetable. They also provided a narrow definition of fruit and vegetables that has specific conditions relating to macronutrient content, processing and serving sizes, but this definition is not practical for use in relation to epidemiological studies.

The culinary term *fruit* refers to the edible part of a plant, tree, bush or vine that contains the seeds and pulpy surrounding tissue and has a sweet or tart taste. In essence, culinary fruits are the subset of botanical fruits that remains after excluding cereal grains (wheat, rye, oats, barley), nuts, seeds and fruits used as vegetables. Fruits are used as a breakfast beverage or side-dish (for example, orange juice, berries, grapefruit, melon), lunch side-dish or dessert, snack food between meals or dinner dessert. Raw and canned fruits are also used as appetizers, salad ingredients and side-dishes.

The culinary term *vegetable* refers to edible part(s) of a plant consumed raw or cooked, generally with a main dish, in a mixed dish, as an appetizer or in a salad. Vegetables include edible stems and stalks, roots, tubers, bulbs, leaves, flowers, some fruits, pulses (mature beans and peas), fungi (mushrooms, truffles), algae (seaweed) and sweet corn and hominy (cereal grains used as vegetables). The culinary term *vegetable* excludes other cereal grains, nuts, peanuts (a type of pulse) and culinary fruits. The distinction as to which botanical fruits are considered to be culinary vegetables depends on cultural use in meal patterns and the flavours they impart. Botanical fruits used as vegetables (e.g., eggplant, okra, zucchini) tend to be savory in taste, while those used as fruits are generally sweet (due to a higher sugar concentration) or tart as in cranberries, lemons and limes (due to a higher acid content).

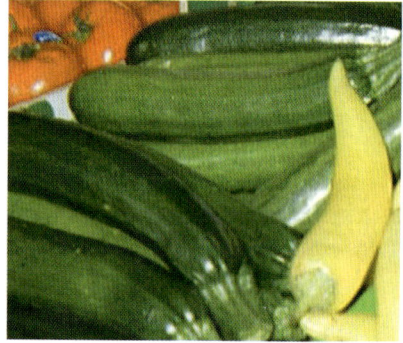

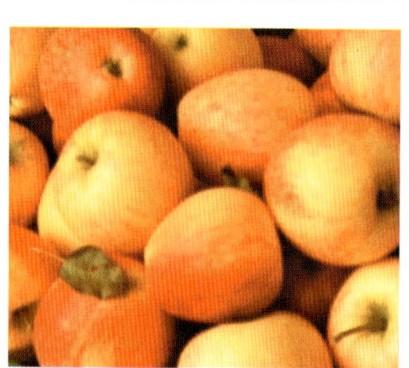

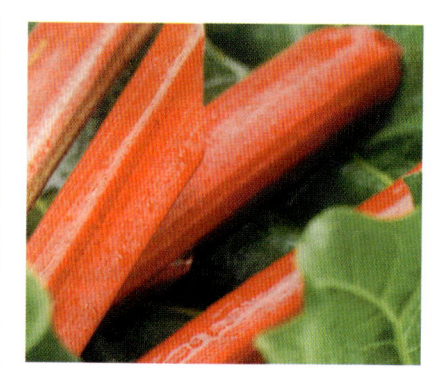

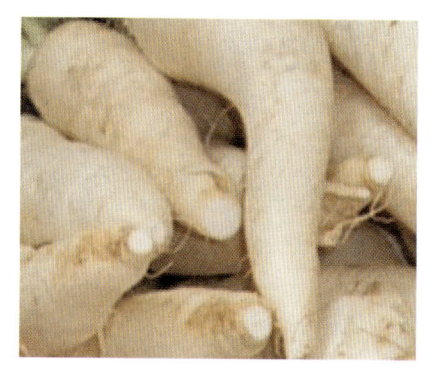

Definitions and classifications for fruit and vegetables

Cultural differences in culinary definitions

Culinary distinctions as to which plant parts are used as fruits and vegetables (and which are designated as fruits and which as vegetables) are based on traditional use and tend to be imprecise, varying within and between cultures. Information about which foods serve as fruits and vegetables is generally presented in books on cookery and in food guides that are developed for consumers by government public health agencies or by professional nutrition associations. Food guides are used by nutrition educators to communicate the types and quantities of foods that should be consumed on a daily basis to meet nutrient needs, prevent deficiency diseases and lower the risk for diet-related chronic diseases.

A recent comparison of food guides used in Australia, China, Canada, Germany, Korea (Republic of), Mexico, the Philippines, Portugal, Puerto Rico, Sweden, the United Kingdom and the United States (USA) revealed that despite the cultural differences in dietary patterns, food groupings (cereal grains, vegetables, fruit, meat and meat substitutes, dairy products, fats and sweets) are generally similar (Painter et al., 2002). Fruit and vegetables appear as a single group in six food guides (Canada, China, Korea, Portugal, Mexico and the United Kingdom), but are separate groups in the other guides. All the guides separate nuts, seeds and cereal grain products from fruit and vegetables.

There are differences in the placement of starchy root and tuber vegetables and pulses between the guides. Six of the guides (Australia, Canada, China, the Philippines, Puerto Rico and the USA) group potatoes in the vegetable group. Germany, Korea, Mexico, Portugal and the United Kingdom group potatoes in the grain group, but place other root and tuber vegetables such as turnips and parsnips in the vegetable group. Potatoes might be grouped with grains because, like grain products, they are starchy, inexpensive, readily available and commonly consumed. The Swedish food guide has a separate food group for potatoes and other root vegetables and recommends that root vegetables be the foundation for a daily inexpensive diet supplemented with other vegetables that vary from day to day and between seasons.

Seven of the guides place pulses in the meat group because of their protein content; Australia, Germany and Sweden put pulses in the vegetable group because of their vitamin, mineral and dietary fibre content. The US food guide places immature pulses in the vegetable group and mature pulses in the meat, poultry and fish group. The Chinese guide places pulses (primarily soybeans and soymilk) in the milk and dairy products group. A food guide for vegetarians and vegans (Venti & Johnston, 2002), places beans in a protein group and provides separate groups for dark green leafy vegetables and dried fruit to encourage use of sources of iron and other minerals that are usually obtained from meat.

Foods derived from fruit and vegetables such as preserves, jams and jellies, sugared fruit pieces used as candies, and sweet cucumber pickles fit into the sweets or sugars group of food guides. Food guides do not have groupings for mixed dishes or desserts that contain fruit or vegetables, for condiments or snack foods that are derived from fruit or vegetables, or for herbs and spices.

Summary of definition issues

Botanical definitions for fruit and vegetables are more precise than culinary definitions. However, culinary definitions are based on cultural uses of foods and are more commonly under-

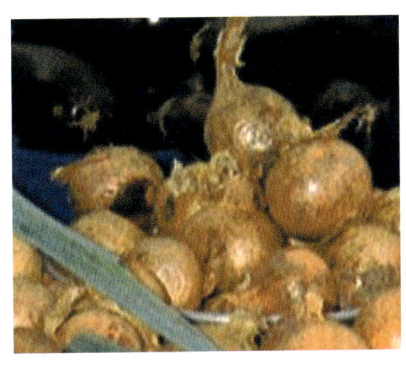

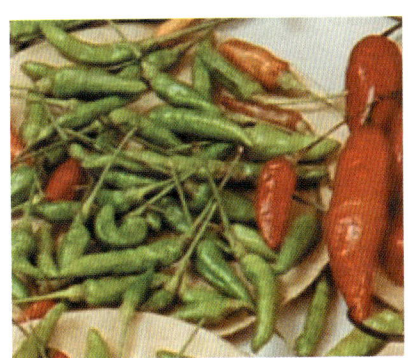

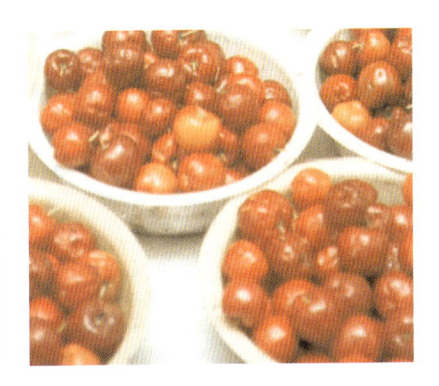

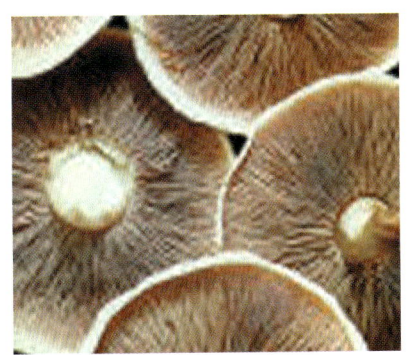

3

stood by nutrition researchers and by participants in epidemiological studies. The following botanical and culinary issues may affect the grouping of fruits, vegetables, mixed dishes and desserts containing fruits and vegetables, and foods derived from fruits and vegetables:

- Mushrooms (fungi) and seaweed (algae) are commonly considered to be vegetables because of their culinary use. However, botanically, they may or may not be considered to be derived from plants, depending on the scheme used to classify organisms into kingdoms.
- In some cultures, potatoes and other starchy root and tuber vegetables (e.g., taro) are separated from other vegetables and considered to be a separate group or part of the grain group.
- Pulses (mature beans and peas) may be considered as meat alternatives (substitutes) rather than vegetables (or in addition to being vegetables) in some cultures. Products derived from soybeans such as tofu and soy-based meat substitutes are often grouped with high-protein foods (meat, fish, poultry, eggs, nuts and seeds), rather than with vegetables. Soymilk is usually classified in the milk group, with the assumption that it is fortified with calcium.
- Peanuts (groundnuts) are a type of pulse with various cultural uses (e.g., snack food, part of a main dish, boiled side-dish, peanut butter, or peanut sauce). Peanuts are usually considered to be nuts and grouped with the high-protein foods.
- Fresh or sweet corn and hominy are cereal grains, but are generally used as vegetables (i.e., side-dishes with a dinner meal). Mature corn (also known as field corn or maize) is generally used as a cereal grain in the form of corn grits, corn meal or corn flour. Corn meal and flour are used to make cornbread, tortillas and tortilla chips.
- Although most fruits and vegetables are low in fat, several (avocados, coconut, olives) have higher fat content and varied uses in cuisines. Food guides do not provide sufficient detail to indicate where these foods are grouped. Avocados and olives may be grouped with fruit, vegetables or fats. Coconut may be grouped with nuts, fruit (e.g., cut or shredded in a fruit salad) or vegetables (e.g., used in stews mixed with meats and other vegetables).
- Herbs (e.g., coriander, parsley) include the stems and leaves of plants, and some vegetables (e.g., garlic and chili peppers) are used as spices or garnishes. Herbs and spices are not included in food guides, mainly due to the small amounts used, but they may contribute important food components and should not be ignored in terms of dietary assessment.
- Fruits and vegetables that are part of mixed dishes (i.e., main dishes or desserts) may be overlooked when assessing total fruit and vegetable intake. Food guides do not have groupings for mixed dishes (meat and vegetable casseroles, stews, stir-fries) or desserts that may contain fruits or vegetables (chocolate-covered raisins, fig bars, fruit pies, pumpkin pie, carrot cake).
- Some food products derived from fruit and vegetables may not retain the nutritive value of the original fruit and vegetable and may contain added fat or sugar. Food guides usually group jams, jellies, and fruit drinks (lemonade, fruit punches) with the sweets or sugars food group, but it is not clear where potato crisps, fried potatoes or pickled fruits or vegetables are grouped.

Subgroup classifications for plants, fruit and vegetables

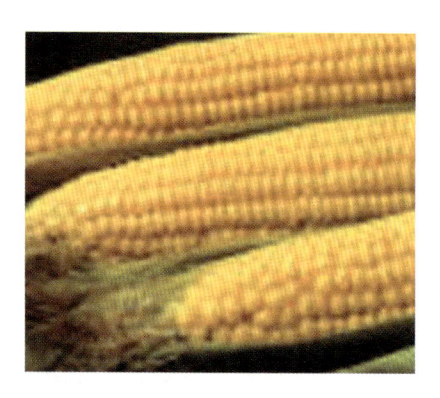

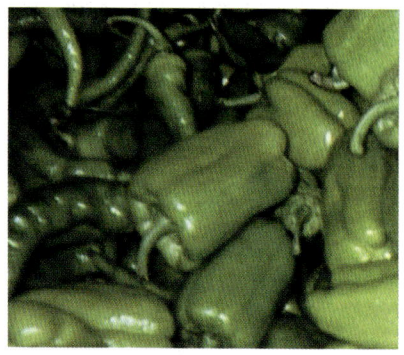

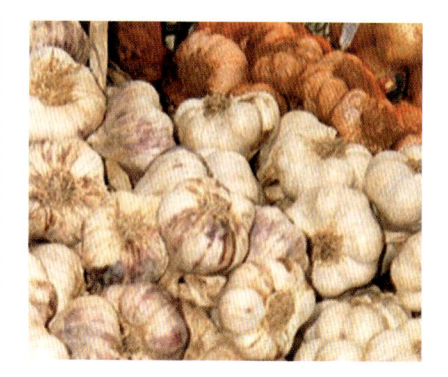

Subgroup classifications for plants, fruits and vegetables according to their content of food components can be useful for epidemiological studies. Because most fruit and vegetables have low calorie, fat, saturated fat and sodium content and are devoid of cholesterol, the classifications may focus more on vitamins, minerals and other bioactive components. Such classification is complicated by the large number of food components in fruit and vegetables, and by the facts that not all the components have yet been identified and that not all fruits and vegetables have been analysed to determine the level of the components that have been identified. Some components (dietary fibre, potassium, plant sterols) are present in most fruit and vegetables, while others (vitamin C, carotenoids, folacin (folic acid), iron, zinc, magnesium, calcium, flavonoids) occur mainly in specific fruits and vegetables. For many of the food components, the published data have not yet been aggregated and summarized and therefore have not been incorporated into food composition databases.

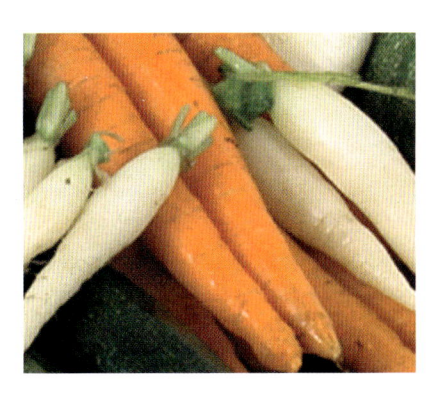

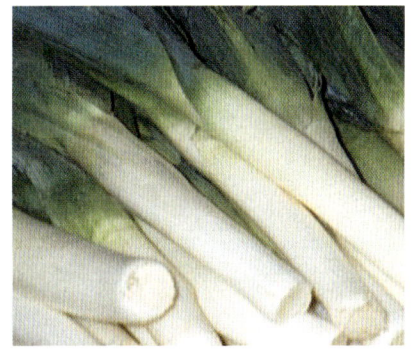

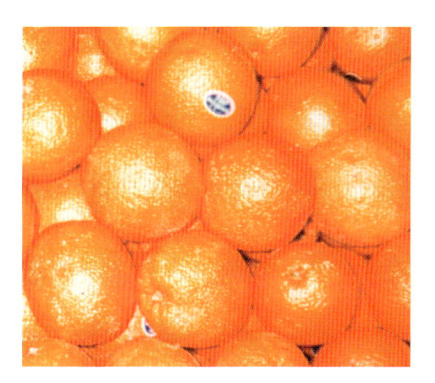

Table 1 lists selected vitamins and other bioactive components and their fruit and vegetable sources. Current food composition databases provide information about fruit and vegetable sources of β-carotene (dark green leafy vegetables, deep yellow and orange fruits and vegetables), vitamin C (citrus fruits, dark green leafy vegetables, cantaloupe) and folacin (dark green leafy vegetables, oranges, pulses). Food composition data and databases are beginning to be developed for other bioactive components such as glucosinolates, indoles and isothiocyanates in cruciferous vegetables (Fahey *et al.*, 2001); flavonols, flavones and other flavonoids (Hertog *et al.*, 1992, 1993b; Häkkinen *et al.*, 1999; Peterson & Dwyer, 2000; Sampson *et al.*, 2002); flavonoids and phenolic acids in fruit juices (Spanos & Wrolstad, 1992); flavonoids and carotenoids in citrus fruits (Ranganna *et al.*, 1983); carotenoids (Mangels *et al.*, 1993); isoflavones (Coward *et al.*, 1993; Wang & Murphy, 1994; USDA, 1999a); isoflavones, coumesterol and lignans (Boker *et al.*, 2002); phytoestrogens (Reinli & Block, 1996; Pillow *et al.*, 1999); and lemonoid glucosides in citrus juices (Fong *et al.*, 1989).

Several subgroup classifications for plants, fruits, and vegetables are considered below, to assess how they relate to the presence of nutrients and bioactive food components. The subgroups include botanical families and growing conditions for classifying plants and botanical fruit development terms for classifying fruit. Fruit and vegetable subgroups used for reporting food supply and consumption data are presented, as are subgroups based on edible parts, colour and processing and preparation.

Botanical families

Botanical classification of plants is based on the physiological characteristics of plant development, organization and structure. The 11 levels of botanical classification are kingdom, division, class, subclass, order, family, genus, species, variety, cultivar and strain. As an example, the 11 classification terms for the Gray zucchini summer squash are, respectively, Plant, Spermatophyta, Angiospermae, Dicotyledonae, Cucurbitales, Cucurbitaceae, Cucurbita, Pepo L., Melopepo Alef., Zucchini, and Gray (Yamaguchi, 1983). Botanical classification is useful for biologists to establish plant origins and relationships and to help identify plants across different cultures and languages; it is also useful for horticulturists because plants within a family may have similar climatic requirements, economic uses, and disease and insect controls. The usefulness of botanical classification in dietary assessment is less clear, because foods derived from the same botanical family may or may not contain similar levels of bioactive food components.

The plant kingdom (using the traditional two-kingdom scheme) has four divisions, of which three (Thallophyta, Pteridophyta and Spermatophyta) contain foods consumed by humans *(Encyclopedia Britannica,* 1974). Most human foods are within the Spermatophyta (seed

IARC Handbooks of Cancer Prevention Volume 8: Fruit and Vegetables

Table 1. Selected vitamins and other bioactive components in fruit and vegetables[a]

Vitamins

Folacin:
Avocado, orange; asparagus, black bean, black-eyed pea, Brussels sprout, chickpea, chives, endive, green pea, kidney bean, lentil, mustard greens, navy bean, okra, pinto bean, soybean, spinach, turnip greens

Vitamin C:
Blackberry, blueberry, cantaloupe, cranberry, elderberry, grapefruit, kiwi fruit, lemon, lime, mango, orange, papaya, peach, raspberry, strawberry, tangerine; broccoli, Brussels sprout, cabbage, cauliflower, kale, kohlrabi, spinach, sweet red/green pepper, tomato

Other bioactive components

Allyl sulfides:
   Allicin:
   Chives, garlic, leek, onion, shallot

Capsaicin:
Chili pepper

Carotenoids:
   α-carotene:
   Carrot, pumpkin, sweet potato
   β-carotene:
   Apricot, cantaloupe, guava, mango, peach, persimmon, red/pink, grapefruit; Arugula, asparagus, beetgreens, broccoli, Brussells sprouts, cabbage, carrot, cassava leaves, chicory, chili pepper, collards, cress, dandelion greens, fiddlehead greens, kale, mustard greens, pak-choy, pumpkin, sweet redpepper, romaine, spinach, sweet potato, Swiss chard, tomato, turnip greens, winter squash
   β-cryptoxanthin:
   Apple, apricot, avocado, cantaloupe, carambola, grape fruit, jackfruit, kiwifruit, kumquat, mango, olive, orange, papaya, passion fruit, peach, persimmon, plum, tangerine, watermelon; broccoli, corn, pumpkin, red pepper, tomato, winter squash
   Lycopene:
   Guava, red/pink grapefruit, watermelon; tomato
   Lutein:
   Kiwifruit, orange, tangerine, watermelon; asparagus, broccoli, Brussels sprouts, cabbage, carrot, collards, corn, kale, lettuce, potato, pumpkin, spinach, sweet red pepper, tomato, turnip greens

   Zeaxanthin:
   Orange, persimmon; collards, corn, kale, lettuce, pumpkin, red pepper, spinach, tangerine, turnip greens

Flavonoids[b]:

Anthocyanins:
Apple, blackberry, blackcurrant, blueberry, cherry, chokecherry, cranberry, elderberry, nectarine, peach, plum, raspberry, pomegranate, red grape, red/green pear, strawberry; asparagus, carrot, red cabbage, red onion, redbean; red wine

Flavanols:
Apple, apricot, nectarine, peach, pear, red grape, strawberry; green bean
   Catechins: Apple, blackberry, cranberry, elderberry, red-purple grape
   Epicatechin: Apple, red-purple grape
   Proanthocyanidins: Apple, blueberry, cranberry, red-purple grape, strawberry

Flavanones:
Grapefruit, lemon, orange; tomato
   Hesperidin: Grapefruit, lemon, lime, orange, tangerine
   Naringenin: Grapefruit
   Neohesperidin: Grapefruit, orange

Flavones:
Grapefruit, lemon, orange; carrot, celery, parsley sweet red/green pepper
   Apigenin:
   Carrot, celery
   Luteolin:
   Sweet red/green pepper

Flavonols:
Orange, red-purple grape; broccoli, Brussels sprouts, cauliflower, onion, turnip greens
   Quercetin: Apple, apricot, bilberry, blackberry, blackcurrant, blueberry, cherry, cranberry, elderberry, grapefruit, lemon, mango, peach, pear, plum, raspberry, red bilberry, redcurrant, red-purple grape, strawberry, whitecurrant; broccoli, cabbage, chives, corn, endive, kale, lettuce, pepper, red cabbage, red onion, string bean, sweet potato, tomato
   Myricetin: Apple, bilberry, blackcurrant, blueberry, cranberry, red-purple grape, red bilberry, redcurrant, whitecurrant; carrot
   Kaempferol: Apple, apricot, bilberry, blackberry, blackcurrant, cherry, cranberry, mango, peach, pear, plum, raspberry, red bilberry, redcurrant, red/pink grapefruit, red-purple grape, whitecurrant; broccoli, Brussels sprouts, cabbage, chives, endive, green bean, horse radish, kale, lettuce, leek, red onion, tomato
      Isorhamnetin: Apple, blackberry, cherry, pear
      Rutin: Apple, blackcurrants, cantaloupe; asparagus

Table 1 (contd)

Isoflavones: Green bean, legumes, soybean
    Genistein: Currants; alfalfa sprouts, legumes, soybean
Daidzein: Currants; legumes, soybean
Daidzin: Soybean
Genistin: Soybean
Glycitin/Glycitein: Soybean
Biochanin A: Legume
Coumestrol: Legumes, soybean
Formononetin: Legumes

Glucosinolates, indoles and isothiocyanates:
Bok choy, broccoli, Brussels sprouts, cabbage, cauliflower, collard greens, kale, napa cabbage, turnip

Glutathione:
Cantaloupe, grapefruit, orange, strawberry; asparagus, spinach

Lignans:
Banana, cantaloupe, cranberry, orange, pear, peach, pomegranate, strawberry; asparagus, bok choy, broccoli, cabbage, carrot, cauliflower, iceberg lettuce, lentil, napa cabbage, onion, potato, pumpkin, rutabaga, soybean, summer squash, sweet red/green pepper, tomato, turnip, winter squash

Phenolic acids:
Apple, citrus fruit; olive
    Cinnamic acids
        Caffeic acid: Apple, gooseberry, grape, olive, raspberry, strawberry; broccoli, Brussels sprout, carrot, endive, red onion, savoy cabbage, sweet potato, tomato
        Chlorogenic acid: Apple, apricot, blackberry, blueberry, cherry, cranberry, grape, plum, pomegranate, strawberry; cabbage, carrot, sweet red/green pepper, tomato
        Ferulic acid: Apple, blackberry, blueberry, cantaloupe, grapefruit, plum, raspberry, strawberry; Brussels sprout, corn, endive, red onion
        para-**Coumaric acid:** Apple, blueberry, cherry, gooseberry, plum, red-purple grape, strawberry; Brussels sprout, cabbage, carrot, savoy cabbage, sweet red pepper, tomato
    Ellagic acid:
    Blackberry, blueberry, boysenberry, cranberry, elderberry, marionberry, pomegranate, red/black raspberry, red grape, strawberry

Gallic acid: Blackberry, cherry, mango, pomegranate, red-purple grapes

Citric acid:
Grapefruit, lemon, lime, orange, tangerine

Plant sterols
    β-**sitosterol:** Apple, apricot, avocado, banana, cantaloupe, cherry, fig, grapefruit, lemon, orange, peach, pear, pineapple, plum, pomegranate, red grape, strawberry, watermelon; asparagus, Brussels sprout, carrot, cauliflower, cucumber, eggplant, lettuce, okra, onion, pea, potato, pumpkin, radish, soybean, tomato
    Campesterol:
    Apple, apricot, banana, fig, grapefruit, lemon, pineapple, orange, peach; asparagus, Brussels sprout, carrot, cauliflower, lettuce, okra, onion, pea, radish, soybean, tomato
    Phytosterol:
    Pulses
    Saponins:
    Asparagus, beet, garlic, spinach
    Stigmasterol:
    Banana, fig, grapefruit, lemon, orange, peach; asparagus, carrot, cauliflower, eggplant, lettuce, okra, pea, potato, soybean, tomato

Pectin:
Apple, cherry, pear

Resveratrol:
Blueberry, red-purple grape

Rutin:
Cantaloupe; asparagus

Salicylates:
Apricot, cantaloupe, cherry, date, grape, guava, orange, pineapple, raisin, raspberry, strawberry; Chili pepper, endive, radish, sweet green pepper, zucchini

Terpenes/terpenoids:
Lemon, lime, orange, pink grapefruit
    Limonene:
    Grapefruit, lemon, orange, tangerine; carrot, celery

---

[a] Fruits are listed first, followed by a semicolon and the listing of vegetables.
[b] There are over 4000 flavonoid compounds, but far fewer have been identified in commonly consumed foods; most of them are within the six classes listed here.
Sources: Smith *et al.*, 1995; Perry *et al.*, 1996; USDA, 1998, 1999a, 2002; Holden *et al.*, 1999; Barratt-Fornell & Drewnowski, 2002; Mayo Clinic *et al.*, 2002; McCann *et al.*, 2002; Pennington, 2002; World Health Organization & Tufts University School of Nutrition and Policy, 2002

plants) division. Of the two classes within the Spermatophyta (Gymnosperm and Angiosperm), almost all human foods are in the Angiosperm (flowering) class. Within the two Angiosperm subclasses (Monocotyledonae and Dicotyledonae), there are approximately 93 orders and 432 families (20 orders and 67 families for the Monocotyledonae and 73 orders and 365 families for the Dicotyledonae). Even though only a small percentage of available plants are used as human foods, hundreds of different types of fruit and vegetable are consumed across the world and consideration of the various cultivars and strains for each fruit and vegetable increases the number of available fruit and vegetables into the thousands.

Table 2, which lists the subclasses, orders, and families of Spermatophyta that are used as human foods and provides examples of food plants within each family, illustrates the complexity of the botanical classification. Various food components in fruit and vegetables are concentrated in some families, but are also widely and variously distributed among the families. Peterson and Dwyer (1998) reported that botanical classifications may be helpful in ascertaining the likely presence of flavonoids in foods when food composition data are not available; however, they noted that quantitative estimates are likely to be imprecise.

Table 3 lists 16 botanical families that are sources of food components (as identified from Table 2) and lists some of the fruits and vegetables within these families. The asparagus (Asparagaceae), olive (Oleaceae), grape (Vitaceae) and morning glory (Convolvulaceae) families contain only one type (or main type) of food, and each has a unique food component profile. Individual families that contain fruits and vegetables with somewhat similar food component profiles include rue (Rutaceae), rose (Rosaceae), cabbage (Cruciferae), amaryllis (Amaryllidaceae), goosefoot (Chenopodiaceae), heath (Ericaceae), legume (Leguminosae) and sunflower (Asteraceae). Foods within the gourd (Cucurbitaceae), nightshade (Solanaceae), carrot and laurel families do not contain similar food component profiles. The gourd family includes cantaloupe (vitamin C and β-carotene), watermelon (lycopene) and pumpkin and deep yellow winter squash (β-carotene). Other members of the gourd family (honeydew melon, summer squash, and non-yellow winter squash) do not serve as major sources of these or other food components. The nightshade family includes chili peppers (β-carotene, capsaicin); sweet peppers (vitamin C, lycopene if red); tomatoes (vitamin C, β-carotene, lycopene); and eggplant and white potatoes (not major sources of food components). The laurel family includes avocado (folacin, vitamin B6) and plants that are sources of herbs or spices (cinnamon, sassafrass, sweet bay). The carrot family includes carrot (α- and β-carotenes); the stalk vegetable celery; the root vegetables celeriac and parsnip; and plants used as herbs (anise, caraway, coriander, dill, fennel, parsley).

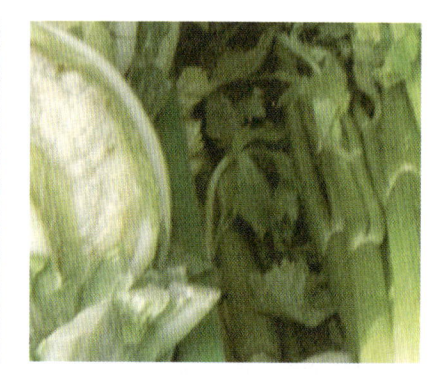

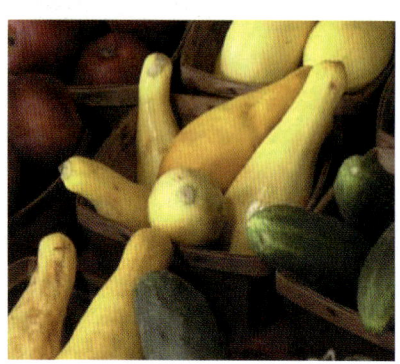

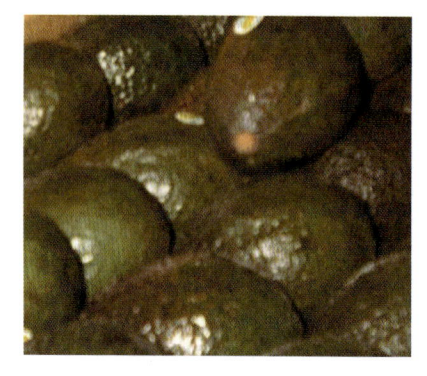

Thus, although, some botanical families have some fruits and vegetables with similar food components, not all foods within a family may be reliable sources of a given food component. Another issue that makes the use of botanical families somewhat difficult for classifying fruits and vegetables as foods is that different parts of some plants may be eaten separately and have different food components (e.g., beet roots and greens, turnip roots and greens, broccoli stems and flowers, chive bulbs and green tops). Botanical classification applies to the entire plant and is not

Definitions and classifications for fruit and vegetables

specific for the different parts of a plant that are consumed.

Growing conditions

Plants may be classified according to habitat, i.e., whether they grow in water or in soil, and the soil-growing plants may be further classified according to whether they grow in areas that are desert (low humidity, high temperature), tropical (high humidity, high temperature) or temperate (moderate humidity and temperature) (Yamaguchi, 1983). Aquatic plants include lotus, taro, water chestnut, water convolvulus and watercress. Desert plants include cactus and some desert cucurbits (buffalo gourd). Tropical plants include avocado, banana, breadfruit, carambola, cassava, date, durian, guava, mango, papaya, passion fruit, pineapple and winged beans (goa beans). Plants grown in temperate areas may be divided according to their growing season. Cool-season crops, which are adapted to mean monthly temperatures of 16–18°C (60–65°F), include artichoke, asparagus, Brussels sprout, broccoli, cabbage, carrot, cauliflower, celery, chard, endive, garlic, kale, lettuce, mustard, onion, parsnip, pea, radish, spinach, turnip and white potato. Warm-season crops, which are adapted to mean monthly temperatures of 18–30°C (65–86 °F) and are intolerant of frost, include cantaloupe, cucumber, eggplant, lima bean, okra, pepper, snap bean, squash and pumpkin, sweet corn, sweet potato, tomato and watermelon.

Several foods within the tropical plants (avocado, mango, papaya), the cool-season plants (Brussels sprout, broccoli, cabbage, carrot, cauliflower, chard, endive, garlic, kale) and the warm-season plants (pumpkin, sweet potato, tomato, watermelon) contain a range of vitamin and bioactive components. However, it appears that classification by growing season, habitat, or climate is not directly related to food component composition and not very useful for nutritional epidemiology. Classification by growing conditions might have some use for population studies where fruits and vegetables are locally grown and are of limited variety. Such a classification is less useful for populations with access to national and international food commerce and commercial methods of food preservation (freezing, canning), processing and preparation.

Fruit development from flowers

In addition to the botanical classification of whole plants (Table 2), there is a botanical classification of fruits according to how they develop from their flowers. Fruits typically have three regions, the exocarp, which is the skin (peel) or outermost layer of the fruit wall; the mesocarp or middle region; and the endocarp, which is the innermost area around the seeds (Stern, 1988). Fruits with a mesocarp that is dry at maturity are classified as *dry fruits* (cereal grains, beans, peas, and nuts), and fruits with a mesocarp that is at least partly fleshy at maturity are classified as *fleshy fruits* (all others). Fleshy fruits may be *simple, aggregate or multiple*.

Simple fleshy fruits develop from a flower with a single pistil; the ovary alone may develop into the fruit, or other parts of the flower may develop with it. Simple fleshy fruits include *drupes, pomes* and *berries*. Drupes have a single seed enclosed by a hard, stony pit, as in the apricot, cherry, coconut, date, nectarine, olive, peach and plum. In pomes, the flesh comes from the enlarged receptacle that grows up around the ovary, and the endocarp around the seeds is papery or leathery, as with the apple, pear and quince. Berries develop from a compound ovary and usually contain more than one seed. The three types of berry are *true berries*, *pepos* and *hesperidiums*. True berries are fruits with a thin skin that is soft at maturity, as in avocado, blueberry, cranberry, date, eggplant, gooseberry, grape, persimmon, red/green pepper and tomato. Pepo berries have a relatively thick rind and include cantaloupe, cucumber, pumpkin, squash and watermelon. Hesperidium berries have a leathery oil-containing skin, and outgrowths from the inner lining of the ovary wall become sac-like and swollen with juice as the fruit develops. All members of the rue family (grapefruit, kumquat, lemon, lime, orange and tangerine) produce this type of fruit.

Aggregate fruits develop from a single flower with several to many pistils. The pistils develop into tiny drupes and mature as a clustered unit on a single receptacle. Examples are blackberries, loganberries, raspberries and strawberries.

Multiple fruits are formed when a cluster of flowers grouped closely

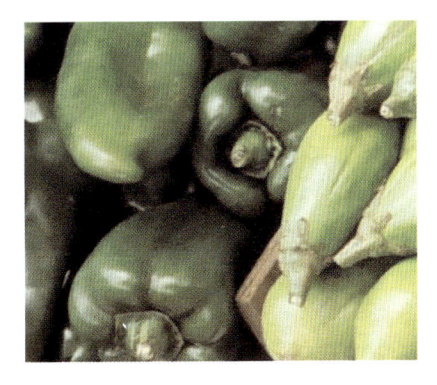

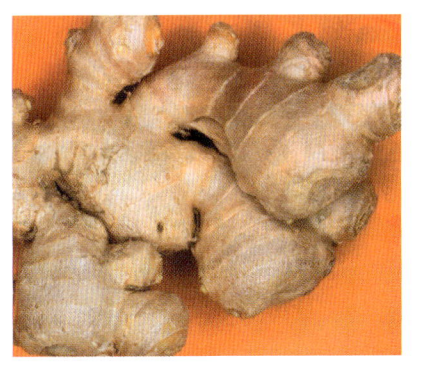

Table 2. Botanical classification of edible angiosperms

Class: Monocotyledons/liliopsida
Subclass: Alismidae
Order: Alisamales
Alismataceae (*Water plantain family*)
 California soaproot, old world arrowhead, sarsaparilla
Subclass: Arecidae
Order: Arales
Araceae (*Arum family*)
 Alocasia, ape, belembe, calalu, cocoyam, dasheen, giant swamp taro, giant taro, tannia, taro, yautia
Order: Arecales
Palmae/Arecaceae (*Palm family*)
 Coconut, date, palm cabbage, palm heart, palmito
Subclass: Commelinidae
Order: Bromeliales
Bromellaceae (*Pineapple family*)
 Pineapple
Order: Cyperales
Cyperaceae (*Sedge family*)
 Water chestnut (matai)
Order: Poales
Gramineae/Poaceae (*Grass family*)
 Bamboo shoots, barley, corn/maize, oats, rice, rye sorghum, sugarcane, wheat
Subclass: Liliidae
Order: Liliales
Amaryllidaceae (*Amaryllis family*)
 Chinese chive, chive, garlic, Japanese bunching onion, leek, onion, rakkyo, scallion, Welsh onion
Asparagaceae (*Asparagus family*)
 Asparagus
Dioscoreaceae (*Yam family*)
 Chinese yam, nagaimo, winged/water yam, white/Guinea yam, yam
Liliaceae (*Lily family*)
 Tiger lily
Order: Zingiberales
Cannaceae (*Canna family*)
 Queensland arrowroot
Marantaceae (*Arrowroot family*)
 Arrowroot
Musaceae (*Banana family*)
 Banana, plantain
Zingiberaceae (*Ginger family*)
 Ginger, Japanese ginger (mioga)

Class: Dicotyledons/magnoliopsida
Subclass: Asteridae
Order: Asterales
Asteraceae/Compositae (*Sunflower family*)
 Butterhead lettuce, cardoon (edible burdock, gobo), dandelion, endive (Belgian endive, chicory, radicchio), fuki, garland chrysanthemum, globe artichoke, iceberg lettuce, Jerusalem artichoke (sunchoke), loose leaf lettuce, romaine, salsify (vegetable oyster, oyster plant)

Order: Dipsacales
Caprifoliaceae
 Elderberry
Order: Lamiales
Lamiaceae/Laminariaceae (*Mint family*)
 Basil, marjoram, oregano, peppermint, rosemary, sage, spearmint, thyme
Order: Polemoniales
Boraginaceae (*Borage family*)
 Borage
Convolvulaceae (*Morning Glory family*)
 Sweet potato, water convolvulus (*water spinach*)
Order: Scrophulariales
Solanaceae (*Nightshade family*)
 African eggplant, chili/hot pepper (red, green), eggplant (aubergine), garden huckleberry (wonderberry), jilo, naranjillo (lulo), pepino, pimento pepper, sweet/bell pepper (red, green, orange, yellow), tobasco pepper, tomatillo, tomato (red, green, yellow), white/Irish potato
Subclass: Caryophyllidae
Order: Caryophyllales/Chenopodiales
Aizoaceae (*Carpetweed family*)
 New Zealand spinach
Amaranthaceae (*Amaranth family*)
 Amaranth, tampapa (*Chinese spinach, edible amaranth*)
Basellaceae (*Basella family*)
 Malabar nightshade (*malabar spinach*)
Catacaeae (*Cactus family*)
 Prickly pear (Indian fig, nopal, nopalitos, Sharon's fruit)
Chenopodiaceae (*Goosefoot family*)
 Beet (greens and root), orach (mountain spinach), spinach, Swiss chard
Portulacacea (*Purslane family*)
 Purslane
Order: Polygonales
Polygonaceae (Buckwheat family)
 French sorrel, garden sorrel, rhubarb (pieplant)
Subclass: Dilleniidae
Order: Capparales
Cruciferae/Brassicaceae (*Cabbage family*)
 Arugula (Italian cress, garden rocket), bok choy (Chinese cabbage), broccoli, broccoli raab (rapa, Italian turnip), brown mustard (Chinese spinach), Brussels sprouts, cabbage, cauliflower, collards, garden cress, horseradish, Indian mustard, Japanese horseradish, kale, kohlrabi, maca, mustard greens, mustard spinach, napa cabbage (Chinese cabbage), pak choi (Chinese mustard), radish, rocket salad (sea rocket), rutabaga (Siberian kale, hanover salad), turnip (turnip greens), upland cress (winter cress), watercress cress, garden cress)
Order: Cucurbitales
Cucurbitaceae (*Gourd family*)
 Bitter melon (balsam pear, bitter cucumber, bitter gourd), calabash gourd (zucca melon, white flowering gourd), cantaloupe (musk-melon), chayote, Chinese okra (vegetable

Definitions and classifications for fruit and vegetables

Table 2 (contd)

gourd), cucumber, dishcloth gourd (sponge gourd, loofa), honeydew melon, snake gourd (serpent gourd), summer squash (e.g., zucchini), watermelon, wax gourd (Chinese winter melon, preserving melon), West India gherkin, winter squash (e.g., pumpkin)

Order: Ebenales
Ebenaceae (*Ebony family*)
    Persimmon
Sapotaceae
    Sapotes

Order: Ericales
Actinidiaceae (*Actinidia family*)
    Kiwi (kiwi fruit, Chinese gooseberry)
Ericaceae (*Heath family*)
    Blueberry, cranberry, lingonberry

Order: Euphorbiales
Euphorbiaceae (*Spurge/Castor Bean family*)
    Cassava (manioc, tapioca, yucca), Chinese artichoke, shiso

Order: Malvales
Bombacaceae (*Bombax family*)
    Durian
Malvaceae (*Mallow/Cotton family*)
    Egyptian mallow, okra (lady's finger, gumbo), roselle (Jamaican sorrel)
Tiliaceae (*Basswood/Lindin family*)
    Jew's mallow

Order: Passiflorales
Caricaceae (*Carica family*)
    Papaya (tree melon)
Passifloraceae (*Passionflower family*)
    Passion fruit (granadilla)

Order: Theales
Theaceae (*Tea family*)
    Mangosteen

Subclass: Hamamelididae
Order: Urticales
Moraceae (*Mulberry family*)
    Breadfruit, fig, jackfruit, mulberry

Subclass: Magnollidae
Order: Laurales
Lauraceae (*Laurel family*)
    Avocado, cinnamon, sassafrass, sweet bay
Order: Magnoliales
Annonaceae (*Custard apple family*)
    Cherimoya (custard apple)
Order: Nymphaeales
Nymphaeceae (Water Lily family)
    Lotus root (East Indian lotus)

Subclass: Rosidae
Order: Cornales/Umbellales
Araliaceae (*Aralia/Ginseng family*)
    Udo
Umbelliferae/Apiaceae (*Carrot/Parsley family*)
    Anise, arracacha, caraway, carrot, celeriac, celery, coriander, dill, fennel (sweet anise), Florence fennel, mitsuba, parsley, parsnip

Order: Fabales
Leguminosae/Fabaceae (*Legume family*)
    Adzuki beans, alfalfa, asparagus beans, bambara ground nuts, black beans, broad beans (horse beans, field beans, fava beans), carob, chickpeas (garbanzo beans), cluster beans (guar), cowpeas, edible-podded peas (e.g., sugar peas, China peas), Egyptian lupines, fenugreek, green/garden peas, hyacinth beans (chickling peas), jack beans, jicama (yam bean), kidney beans, lentils, lima beans, mat beans, mung beans, peanuts (ground nuts), potato beans, ricebeans, scarlet runner beans, snapbeans (includes green beans, string beans, wax beans, yellow snap beans, romano beans, haricots), soy beans, sword beans, tamarind (Indian date), winged beans (goa beans)

Order: Geraniales
Malpighiaceae
    Acerola (Barbados cherry, West Indian cherry)
Oxalidaceae
    Carambola

Order: Myrtales
Myrtaceae (*Myrtle family*)
    Feijoa (pineapple guava), guava
Punicaceae (*Pomegranate family*)
    Pomegranate

Order: Oleales
Oleaceae (*Olive family*)
    Olives

Order: Rhamnales
Rhamnaceae (*Buckthorn family*)
    Jujube (Chinese date, red date)
Vitaceae (*Grape family*)
    Grapes

Order: Rosales
Rosaceae (*Rose family*)
    Apple, apricot, blackberry (brambleberry, dewberry), cherry (sweet cherry), loganberry, loquat (may apple, Japanese medlar, Japanese plum), nectarine, peach, pear, plum, quince, raspberry, strawberry

Order: Rutales
Anacardiaceae (*Cashew family*)
    Mango
Rutaceae (*Rue family*)
    Calamondin, grapefruit, kumquat, lemon, lime, orange, pummelo (pomelo, pommelo, Chinese grapefruit, shaddock), tangerine

Order: Sapindales
Sapindaceae (*Soapberry family*)
    Longan, lychee (litchi), rambutan

Order: Saxifragales
Saxifragaceae (*Saxifrage family*)
    Currants (red, pink, white, black, Asian), gooseberry

Sources: Masefield *et al.*, 1969; *Encyclopedia Britannica*, 1974

IARC Handbooks of Cancer Prevention Volume 8: Fruit and Vegetables

Table 3. Foods and food components listed by botanical families

Family	Foods in family	Food components
Amaryllis	Chive, garlic, leek, onion, scallion	Allyl sulfides
Asparagus	Asparagus	Folacin, lignans, β-sitosterol, campesterol, vitamin B6
Cabbage	Arugula, bok choy, broccoli, Brussels sprout, cabbage, cauliflower, collards, garden cress, kale, kohlrabi, mustard greens, mustard spinach, napa cabbage, pak choi, radish, rutabaga, turnip, watercress	β-Carotene, lutein, folacin (collards, kale), magnesium, calcium, quercetin, kaempferol, glucosinolates, indoles, isothiocyanates, lignans, caffeic acid, *para*-coumaric acid, chlorogenic acid, vitamin C
Carrot	Anise, caraway, carrot, celeriac, celery, coriander, dill, fennel, parsley, parsnip	α- and β-Carotene, lutein, apigenin, lignans, β-sitosterol, campesterol (all in carrot)
Goosefoot	Beet greens and root, spinach, Swiss chard	β-Carotene, lutein (spinach), zeaxanthin, folacin, magnesium, calcium, glutathione (spinach), vitamin C
Gourd	Bitter melon, calabash gourd, cantaloupe, chayote, cucumber, honeydew melon, summer squash, watermelon, winter squash	β-Carotene (cantaloupe, pumpkin, orange-yellow squash, lycopene (watermelon), vitamin C (cantaloupe)
Grape	Red-purple grapes, green grapes	Anthocyanins, catechins, proanthocyanidins, quercetin, myricetin, ellagic acid, gallic acid, resveratrol (all in red-purple grapes)
Heath	Blueberry, cranberry, lingonberry	Anthocyanins, proanthocyanidins, quercetin, ellagic acid, vitamin C
Laurel	Avocado, cinnamon, sassafrass, sweet bay	Folacin, β-sitosterol, *para*-coumaric acid, chlorogenic acid, ferulic acid, caffeic acid, gallic acid, glutathione, vitamin B6 (all in avocado)
Legume	Black beans, broad beans, carob, chickpeas, cowpeas, green peas, jicama, kidney beans, lentils, lima beans, mung beans, peanuts, snap beans, soybeans	Folacin, iron, isoflavones, protein, starch, vitamin B6
Morning glory	Sweet potato, water convolvulus	α- and β-Carotene (sweet potato)
Nightshade	Chili pepper, eggplant, sweet red/green pepper, tomato, white potato	Capsaicin (chili pepper), β-carotene (chili pepper), lycopene (tomato), luteotin (sweet pepper), lignans, vitamin C (tomato, sweet pepper)
Olive	Olives	Monounsaturated fatty acids, β-cryptoxanthin, phenolic acids
Rue	Grapefruit, lemon, lime, orange, tangerine	Lycopene (red grapefruit), hesperidin, neohesperidin, citric acid, β-sitosterol, campesterol, salicylates (orange), limonene, vitamin C
Rose	Apple, apricot, blackberry, cherry, loganberry, loquat, nectarine, peach, pear, plum, quince, raspberry, strawberry	β-Carotene (apricot, nectarine, peach), anthocyanins, quercetin, kaempferol, isorhamnetin, caffeic acid, ellagic acid, β-sitosterol, campesterol, pectin, salicylates, vitamin C
Sunflower	Butterhead lettuce, endive, globe artichoke,	Kaempferol, stigmasterol, lignans iceberg lettuce, Jerusalem artichoke, loose leaf lettuce, romaine, salsify

Definitions and classifications for fruit and vegetables

together consolidates into a mass during ripening. For example, each of the many sections that make up a pineapple is a developed flower, and each one is attached to the center core, which has a woody stem structure. Other multiple fruits are fig, mulberry and osage orange.

Classification of fruits based on development from flowers is not likely to be useful for epidemiological studies because the classes are not specific for food component content. One exception is the hesperidium berry class, which contains the rue family (citrus) fruits. Classification by fruit development would be confusing for nutritionists and survey participants because the botanical term *berries* is used for some fruits that are not commonly considered to be berries, such as avocado, banana, cantaloupe, cucumber, date, grapefruit, kumquat, lemon, lime, orange, squash, tangerine and watermelon. Fruits that are commonly referred to as *berries* are found in the true berry and aggregate fruit classes.

Food supply and consumption data

Government agencies often use fruit and vegetable classifications for reporting national food supply (availability) and food consumption data. For example, the United States Department of Agriculture (USDA) Economic Research Service (ERS) reports national food supply data (i.e., *per capita* food availability) for fruit and vegetable classes (USDA, 1999b; United States General Accounting Office, 2002) and the USDA Agriculture Research Service (ARS) uses these same classes to report summarized results from national food consumption surveys (Krebs-Smith & Cantor, 2001). The classifications are based on fruit and vegetable type as well as on processing methods. For fruits, there are four type classes (citrus, melons, berries and other) and five processing classes (fresh, juices, canned/chilled, dried and frozen). For vegetables, there are five type classes (dark green leafy; deep yellow/orange; starchy; dry beans, peas, and lentils; and other) and four processing classes (fresh, canned, frozen and dehydrated). Although these classes are broad, they provide rank orders for individual fruits and vegetables, so that the most commonly consumed foods can be identified.

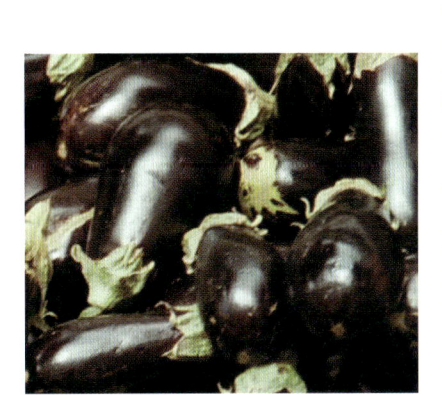

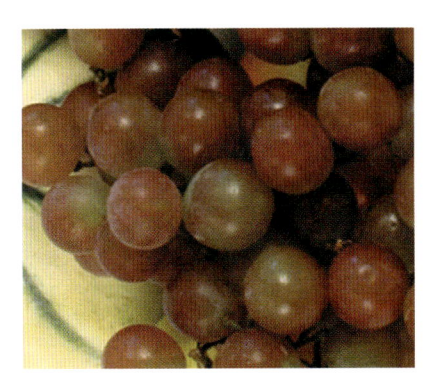

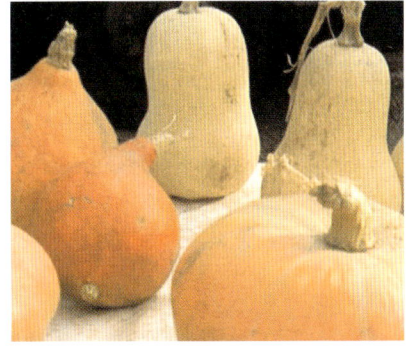

Edible parts of plants

Classification by edible part attempts to group fruits and vegetables by the part of the plant, bush, vine or tree that is used as food (Table 4). This classification is useful because of the similar nutrient composition of some plant tissues (e.g., leaves, stalks and stems, roots and tubers, and pulses). This type of classification is found in some food composition databases. The similarity in nutrient content among some plant parts is due to the functions of these tissues. Stem and stalk vegetables (e.g., celery, rhubarb) are usually high in dietary fibre, which serves to support the structure of the plant. Leaves, especially the dark green ones, tend to be the most metabolically active and most nutritious part of plants and are usually good sources of dietary fibre, folacin, carotenoids, vitamin C, flavonoids, and minerals such as iron, zinc, calcium and magnesium. Pulses (mature beans and peas) are high in protein, starch, isoflavones, vitamin B6, folacin, iron and other minerals. Bulbs (chives, garlic, onion, shallots) are noted for allicin. Enlarged roots and tubers are storage organs for plants and usually have high starch content; they may serve as inexpensive sources of energy (potatoes, sweet potatoes, taro). Other roots and tubers are lower in energy content (e.g., Jerusalem artichokes, parsnips, turnips) and may provide specific food components (e.g., α- and β-carotene in carrots). Fruits, which are grouped as vegetable fruits, citrus, berries, melons, and other, are more variable in nutrient content; some are especially high in vitamin C and/or β-carotene.

Colour

The main pigments responsible for colour in fruit and vegetables are chlorophyll (green), various carotenoids (yellow, orange and red) and anthocyanins, a type of flavonoid (red, blue and purple). Variations in colour between different fruits and vegetables and between various cultivars of a fruit or vegetable result from the different concentrations of pigments. Carotenoids and anthocyanins function as antioxidants. Although chlorophyll does not appear to be useful in human physiology, foods that are high in chlorophyll are usually also high in β-carotene. (The yellow-orange colour of β-carotene is masked by the green chlorophyll). The carotenoids most extensively investigated in relation to human health are α-carotene, β-carotene, β-cryptoxanthin, lycopene, lutein and zeaxanthin (IARC, 1998). α- and β-carotene, β-cryptoxanthin, and lutein provide an orange-yellow colour; lycopene red and zeaxanthin yellow. There are over 300 different anthocyanins and about 70 have been identified in fruits and vegetables. Their colours range from crimson or magenta red to violet or indigo purple or blue.

Colour classifications for fruit and vegetables have been used to help consumers select a wider variety of these foods in their daily diets (Mangels *et al.*, 1993; Heber & Bowerman, 2001; Joseph *et al.*, 2002; National Cancer Institute, 2002).

Table 5 lists some common green, orange, red and blue fruits and vegetables by colour, the pigment(s) responsible for their colour, and other components that are present in these foods. In relation to food consumption, colour may be a useful indicator of the presence of some food components in fruit and vegetables, but may not be specific for a bioactive component. For example, red could be due to anthocyanins or lycopene. White is indicative of the allyl sulfides in garlic and onion, but other white vegetables such as potatoes, parsnips and turnips do not contain these protective components. As indicated in Table 5, fruits and vegetables that contain the pigments chlorophyll, anthocyanins or carotenoids may not have similar profiles with respect to other food components such as vitamin C, minerals and phenolic acids. Some green vegetables are sources of carotenoids; some are sources of glucosinolates, indoles and thiocyanates; and some (iceberg lettuce, green peas, green beans) do not contain these food components.

Some fruits and vegetables have a peel with a colour that is different to the underlying tissue. The peel constitutes only a small part by weight of the fruit or vegetable and the peel may not be consumed. Thus, reliance on peel color could be misleading with regard to food component content. Examples are summer squash with yellow or green peel; cucumber with green peel; eggplant with purple peel; potatoes with red peel; and apple with red, green, or yellow peel. Another issue is that there are many different cultivars for each fruit and vegetable, and the cultivars may vary by colour and hence by their concentration of pigments. For example, most cultivars of cherries are red, but some are white and others are yellow. Sweet potatoes show variation in β-carotene concentration among the orange, yellow-white and purple cultivars (Huang *et al.*, 1999).

Processing and preparation

The usefulness of processing terms for classifying fruits and vegetables depends on their association with food component concentrations. The terms *fresh, juice, canned/chilled, dried* and *frozen* for fruits and *fresh, canned,*

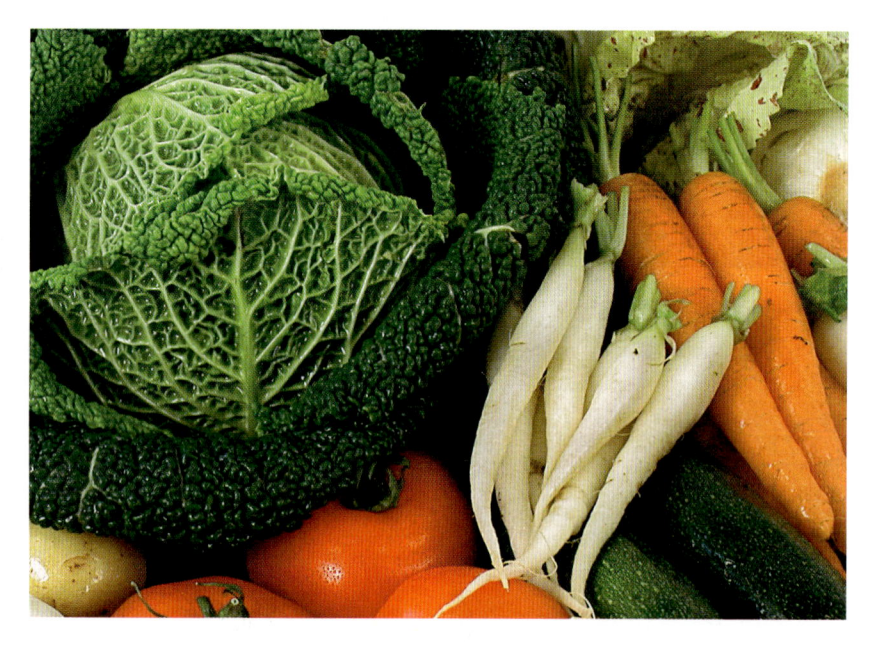

Definitions and classifications for fruit and vegetables

Table 4. Classification of fruits and vegetables by edible parts

Flowers/flower buds with stems/stalks
Asparagus; broccoli; broccoli raab; Chinese broccoli; cauliflower; globe/French artichoke; green cauliflower; pumpkin flower

Stems and stalks
Cardoon; celery; fennel bulb; green/spring onion (scallion); kohlrabi; leek; rhubarb

Leaves
Amaranth leaves; arugula; balsam pear leafy tips (bitter melon/bitter gourd); beet greens; borage; Brussels sprouts; butterbur (fuki) leaves; Chinese cabbage (pak-choi, pe-tsai); cabbage (green, red, savoy, swamp/skunk); chard (Swiss chard); chicory greens; chicory, witloof; chrysanthemum leaves; collards; coriander/cilantro; cornsalad; cowpeas, leafy tips; dandelion greens; dock/sorrel; endive; eppaw; fiddlehead ferns; garden cress; garland chrysanthemum; grape leaves; horseradish tree, leafy tips; jew's mallow; jute, potherb; kale; kale, scotch; lambs-quarters; lettuce (butterhead, iceberg, looseleaf/leaf, romaine/cos); malbar spinach; mustard greens; mustard spinach/tendergreen; New Zealand spinach; pumpkin leaves; purslane; radicchio; salsify (oyster plant, vegetable oyster); spinach; sweet potato leaves; taro leaves; tree fern; turnip greens; vinespinach; watercress; winged bean leaves

Pulses
Adzuki beans; black beans; black turtle beans; broadbeans (fava beans); chickpeas (garbanzo beans, bengal gram); cowpeas (blackeye peas, crowder peas, southern peas); catjang; cranberry (roman) beans; French beans; great northern beans; hyacinth beans; kidney beans; lentils; lima beans; lima beans, baby; lupins; mothbeans; mung beans; mungo beans; navy beans; peas, green; peas, split; pigeon peas (red gram); pink beans; pinto beans; shellie (shell) beans; soybeans; white beans; winged beans; yardlong bean; yellow beans; winged beans

Roots (part of the plant below the ground that holds the plant in place, draws water and nourishment from the soil, and stores food)
Arracacha; arrowroot; beet (beetroot); burdock root; carrot; cassava; celeriac (celery root); chicory root; jicama (yambean); lotus root; parsnip; radish; radish, oriental; radish, white icicle; rutabaga (swede); salsify; sweet potato; turnip; wasabi root

Tuber (short, thickened, fleshy part of an underground stem)
Jerusalem artichoke (sunchoke); Hawaiian mountain yam; poi (taro root paste); potato (brown-, red-, white- skinned and russet); Tahitian taro; yautia (tannier); yam

Shoots/sprouts
Alfalfa sprouts; bamboo shoots; kidney bean sprouts; lentil sprouts; mung bean sprouts; navy bean sprouts; pea sprouts; pokeberry shoots (poke); radish seed sprouts; soybean sprouts; taro shoots

Bulbs (underground bud with roots and short stem covered with leafy layers)
Chives; garlic; leek; onion; onion, Welsh; shallot

Fruits used as vegetables
Avocado, balsam pear (bitter melon, bitter gourd); breadfruit; calabash/white-flowered gourd; cucumber; dishcloth gourd (towel gourd); eggplant (aubergine); snap beans, green, yellow; hominy, white/yellow; horseradish tree pods; okra (lady's finger, gumbo); pepino; chili/hot peppers (ancho, banana, Hungarian, jalapeno, pasilla, pimiento, serrano); sweet/bell peppers, green/red/yellow; plantain; sesbania flower; snow peas (edible podded peas); summer squash (chayote, crookneck, marrow, scallop, straightneck, zucchini); sweet corn; tomatillo; tomato (green, orange, red, cherry, Italian, plum, yellow); waxgourd (Chinese preserving melon); winter squash (acorn, butternut, hubbard, pumpkin, spaghetti); zucca melon

Fruits – citrus
Grapefruit (pink, red, white); lemon; lime; mandarin oranges; orange; tangerine

Fruits – berries
Blackberry; blueberry; boysenberry; cranberry; elderberry; gooseberry; loganberry; mulberry; oheloberry; raspberry; strawberry

Fruits – melons
Cantaloupe (muskmelon); casaba melon; honeydew melon; watermelon

Fruits – other
Abiyuch; acerola (West Indian cherry); apple; apricot; Asian pear, banana; carambola (star fruit); carissa (natal-plum); cherimoya; cherry (sour, sweet); crabapple; currants (black, red, white, zante); custard apple (bullock's heart); date; durian; feijoa; fig; grape, red/green; groundcherry; guava; guava, strawberry; jackfruit; java plum; jujube; kiwi fruit (Chinese gooseberry); kumquat; lychee (litchi); longan; loquat; mammy apple (mamey); mango; mangosteen; nectarine; papaya; passion fruit (grandilla), purple; peach; pear; persimmon, Japanese; persimmon; pineapple; pitanga (Surinam cherry); plum; pomegranate; prickly pear; prune; pummelo; quince; rambutan; rose apple; roselle; rowal; sapodilla; sapote; soursop; sugar apple; tamarind

Table 5. Pigment in fruits and vegetables

Colour	Food	Pigment(s)	Other food components
Dark green	Kale	Chlorophyll, β-carotene, lutein	Calcium, iron, magnesium, quercetin, kaempferol, glucosinolates, indoles, isothiocyanates, vitamin C
Dark green	Spinach	Chlorophyll, β-carotene, lutein	Folacin, calcium, iron, magnesium, glutathione, saponins, vitamin C
Green	Asparagus	Chlorophyll, β-carotene, lutein, anthocyanin	Folacin, glutathione, lignans, saponins, rutin
Green	Broccoli	Chlorophyll, β-carotene, lutein	Quercetin, glucosinolates, indoles, isothiocyanates, lignans, caffeic acid, vitamin C
Green	Brussels sprout	Chlorophyll, β-carotene, lutein	Glucosinolates, indoles, isothiocyanates, *para*-coumaric acid, caffeic acid, ferulic acid, vitamin C
Green	Cabbage	Chlorophyll, β-carotene, lutein	Quercetin, kaempferol, glucosinolates, indoles, isothiocyanates, chlorogenic acid, vitamin C
Green	Kiwi fruit	Chlorophyll, β-cryptoxanthin, lutein, zeaxanthin	Vitamin C
Deep orange-yellow	Apricot	β-Carotene	Quercetin, chlorogenic acid
Deep orange	Cantaloupe	α-Carotene, β-carotene	Glutathione, ferulic acid, rutin, vitamin C
Deep orange	Carrot	α-Carotene, β-carotene, β-cryptoxanthin, lutein	Apigenein, myricetin, caffeic acid, *para*-coumaric acid, chlorogenic acid, limonene
Deep orange	Mango	β-Carotene, β-cryptoxanthin, anthocyanins	Quercetin, kaempferol, gallic acid, vitamin C
Deep orange	Pumpkin	α-Carotene, β-carotene, lutein, zeaxanthin	Lignans, ferulic acid
Deep orange	Sweet potato	β-Carotene	Quercetin, caffeic acid, chlorogenic acid
Orange	Orange	β-Cryptoxanthin, lutein, zeaxanthin	Hesperidin, glutathione, β-sitosterol, limonene, vitamin C
Orange	Tangerine	β-Cryptoxanthin, lutein	Limonene, vitamin C
Yellow	Corn	Lutein, zeaxanthin	Quercetin, ferulic acid
Red	Cherry	Anthocyanins	Quercetin, kaempferol, chlorogenic acid, *para*-coumaric acid, gallic acid

Table 5 (contd)

Colour	Food	Pigment(s)	Other food components
Red	Cranberry	Anthocyanins	Catechins, epigallocatechin gallate, proanthocyanidins, quercetin, myricetin, kaempferol, lignans, ellagic acid, chlorogenic acid, vitamin C
Red	Pomegranate	Anthocyanins	Lignans, ellagic acid, chlorogenic acid, gallic acid
Red	Raspberry	Anthocyanins	Quercetin, kaempferol, caffeic acid, ellagic acid, ferulic acid, salicylates, vitamin C
Red	Red onion	Anthocyanins	Allicin, quercetin, kaempferol, caffeic acid, ferulic acid
Red skin	Red-skinned apple	Anthocyanins	Quercetin, myricetin, ferulic acid, pectin, rutin
Red	Strawberry	Anthocyanins	Glutathione, lignans, ellagic acid, caffeic acid, ferulic acid, vitamin C
Red	Tomato	Lycopene, β-carotene	Quercetin, kaempferol, *para*-coumaric acid, chlorogenic acid, vitamin C
Red-pink	Red-pink grapefruit	β-Carotene, lycopene	Hesperidin, naringenin, quercetin, kaempferol, glutathione, ferulic acid, limonene, β-sitosterol, vitamin C
Red	Sweet red pepper	β-Carotene, lutein	*para*-Coumaric acid, chlorogenic acid, vitamin C
Blue-black	Blackberry	Anthocyanins	Catechins, quercetin, kaempferol, chlorogenic acid, ellagic acid, ferulic acid, gallic acid, vitamin C
Blue	Blueberry	Anthocyanins	Proanthocyanidins, quercetin, myricetin, kaempferol, chlorogenic acid, *para*-coumaric acid, ferulic acid, resveratrol, vitamin C
Blue	Elderberry	Anthocyanins	Catechins, quercetin, ellagic acid, vitamin C
Red-purple	Red-purple grape	Anthocyanins	Catechins, epicatechin, proanthocyanidins, quercetin, myricetin, kaempferol, chlorogenic acid, caffeic acid, gallic acid, *para*-coumaric acid, resveratrol
Purple	Plum	Anthocyanins	Chlorogenic acid, *para*-coumaric acid, ferulic acid

Source: Barratt-Fornell & Drewnowski, 2002; Joseph *et al.*, 2002; National Cancer Institute, 2002; Pennington, 2002.

frozen and *dehydrated* for vegetables were presented earlier in this chapter. Current methods of commercial processing, such as the freezing and canning of fruit and vegetables appear not to significantly alter the nutrient content of these foods, although there may be some loss of components such as vitamin C and folacin. Often the cultivars used for freezing and canning are different from those sold in markets as the raw product. Thus, differences in nutrient profiles between a raw and processed food may be due to differences in cultivar as well as the effects of processing. The drying of fruit and vegetables removes water and probably also some volatile nutrients, reducing the volume and weight of the product and concentrating the remaining food components. The juicing of fruit and vegetables usually removes the pulp, which contains dietary fibre, and may concentrate other nutrients on a weight basis. The cultivars used for commercial juicing may be different from those available in the market as raw fruit and vegetables, so again food component levels may be different. Some commercial orange and grapefruit juices are fortified with calcium, giving significantly higher levels than in unfortified juices.

Fruit and vegetable juices and dried fruit offer different levels of nutrients and bioactive components on a weight basis compared with their fresh, canned and cooked counterparts. For example a serving of orange juice might constitute the juice from two or more oranges; dried plums will weigh less than the fresh. For dark green leafy vegetables, the quantity (weight) consumed could vary considerably between the raw and the cooked. For example, a given volume of raw spinach yields only about half that volume of cooked spinach. Processing and preparation may remove peels from fruits and vegetables and may add other ingredients (fat and sugar) as in frying vegetables, preparing vegetables in a cream or butter sauce, adding mayonnaise or salad dressing to potatoes or salads, canning fruit in a sugar syrup or juice, or preparing pickled vegetables in a salt brine.

Classification of fruits and vegetables by processing and preparation methods could be especially important in cultures where there is reliance on a limited number of local crops and the processing techniques alter the composition so as to limit the intake of critical food components. For populations that have access to a wide variety of fruit and vegetables and a range of processing and preparation methods, these methods are not likely to be useful as classification terms.

Considerations for epidemiological studies

Fruit and vegetable groupings used in dietary assessment tools

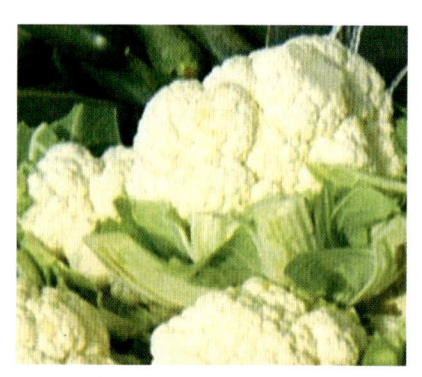

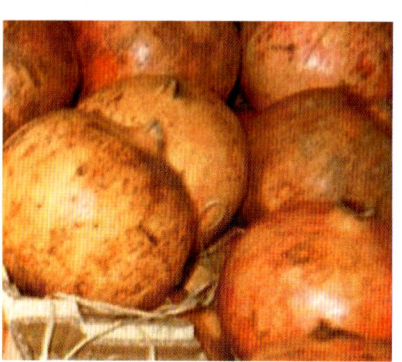

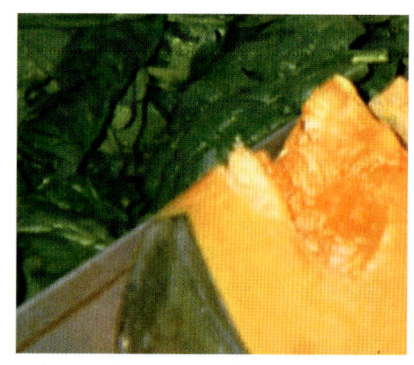

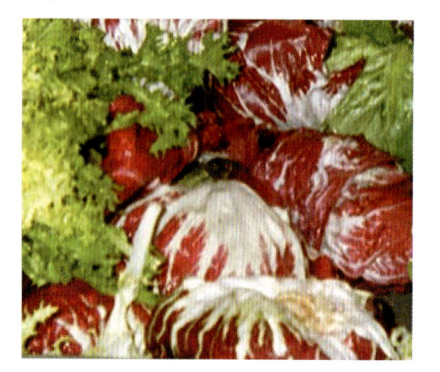

The various instruments used to assess dietary intakes in epidemiological studies are discussed in Chapter 2, which covers the advantages and disadvantages of various methods as well as the estimation of associated measurement errors. Dietary assessment tools are mentioned in this chapter with respect to aspects of fruit and vegetable definitions and classifications. The definitions and classifications for fruit and vegetables vary between epidemiological studies because of differences in the purposes of the study and the dietary patterns of the population being evaluated. Table 6 provides examples of several fruit and vegetable groupings based on plant part, colour and/or botanical family that have been used to collect and/or report information from epidemiological studies. The table provides information on botanical families, important food components and some considerations with respect to food processing. The list does not cover all fruits and vegetables, e.g., it does not include some commonly consumed fruits such as apples, pears and bananas. Open-ended dietary assessment tools (e.g., 24-hour recalls or food records) allow flexibility in terms of identifying and classifying fruit and vegetable consumption because the investigators may organize the results as desired after the survey has been completed. Food frequency questionnaires (FFQs) require *a priori* decisions as to which foods are to be listed on the questionnaire and how the foods are organized into groups.

There are many similarities between available FFQs with respect to questions asked about fruit and vegetable consumption. Differences include the number of fruits and vegetables that are listed; which foods are considered to be fruits and which vegetables; the placement of certain fruits and vegetables in other food groups; and the listing and placement of foods that contain fruit and vegetables or are derived from these foods. For example, fruit and vegetables that are used as dietary staples (i.e., as a main source of energy) for a population may not be considered to be fruits or vegetables. These foods include pulses (mature beans and peas), bananas, plantain, white potatoes, sweet (yellow) potatoes and taro. Soybeans are usually considered with pulses; however, soybean products (tofu, miso, temph, soy-based meat analogues, soymilk) are generally grouped elsewhere. FFQs usually ask questions about mixed dishes containing fruit or vegetables (casseroles, stews, stir-fries; pasta, rice and pizza with tomato sauce; soups with vegetables; and pies containing fruit, pumpkin or sweet potato) separately from questions about fruit and vegetables. For a number of fruit and vegetable foods, decisions about placement and grouping in FFQs may be made according to how they are usually used in dietary patterns. Examples of these foods are tomato ketchup, paste, puree, sauce and salsa; fried potatoes; soups containing tomatoes, pulses, or other vegetables; garlic and onion (used as garnish versus vegetable); coconut; sauerkraut; pickled fruits and vegetables; and olives. Potato crisps, jams, jellies, preserves and candied fruit are usually not counted as vegetables or fruits in FFQs.

Fruit and vegetable groupings familiar to survey participants

Because food guides and related dietary guidance information are provided to children and teenagers in schools and to the general public from government health and/or agricultural agencies and from health professionals (dietitians, nurses, physicians), many survey participants are likely to be familiar with the food groups presented in these materials. Dietary guidance materials emphasize the weekly or biweekly consumption of dark green leafy vegetables and/or deep yellow-orange fruits and vegetables as a source of the vitamin A precursor, β-carotene; daily consumption of citrus fruit or juice for vitamin C; and daily consumption of protein sources such as meat and meat substitutes, which include beans, peas, and soy products. Thus, the public is usually exposed to and has some understanding of several fruit and vegetable groups depicted by colour, plant part and/or botanical family.

Dark green leafy vegetables represent both the plant part and colour; deep orange/yellow fruits and vegetables represent colour; and citrus fruits and pulses represent both botanical families and plant parts. Consumers are also generally familiar with the plant part groupings of berries, melons and starchy root/tuber vegetables and with processing terms such as fresh, frozen, canned and dried. Cabbage family vegetables are likely to be familiar to survey participants because of media attention over the past 10–15 years. Consumers who are especially interested in food and health may also have read or heard about bioactive components in garlic, onions, tomatoes, tomato products, watermelon, grapes, cherries and blueberries. Consumer knowledge of fruit and vegetable groupings might be used to advantage by researchers in designing epidemiological studies.

Table 6. Some fruit and vegetable groupings used to collect or report information in epidemiological studies

Suggested groupings	Botanical family and foods	Important components	Processing considerations; Notes
Dark green leafy vegetables	*Goosefoot:* beet greens, spinach, Swiss chard Cabbage: collards, kale, mustard greens, mustard spinach, turnip greens	β-Carotene, folacin, magnesium, calcium	Separate questions for raw and cooked because of changes in weight and volume
Cabbage family (some green leafy vegetables, stem and flower vegetables)	*Cabbage:* arugula, bok choy, broccoli, Brussels sprouts, cabbage, cauliflower, collards, kale, mustard greens, napa cabbage, pak choi	Glucosinolates, isothiocyanates, indoles	Separate questions for coleslaw and sauerkraut; some overlap with dark green leafy vegetables (collards, kale)
Lettuce	*Sunflower:* butterhead lettuce, endive, iceberg lettuce, loose leaf lettuce, romaine		May be commonly consumed
Deep orange-yellow fruits and roots	*Gourd:* cantaloupe, pumpkin *Carica:* papaya *Rose:* apricot, nectarine, peach *Carrot:* carrot *Morning Glory:* Sweet potato *Cashew:* mango	β-Carotene, α-carotene (carrot, pumpkin, sweet potato)	
Citrus family fruits and juices	*Rue:* clementine, lime, lemon, grapefruit, orange, tangerine, clementine	Hesperidin, naringenin (grapefruit), neohesperidin (grapefruit, orange), limonene, vitamin C	Separate questions for citrus fruit juices and juices fortified with calcium
Tomatoes, tomato products, and several red fruits	*Nightshade:* tomato *Gourd:* watermelon *Rue:* red-pink grapefruit *Myrtle:* guava	β-Carotene, lycopene, vitamin C	Separate questions about tomato juice, tomato sauce, ketchup, salsa, pizza, tomato soup and pasta with tomato sauce
Red cherries, berries, several vegetables	*Rose:* cherry, raspberry, strawberry *Health:* cranberry *Nightshade:* red sweet pepper, red chili pepper *Goosefoot:* beets *Legume:* red beans *Brassica:* red cabbage *Allium:* red onion	Anthocyanins, quercetin, phenolic acids (berries)	
Blue-black berries and red-purple grapes	*Rose:* blackberry, loganberry *Heath:* blueberry, lingonberry *Saxifrage:* gooseberry *Grape:* red-purple grape	Anthocyanins, quercetin, phenolic acids; red-purple grapes also have proanthocyanidins, catechins, myricetin, resveratrol, vitamin C	Separate question for juices; separate questions for grapes of other colours

Definitions and classifications for fruit and vegetables

Table 6 (contd)

Suggested groupings	Botanical family and foods	Important components	Processing considerations; Notes
Allium family bulbs	*Amaryllis:* chives, garlic, leeks, onion, shallots	Allyl sulfides	Clarify if garlic and onion are consumed as a vegetable, garnish, powder or salt
Legume family	*Legume:* black beans, broad beans, chickpeas, cowpeas, edible-podded peas, green peas, hyacinth beans, kidney beans, lentils, lima beans, soybeans	Iron, isoflavones, protein, starch, vitamin B6	Include beans in mixed dishes (chili, burritos, soups), tofu, soy-based meat substitutes, and other soy products
Starchy vegetables	*Nightshade*: potato *Grass*: corn, hominy *Arum:* taro *Yam:* yam	Calories, starch, phenolic acids	Separate questions for deep-fried potatoes or potatoes made with sauce or mayonnaise

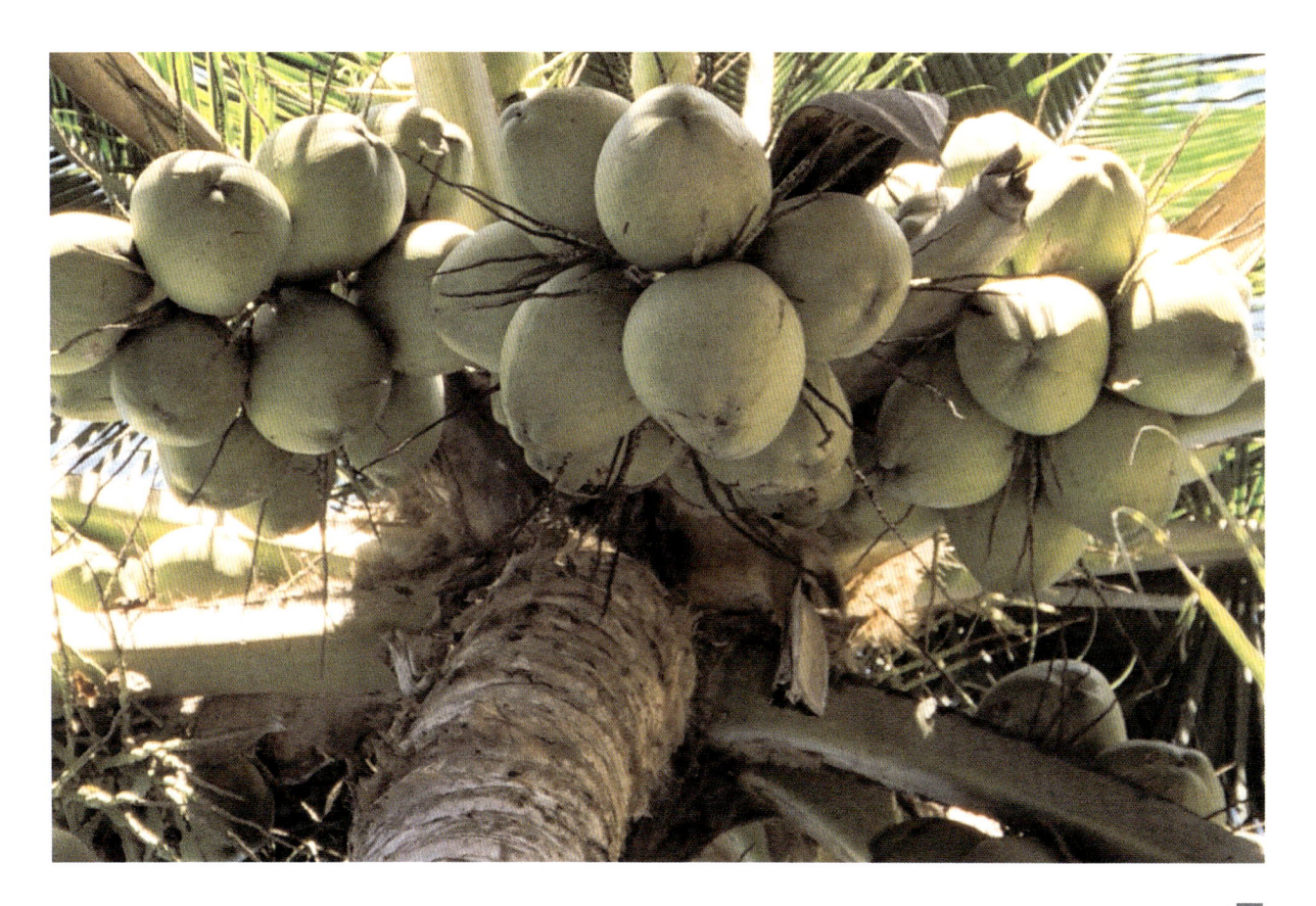

Chapter 2
Measuring intake of fruit and vegetables

This chapter describes methods for estimating fruit and vegetable intake: household measures, questionnaire measures of usual or habitual intake and recording of actual or current intake (Table 7). These methods are used for various purposes, including nutrition surveillance, epidemiological research (case–control and cohort studies) and methodological research for validation of other dietary methods. They can also be used in clinical trials and intervention studies as well as for clinical evaluation.

Household measures of food availability

Household dietary surveys, household budget surveys and food balance sheets are used at the national or population level to estimate intake for nutrition surveillance and monitoring. They provide a broad view of the availability and consumption of fruit and vegetables. These survey methods provide what are technically considered crude measures of dietary intake, expressed at the household or per capita level.

Household dietary surveys
This method involves the compilation of an inventory of all foods present in the household at the beginning and at the end of the survey, complemented by the report of the amounts of foods purchased or otherwise obtained or consumed elsewhere and of the amount of edible food wasted or otherwise disposed of in the intervening survey period (Cresta et al., 1969; Burke & Pao, 1976). The data may be recorded by weight and/or estimated on the basis of household measures and units, or as a combination. This method, fairly common in the past, is now more rarely used. The information obtained refers to the household and is expressed as per capita consumption. Expressing total consumption on the basis of consumption units, determined according to the estimated energy requirements of the individual members of the household, can provide some approximation of individual consumption. This procedure however ignores perforce the possible non-proportional distribution of various foods among the members of a household, and no statistical method can fully correct for this.

Household budget surveys
Another source of information on nationally representative dietary patterns is household budget surveys (HBS) (Trichopoulou et al., 1999). These surveys are regularly conducted in most of the developed countries and in several developing ones. The sampling unit is the household, and the surveys are conducted principally for the purpose of monitoring the expenditure of families. Purchases of food are recorded as part of the overall purchases of the family and translated at a second stage into amounts. In some countries, foods are reported also as quantities. Socio-demographic information is also obtained, such as the educational level and employment of the head and other members of the family, the composition of the household, the urban, rural or semi-urban location of the household. Since each country has its own procedures and protocols for these surveys, the disparity of the collected data precludes comparison between countries. The diversity concerns not only the sampling methods but also the duration of the survey period, the number and details of the foods recorded, the inclusion or omission of foods consumed outside the home and the level of aggregation of individual food items into larger groups. In 1993, the European Commission funded a project (DAFNE, DAta Food NEtworking) that undertook to create an European data bank on food availability for human consumption, exploiting HBS data. In 1998, DAFNE harmonized the HBS of 10 European countries (Belgium, Germany, Greece, Hungary, Ireland, Luxembourg, Norway, Poland, Spain, United Kingdom), thus making available a set of data that provides an insight into national food habits and their distribution on the basis of socio-economic, educational and demographic parameters.

Food balance sheets
The food balance sheets (FBS) of the United Nations Food and Agriculture Organization (FAO) provide a unique set of data on food intake, collected

Table 7. Methods for estimation of dietary fruit and vegetable intake in different settings

Method	Measurement of consumption	National surveillance	Observational epidemiology[a]	Validation for FFQ
Household measures of food availability				
Household dietary surveys	Food inventory (disappearance)	V		
Household budget surveys	Expenditure	V		
Food balance sheets	Food disappearance	V		
Questionnaires of usual intake for individuals				
Diet history	Usual intake (past, time varies)		v	
FFQ—long	Usual intake (past, time varies)	v	V	
FFQ—brief	Usual intake (past, time varies)	v	v	
Recording of actual intake				
24-hours recall	Actual intake (specific time-point)	V	v	V
Food record	Actual intake (specific time-point)	V	v	V

[a] Case–control and cohort studies
v, occasionally used; V, frequently used

year after year with a unified and consistent method. Details of this method are available on the internet (http://www.fao.org/waicent/faostat/agricult/fbs-e.htm). The information provided by FBS is in fact an estimate of the quantity of the various food commodities available for human consumption, after accounting for post-harvest losses. Post-harvest losses are particularly important for perishable foods, including fruit and vegetables, especially in developing countries. However, they do not account for wastage of edible foods at the household level. Thus, FBS data are more correctly referred to as disappearance or availability figures. The information is at a country level and provides no insight into intra-country differences in food consumption, between either socioeconomic groups or diverse ecological or geographical zones, nor into seasonal variations of the total food supply. A serious limitation of the FBS is the level of aggregation. The category "Vegetables", for example, includes a great variety of specific vegetable commodities, but it is not possible to retrieve any information on these.

The accuracy of FBS depends on the reliability of the underlying basic statistics on the supply and utilization of foods transmitted by each country, and varies therefore between countries. The developing regions of the world tend to have poorer statistics, and their FBS therefore have a larger margin of uncertainty.

Despite these limitations, FBS have the advantage that – having been regularly tabulated every year with a unified and unchanging technique since 1961 – they are the only source of information on worldwide time trends and country differences.

Methods to measure dietary intake at the individual level

Two main approaches are used to estimate dietary intake at the individual level. Questionnaires can be used to obtain information on usual intake during the preceding months or years either as quantities and frequencies of specific foods consumed (quantitative food frequency questionnaires) or the frequencies only (food frequency questionnaires). Alternatively, subjects are asked to report from memory the precise amounts of different foods actually eaten over the last 24 hours (24-h diet recall method) or to record all that they eat at the time of consumption (food consumption diaries or weighed food consumption records).

Questionnaire methods

Comprehensive descriptions and discussions of these methods as well as summaries of strengths and weaknesses of each method have been published (Margetts & Nelson, 1991; National Cancer Institute, 1994; Thompson & Byers, 1994; Willett, 1998a, b).

The most commonly used methods to assess dietary intake in cohort and case–control studies of cancer are food frequency questionnaires (FFQ) and the diet history. In cohort studies, the aim is to assess habitual current diet. In case–control studies, the aim is to assess habitual diet during a reference period before the onset of disease. In order to ascertain individual exposure to fruit and vegetables and other dietary components, information on intake needs to be obtained. However, accurately quantifying and classifying an individual's exposure is complex; measures that provide an estimate of usual intake are designed to minimize the effect of intra-individual variation.

The questionnaires used have differed widely between studies. They vary in the length of the food list, the number of questions, the fruits and vegetables included, how the instrument is structured, what other dietary information is obtained, the method used to address portion sizes and quantification of the data. There is no universally accepted questionnaire, standard interview, database or calculation system for use in epidemiological studies. Most FFQs or diet history questionnaires and interview methods are study-specific, being tailored to specific research questions and to the population being studied. Dietary methods are continually being refined based on methodological research. The many resulting variations in methods can affect estimates of dietary intake of fruits and vegetables in epidemiological studies and their relation to disease outcome.

During surveys with the FFQ and diet history, individuals provide information about intake of specific foods, food groups, dietary practices and/or food preparation methods. The information may be obtained by interview, by self-administered questionnaire or through a combination of these methods. The respondent may be the designated participant or a surrogate respondent. The data obtained are then reduced to summary measures using defined algorithms and food and nutrient databases.

Diet history

A diet history is information about usual intake of the individual's whole diet, usually obtained by interview (Burke, 1947). Detailed information is collected for a specified time period on the type, amount and frequency of foods eaten as well as food preparation practices. Typically a food list is used. Recipe information may be obtained, as well as meal-by-meal information about the time, place and content of meals. There is often a crosscheck feature to ensure complete determination of intake and to check for potential overreporting or double counting by the participant. Data may be collected in written form or directly on a computer using a special program (McDonald et al., 1991).

The strength of this method is that detailed quantified information is collected about usual dietary intake for an extended period of time. Compared with data from the recording and recall methods described later, a diet history covers a longer period of time and provides estimates of usual intake. It provides information on specific fruits and vegetables and about seasonal intake, as well as their consumption in mixed dishes. The method is time-consuming for the respondent and the investigators, but may be less conceptually demanding for respondents than food records or FFQs.

Food frequency questionnaire

Food frequency questionnaires (FFQs) have been the most commonly used method to assess dietary exposure in cohort and case–control studies. Respondents are asked to report their usual daily, weekly or monthly frequency of consumption of each item on a list of specific foods over a recent period of about a year. FFQs were developed during the 1950s and 1960s as the most cost-effective method for large epidemiological studies. Initial versions of the FFQ were designed only to rank individuals according to their relative level of dietary consumption expressed in quantiles, and only the frequency of food consumption was requested of the study subjects. Such questionnaires are reported as non-quantitative FFQs. During the 1980s and 1990s, variants of the FFQ were developed to allow its use in different study contexts and populations and to improve the estimation of individual absolute intake. Different questionnaire designs including standard or individual portion size estimates for all or selected items of the food list can lead to inconsistent reporting. These questionnaires may be described as "semi-quantitative" or "quantitative" FFQs (or dietary questionnaires). Over the last 20 years, there has been a clear methodological shift in epidemiological research from basic FFQs to more quantitative questionnaires, including the so-called dietary history questionnaires (see above).

The FFQ is usually self-administered in cohort studies. Respondents may receive the questionnaire along with any associated instructions and visual aids by mail and are asked to complete it at home and return it by mail. They may also complete the questionnaire at a research study centre; in this case verbal instructions can be provided and the questionnaire may be reviewed and clarified before the participant leaves the centre. In case–control studies, an FFQ may be administered by interviewers.

A core feature of the FFQ is usually a closed list of foods. The length of the list varies considerably between studies. The items included on the list depend on the nature of the investigation (particular foods and nutrients may be of interest); it must be borne in mind that a very detailed questionnaire places a heavy demand on the respondents. In cancer epidemiology, there are hypotheses about the effects of overall intake of fruit and vegetables as well as regarding the effects of individual fruits, vegetables or subcategories. Inaccurate estimates of intake can result from an incomplete listing of fruits and vegetables, while if key fruits or vegetables are neglected or if fruits or vegetables are grouped inappropriately (see Chapter 1), important information regarding intake may be lost.

Krebs-Smith et al. (1995) compared data from three surveys in the USA, in which FFQs had different numbers of questions relating to intake of fruit and vegetables. The values for median frequency of total fruit and vegetable intake differed between the surveys, and were associated with the number of questions asked. This pattern was also apparent for total fruit and total vegetables. The pattern did not appear to be accounted for by survey year, differences in the seasons covered or differences in the distribution of subjects by age and sex. In one of the surveys, the responses to a summary question "About how many servings of fruits and vegetables do you eat per day or per week?" indicated a median frequency of consumption substantially lower than that obtained by summing the responses to all individual questions about fruit and vegetable intake. In a pooled analysis of cohort studies of breast cancer and intake of fruit and vegetables, there was a more than four-fold variation between studies in the number of questions about fruit and vegetable intake (Smith-Warner et al., 2001a). The median intake increased with the number of items on the questionnaire. Thus, the number of questions asked is a potential source of heterogeneity between studies, and has implications for the categorization of reported intakes if data from different studies are combined.

Some FFQs provide only a list of foods, without portions specified. Others provide a portion size with each item and the respondent reports the frequency of intake of such a portion. Estimates of servings of food/food groups and nutrient intake are obtained by summing the reported frequencies (and the nutrient levels for each) over all foods. Intake is usually expressed as a mean number of servings per day or as a mean nutrient amount per day (Thompson & Byers, 1994; Willett, 1998a).

The portion sizes typically reflect some standardized approach with common household units (such as cups, ounces or grams) as reported in nutrient databases, although in some cases they may reflect typical local portion sizes. Some FFQs allow the respondent, for each item, to choose a portion size from a list or to record his or her own portion size. FFQs may incorporate questions regarding usual portion sizes for some food items. For studies of fruit and vegetables, this may be particularly important in populations that are relatively well fed and that have access to a wide variety of foods. In general, the ranking of individuals according to intake of specific nutrients seems to be determined largely by reported frequency of intake, with little contribution of inter-individual variation in portion size (Samet et al., 1984; Humble et al., 1987; Hunter et al., 1988; Flegal & Larkin, 1990; Tjonneland et al., 1992; Noethlings et al., 2003), although there are exceptions (Clapp et al., 1991; Block, 1992).

In a study in which cognitive interviewing was used, respondents tended to skip portion-size questions after completing frequency questions (Subar et al., 1995). In a study of women in Sweden who were randomly allocated to receive different questionnaires, mean frequency of consumption was significantly lower for vegetables (and other foods) when portion size questions were included (Kuskowska-Wolk et al., 1992). Moreover, there was an adverse effect on response rate. In an investigation of the validity of using pictures to estimate portion size, 103 volunteers were offered standard dishes, and the weight of the food eaten was compared with weight estimated by recall the next day with the aid of pictures (Faggiano et al., 1992). There was a tendency to overestimate portion size among those who ate smaller portions and to underestimate portion size among those who ate larger portions. However, Blake et al. (1989) reported that there were no differences in the ability to estimate portion size between normal-weight and overweight subjects.

It is difficult with FFQs to capture information about fruit and vegetable intake consumed in the form of mixed dishes. Such dishes may be listed as "mixed dishes", pasta dishes, soups, vegetable soups, stews, casseroles, Chinese dishes, ethnic foods, salads etc. The actual fruit and vegetable content of these items varies greatly and no estimate of specific fruits and vegetables will be available. In many cuisines, mixed dishes contribute a large proportion of fruit and vegetable intake. The FFQ method requires respondents to integrate the fruit and vegetable intake from these foods into their report of the separate fruit and vegetable items.

Respondents are asked to report their usual intake for a specified time period. The time frame used is often one year, but varies between studies from as little as one month up to 3–10 years. It is assumed that intake over a recent one-year period reflects longer-term intake.

FFQs can be structured in several ways, most commonly by food group, but sometimes by meal. Cognitive testing indicates that many individuals, when asked to report their usual intake of fruit and vegetables, do so by recalling a typical day (Thompson et al., 2000). When 874 subjects in the USA were randomly assigned to receive one of two brief questionnaires designed for surveillance of fruit and vegetable intake, the questionnaire subdivided to assess intake in different parts of the day gave the best agreement with true habitual intake estimated on the basis of two 24-hour recalls (Thompson et al., 2000). In a study in France of two groups of 20 volunteers, Boutron et al. (1989) compared data on intake of foods and nutrients obtained with two interviewer-administered questionnaires, one structured by meals and the other by broad food groups, and a 14-day dietary record. The questionnaire structured by meals gave better correlation with the dietary record than the questionnaire structured by food groups, when the data were analysed either in terms of the relative ranking of subjects or in terms of correlation with absolute intake.

Two other aspects of FFQ structure are whether food items are grouped or listed separately and whether closed or open-ended questions are used (Kuskowska-Wolk et al., 1992; Tylavsky & Sharp, 1995; Subar et al., 2000; Thompson et al., 2002).

Brief food frequency questionnaires
Brief food frequency questionnaires are sometimes used, containing a very abbreviated list of foods. The questionnaire may focus on a specific food group or a limited number of food groups or food items. The food list may comprise groupings of foods and be aimed at characterizing some major dietary components such as fat. Respondents are asked to report their usual frequency of intake for the specified time period, as described above. Such instruments have been used to estimate fat and calcium intake, as well as intake of servings of fruit and vegetables (Block et al., 1990, 2000; Willett, 1998a). As a part of the Behavioral Risk Factor Surveillance System (BRFSS), the US Centers for Disease Control and Prevention (CDC) use a brief telephone-administered questionnaire to assess fat intake with 13 questions and fruit and vegetable intake with six questions (Serdula et al., 1993). In efforts to assess changes in fruit and vegetable intake in response to intervention programmes, a variety of brief questionnaires addressing fruit and vegetable intake have been developed and validated in conjunction with 5-A-Day research programmes (see Chapter 3) and community campaigns (Domel et al., 1993a). Brief methods have been developed in efforts to apply a common measure across studies, reduce cost and participant burden, and to enhance the number and type of individuals who can be reached. Kristal et al. (2000) compared the validation data from these studies in which 24-hour dietary recalls, food records or serum carotenoid concentrations were used as criterion measures. The validation studies differed in distributions of participants' age, race/ethnicity, sex and socioeconomic status. Mean intakes of total fruit and vegetables based on the 5-A-Day brief method were consistently lower than those from either a much longer FFQ (3.11 versus 4.06), 24-h recalls (3.32 versus 4.07) or food records (3.11 versus 3.46; all $p < 0.01$), and this was due primarily to underestimation of vegetable intake with the brief FFQ method.

These methods have many limitations in the context of epidemiological investigations aimed at understanding associations between fruit and vegetables and cancer risk. They yield very limited information about intake of specific food items crucial to hypotheses about diet and cancer. If they are limited to a single nutrient or food group, information on the total diet and other potential dietary confounders is not available. Because they focus on a few items (particularly fat, fruit and foods that receive a great deal of media attention regarding health consequences), brief questionnaires may suffer from biased reporting based on the subjects' perceptions of what they ought to eat (social desirability bias) and general overreporting of fruit and vegetable intake.

Recording-based measures of actual intake
The 24-hour dietary recall
The aim of the 24-hour dietary recall is to estimate actual dietary intake. An interview is conducted either in person or by telephone, often by a dietitian. The respondent is asked to recall and then report all foods and beverages consumed in the previous 24 hours (sometimes in the preceding day). Respondents are asked to report the amount they consumed typically in household units or weights if known and to provide information about food preparation, brand names and recipes. Photographs of portion sizes may be used. Respondents are asked to report any items added to foods such as condiments, salt, sugar or fats. The interview is usually structured with probes to help the individual remember foods consumed and to provide detailed descriptions of these foods. Data may be recorded using paper forms and subsequently coded and entered on a computer or may be directly entered on the computer with the help of specialized software.

Because the recall covers a recent time period, issues related to memory are reduced. Respondents are not required to be literate and the burden on them may be much lower than with self-administered dietary methods. This generally improves the participation rate. A major strength of the 24-hour recall is that detailed information about all fruit and vegetables and other foods consumed and their specific form (cooked, raw) can be obtained (assuming that a comprehensive food data-base is used). The major limitation regarding fruit and vegetable intake is the short time period covered, since there is considerable day-to-day and season-to-season variation in both the types and the amounts of fruit and vegetables consumed. When only one day of intake is sampled, this approach does not provide a reliable estimate of an individual's intake over longer periods (Beaton et al., 1979, 1983; Todd et al., 1983). Obtaining repeat 24-hour recalls reduces this problem greatly.

The 24-hour recall method was used in some early case–control and cohort studies, before development and widespread use of FFQs, and in clinical trials where the primary purpose of the dietary data was to characterize group intakes. Dietary recall data from clinical trials have been used to evaluate cohorts for subsequent investigations related to diet and cancer.

Food records
Food records are detailed meal-by-meal recordings of the types and quantities of food and drink consumed during a specified period, typically 3–7 days. For a weighed record, or weighed inventory record, the subject weighs all foods consumed during the specified period. A variant of this method does not require the subject to weigh the foods, but to report quantities in terms of household measures or using food models or photographs. This provides detailed information on actual food intake. By having respondents record their intake at the time of consumption, recall problems are minimized and more details about each food item may be available. Such methods may place a considerable burden on the subjects, limiting their application to literate respondents who are highly motivated, and may therefore introduce selection bias, while compliance may produce alterations in diet (Bathalon et al., 2000).

Quantification of fruit and vegetable portions

In general, recalling and reporting sizes of portion sizes of foods consumed is a difficult cognitive task; respondents often have difficulty in estimating weights, volumes and dimensions (Thompson et al., 1987; Smith et al., 1991). Methods to help respondents with reporting and quantification have been developed and good questionnaire design can also improve estimation of fruit and vegetbale intake. Respondents may, depending on the method used, report consumption in units they are most comfortable with or they may have to convert their concept of portion size to those used on a questionnaire. They also may have to adjust their frequency reporting to those specified. Fruits and vegetables vary greatly in size, shape and seasonal availability, how they are prepared and the form consumed. Quantities for fruits and vegetables can be obtained as servings as defined by the respondent, in household units such as cups, or in pieces such as one apple, with dimension descriptions or by weight.

There are many differences between how fruit and vegetables are eaten that affect portion size specification and quantification. Because of the ways fruits are prepared and eaten, they may be easier than vegetables to remember and to quantify. Fruits are often eaten as the single item or combined with other fruits as in a fruit salad or fruit cup. Although pieces of fruit vary in size, there is some uniformity due to modern horticultural and retailing practices for grading and selling fruit based on size. Furthermore, fruit is often consumed as fruit juice, again a discrete item that may be easy to recall and quantify. When juice is sold in individual portions, there is also some standardization of the amount sold. Because fruits are often eaten in specific contexts such as a snack or as a dessert, they may be easier to recall and quantify than vegetables.

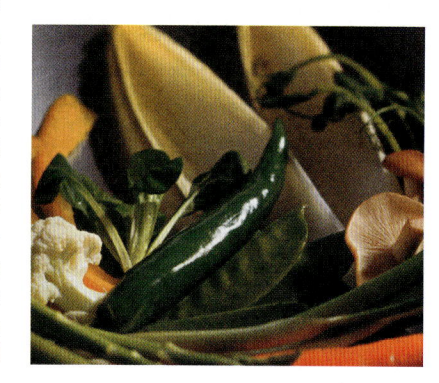

Vegetable consumption varies much more. As noted in Chapter 1, there is a wide variety of vegetables consumed by humans and even what is defined as a vegetable varies according to the cultural and research settings. Food preparation and culinary practices vary greatly for vegetables and this affects how they can be quantified. Vegetables may be consumed as a single item (a carrot, corn, artichoke, potato), but are commonly served after some preparation (chopping, slicing, cooking etc.) and as mixtures (soup, stew, pasta dishes, stir fry); many are included in recipes in forms that may not be easily identified by respondents (tomato sauce, chopped onion or garlic). They may also be served as accompaniments to foods in sauces, relishes or sandwiches. These varied ways of serving and eating vegetables make recall and quantification more difficult for respondents and complicate conversion of data from diet assessments to food consumption amounts (either servings or weights) to be used in statistical analyses. There are many nutrients and phytochemicals of interest in cancer epidemiology and even small amounts of specific fruits or vegetables may contribute importantly to total intake of these. If important sources in the diet are not identified, it may be impossible to adequately classify individual exposure.

Visual aids have been developed to help respondents estimate the amount of foods consumed or the portions typically eaten, including for fruit and vegetables (Margetts & Nelson, 1991; Riboli & Kaaks, 1997). Such visual aids can be used in conjunction with any dietary assessment method. Three-dimensional aids such as food models, actual plates, cups, glasses, spoons or portions of real food displayed in service ware may be shown to respondents during an interview. Two-dimensional printed aids are used in many settings and frequently with FFQs and dietary recalls conducted by telephone. These may be diagrams of food portions (such as portions of meat) or household utensils (measuring cups or spoons) and dishes with portion size indications noted, or be pictures of actual foods on or in appropriate service ware; these may include pictures of several different portion sizes. One study found no great difference between mean intakes reported with use of three-dimensional aids compared with those obtained using two-dimensional diagrams (Posner et al., 1992). A benefit of photographs is they can show regional foods and can display foods in a familiar context, both of which may improve recall and quantification, and this approach has been used with good results in several studies (Pietinen et al., 1988). Visual aids may be used in the interview setting or be provided to participants (by mail or other means) to refer to when they are completing a questionnaire or record.

Some research protocols use more extensive procedures and ask respondents to either measure typical amounts of foods they consume, measure the volume of their usual service ware or weigh their foods before consumption. Training of respondents on how to estimate and report their intake has been shown to improve reporting and portion estimation (Bolland et al., 1988).

Measurement error and validity

Sources of error

Many factors affect the accuracy with which the intake of fruit and vegetables can be measured and contribute to measurement error. Respondent factors and factors associated with the measurement techniques are the two main sources. Respondent factors that may contribute to error include: memory, socio-demographic factors such as age, gender, education, literacy, ethnicity, occupation, cultural background, disease or health status, knowledge and attitudes. Even individuals able to accurately recall their food intake may be influenced by factors such as social desirability that affect how and what intake they report. For fruit and vegetables, respondents may overreport consumption because high intake of these foods is perceived as healthy (Margetts & Nelson, 1991; Hankin & Wilkens, 1994; Willet & Lenart, 1998).

Dietary changes during prospective studies need to be considered in the design and analysis of longitudinal studies, particularly very long ones. In the Potsdam cohort of the EPIC study, 47% of the participants reported making some type of dietary change during the first two years of the study (Bergmann & Boeing, 2002). The reported changes tended to be consistent with dietary guidelines; increased fruit and vegetable consumption and lower fat intake were the most common changes noted.

Method-related errors can arise through aspects of questionnaire construction (composition of the food list, specification of portion sizes, grouping of foods into a single item, the order of questions) and the database used to calculate nutrients, food group coding and fruit and vegetable classifications (Margetts & Nelson, 1991).

Validity

A major issue is whether a study aimed to rank individuals according to relative dietary intake or to provide a measure of absolute intake of fruit and vegetables. There continues to be debate about whether FFQs (and to some extent diet history interviews) can accurately assess absolute intake of foods, or can only classify individuals in terms of their relative intake (Block, 2001; Byers, 2001; Willett, 2001d). Validation studies have been used to investigate the extent of misclassification, and this information has sometimes been used to adjust for misclassification within studies (Rosner & Gore, 2001).

Because there is no gold standard for validation of diet methods (Mertz, 1992), a variety of reference methods have been used in validation studies, including 24-hour diet recalls, food consumption records and biological markers (Bingham et al., 1997; Ocké et al., 1997b; Pisani et al., 1997; Riboli & Kaaks, 1997; Smith-Warner et al., 1997; Field et al., 1998; Thompson et al., 2000).

In relation to relative intake, there have been many studies of the reproducibility of dietary instruments, that is, the extent to which different methods applied to the same individuals result in the same ranking of individuals. In order to check that a method is not "consistently wrong", there is a need to compare it with a reference method, usually repeated food records or 24-hour diet recalls.

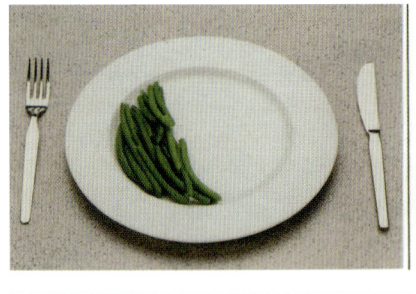

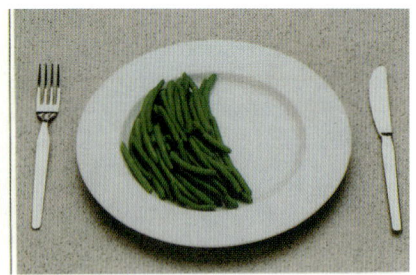

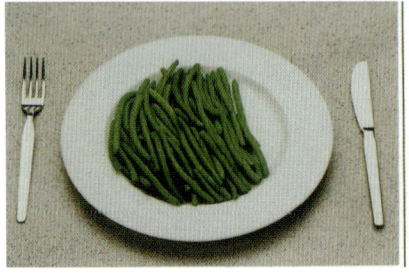

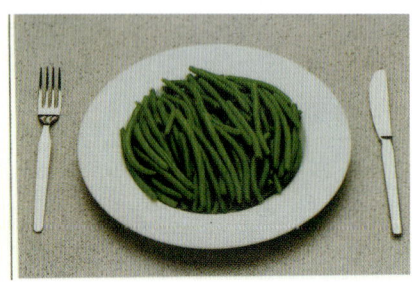

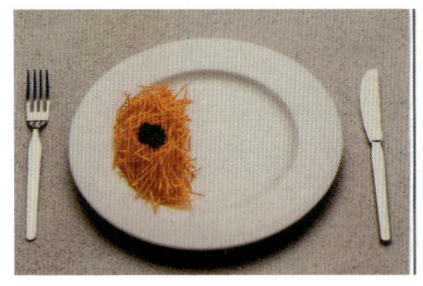

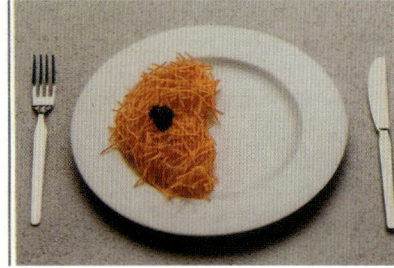

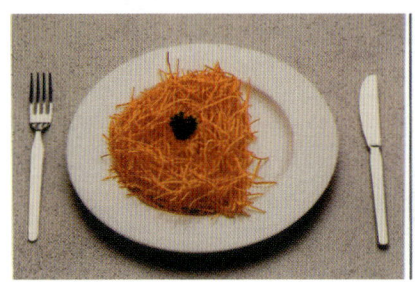

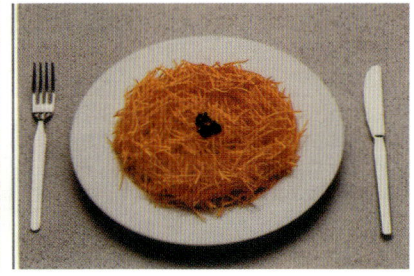

IARC Handbooks of Cancer Prevention Volume 8: Fruit and Vegetables

Examples of food portion sizes from a dietary questionnaire (EPIC), Lyon

The majority of validation studies have compared questionnaire estimates of food consumption or nutrient intake with assessments of current or very recent diet by the reference method. Such an approach is satisfactory for a cohort study investigating the relationship between diet current at the time of assessment and future disease. However, in case–control studies, the relationship between disease and past diet is under investigation, so that, in theory, the reference method should have been applied in the past. In practice, this has rarely been done, and the investigator is forced to make assumptions about the relationship between current and past diet. In studies of chronic disease such as cancer, an additional difficulty is that the disease process itself may have an effect on diet.

Besides various interview and questionnaire methods to assess individuals' intake of fruit and vegetables, biochemical markers of dietary intake have also been proposed (Kaaks et al., 1997a; Hunter, 1998; Crews et al., 2001). Examples of such markers are vitamin C and different types of carotenoid, which can be measured in blood or in adipose tissue (carotenoids only). Measurements of biomarkers can provide complementary information to help assess the performance of different dietary methods, as they should be more objective, depending less on subjects' memory or overall response or cooperation in a study. However, despite initial hopes that markers could be identified that would correlate highly with subjects' true intake of specific dietary compounds or of specific foods, many studies have shown rather weak correlations (Kaaks et al., 1997a; Polsinelli et al., 1998; McEligot et al., 1999; Crews et al., 2001; El Sohemy et al., 2002). Although there may be exceptions (e.g., blood lycopene level as a specific marker of tomatoes and tomato products), these low correlations make markers less attractive than traditional dietary assessment methods as the main exposure assessment method for epidemiological studies (see Chapter 4). Nevertheless, markers can be of some use as an additional reference measurement in validation studies (see also below).

Effects of dietary measurement error

Dietary intake assessments are generally imperfect and generally contain errors. The overall measurement error

– simply defined as the difference between individuals' measured and true intake levels – can be decomposed into systematic and random components (Kaaks *et al.*, 1994a; Willett, 1998c; Kipnis *et al.*, 1999).

Constant or proportional scaling biases may occur when, on average, study subjects tend to over- or underestimate intake by, respectively, a constant amount or by an amount that is proportional to the subjects' true intake levels. This type of error may cause bias in relative risk estimates for quantitative differences in dietary intake levels expressed on an interval scale. In addition, between-population differences in scaling errors may complicate the pooling of data across different populations (Kaaks *et al.*, 1994b). Scaling errors, however, will not affect relative risk estimates for subjects classified into diferent quantile categories of the population distribution of intake levels.

In contrast to scaling errors, random (between-subject) error components are neither constant nor structurally related to subjects' true intake level (Kaaks *et al.*, 1994a) and generally tend to lead to underestimation ("attenuation") of measures of association between diet and disease, with a substantial loss of statistical power to detect these associations. The underestimation of relative risk and associated loss of statistical power depend on the correlation, ρ_{QT}, between the questionnaire measurements of intake and the true habitual intake levels. Assuming that both true and measured intake levels follow an approximately normal distribution, the relationship between the relative risk observed for quantile categories (e.g., quartiles or quintiles) of intake measurements and the relative risk for the same quantile categories of true intake levels can be written as (de Klerk *et al.*, 1989)

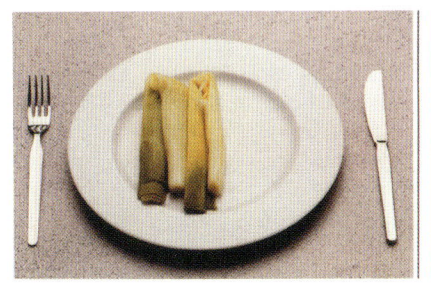

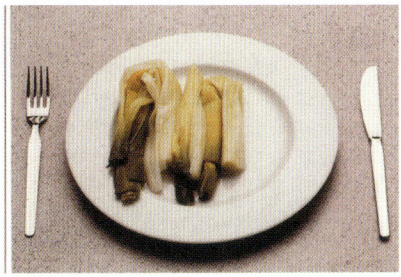

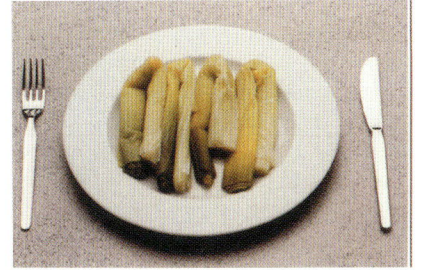

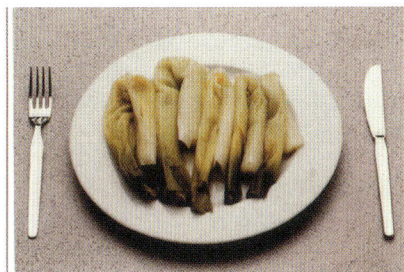

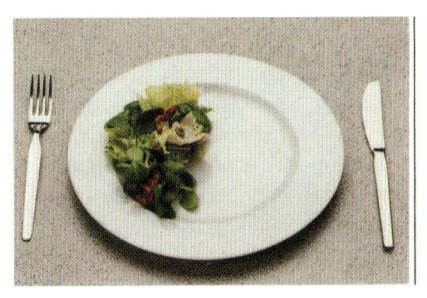

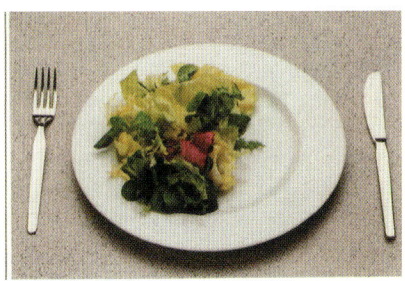

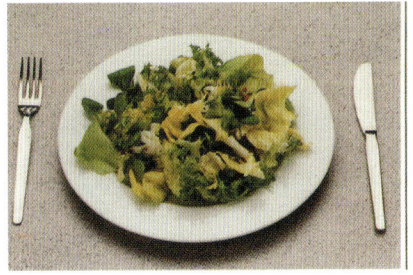

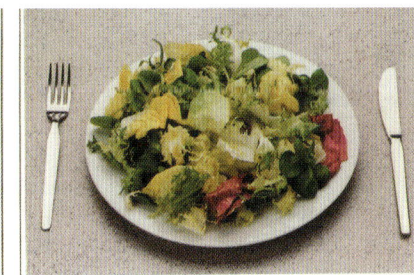

$$RR_O = (RR_T)^{\rho_{QT}} \quad [1]$$

From this mathematical relationship [1] of estimated versus true relative risks for given proportions (e.g., quintiles) of the population ranked into low and high intake levels, it follows that estimates of population attributable risk, as well as relative risk, will also be biased by random measurement error.

Relative risks estimated for a quantitative difference in intake levels expressed on an absolute (interval) scale (e.g., relative risk for a 100 gram increase in total vegetable intake) will be also biased by random error. Here, the mathematical relationship between true and estimated relative risks can be written as

$$RR_O = (RR_T)^{\rho'_{QT}} \quad [2]$$

Approaches to evaluating impact of dietary assessment error

To correct for attenuation bias in measures of diet–disease associations, the correlation coefficient ρ_{QT} can be estimated in validation studies and, using either equation [1] or [2], corrected relative risk estimates can be obtained from initial, 'crude' estimates based on questionnaire assessments (de Klerk et al., 1989; Rosner et al., 1989; Kaaks et al., 1995). Especially within prospective cohort studies, validation studies have been increasingly included as a standard part of the overall design (Willett et al., 1985; Colditz et al., 1986; Goldbohm et al., 1994; Margetts & Pietinen, 1997; Stram et al., 2000; Hankin et al., 2001; Slimani et al., 2002). Validity is estimated for measurements obtained by a given questionnaire within a specific study context, rather than for the method itself, which may not perform the same way in other contexts. It is crucial that validity studies be conducted in a representative subsample of the main study population.

Most validation studies have been based on a comparison with repeated daily intake methods for a number of days. The correlation ρ_{QT} can then be estimated by

1. calculation of a crude correlation coefficient ρ_{QR} between questionnaire measurements and individuals' average intake estimates from several days of food consumption records;
2. estimation of the residual error variance in the reference measurements (average food consumption records) themselves, and calculation of an attenuation coefficient by which the estimate ρ_{QR} would need to be corrected, to yield a more unbiased estimate of ρ_{QT} (Rosner & Willett, 1988).

The second step of this estimation procedure should correct for residual random error in the reference measurements. In the early 1990s, this approach of estimating ρ_{QT} was extended, using models in which subjects' true dietary intake levels are considered a 'latent variable' (Plummer & Clayton 1993a, b; Kaaks et al., 1994a).

The most important assumption that underlies any type of validity study is that different types of measurement being compared – from questionnaires, recording methods or biomarkers – will be correlated exclusively because they all measure the same underlying latent variable (true intake). This means that random errors must be uncorrelated between the different types of measurement compared (Plummer & Clayton 1993a, b; Kaaks et al., 1994a, 2002). Unfortunately, there is increasing evidence that generally errors may not be entirely independent between questionnaire assessments of habitual dietary intake and measurements obtained by a recording method, assessing actual food consumption on a number of days. In particular, it has been shown that individuals vary systematically in their tendency to over- or underreport dietary intakes, not only when using the same measurement method, but even when different questionnaire and/or recording methods are used (Livingstone et al., 1990; Black & Cole, 2001; Livingstone & Black, 2003). Thus, errors that are random between individuals may be partially systematic within subjects ("subject-specific biases") and this will result in positive correlations between random errors in different intake measurements from the same individual. A positive correlation between random errors of questionnaire measurements and the reference measurements used tends to cause overestimation of ρ_{QT}. On the other hand, a positive correlation between random errors of replicate dietary intake records, as the reference, can lead to incomplete adjustment for attenuation bias in estimates of ρ_{QT}. In practice, it is difficult to predict the balance between the two possible and opposite biases in estimating ρ_{QT} (Kipnis et al., 2001; Kaaks et al., 2002). This problem of correlated measurement errors can only be partially, if at all, overcome by the use of available biomarkers, depending on the type of nutrient of food group considered (Plummer & Clayton, 1993a,b; Kaaks et al., 1994a, 2002; Kipnis et al., 2001).

Estimated validity of measured fruit and vegetable consumption

Table 8 shows the estimated correlation ρ_{QT} for total fruit and total vegetable intake, from a number of validity studies. Correlation coefficients were within a range of about 0.30 to 0.76, and were generally estimated with rather wide confidence intervals, due to the limited size of studies (generally 50–150 subjects). From equation [2], it can be estimated that, with a correlation of $\rho_{QT} = 0.30$ and a true relative risk of 3.0 between highest and lowest exposure categories (e.g., quintiles of the intake distribution), the observed relative risk would be as low as 1.10. For a correlation of $\rho_{QT} = 0.7$, the estimated relative risk would be less attenuated but still only 1.7. Thus, as illustrated by this numerical example, there will generally be considerable attenuation bias in relative risk estimates for quantile categories of intake and this may lead to substantial loss of statistical power to detect a real association.

Table 8. Estimated validity of fruit and vegetable intake for questionnaires (FFQ) for selected study populations

Population, reference	No. items on FFQ	Reference method	No. repeated measures	Type of correlation*	N	Men Fruit	Men Vegetables	N	Women Fruit	Women Vegetables
The Netherlands cohort, Goldbohm et al., 1994	150 (21 veg., 8 fruits)	Diet records	3, 3 days	S, c	107 (59 M + 48 W)	0.60	0.38	–	–	–
Hawaii cohort, Hankin et al., 1991	Diet history (47)	Food records	4, 1 week	ICC	128	0.60	0.39	134	0.34	0.19
EPIC – France, van Liere et al., 1997	Diet history (101)	24-h DR	12	S, c	–	–	–	115	0.44	0.50
EPIC – Germany, Bohlscheid-Thomas et al., 1997; Kaaks et al., 1997	158	24-h DR	12	S, c	49	0.33	0.39	55	0.45	0.53
EPIC – Italy, Pisani et al., 1997	47	24-h DR	12	S, c	47	0.56	0.30	150	0.39	0.45
EPIC – Netherlands, Ocké et al., 1997b	79	24-h DR	12	S, c	63	0.68	0.38	58	0.56	0.31
EPIC – Spain, The EPIC group of Spain, 1997	Diet history (17)	24-h DR	12	P, c	46	0.76	0.73	45	0.66	0.65
EPIC – Sweden, Kaaks et al., 1997b	130	24-h DR	12	S, c	44	0.72	0.42	559	0.62	0.49
Health professionals cohort, Feskanich et al., 1993	122	Diet records	2, 1 week	P, d	127	0.75#	0.46#	–	–	–
Minnesota Cancer Prevention diet intervention trial, Smith-Warner et al., 1997	153 (33 veg, 18 fruits)	Diet records	5, 3 days	P, d	101 (71 M + 30 W)	0.67	0.32	–	–	–
Finnish lung cancer intervention trial, Pietinen et al., 1988	276	Food records	12, 2 days	P, d	158	0.69	0.58	–	–	–

*: S, Spearman; P, Pearson; ICC, intraclass correlation coefficient; c, crude; d, deattenuated
Median of reported values for individual fruits or vegetables DR, dietary recall

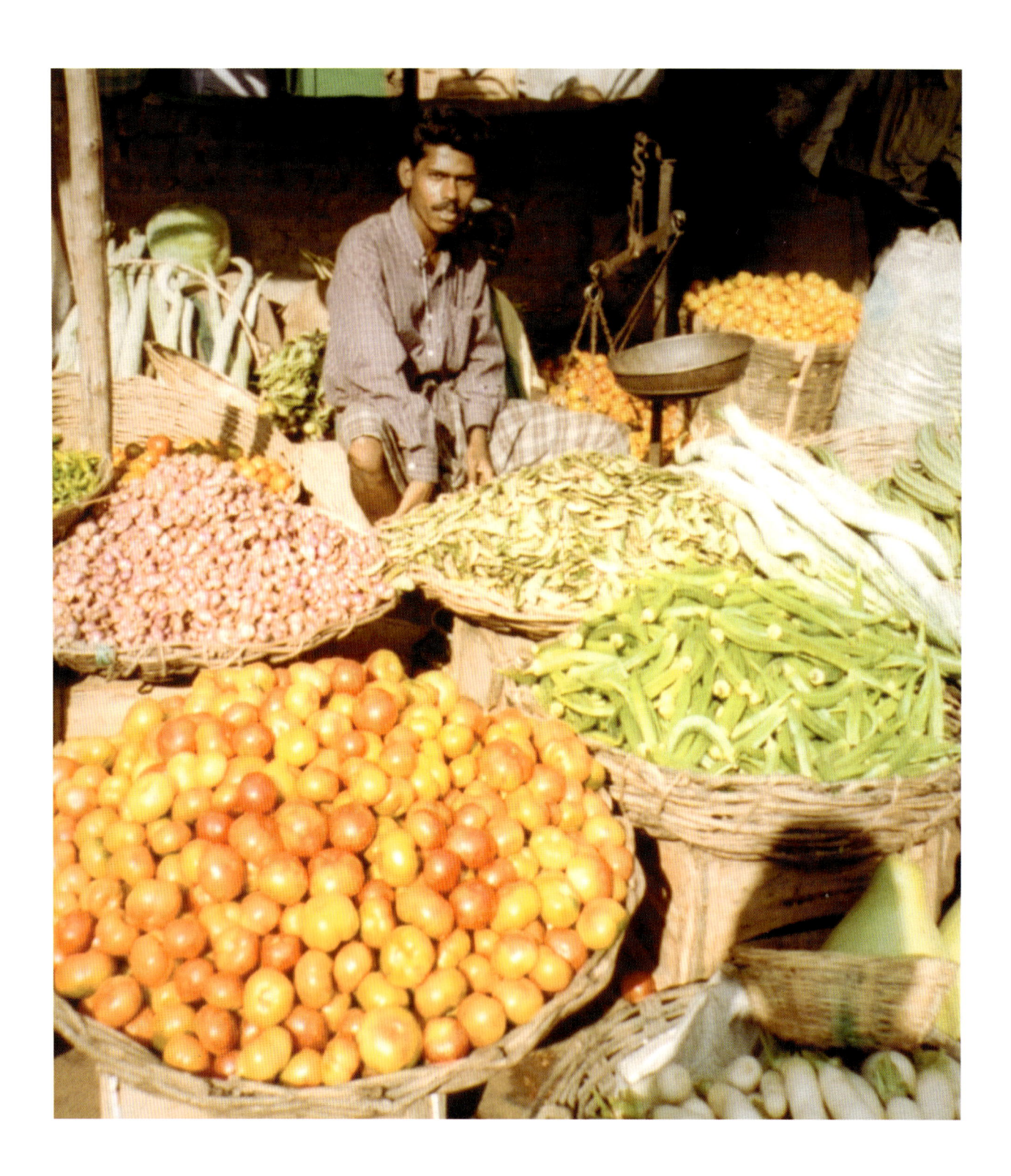

Chapter 3
Consumption, availability and food policies

Fruit and vegetable consumption

This section reviews quantitative information on consumption of fruit and vegetables from published and unpublished surveys. Most of the survey results were published in the international scientific literature, but some were retrieved from national journals with limited circulation and from government reports. Studies and reports presenting information on the frequency of consumption only were excluded. Another selection criterion was the level of representativity of the study sample, at the national or subnational level, although in special cases, data on smaller, selected groups of populations were retained for the purpose of highlighting specific points. The review focuses on surveys conducted in the last couple of decades; earlier data are considered only if they are of special significance or if they document specific aspects, such as time trends.

In view of the paucity of information on food consumption in the developing regions of the world, recourse was made to the series of Nutrition Country Profiles (NCPs) of the Food and Agriculture Organization (FAO) to obtain a glimpse, albeit crude, of the situation in these countries. NCPs are prepared in a standard format and provide information on the food and nutritional situation in individual countries. Data are derived from the UN agencies' global data banks, complemented by information from national institutions and independent experts from the countries. The quality of the information on food consumption is highly variable between countries, but is mostly rather crude. Only overall fruit and vegetable consumption data are reported, and little, if any, methodological information (sampling technique, survey methods, individual food items included under either category, general context of the survey) is provided. Some surveys used the household budget survey method, others used food frequency questionnaires, yet others used weighed or estimated food intake records over a variable number of days (for more information, see http://www.fao.org/es/esn/nutrition/profiles_en.stm). Finally, the FAO food balance sheets (see Chapter 2) were used to obtain an overview of the situation worldwide, as well as to detect trends over time (FAOSTAT, 2000).

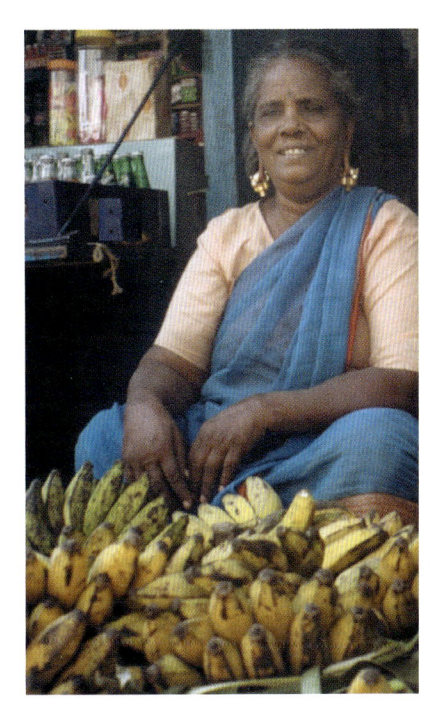

From the above, it is apparent that the data reported in this chapter have been generated by a variety of methods, some of which are known to provide only a crude estimate of dietary intake. A detailed description of the diverse approaches is provided in Chapter 2. The limitations encountered in trying to provide a general picture of the consumption of fruit and vegetables are detailed below, and should be kept in mind when considering the data and drawing conclusions.

Categories of fruit and of vegetables

The presentation of data-sets on consumption of fruit and vegetables as aggregated groups is an important issue that can seriously limit their comparison and interpretation. In some cases, only values for combined fruit and vegetables are provided. More frequently, separate values are given for the two categories, but these are not homogeneous across studies, as they may or may not include individual items such as potatoes, starchy fruit (e.g., bananas), dry and/or fresh pulses, or fruit and vegetable juices. Unfortunately, it has not been possible to fully harmonize the data and the errors introduced when comparing two non-identical food aggregations can be neither corrected nor controlled for. Indeed, the most serious and widespread limitation is that reports only seldom specify the individual fruit and vegetable items included in or excluded from their analyses. Examples of detailed descriptions of the food items included within the fruit and vegetable categories are the CSFII surveys (USDA Food Surveys Research Group, 2003a) and the multicentre European Prospective Investigation into Cancer and Nutrition (EPIC) (Agudo et al., 2002). The lack of detail in the reports from developing countries may be accounted for by the fact that the focus of these surveys has been food security and therefore the emphasis was placed on staple foods rather than the low-energy content fruits and vegetables. However, a similar paucity of data on food groupings is shared by several reports from developed countries.

The problem is compounded by the loose and sometimes imprecise use of botanical classification of fruit and vegetables. Thus, "roots and tubers" may or may not be included in the vegetable category; potatoes are sometimes, but not always, included in "roots and tubers"; olives may be specified as fruits; starchy fruits and vegetables (bananas, yams, breadfruit) may or may not be listed in their respective categories; the category of pulses is sometimes given separately but it is almost never specified whether fresh pods are included or not in the vegetable category. The term "legumes" is used in a loose manner, especially in the non-English literature, where it sometimes refers to fresh vegetables in general. Fruit and vegetable juices and nectars may or may not be listed separately, as may canned and preserved fruits. This may introduce a large margin of uncertainty around the reported values. A further problem is the fact that certain items are country-specific. Thus, inclusion or exclusion of a food item here was determined with the purpose of maximizing the comparability of the datasets. As a rule, potatoes, pulses and canned beans were excluded from the vegetable category, while "beans", "peas", "fresh legumes" and "canned vegetables" were included. "Other root vegetables" were also included. Olives were excluded. For the category of fruit, the following items were excluded: jams, preserves, dates, bananas, plantains, nuts and dry fruits. The fruit category includes fruit juices, fruit nectars and canned fruits. An exception was made with the food balance sheet data, where bananas were included in the fruit category, in view of the important position of bananas in the diet of large regions in Africa and Latin America. This inclusion is not based on evidence of any potential health-protective effect.

In conclusion, an attempt was made to harmonize the categories of fruit and vegetables across the various surveys. However, this process has been possible only to a limited extent and no presumption can be made about the homogeneity of the categories in the various studies.

Age and sex groupings

Another factor that limits the comparability of food intake data from the various sources derives from the disparity in the sex and age composition of the study samples. Often data are given as averages for both sexes combined. In some cases, age groups do not overlap, in other cases the range is wide and no information on the median or mean age of the entire group is provided. While age has a bearing on the total volume of food consumed as well as on total energy intake (increasing with age from childhood to maturity and levelling off later to fall in advanced old age), it cannot be assumed that the same pattern applies to the intake of fruit and vegetables. Indeed, an age-associated increase in fruit and vegetable consumption can be seen in some but not all data-sets. More important might be the possible change in the spectrum of individual food items consumed at various ages. A clear case is that of consumption of fruit juices and nectars that increases sharply in the second to third years of life, remains high during childhood, and then declines with advancing age.

National surveys

Nationally representative data on fruit and vegetable consumption were available for 21 countries including China, India, Israel and the Philippines. The remaining 17 countries include 14 within the WHO European Region and Australia, Japan and the USA.

Figure 1 shows the data obtained in Australia (McLennan & Podger, 1999), the Baltic republics (Pomerleau et al., 2001), Belgium (Kornitzer & Bara, 1989), China (Institute of Nutrition and Food Hygiene, 2002), Denmark (National Food Agency of Denmark, 1990), Finland (National Public Health Institute of Finland, 1998), France (Volatier & Verger, 1999), India (Department of Women & Child Development, 1998), Ireland (Irish Nutrition & Dietetic Institute, 1990), Israel (D.N. Kaluski, personal communication), Italy (Turrini et al., 2001), Japan (Office for Life-style Related Disease Control, 2002), the Netherlands (Netherlands Nutrition Centre, 1998), Norway (Johansson & Sovoll, 1999), the Philippines (Food and Nutrition Research Institute, 2001), Spain (Instituto Nacional de Estadistica, 1991), Sweden (Becker, 2001), the United Kingdom (Gregory et al., 1990) and the USA (USDA Food Surveys Research Group, 2003b).

Consumption, availability and food policies

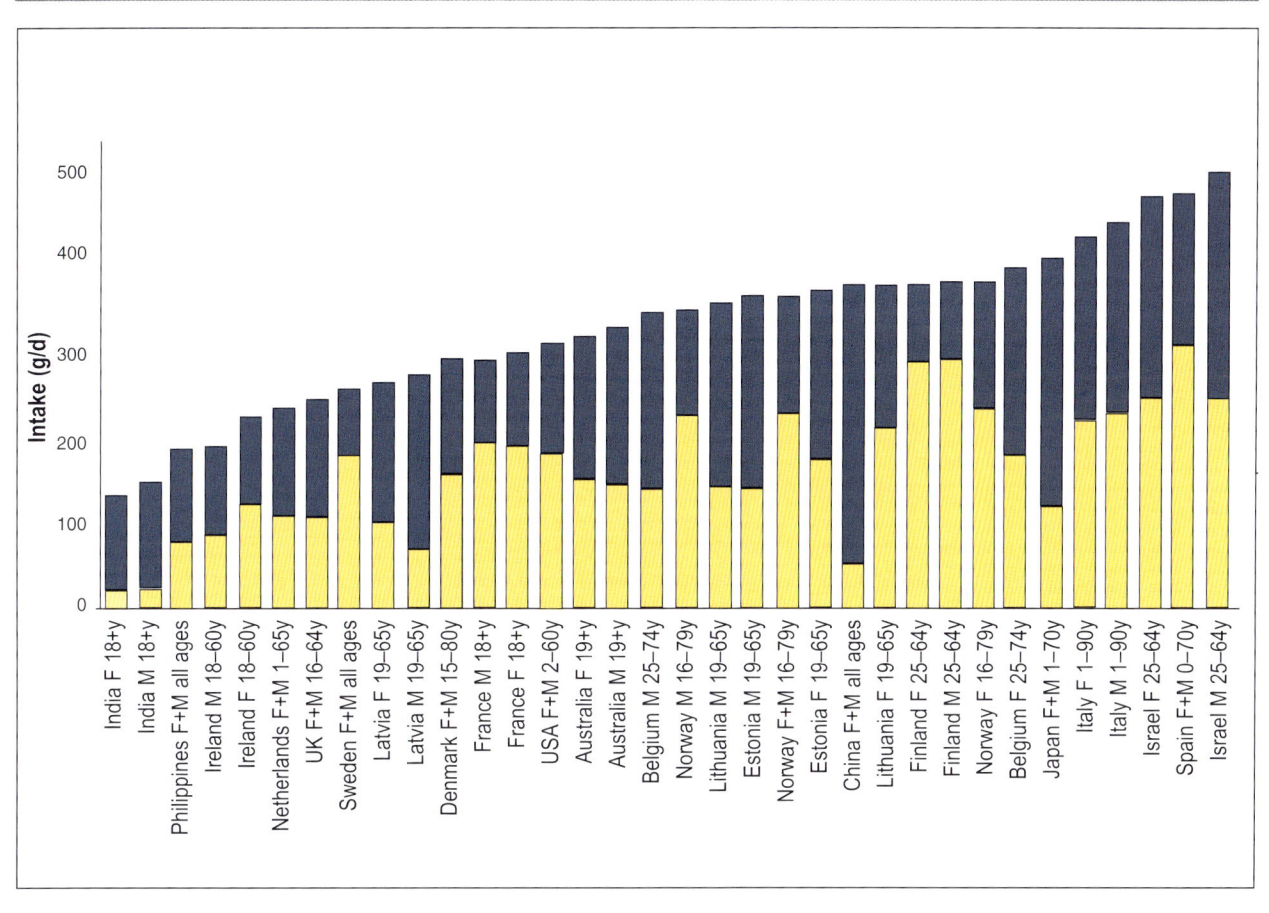

Figure 1 Overview of the fruit (yellow) and vegetable (blue) consumption in 21 selected countries, as reported by the most recently conducted national surveys

There are obvious limitations to this comparison, such as the different age ranges used, the survey methods, the dates of the survey and the items included in the categories of fruit and vegetables. Where the data permitted, values shown in Figure 1 are for adults, but in some cases the range includes children and/or the elderly. About half of the surveys give data for men and women separately.

The picture that emerges shows a wide disparity in intake across countries, with a four-fold difference between the lowest intake of just over 100 g of fruit and vegetables per day in India and the highest intake of almost 500 g/d in Israel, a difference in intake of well over 300 g/d. Developing countries have the lowest intake, for example 128–148 g/d in India and 183 g/d in the Philippines. In most European countries, consumption is between 250 and 350 g/d of total fruit and vegetables, but there is wide diversity between European regions. Japan has one of the highest levels of overall consumption (almost 400 g/d), while the USA and Australia have about 300 g/d. Fruit consumption in individual countries appears to fluctuate independently of vegetable consumption and may represent between less than a fifth of the total intake (India, China) up to more than half (Finland, Spain). There seems to be a slight tendency for developed countries to have higher proportions of fruit consumption. In particular, Scandinavian countries (Norway, Sweden, Finland) have very high fruit intake.

Selected multi-centre studies

A multi-country survey on the prevalence of non-insulin-dependent diabetes mellitus and related risk factors was carried out in Algeria, Bulgaria, Egypt, Greece and Italy on small homogeneous groups of non-diabetic men and women aged 35–60 years (Karamanos et al., 2002) (Figure 2). Food consumption was assessed by a validated dietary history method. The results indicate that consumption of fruit and vegetables is similar in North African countries and in European Mediterranean countries, with intakes ranging from 416 g/d to 501 g/d of total fruit and vegetables. The data from Italy are in good agreement with the national results. Interestingly, the highest intake was recorded in Bulgaria (536–594 g/d). For all countries except Egypt, fruits represented half or more of the total amount.

The multi-country SENECA project (Survey in Europe on Nutrition and the Elderly, a Concerted Action) collected information on the diet of elderly people (born between 1913 and 1918) in 11 European countries in an initial survey in 1988–89 and in a follow-up in 1993 on a smaller sample. Dietary intake was assessed by a three-day food record in household measures, followed by an interview with a dietitian to establish the weight of portion sizes. The method was strictly standardized across all study sites, affording a set of uniquely comparable data. The data reviewed here are those for people aged 74–79 years in Belgium, Denmark, France, Greece, Italy, the Netherlands, Poland, Portugal, Spain, Switzerland and the United Kingdom (Trichopoulou et al., 1995b; Schroll et al., 1996, 1997).

A surprisingly high consumption of vegetables was recorded everywhere, but potatoes and other roots were included in the vegetable category, thus inflating the total amount to a degree that differs depending on the study site. The proportion covered by potatoes appears to range roughly from over two thirds in Denmark and Poland to less than one third in Italy and one French site (Schroll et al., 1996). Therefore, these data should be considered only within the context of the SENECA project. For women and men, the highest overall consumption of fruit and vegetables was recorded in Spain (766 g/d for women, 935 g/d for men), followed by Portugal and France, Belgium, the Netherlands, Greece and Italy. The lowest intakes were recorded in Denmark (347 g/d for women and 371 g/d for men) and Switzerland (about 420 g/d for both men and women). Fruit consumption was also highest in Spain (about 550 g/d) and lowest in Denmark (120 g/d), and followed a pattern of increasing consumption from northern to southern Europe. In most sites, fruits represented well under half of the overall amount of fruit and vegetables consumed, but reached about 50% in Greece and Portugal and over 60% in Italy and Spain (Schroll et al., 1997). For Denmark, the Netherlands, Spain and Switzerland, data are available on the same subjects assessed four years earlier (Schroll et al., 1997). The changes over the intervening four years were negligible and within the methodological error.

The dietary pattern of 519 878 healthy adult men and women was assessed by food frequency questionnaire in 27 cohorts recruited in ten European countries within the framework of the EPIC project. Details on the background, rationale and design of the study, on population characteristics, the selection process, data collection and some preliminary results are given elsewhere (Riboli, 1992; Slimani et al., 2000, 2002; Riboli et al., 2002), along with detailed information on the food items included in the categories of fruit and vegetables. The diet of a subsample of 35 955 men and women aged 35–74 years (mean age, 55 years for women, 57 years for men) randomly selected from each EPIC cohort was assessed by a standardized 24-hour recall method (Agudo et al., 2002). The cohorts are located in Denmark (two sites), France (four sites), Germany (two sites), Greece (one site), Italy (five sites), the Netherlands (two sites), Norway (two sites), Spain (five sites), Sweden (two sites) and the United Kingdom (two populations). Men and women participate in the study in 19 centres, and only women in eight. The data presented are adjusted for age, season and day of the week, thus providing an internally comparable set of data (Figure 3), although these data differ

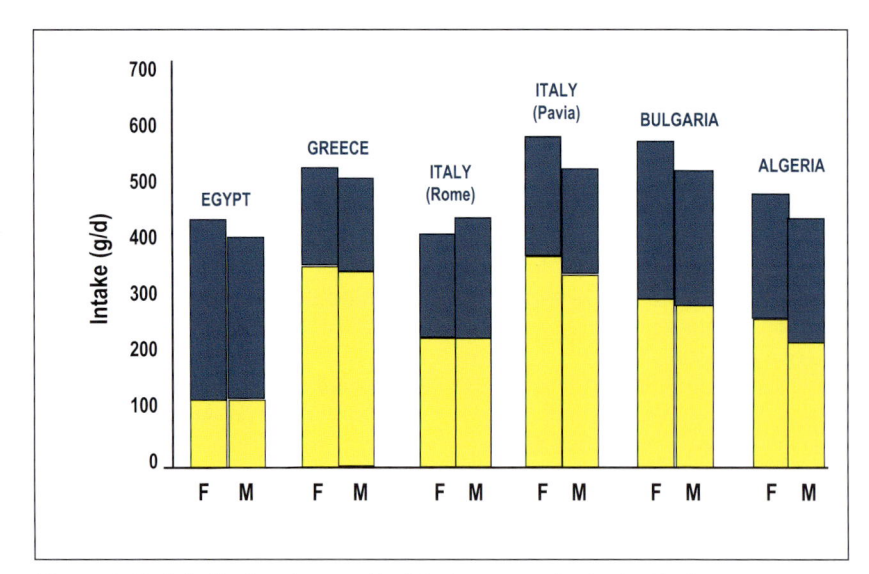

Figure 2 Fruit (yellow) and vegetable (blue) consumption in the Mediterranean countries participating in the Mediterranean Group for the Study of Diabetes (MCSD)

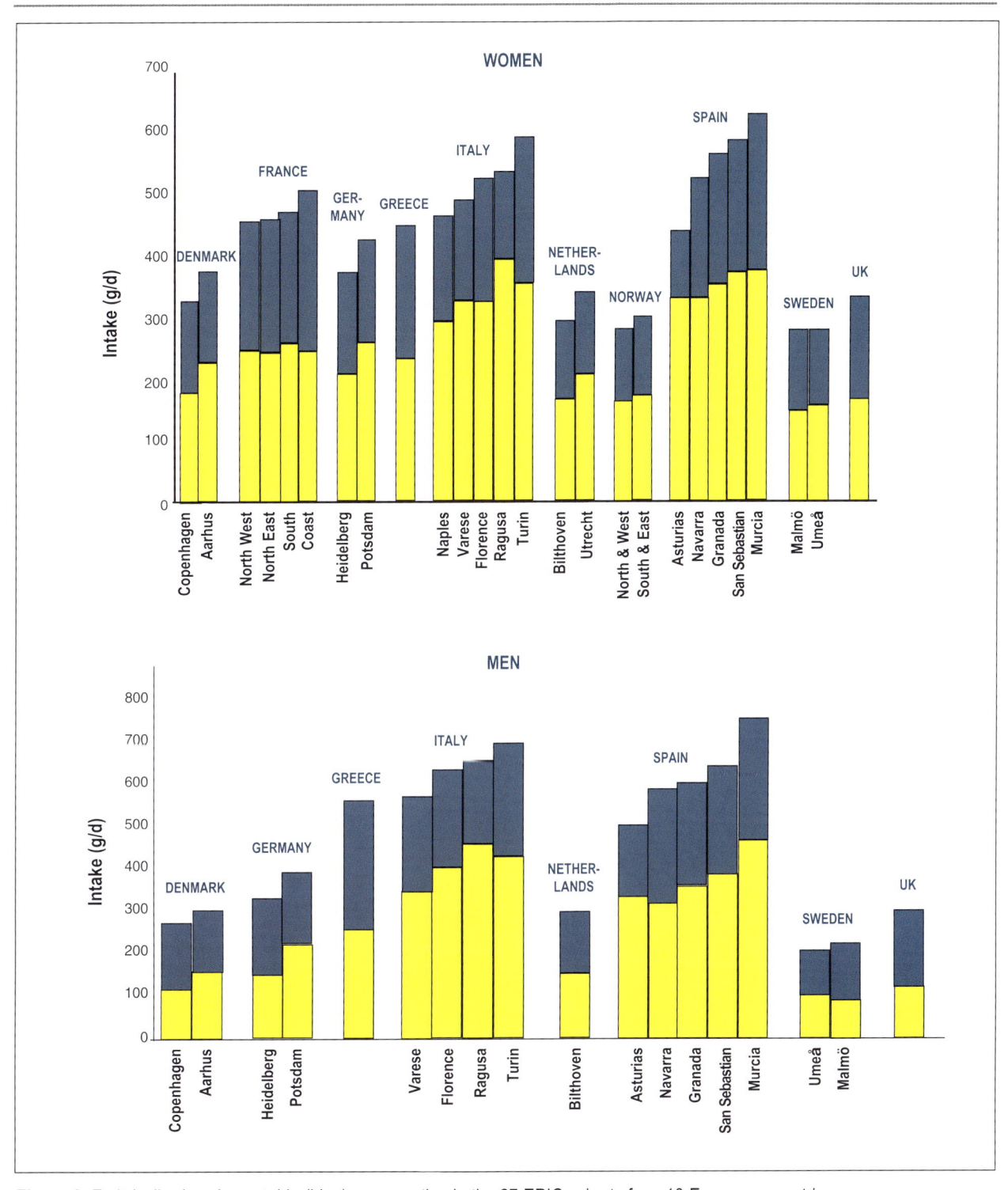

Figure 3 Fruit (yellow) and vegetable (blue) consumption in the 27 EPIC cohorts from 10 European countries

only very slightly from the unadjusted values. For both sexes, the highest overall consumption of fruit and vegetables was seen in Spain (721 g/d for men in Murcia) and Italy, while the lowest consumption was found in Sweden (225 g/d for men in Umeå), followed by the Netherlands, Norway, the United Kingdom and Denmark. Where the information is available, women seem to consume similar amounts of fruit and vegetables to men, except in Greece, Italy and Spain, where men have appreciably higher consumption.

Besides the notable variations in total intake between countries, there are also wide variations within countries, particularly in those countries where consumption is highest (Italy, Spain). The intake of fruit generally represents about half the total intake, but rises to two thirds in countries where the total intake is high. Thus, the lowest consumption of fruit was recorded in Sweden (122–159 g/d) and the highest in Spain (454 g/d) and Italy (448 g/d). The data from this study indicate that the countries with the highest total intake have the largest within-country variation and the highest consumption of fruit. Similar high variability is shared by other studies, and is reflected in the large difference between the intake of individual consumers and the mean intake of the entire group.

The European DAFNE project, designed to harmonize the data of the household budget surveys of diverse countries, produced comparable data for ten European countries: Belgium, Germany, Greece, Hungary, Ireland, Luxembourg, Norway, Poland, Spain and the United Kingdom. All surveys were conducted between 1987 and 1995 (Naska *et al.*, 2000). Despite limitations inherent to the nature of the data (level of aggregation of the data, household level of the information, foods being reported as crude values rather than as edible portion, possible stores present in the household, data representing availability rather consumption), the harmonized household budget surveys permit cross-country comparisons. Fruit and vegetable availability ranged from 217 g/d in Ireland, almost equally divided between the two categories, to the values recorded in Spain (463 g/d) and in Greece (613 g/d), which include higher proportions of fruit. As data for eastern Europe are scarce, it is interesting to note the values recorded in Poland (302 g/d in 1988) and Hungary (354 g/d in 1991), the difference being mainly a result of higher availability of fruit in Hungary than in Poland. The highest availability of fruit is again recorded in Greece (346 g/d) and Spain (283 g/d). Data from Greece for 1988 and 1994 show an unexpected decline in availability of both fruit and vegetables, which dropped from 613 g/d in 1988 to 496 g/d in 1994. On the whole, the ranking of the DAFNE data on the basis of fruit and vegetable availability is in good agreement with the results of national surveys (Figure 1) and the EPIC (Figure 3) and SENECA studies on food consumption, with Ireland and the United Kingdom at the lower end and Greece and Spain at the higher end.

Developing countries

For a small number of developing countries, information on fruit and vegetable consumption was retrieved from the Nutrition Country Profiles series (FAO NCPs). Data for Iran, Mali, Morocco, Pakistan, Sri Lanka, Turkey, Venezuela and Viet Nam are shown in Figure 4. The data available do not separate fruit and vegetable consumption. While the quality of the data may be questionable, the picture that emerges is one of great disparity between countries. Asian countries (Pakistan, Sri Lanka, Viet Nam), Mali and Venezuela are at the lower end of the spectrum, with intakes below 200 g/d. At the higher end of the spectrum, the Middle Eastern and North African countries (Morocco, Turkey and Iran) have intakes of over 350 g/d.

Availability and time trends in large regions

The food balance sheets of the FAO (FAOSTAT, 2000), collected with a unified and unchanging technique since 1961, offer a unique opportunity to examine time trends worldwide. The data are more correctly referred to as disappearance or availability figures, and thus are not directly comparable with the data obtained from dietary surveys. An additional difference is that bananas are included in the fruit category.

Figures 5 and 6 provide an overview of the availability of fruit and vegetables in major regions of the world and of changes over the last 40 years. A six-fold difference in fruit and vegetable availability is apparent across the world (Figure 5). The four regions in sub-Saharan Africa have the lowest levels overall, with countries in eastern Africa having less than 100 g/d. Western Europe, the Asian Near East and North America at the upper end have over 600 g/d.

In most developing regions, the availability of vegetables is higher than that of fruit, except in those regions where bananas represent a large percentage of the fruit (central Africa, Latin America and the Caribbean). In contrast, in the developed regions where the total availability of fruit and vegetables is highest (western Europe and North America), there is similar availability of fruit and of vegetables. Eastern European countries have very low intake of fruit compared with that of vegetables and compared with western Europe.

Different trends over time are observed between regions. In eastern and central Africa, availability of both

Consumption, availability and food policies

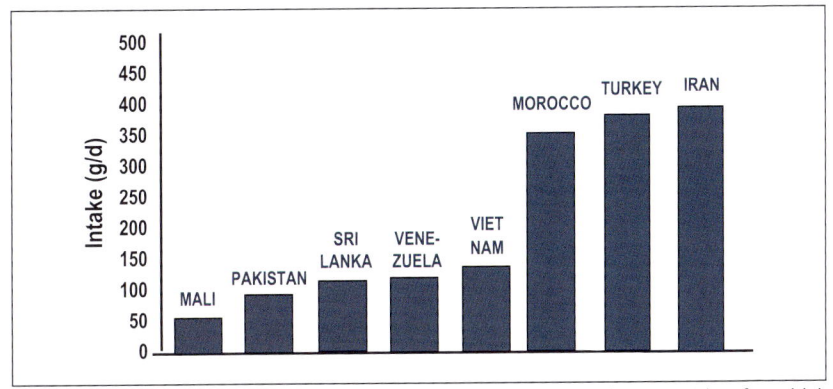

Figure 4 Total fruit and vegetable intake in selected developing countries for which recent, nationally representative data were available

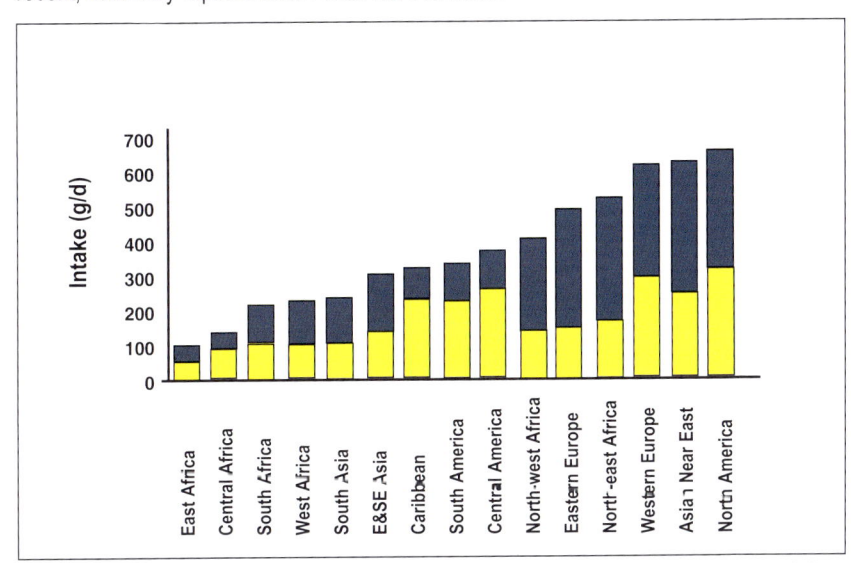

Figure 5 Fruit (yellow) and vegetable (blue) availability in large regions around the world. Data retrieved from the FAO Food Balance Sheets (FAOSTAT, 2000). To smooth out yearly fluctuations, five-year averages for 1996–2000 are shown.

fruit and vegetables decreased steeply, particularly in the last 20 years (Figure 6A). Total values for Latin America and the Caribbean and values for vegetables in southern Africa and for fruit in western Africa did not change over the period examined (Figures 6A and D). In contrast, a large number of regions show steady increases in both fruit and vegetable availability, the greatest increase occurring during the 1970s and early 1980s. These regions include developed countries such as those of North America and Europe (Figure 6C), but also countries 'in transition' such as northern Africa and the Near East (Figure 6B). A decrease in fruit and vegetable availability is seen in Japan, while most other countries in southeast Asia show a small increase over time (Figure 6E).

Variations within countries

Inspection of the standard deviations and quantile distributions of fruit and vegetable intakes reveals great interindividual variation in patterns of consumption. Figure 7 displays within-country variations of fruit and vegetable intake in selected developed countries. The largest interregional difference is seen in the USA (USDA Food Surveys Research Group, 2003c), where it reaches 112 g/d, followed by Finland (87 g/d in men). Elsewhere, the differences are smaller, ranging between 36 g/d in Norway and 67 g/d in Finland for women. In those countries for which data are available, there appear to be larger differences between men than between women. In the United Kingdom, a four-fold difference was found between the 1st and the 4th quartiles in the amount of fruit and vegetables consumed by adults: 105 and 448 g/d respectively (Billson et al., 1999). In the data from the EPIC project (Agudo et al., 2002), the range observed within one country varies from non-existent or minimal (Sweden or Norway) up to 200 g/d as seen across the five sites in Spain (Figure 3). The SENECA study confirms the persistence of within-country variation in the elderly (data not shown).

Within-country diversity in intake also exists in developing countries, although the available evidence is scanty. Data from Iran show a difference of about 400 g/d between the lowest and highest intakes (222 g/d in Baluchistan and 647 g/d in Markaz, respectively; FAO NCPs). In Brazil, fruit and vegetable consumption varies from 236 g/d in Curitiba to almost 700 g/d in Rio de Janeiro (FAO NCPs). In India, amazingly large variations have been described, cutting across all strata of society and possibly reflecting diversity in production and access (Department of Women & Child Development, 1998). Figure 8 shows regional differences in fruit and vegetable consumption in India for different levels of education attained. Intakes range from less than 70 g/d to

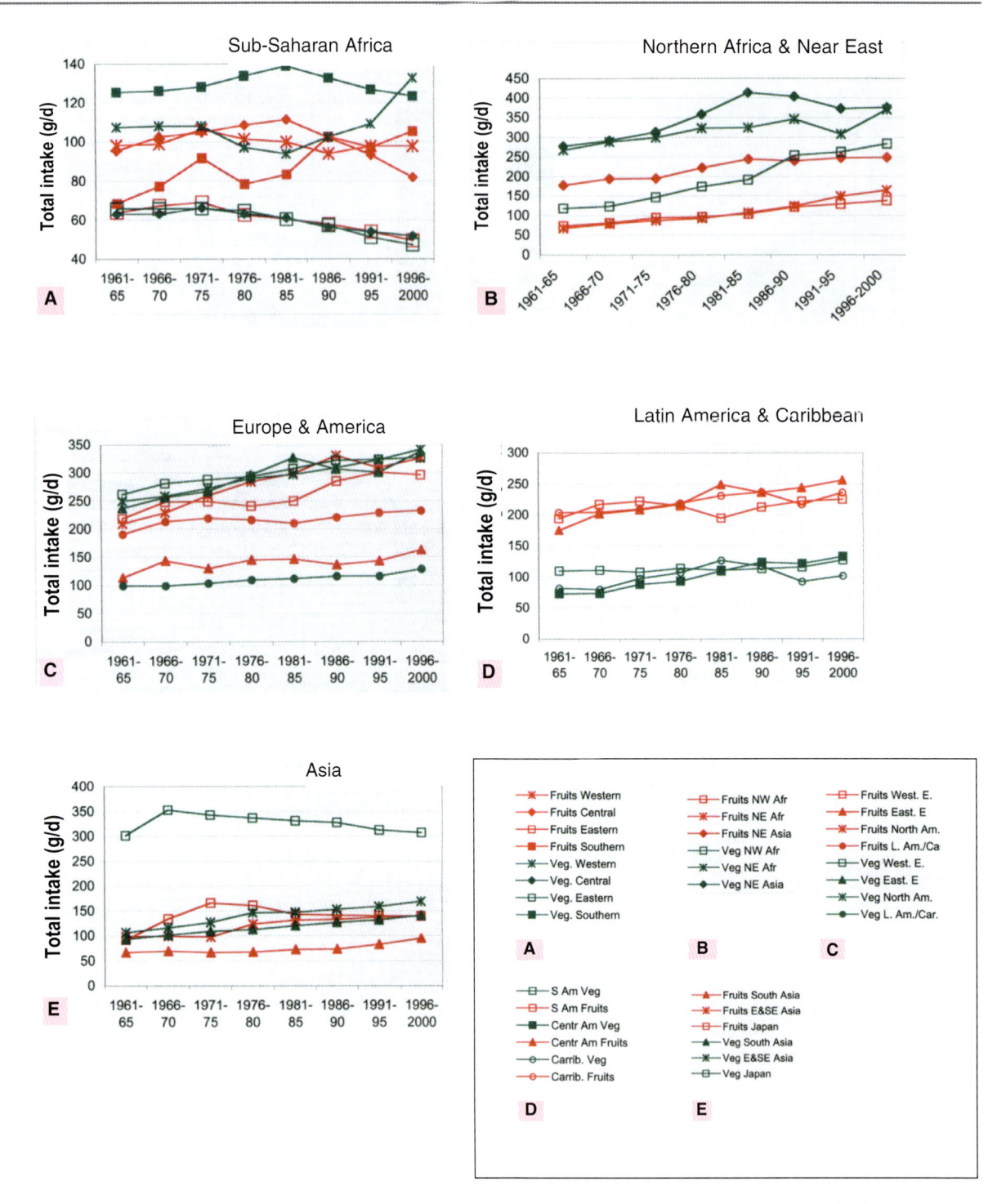

Figure 6 Time trends in fruit and vegetable consumption in large regions worldwide: Data retrieved from the FAO Food Balance Sheets (FAOSTAT, 2000). Except where mentioned, the same regions as for Figure 5 were selected.

over 200 g/d among illiterates and from 75 g/d to over 300 g/d among the college-educated. A 3–4-fold interregional difference is observed at all levels of education attained, from illiteracy through primary, secondary and high school to college education (see also below).

A large number of factors may account for the diverse food patterns observed within a country. For some countries, separate data are available for urban and rural populations. Almost everywhere, urban populations tend to consume more fruit and vegetables than rural ones, but the difference is often negligible (FAO NCPs). A national survey conducted in Turkey in 1984 indicated an average consumption of 408 g/d of fruit and vegetables, with an urban/rural difference of 425 g/d versus 392 g/d (FAO NCPs). The survey also revealed a seasonal trend, with values of 518 g/d in summer and 482 g/d in winter. In Iran, the urban/rural difference was very marked, 523 g/d versus 389 g/d (FAO NCPs). Data from India (Department of Women & Child Development, 1998) and Pakistan (FAO NCPs) indicate very small, non-significant urban/rural differences. In China, a difference of 65 g/d was reported, from 345 g/d in the rural population to 410 g/d in the cities, the difference being related predominantly to fruit consumption (FAO NCPs; Institute of Nutrition and Food Hygiene, 2002). In Chile, in contrast, a nationwide survey in 1969 recorded intakes of relatively high amounts of fruit and vegetables (about 435 g/d), while later surveys conducted mostly in the Santiago area found lower intakes (around 300 g/d) (FAO NCPs). Similarly in Ireland, intakes were slightly higher (30 g/d) in the rural population, among both men and women (Irish Nutrition & Dietetic Institute, 1990).

Another very likely determinant of fruit and vegetable intake is income. In the USA, intake is positively income-associated in both sexes and at all ages (USDA Food Surveys Research Group, 2003d) (Figure 9). The greatest effect appears to be in adolescent women, with a difference of about 100 g/d between the strata of highest and lowest income; for the other age groups the difference between the poorest and the richest amounts to 35–60 g/d. National data from the 1992 survey in China also indicate an appreciable positive income-associated gradient in total intake of fruit and vegetables, the higher-income group

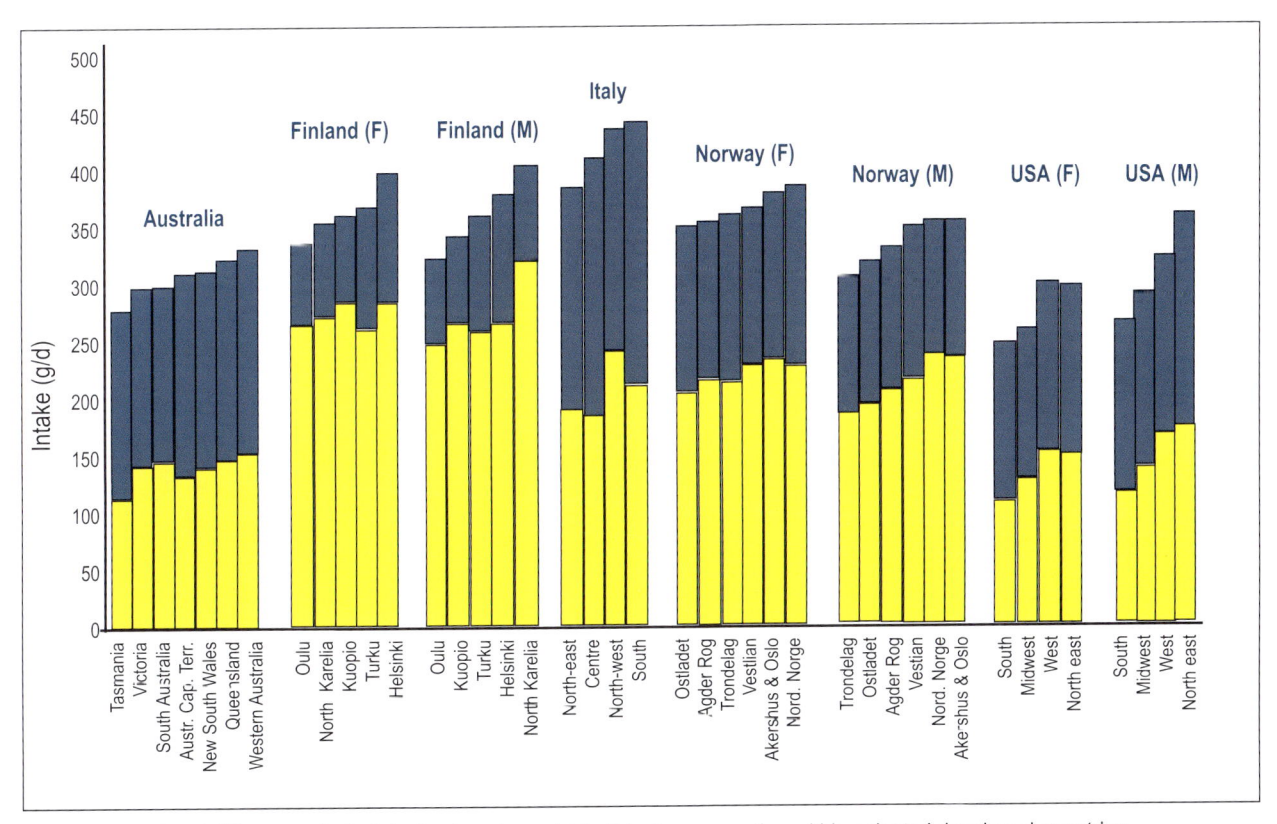

Figure 7 Regional differences in fruit (yellow) and vegetable (blue) consumption within selected developed countries

consuming three times more fruit than the lower-income group, while the difference in vegetable consumption was minimal (Institute of Nutrition and Food Hygiene, 2002).

Educational level, taken as a proxy for socioeconomic status, has been shown in several surveys to influence fruit and vegetable intake. The national data from India (Department of Women & Child Development, 1998) indicate that only part of the variation in fruit and vegetable consumption across the country can be accounted for by educational level (Figure 10); the differences in intake between regions are greater than those associated with the education attained within any given state, which reach a maximum of 183 g/d (2.5-fold) in Daman & Diu. The clear positive association with educational level found in several states (7/17) appears to be independent of the absolute intake, as it occurs in regions of both low and high total intake. In other regions, education was not associated with fruit and vegetable consumption. In yet other regions, fruit and vegetable intake steeply increases only at college educational level (Meghalaya, Chandigarh, Dadra & Nagar Daveli, Daman & Diu). Thus, the amount of fruit and vegetables consumed by the college-level households in certain states may be lower than that of illiterate households in other states.

A positive association between educational level and consumption of fruit and vegetables has also been found in developed countries, such as the USA (Devine et al., 1999; Xie et al., 2003) and Australia (Turrell et al., 2002). In Europe, the situation seems to be less clear, as the DAFNE data do not confirm a positive trend in the total amount consumed with increasing level of education. For the total consumption of fruit and vegetables, the trend, albeit slight, is for consumption to be higher at the lower levels of education (elementary level or less), a decrease of consumption in the secondary level of education, and an increase again at the university education level. However, looking at consumption of fruit and vegetables separately reveals an inexplicable decrease of fruit consumption with increasing education in Spain, but an increase in Greece. The other three countries for which values are available, Poland, Hungary and Belgium, present a U-shaped trend. Vegetable consumption decreases with education in Greece, Hungary and Poland, while the relationship with education is less clear in Belgium and Spain.

These data are generally not adjusted for possible confounders, so that the relationship between intake and various parameters may be confounded by lifestyle covariant parameters such as smoking, alcohol-drinking habits or culture as well as by the ecological niche. Care must therefore be exercised in interpreting these associations. For example, stratification by ethnic group (Mexican American, other Hispanic origin, non-Hispanic blacks and non-Hispanic whites) in the USA has revealed differences in the pattern of fruit and vegetable consumption (USDA Food Surveys Research Group, 2003e). Although the differences are neither systematic nor very large, it appears that non-Hispanic blacks, who are likely to have lower educational attainment and lower income, tend also to be lower consumers. In Ireland, the unemployed and the unskilled have systematically lower consumption than "professionals" and "non manuals" (Irish Nutrition & Dietetic Institute, 1990).

Such diverse behaviour and the variety of forces responsible for it have

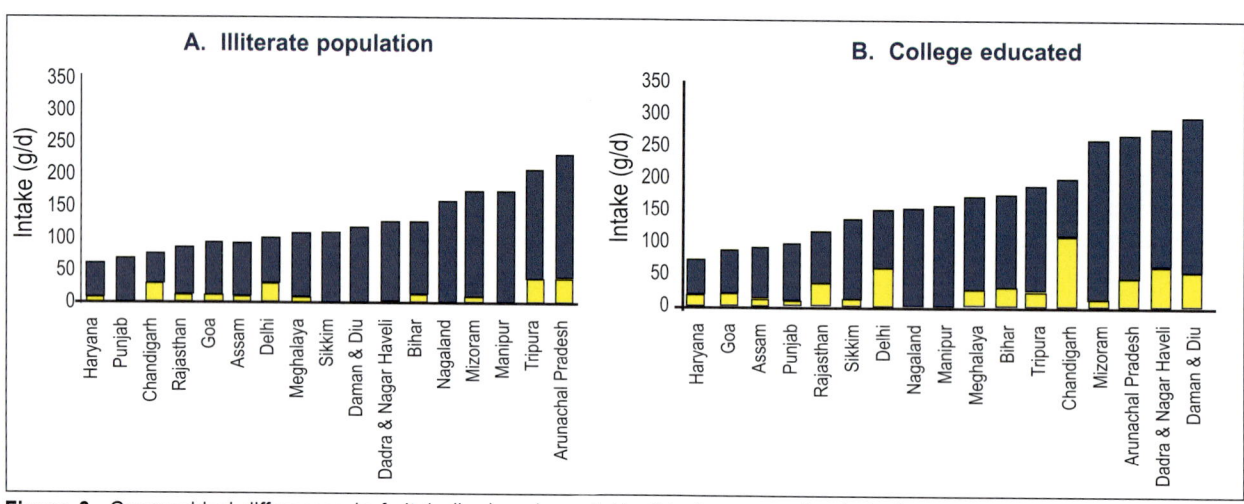

Figure 8 Geographical differences in fruit (yellow) and vegetable (blue) consumption in India, according to the education level attained

Consumption, availability and food policies

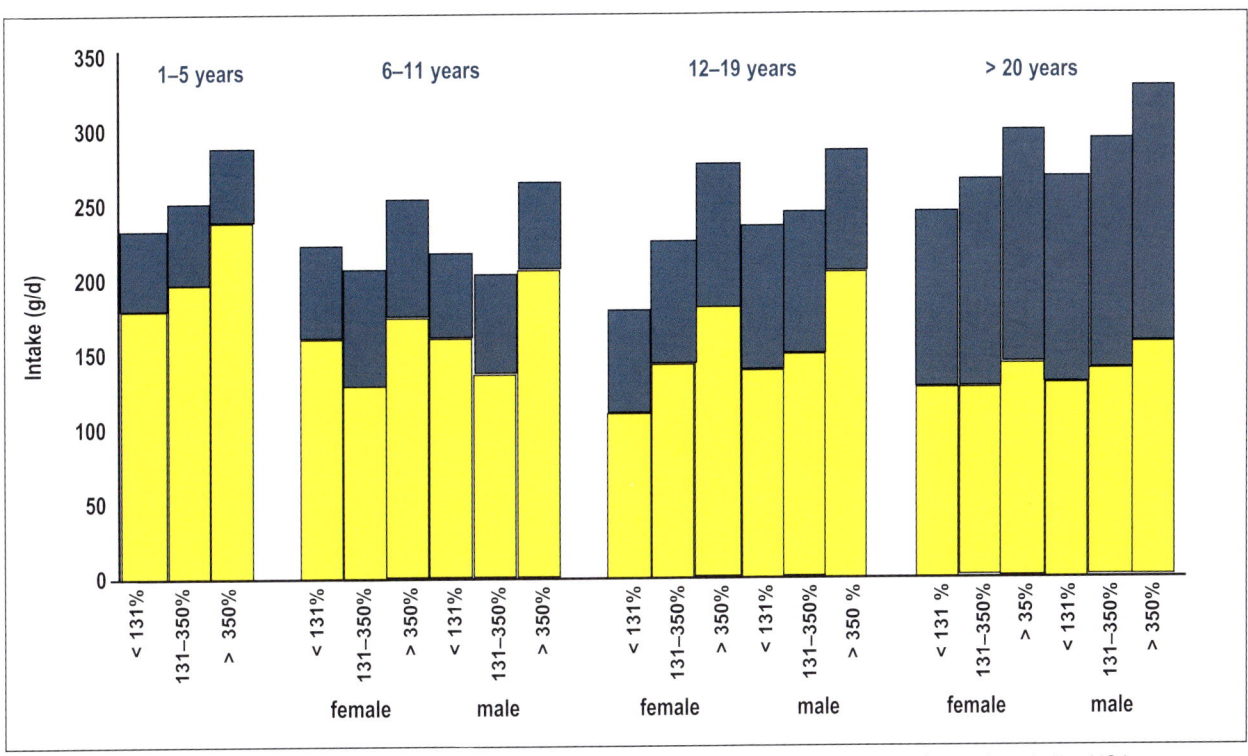

Figure 9 Differences in fruit (yellow) and vegetable (blue) consumption by household income and age class in the USA

started to be investigated, and are revealing that consumers' choices are shaped by an amazingly wide and complex array of factors, that include market forces, physical access, price, traditions, availability and many others.

Nutrition and food policies and special campaigns

Historical perspective

Nutritional research, programmes and food policy have shifted focus over the last hundred years. In the early 1900s, the focus was on identifying and preventing nutrient deficiency diseases, while in the 1940s and 1950s, attention moved to the identification of nutrient requirements. Subsequently, investigations were directed to the role of diet in maintaining health and reducing the risk of cancer, heart disease, osteoporosis and other noncommunicable diseases. During the 1970s and 1980s, dietary fat was a major focus of research and policy, and later in this period the roles of dietary fibre and antioxidants were addressed. More recent epidemiological, clinical and laboratory research has been focused on foods and food groups, particularly fruit and vegetables. During the past 25 years, research findings suggesting an inverse association between fruit and vegetables and cancer have contributed to the development of international and national policy statements about cancer and the consumption of fruit and vegetables.

Doll and Peto (1981) estimated that approximately 35% of cancer deaths were related to diet (from 10 to 70%, depending on the type of cancer). Since then, a growing body of evidence has suggested that higher levels of fruit and vegetable consumption are associated with reduced risk of some cancers (see Chapter 4).

Several comprehensive reviews of data regarding diet in relation to cancer, chronic disease and health concerns in general have identified foods, nutrients and other dietary components as being potentially important for cancer prevention (Assembly of Life Sciences, 1982; National Cancer Institute, 1986; James, 1988; US Public Health Service and Office of the Surgeon General, 1988; WHO, 1990, 2003). These also provided estimates of the potential effects of cancer-prevention efforts and recommendations and priorities for dietary change, including reducing the intake of total fats, especially saturated fat, maintaining desirable weight and improving diet quality. The earlier dietary guidelines included

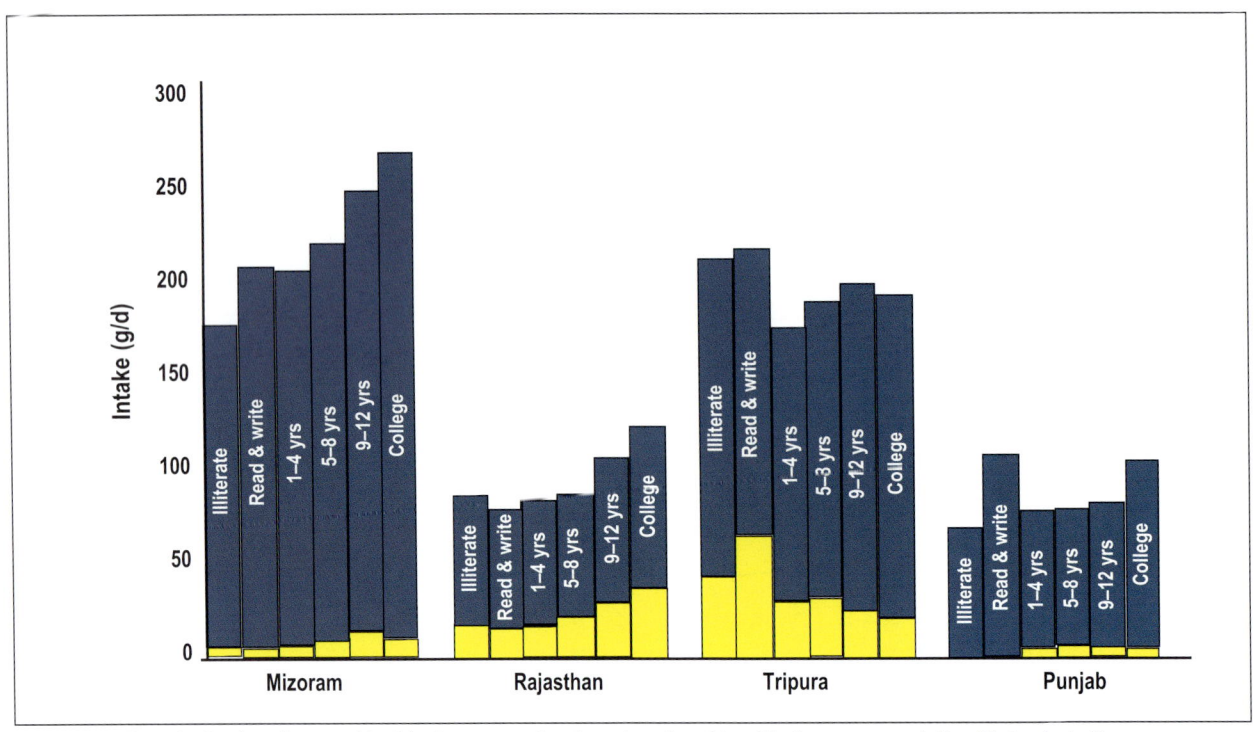

Figure 10 Fruit (yellow) and vegetable (blue) consumption by educational level in four representative States in India

few specific recommendations for fruits and vegetables. In the USA, the National Research Council (1989) provided a quantitative recommendation to "every day eat five or more servings of a combination of vegetables and fruit, especially green and yellow vegetables and citrus fruits". The recommended number of servings of fruit and vegetables was derived by calculating nutritionally balanced diets that would meet the overall dietary recommendations (Cronin et al., 1987). These reports taken together provided a focus on dietary patterns containing a variety of foods, rich in plant foods including fruits, vegetables, cereals and whole grains, while being generally low in energy, fat, especially saturated fat, cholesterol and sodium.

Current policy and dietary guidelines

Over the years, nutrition and dietary guidelines have moved from focusing solely on nutrient intakes and nutrient adequacy to recommendations that are more food-based and aimed towards health maintenance and food safety. In 2002, the WHO issued guidelines and policies for national cancer control programmes (WHO, 2002). These emphasized improved diet and increased fruit and vegetable intake as essential parts of the approach to cancer prevention. A joint WHO/FAO Technical Report (WHO, 2003) made it clear that a growing epidemic of chronic diseases, including obesity, diabetes mellitus, cardiovascular disease, hypertension and stroke, and some types of cancer, afflicting both developed and developing countries, is related to dietary and lifestyle changes, often linked to industrialization, urbanization, economic development and market globalization. While standards of living and food availability have improved, there have also been negative consequences in terms of unfavourable dietary patterns and decreased physical activity. Fruit and vegetable intake still varies considerably between countries, in large part reflecting the prevailing economic, cultural and agricultural environments. The WHO/FAO report emphasized the need for concerted efforts to improve diet, with increasing intake of fruit and vegetables, and for a lifelong approach to healthy eating.

Recent reports from international and nongovernmental organizations have included recommendations for fruit and vegetable intake, as summarized in Table 9. The World Cancer Research Fund review (WCRF/AICR, 1997) estimated that "a simple change, such as eating the recommended five servings of fruit and vegetables each day, could by itself reduce cancer rates more than 20 percent". The first recommendation of the American Cancer Society's Guidelines on Nutrition and Physical Activity for Cancer Prevention (Byers *et al.*, 2002) is to "eat a variety of healthful foods with an emphasis on plant sources" and specifically to "eat five or more servings of a variety of vegetables and fruits each day". The WHO/FAO Expert Consultation on Diet, Nutrition and the Prevention of Chronic Disease (WHO, 2003) recommends consuming at least 400 grams of fruit and vegetables per day.

Programmes to implement dietary guidelines and nutrition policy

National and regional health organizations translate these international policy statements into food-based dietary guidelines that reflect the cultural food patterns and the prevalence of noncommunicable diseases in individual populations (WHO, 1998). Such guidelines aim at disease prevention, taking into account local economic, food availability and food safety considerations (Becker, 1999; Löwik *et al.*, 1999; Valsta, 1999; US Department of Health and Human Services, 2000).

The WHO European Regional Office has provided Member States with a Regional Food and Nutrition Action Plan, which refers to fruit and vegetable consumption as a priority (WHO/EURO, 2000). WHO also provides information and assistance for developing food-based guidance systems (WHO, 1998).

The International Conference on Nutrition in 1992 called upon countries to develop national food and nutrition action plans (http://www.fao.org/-es/esn/nutrition/ICN/ICNCONTS.htm). To date about 150 countries have such plans and another 20 have them under development. Many of these plans in developed countries, and to a lesser extent in developing countries, include goals for prevention of noncommunicable diseases through population-based dietary strategies.

The EURODIET project (1998–2000) established a broad network and a strategy and action plan for the development of European dietary guidelines and outlined ways for effective promotion of diet and healthy lifestyles in European Union member states (Kafatos & Codrington, 2003). Other groups of countries also work together to develop nutrition plans, dietary guidelines and educational efforts. The examples in Figures 11–14 show how food-based dietary guidelines for different countries or regions translate the recommendations for fruit and vegetable intake and how they reflect cultural food patterns. Other pictorial representations of dietary guidelines have been reported (Painter *et al.*, 2002).

Recommended amounts of fruit and vegetables

Recommendations for fruit and vegetable intake are fairly similar across international and national guidelines, and are generally designated as servings of fruit and vegetables per day specified in household units, serving sizes or grams. Most publications specify consuming at least 400 grams or five or more servings daily of fruit and vegetables, with a range for the daily intake provided to allow for varying energy intakes. Several guidelines make separate

Table 9. International and national recommendations for fruit and vegetable intake

Agency (reference)	Recommendations	Fruit and vegetables	Suggestions for implementation
World Cancer Research Fund/ American Institute for Cancer Research (WCRF/AICR, 1997)	Promote year-round consumption of a variety of fruit and vegetables, providing 7% or more total energy	400–800 g/day or 5 servings/day or more. Not included: pluses/fruit and vegetables (tubers, starchy roots and plantains	
American Cancer Society (Byers *et al.*, 2002)	Eat a variety of healthful foods, with an emphasis on plant foods	5 servings/day or more	Include vegetables and fruits at every meal and for snacks. Eat a variety of vegetables and fruits. Limit french fries, snack chips and other fried vegetable products. Choose 100% juice if you drink fruit or vegetable juices
WHO (WHO, 2003)		400 g/day or more Not included: tubers	

recommendations for fruit and vegetables (Chinese Nutrition Society, 2000; see Figure 14).

Guidelines differ in what items are included in the food list for fruits and vegetables or in what are "counted" as a fruit or vegetable (see Chapter 1). There are also differences in what specific types of preparation or manufacture of fruits and vegetables are encouraged or emphasized. Potatoes may or may not be included in the food list for fruit and vegetables. For example, the World Cancer Research Fund report (WCRF/AICR, 1997) does not include potatoes (or other starchy roots or plantains) in its list of fruits and vegetables, nor do the food guides for several countries (Denmark, Germany, Ireland, the Netherlands) (Flynn & Kearney, 1999; Haraldsdottir, 1999; Hermann-Kunz & Thamm, 1999; Löwik et al., 1999). Potatoes are included in the food lists for fruit and vegetables of Australia, the USA and the American Cancer Society (Miller et al., 1997; US Department of Health and Human Services, 2000; Byers et al., 2002).

Soy products are usually not included as fruit and vegetables, but other legumes may be included. Pickled vegetables and fruit-based-jams, jellies, preserves, candies and fruit-based soft drinks are frequently not included on the lists of fruits and vegetables. To ensure compatibility with guidelines that address fat intake, some fruit and vegetable dishes that are prepared with fat, salt or sugar may be excluded from the food list, or individuals may be cautioned to limit intake of these dishes. Most guidelines indicate that individuals should limit chips, snack chips and other fried vegetables. Many of the national guidelines also encourage consumption of specific fruits and vegetables, such as dark green leafy vegetables, red-orange fruit, citrus fruit and cruciferous vegetables.

Campaigns to increase fruit and vegetable intake

Over the past twenty years, a variety of campaigns have been conducted to inform individuals of the benefits of fruit and vegetable consumption. Health policy objectives and international and national dietary guidelines have served as the foundation for these campaigns (see above). The campaigns have included large national programmes, regional efforts and local programmes to develop and implement dietary guidelines in order to increase fruit and vegetable intake.

The campaigns have used information developed in earlier community intervention studies (Puska et al., 1983; Farquhar et al., 1990; Luepker et al., 1994) and recommendations about implementing community-based

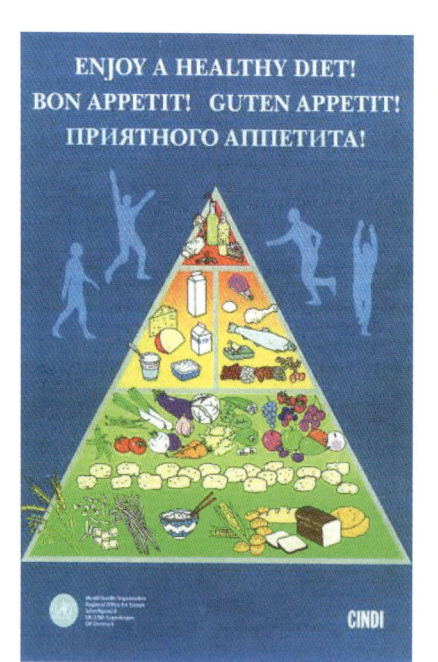

Figure 11 CINDI dietary guide from the WHO Regional Office for Europe (pyramid) (WHO/EURO, 2000). The recommendation is to eat a variety of vegetables and fruits, preferably fresh and local, several times per day (at least 400 g per day)

programmes (WHO, 1998). During the late 1980s, state projects were conducted in California, Australia, Canada, and some European countries to develop programmes and campaigns on fruit and vegetables; these provided valuable experience for further development and national expansion of fruit and vegetable campaigns (Foerster et al., 1995; Miller et al., 1996; Dixon et al., 1998; Farrell et al., 2000). Recent campaigns have expanded social marketing approaches and community-based implementation methods and draw on the scientific credibility of sponsorship by national, state and local health institutions. A major element is partnerships between health agencies, nongovernmental organizations for cancer or heart disease prevention and the fruit and vegetable industry and agricultural groups. The first national initiative was the US National Cancer Institute's 5-A-Day For Better Health Program, initiated in 1991 (see below). The methods in this programme and the experience gained have provided a model for many programmes to develop national partnerships for development and implementation of fruit and vegetable campaigns (National Institutes of Health and National Cancer Institute, 2001). A variety of campaigns conducted predominantly in Europe and North America have focused on the five-a-day theme for recommendation of fruit and vegetable intake. In these, programme partners work together to develop, implement and evaluate interventions. Such campaigns disseminate messages and conduct activities aimed at behavioural change in relation to fruit and vegetable intake, involving a variety of components: media and communications; point-of-sale interventions; community-level programmes, including public health agencies, school-based and worksite programmes; partnership activities with the food industry, retailers and

Consumption, availability and food policies

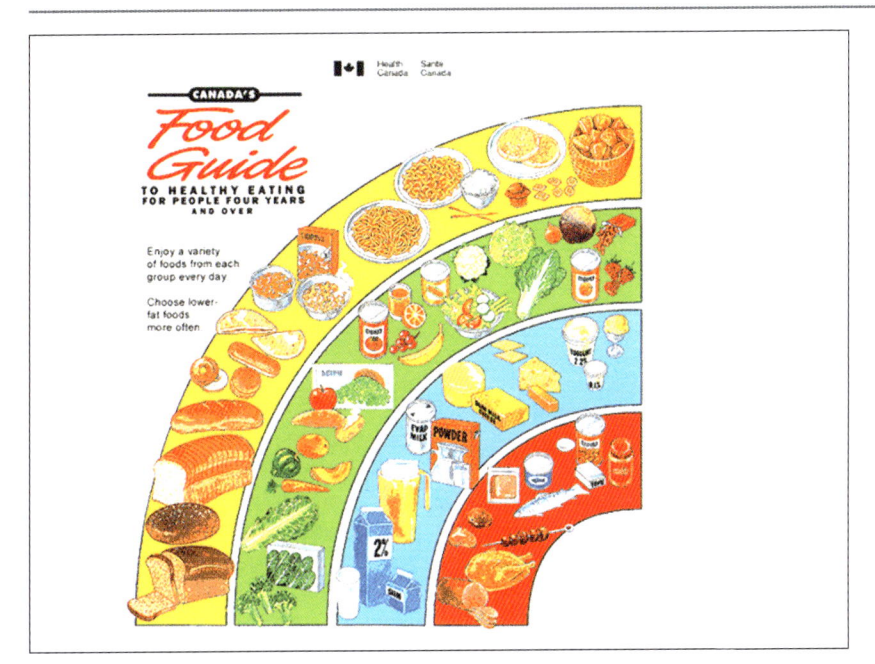

Figure 12 Canada's Food Guide to Health Eating (rainbow) (Health Canada, 2002)
The advice is to eat 5–10 portions of fruit and vegetables per day

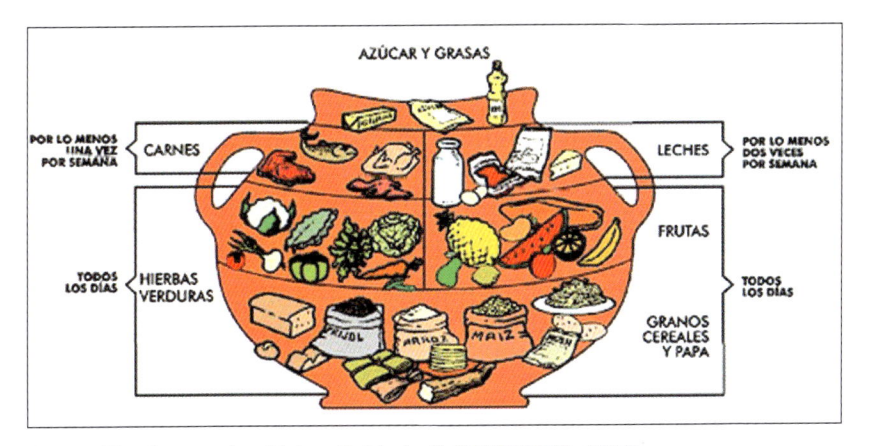

Figure 13 Guatemalan Dietary Guide (pot) (INCAP/OPS, 2000)
The recommendation is to eat fruit and vegetables including leafy vegetables, every day

fruit and vegetable producers; and research efforts. Media components are implemented in complementary ways at the national or state level and at the local level. Examples of such campaigns are described below.

5 A Day Program—USA

The *Eat 5 A Day—for Better Health! Program* originated as a pilot programme in 1988 in the state of California through the California Department of Health. It was initiated nationally in the USA in 1991 by the National Cancer Institute (NCI) as the public side and the Produce for Better Health Foundation (PBH) as the private side (Produce for Better Health Foundation and National Cancer Institute, 1999). PBH is a non-profit organization supported by approximately 1000 donors from the fruit and vegetable industry, supermarkets and other organizations and individuals interested in health promotion. The goal is to increase the average consumption of fruit and vegetables *per capita* to five or more servings every day by providing consumers with information about how to incorporate more servings of these foods into their daily eating patterns and by creating a healthy food environment wherever people eat, in schools, at workplaces or at home.

After a favourable national evaluation of the first decade of the programme in 2000, the National 5 A Day Partnership was formalized and expanded in April 2001. This partnership increased the number of both private and public stakeholders in the US programme. New partners formally added included the Centers for Disease Control and Prevention (CDC), the American Cancer Society (ACS) and several mission areas within the US Department of Agriculture (USDA). These new partners provided more federal and local support. CDC now funds several state 5 A Day research and demonstration projects. USDA has launched a pilot project in four states to bring fresh fruit and vegetables into school classrooms. Coordinators from each of the 50 states, plus all the US Territories and military branches, form the rest of the National 5 A Day Partnership, which is now the largest public–private partnership promoting health in the USA.

The partners are also targeting specific population sectors. NCI targets African American men with a message to *Eat 5 to 9 A Day*. PBH,

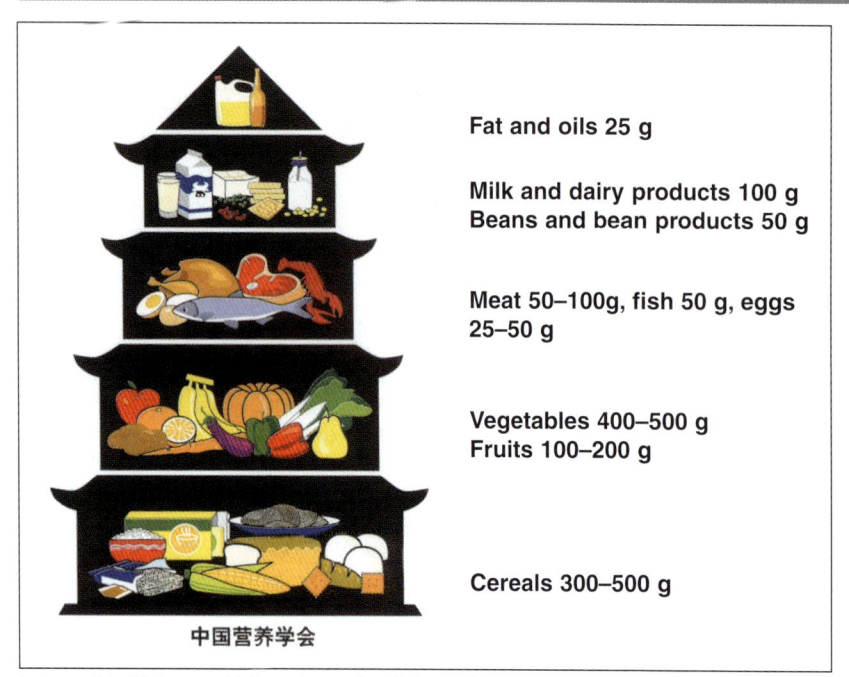

Figure 14 Dietary guidelines from the Chinese Nutrition Society (2000) (pagoda) The recommendation is to eat 400–500 g of vegetables/day and 100–200 g of fruits

focusing on female shoppers, has launched a campaign called *5 A Day The Color Way*. The American Cancer Society's 5 A Day Body and Soul programme is targeting African American women through the black church networks. To reach Spanish-speaking consumers, both NCI and PBH materials have been adapted with appropriate ethnic food choices and visuals promoting *Coma 5 al día y Sea Activo* (Eat 5 A Day and be Active) and *5 A Day—Coma Sus Colores Cada Día!* (5 A Day—Eat Your Colors Every Day!). California 5 A Day has taken the lead in developing many of these materials in their Latino 5 A Day programme.

In all cases, the goal is to promote a positive message about diet and a healthy lifestyle. Eating low-fat meals that include five to nine servings of fruit and vegetables every day is a cornerstone of a healthy life plan. Care is taken not to disparage other food groups, and to promote a colourful variety of vegetables and fruit in culturally appropriate ways and in the context of a low-fat diet; the use of whole grains and minimal use of salt and sugars are also strongly suggested.

NCI and PBH have established criteria to define promotable products that may be promoted as part of the 5 A Day Program. These criteria are intended to keep the 5 A Day Program consistent with US federal nutrition objectives, dietary guidelines and food labelling regulations (US Department of Health and Human Services, 1990, 2000). These criteria are now being re-evaluated to take into account the latest knowledge about fruits and vegetables and new fruit/vegetable products in the US food supply. At the national level, 5 A Day partners also include the United Fresh Fruit & Vegetable Association and the National Alliance for Nutrition and Physical Activity (NANA). The former is a trade organization representing the fresh fruit and vegetable industry, while

NANA is a coalition of over 200 organizations promoting public policy changes to improve both nutrition and physical fitness. NANA leaders include the Center for Science in the Public Interest, American Public Health Association, American Heart Association, American College of Preventive Medicine and many state departments of health. In addition to participating in the NANA coalition, United and PBH are pressing to expand the USDA free fresh fruit/vegetable pilot programme into other schools nationwide.

At the community level, coordinators in each state health department help to implement the 5 A Day programme by targeting their own audiences with their own materials or materials available through the national partners. State and local coalitions involve both the public and private sectors to implement activities at the local level. Local partners include industry as well as local ACS divisions, regional USDA offices, schools and others.

A great strength of the programme has been its focus on organizing and expanding the number and reach of the 5 A Day National Partnership, as much as promoting the actual 5 a day message. The programme has shown the feasibility of health agencies working in partnership with agricultural boards and commissions, fruit and vegetable companies and supermarkets to deliver wide-reaching mass-media messages with modest government resources (National Cancer Institute, 2002).

A survey of 2544 adults conducted in 1997 showed that general awareness of the recommended daily servings of fruits and vegetables had increased from 7.7% in 1991 to 19.2% and knowledge of the 5 A Day programme had increased from 2.0% to 17.8% (Stables *et al.*, 2002). Preli-minary data showed a modest increase in the mean intake of total fruit and vegetables (from 3.75 servings per day in 1991 to 3.98 in 1998) (National Institutes of Health and National Cancer Institute, 2001).

Australia

Several campaigns aimed at improving fruit and vegetable consumption have been conducted in Australia, initiated at the state level. The Western Australia Health Department directed a campaign with the slogan "Fruit 'n' Veg with Every Meal" (Health Department of Western Australia, 1990). Following an evaluation showing a limited impact of this slogan, the department moved in 1991 to using a quantitative message, "2 Fruit 'n' 5 Veg Every Day" (National Health and Medical Research Council, 1991). Surveys conducted in Western Australia identified barriers to increasing consumption of fruit and vegetables including habit, lack of knowledge about the amount of fruit and vegetables to eat for good health, concern about high prices and poor quality, particularly of fruit; and boredom with and lack of preparation ideas for vegetables. On the basis of the Western Australian experience, Victoria conducted a "2 Fruit 'n' 5 Veg Every Day" campaign between 1992 and 1995, placing greater emphasis on formal industry partnerships.

Surveys at the state level indicated increased awareness of the recommended daily amounts of fruit and vegetables, improved attitudes and increased consumption (Dixon et al., 1998; Farrell et al., 2000). A telephone survey of 2602 subjects in November 2000 showed an increase in reported consumption of fresh fruit and vegetables from 4.1 servings per day in 1998 to 4.5 (Reeve, 2000). In addition, respondents were aware of the health benefits of fruit and vegetable consumption and believed they should be eating seven or more servings per day.

Europe

Several campaigns have been conducted in Europe. The European Partnership for Fruits, Vegetables and Better Health (EPBH) is a voluntary network set up in May 2003 involving Denmark, Finland, France, Germany, Holland, Norway, Poland, Slovenia and the United Kingdom. The members are bodies promoting health or fruit and vegetable consumption. National members should ideally include both health organizations and non-profit organizations representing the fruit and vegetable industry, such as growers, importers, shippers, processors, wholesalers and retailers. Where such national partnerships do not exist, countries are encouraged to form such an alliance. The overall objective of EPBH is to assist members to increase the consumption of fruit and vegetables in their countries. This should be achieved by facilitating exchange of documentation and experience on effective strategies and actions and by collaboration and coordination of research activities on fruit and vegetable promotion across Europe. EPBH will formulate and communicate suggestions for policy changes at both national and European levels, coordinate pan-European promotions and actions and stimulate national partnerships between health partners and organizations representing the fruit and vegetable industry.

The EPBH web site (www.epbh. org) provides information on campaigns already implemented in European countries. As an example, the experience in Denmark, including some evaluation results, is summarized below.

In 1998, a broad consensus was reached in Denmark to adopt the message '6 A Day – Eat more fruits and vegetables' as the official national recommendation for fruit and vegetable consumption. A 2002 follow-up report from the Danish Ministry of Food, Agriculture and Fisheries (Fagt et al., 2002) confirmed 600 g/d in addition to potatoes as a recommended target for public health.

Since 1999, the Danish 6 A Day programme has conducted a number of research projects on how to increase fruit and vegetable consumption. A parent-paid subscription programme for fruit in schools was shown to increase students' fruit intake by 0.4 servings per day. Non-subscribers too showed a significant increase in fruit consumption in schools where the programme was introduced (Eriksen et al., 2003).

Supplying free fruit in workplace settings has also proven very effective. In an intervention study, a total of 283 employees at 12 workplaces increased their average fruit intake by 0.7 servings per day and the men's intake of unhealthy snacks was cut in half (Morten Strunge Meyer, Denmark, personal communication). The number of workplaces offering free fruit to employees has greatly increased from 1998 to 2002.

Since 1998, the awareness of 6 A Day has been monitored twice a year. Unpublished data show that 40% of all Danes now know that they should eat 6 A Day or 600 g/d, and 66% have heard or read about the 6 A Day campaign. More important, the average *per capita* intake of fruit and vegetables for adults increased from 279 to 379 g/d from 1995 to 2000/01, according to the national dietary survey (Fagt et al., 2002). Unpublished data from the 6 A Day telephone surveys suggest that this increase took place after the year 2000, when the 6 A Day-campaign was launched (Figure 15).

The 6 A Day research projects have shown that enhancing determinants such as availability and 'ready-to-eat-ness' can be very effective in increasing fruit and vegetable consumption in a population that already knows that fruit and vegetables are good for health. Health information has

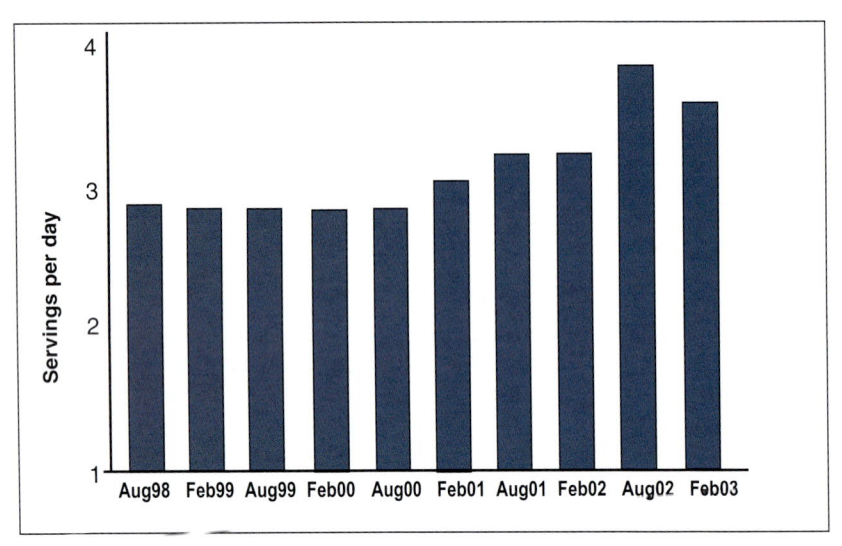

Figure 15 Self reported intake of fruits and vegetables in Denmark
Each bar is based on 500 phone interviews. Potatoes are excluded

not been entirely abandoned, continuing to target, for instance, key professionals, but for interventions to be effective the many and complex determinants must be adequately addressed when developing strategies. 6 A Day's future strategy will have an increased focus on influencing health-oriented public policies and continued strengthening of effective public–private partnerships.

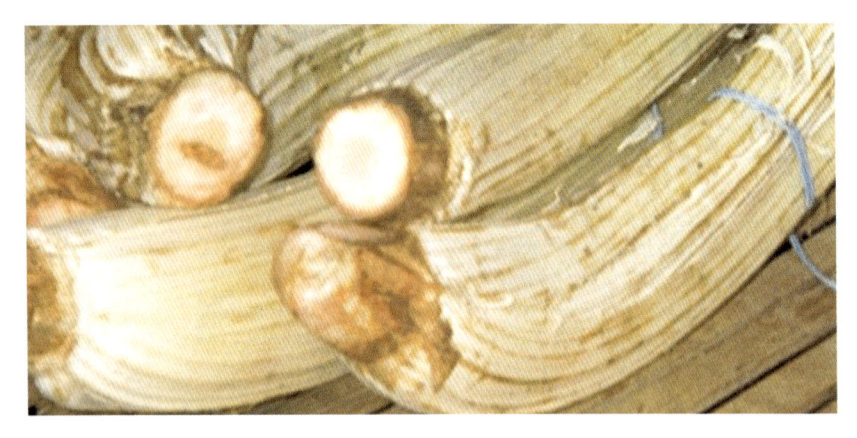

Chapter 4
Cancer-preventive effects

Human studies

The groupings used to evaluate epidemiological studies were:
- Total fruit consumption
- Total vegetable consumption
- Total fruit and vegetable consumption

Where possible, potatoes, pulses and mushrooms were excluded from the evaluations (see also Chapter 1).

The Working Group was concerned that reporting of associations between specific cancers and specific individual foods or subgroups of fruit and vegetables might be subject to publication bias. Few of the studies identified had examined the effects of total intake of fruit and vegetables combined. Therefore the Working Group decided to evaluate the evidence in relation to total fruit and to total vegetables. This approach is conservative in that an effect of any specific fruit or vegetable, or subgroup of them, would be diluted, but would not be conservative if relationships between cancer and fruits and vegetables were due to composite effects of multiple bioactive components.

General issues

In assessing the evidence on the relation between cancer and intake of fruit and vegetables, sources of heterogeneity between studies include:

- differences in study design, with different potential opportunities for bias and confounding to influence results;
- differences in reference period;
- differences in definition of exposure (see Chapter 1);
- differences in dietary assessment instrument and its method of administration (see Chapter 2);
- differences in the extent and control of measurement error;
- differences in the extent to which potentially confounding factors were investigated, and in the adequacy of adjustment for these;
- effect modification;
- differences in methods of statistical analysis;
- chance (and multiple testing);
- differences in study context.

In appraising individual studies, it is important to consider their design, as this affects the biases that may occur and their generalizability. Problems associated with specific designs are addressed in the next section. Problems that affect more than one type of design are discussed in subsequent sections.

Study design
Randomized controlled trials

The definitive method of investigating the efficacy of a potentially preventive intervention is the randomized controlled trial. The particular strength of this design is that, provided the trial is sufficiently large, the distribution of potential confounders, known (measured) and unknown (unmeasured), will differ between the group assigned to receive the intervention and the control group no more than would be expected by chance. In addition, the exposure potentially can be precisely defined, although in the context of fruit and vegetables this would probably apply to the advice (and any measures taken to support this) rather than intake. Blinding (masking) can exclude the possibility that knowledge of the exposure status of the subjects could bias the assessment of outcome. However, subjects cannot be blinded to their intake of foods. For various reasons, such as non-compliance, it is possible that subjects may not receive the exposure to which they have been assigned. The reasons for this may be associated with the outcome of interest. For example, in a randomized trial of the cancer-preventive effect of advice to increase fruit and vegetable intake, there could be a high proportion of non- or poor compliers in the intervention group. In one randomized controlled trial of individualized advice to increase vegetable and fruit intake, drop-outs were more likely to be smokers and of lower socioeconomic status than those who did not drop out (Smith-Warner et al., 2000). As smoking and socioeconomic status are related to cancer outcome, so also is drop-out. It is therefore crucially important that the data are analysed according to the principle of "intention-to-treat", otherwise the effect of randomization in minimizing potential confounding is lost (Peto et al., 1976; Fergusson et al., 2002).

In trials of interventions designed to assess the effects of increasing intakes of fruit and vegetables, randomization should result in similar baseline intakes of fruit and vegetables between the arms of the trial. In theory, the intervention group will augment its intake of fruit and vegetables above the baseline level by a certain amount. However, especially if the intervention is intended to result in increased intake over a prolonged period, measurement of adherence to the intervention is a crucial issue. In addition, changes in intake of fruit and vegetables may bring about other changes such as reduction in meat intake or weight gain, which may have their own effects on cancer incidence, and so complicate interpretation of the effect of the intervention.

In specifying criteria for assessing evidence on which health policies and guidelines are based, several national organizations accord the highest level of evidence to randomized controlled trials (NHMRC, 1999; Briss et al., 2000; SIGN, 2001). Comparisons between such trials and observational evidence have been made for certain topics, but not for consumption of fruit and vegetables (Ioannidis et al., 2001), because few randomized controlled trials of the effects of fruit and vegetables have been conducted. Differences in the estimated magnitude of effect between trials and observational studies are very common and the directions of the differences are difficult to predict (Britton et al., 1998; MacLehose et al., 2000). There are many potential reasons for such differences, including a short period of observation in the trials, trials conducted during an inappropriate period of the natural history of the disease or using end-points with unknown predictive value (especially intermediate end-points, see below), use of a different quantity of fruits and/or vegetables in the trial, or bias or measurement error in the observational studies.

The only randomized controlled trials of the effects of fruit and vegetables in the area of cancer and precancerous lesions have examined the effects of a recommendation to consume a specified amount and/or dietary counselling. Such counselling tends not to be limited to fruit and vegetable intake (there may be, for example, advice to reduce fat intake) and may influence other health-related behaviour. Although trial results can be especially compelling and have widespread implications, caution is needed in generalizing from the results of trials on specially selected groups to the population as a whole.

Cohort studies
In a cohort study, individuals who are disease-free are recruited to participate in the study and are then followed over time to identify those who develop the disease. Information on, for example, socio-demographic factors, medical history and lifestyle factors such as diet is collected at the beginning of the study, before the onset of disease. The cohort design could be regarded as similar to the randomized controlled trial, except that the assignment of exposure is subject-selected rather than randomized. Consequently, (a) it is necessary to measure potential confounders and adjust for them; (b) the distribution of unknown and unmeasured confounders may differ between the groups being compared; (c) it may not be meaningful to analyse the study according to "intention to treat", as any change in exposure (diet) may be highly context-dependent and unlikely to be reproducible in other populations and periods, (d) changes in exposure as a consequence of early symptoms of disease and biases in loss to follow-up that are directly or indirectly related to exposure are potential issues affecting interpretation; and (e) the subjects are not blinded to their exposure status – this may compromise the extent to which assessment of outcome is independent of exposure status.

Large numbers of subjects have to be enrolled in a cohort study in order to have adequate statistical power to determine associations with specific types of cancer. Gains in efficiency, over numbers of subjects analysed or numbers of tests performed on collected specimens, are possible in cohort studies with nested case–control and case–cohort designs, but the requirement for a large cohort size overall is unchanged. Therefore, the methods used for assessment of dietary intake and potentially confounding factors need to be suitable for application to large numbers of subjects. This has implications for the extent of potential measurement error (see Chapter 2). A potential advantage of the cohort design compared with the case–control design is that concurrent measurement of current diet is likely to be better correlated with the true current diet than is retrospective measurement of past diet with the true past diet. Another advantage is that repeated measurements can be obtained, if resources are available. Repeated measurement allows changes in diet and other relevant exposures to be monitored, and also permits development of a summary measure of exposure less subject to random misclassification than a single measure. This gives the investigator a choice of measure of 'diet', including diet at the beginning of the study, more recent intake or a summary measure of repeated exposures.

A strategy for dealing with the possibility that pre-diagnostic changes in diet may bias the observed association between diet and disease is to exclude cases diagnosed in the initial period of follow-up. Investigators often assess whether results are altered by the exclusion of cases identified in the initial period of follow-up, such as the first two years.

Participation bias in a cohort study affects the generalizability of the results, but does not compromise their internal validity. However, it has been suggested that the tendency for the most health-conscious to participate may reduce the variability of dietary intake, making it difficult to detect associations with disease risk (Steinmetz et al., 1994). Over-representation of health-conscious active persons interested in their diet has been noted in dietary surveys (Harris et al., 1989; van't Hof & Burema, 1996; Sidenvall et al., 2002). There is also a possibility that subjects in a cohort study who are knowledgeable concerning effects of diet on health may report their diet in a manner that represents what they believe they should eat, not what they actually eat. This could be a problem of some studies of health professionals.

Bias resulting from differential loss to follow-up by exposure could occur if, for example, both loss to follow-up and fruit or vegetable consumption vary by socioeconomic status. Limited data on loss to follow-up tend to be presented for cohort studies. In a case–control study of lung cancer nested within a cohort study in New York State, USA, although there were some differences in diet between those lost to follow-up (19 of 525 controls, 3.6%) and those whose outcome was known, the results of analyses relating to diet and alcohol were similar including and excluding losses to follow-up (Bandera et al., 2002). In a longitudinal study of cognitive ageing, those who did not return for follow-up had lower educational levels than those who did return (Van Beijsterveldt et al., 2002). In studies in the USA, members of minority groups have tended to have higher drop-out rates than whites (Vernon et al., 1984; Bowen et al., 2000). In a study of black women in the USA, those who were lost to follow-up tended to be less well educated than those who remained in the study (Russell et al., 2001). A related issue concerns the return of incomplete information during follow-up, i.e., item non-response. This has been shown to be associated with subsequent loss to follow-up (Deeg et al., 2002).

In cohort studies, disease rates during follow-up are typically analysed with respect to the values of factors measured at enrolment. Enrolment diet may accurately reflect typical lifetime intake. However, because of the combined effects of measurement errors and changes in the exposure of participating subjects over time, this approach may underestimate the strength of association between habitual level of exposure during the period of follow-up and disease risk. Repeated measurements of baseline exposure in a representative sample of participants in a cohort study can be used to estimate the magnitude of measurement error and correct for it. Repeated measurements taken later in the exposure period can be used to correct for changes in exposure. Using a food frequency questionnaire (FFQ), Goldbohm et al. (1995) observed a high degree of consistency of within-subject dietary patterns relating to fruit and vegetable consumption between five successive annual assessments.

Limited participation at enrolment affects the generalizability of the findings from the study cohort. It does not affect the validity of the study findings.

Case–control studies

In a case–control study, individuals who have recently developed a disease and a sample of individuals without the disease being investigated are recruited and information is then collected on potential risk factors during a specified reference period before the onset of disease. One of the main advantages of the case–control design compared with the cohort design is that the total number of subjects whose diet has to be assessed is much smaller. In theory, this gives more flexibility in the choice of methods for determining diet and potentially confounding exposures than with cohort studies. Thus, for example, data can be collected by in-person interview using a detailed quantitative dietary instrument rather than by self-completed questionnaire.

As in cohort studies, the assignment of exposure is subject-selected rather than randomized, and this raises similar issues with regard to potential bias and confounding. The main potential biases of the case–control design are (a) inappropriate choice of cases or controls, leading to selection bias and (b) misreporting of past diet.

Selection bias
In a number of studies of cancer in relation to fruit and vegetable intake, controls comprised subjects hospitalized with other types of cancer or with a range of other disorders. Hospital-based studies may be attractive for investigations of diseases when it is difficult to characterize the underlying study base (Wacholder et al., 2002). Another possible attraction is that, provided that the diseases of control subjects are of similar severity to that of the cases, recall bias may be minimized (see discussion of recall bias). However, if the conditions for which a subject is hospitalized are themselves related to fruit and vegetable consumption, the measure of association would be distorted (Wacholder et al., 1992).

Selection bias also may occur as a result of differential non-participation between cases and controls. There has been concern about a decline in participation rates (Olson, 2001), especially in population-based studies.

This could result in people selected as population controls being largely those most likely to be at home when contacted. Therefore in studies using population controls, it is critical to ensure as high a response as possible from those eligible in the base population. Information on the potential effects of low participation rates is limited (Madigan et al., 2000).

Differential misclassification of diet – recall bias
Retrospective measurement of diet is likely to be less well correlated with the true diet during the reference period than is the case for concurrent measurement of diet and the true current diet (see Chapter 2). If cases and controls differ in their accuracy of dietary recall, the comparison of the reported diet will be biased.

It has been suggested that the likelihood of recall bias may be greater when recall is poor in general (Coughlin, 1990). However, this was not apparent in a systematic review of empirical studies of recall bias published between 1966 and 1990 (Chouinard & Walter, 1995).

Dietary information obtained from cases and controls by questionnaire or interview was compared with information on the index subject obtained from the next of kin or spouse in two studies in the USA. In one, the responses of 67 men with cancer to a dietary interview were compared with those of their spouses to the same instrument regarding intake of the index subject; a similar comparison was made for 91 male neighbourhood controls and their spouses (Marshall et al., 1980). The study instrument included 27 items to assess vegetable consumption and 11 to assess fruit consumption. The proportion of case–spouse pairs reporting exact agreement regarding vegetable consumption was 59%, compared with 65% for control–spouse pairs, while for fruit consumption the proportions were 49% and 56% respectively. The proportion of case–spouse pairs reporting agreement of vegetable consumption within one category (out of 11 possible categories) was 88% compared with 94% for control–spouse pairs. The corresponding proportions for fruit were 76% and 88%. In the other US study (Herrmann, 1985), the response to a diet interview of 94 cases with colon cancer and their next of kin, and 93 controls selected using an area probability sampling scheme and their next of kin, were compared. The instrument had 31 items relating to consumption of vegetables and 12 relating to fruit. The agreement, over five categories of frequency of consumption, was higher for case–next of kin than control–next of kin pairs both for vegetables (agreement 70% for case–next of kin pairs and 66% for control–next of kin pairs; kappa 0.45 and 0.40 respectively) and fruit (agreement 66% for case–next of kin pairs and 63% for control–next of kin pairs; kappa 0.42 and 0.41 respectively). Although these studies indicate reasonable agreement between the reports of index subjects and proxy subjects, concern has persisted about the quality of data from proxy respondents (Nelson et al., 1990; Lyon et al., 1992).

In other studies, data from self-completed questionnaires or from interviews carried out as part of a survey or enrolment into a cohort study were compared with data obtained from subjects after diagnosis of cancer and from control subjects identified at that time (Table 9). All but one of the studies relating to food groups used FFQs in both assessments. In most of these studies, the data were interpreted as showing little evidence of recall bias (Friedenreich et al., 1991; Holmberg et al., 1996; Lindsted & Kuzma, 1990). Hammar and Norell (1991) noted that there was good agreement between retrospective and original information among subjects who reported that they had not changed their diet between 1967 and 1987. However, this was not the case for those who had changed their diet, and this was a particular issue for those who had changed their diet because of disease. [The ability of some of these studies to detect recall bias may have been limited because of misclassification likely to have resulted from the instruments used, the small size of some of the studies, and correlated errors between the dietary assessments.]

Two studies presented data only on nutrients. Wilkens et al. (1992), in a study in which both assessments of diet were made by interview, found that although there were no marked differences overall between cases and non-cases in the ability to recall past diet, this did not apply in certain subgroups, such as subjects with the longest recall interval (8–10 years), and cases with colorectal cancer or any cases diagnosed with distant stage disease, compared with non-cases. Giovannucci et al. (1993) reported finding no association between breast cancer and intake of total or saturated fat when prospectively collected data were analysed, but a positive association when retrospectively collected data were analysed. However, the prospective analysis related to 392 cases and 786 controls, while the retrospective analysis related to 300 cases and 602 controls. Thus, the difference in results may not be entirely attributable to recall bias; response bias might have contributed. In a study in Finland, Männistö et al. (1999) compared data obtained by FFQ from cases of breast cancer with data from (a) population-based controls and (b) subjects who were referred for the same examinations as cases but who were later diagnosed to be healthy. There was evidence that group (b) differed from group (a) in reporting of milk products,

Table 9. Summary of studies of recall bias in relation to fruit and vegetables and cancer: comparison of data obtained prospectively with those obtained after diagnosis of cancer for cases, and at a similar time for controls

Study	Cases Type	N	Controls Type	N	Prospective method Type	Timing	Retrospective method Type	Timing	Number of items Veg.	Fruit	Results
Lindsted & Kuzma, 1989	Incident, ns	117	Survivors aged <82 years, ns	99	FFQ	1960	FFQ, subset of 1960 instrument	1984	1	1	Spearman rank-order correlation for veg. 0.21 for cases, 0.25 for controls; for fruit 0.26 for cases, 0.23 for controls. Exact and close agreement greater for controls than cases for both veg. and fruit
Lindsted & Kuzma, 1990	Mainly breast, female genito-urinary or colorectal	181	Controls selected randomly from cohort of survivors aged <82 years	225	FFQ	1976	FFQ, subset of 1976 instrument	1984	7 (included 2 categories relating to rice)	7	Spearman rank-order correlation for veg. in range 0.35–0.61 for cases, 0.27–0.65 for controls; for fruit 0.29–0.51 for cases and 0.31–0.46 for controls. % agreement greater for cases than controls for 4/7 veg. categories and 4/7 fruit categories. Over all 35 food groups, case–control difference in recall error was not significant in multivariate analysis that conditioned on dietary changes.
Friedenreich et al., 1991	Breast	325	Selected from 628 participants in mammography screening trial (same study base as cases)		FFQ	1982–85	Self-administered FFQ identical to first except reference period specified as diet at time of first FFQ	1988	17	10	Pearson correlation for veg. 0.50 (95% CI 0.41–0.58) for cases and 0.48 (95% CI 0.42–0.54) for controls; for fruit 0.55 (0.47–0.62) for cases and 0.58 (95% CI 0.53–0.63) for controls
Hammar & Norell, 1991	Colorectal	45	Random sample of original cohort	135	FFQ	1937	FFQ identical to first except reference period specified as diet at time of first FFQ	1987	1	1	Among subjects with high consumption according to the original report, controls tended to under-estimate their previous consumption of fruit/veg. more than cases. Among those with low consumption according to the original report, cases tended to over-estimate their previous consumption more than controls.
Holmberg et al., 1996	Breast	265	Selected from 431 participants in mammography screening (same study base as cases)		FFQ	1987–90, sent out with invitation to participate in screening	Interview	6 mo after screening	9	4	Veg.: 31.3% agreement for cases, 37.3% for controls; kappa 0.16 and 0.08 respectively (0.12 and 0.18 when analysis restricted to subjects who returned complete questionnaires). Fruit 38.5% agreement for cases, 41.9% for controls; kappa 0.23 and 0.18 respectively

and for premenopausal women a difference was apparent also for reporting of tea, sugar, fats and vitamins. Thus the OR of breast cancer in premenopausal women for the highest quintile of vegetable consumption versus the lowest in comparison with group (a) was 1.3 (95% CI 0.5–3.1) and with group (b) 0.6 (95% CI 0.3–1.4).

Investigations of the theoretical impact of recall bias for dichotomous exposures shows that even severe recall bias causes only weak to moderate spurious associations (Drews & Greenland, 1990; Swan et al., 1992; Khoury et al., 1994). However, in a simulation analysis, differential under-reporting of fat and energy intake by cases but not controls substantially altered the association between fat intake and disease risk (Bellach & Kohlmeier, 1998). The direction and magnitude of the effect depended on the type of error structure.

Differences in reference period between types of study

An implicit difference between trials and cohort studies on the one hand and case–control studies on the other lies in the reference period about which data on intake of vegetables and fruit are sought. In trials and cohort studies, the reference period is typically at enrolment, although in some studies data on diet at later time-points in follow-up have been obtained. In case–control studies, data are typically sought for a reference period before diagnosis for cases and for a corresponding period before recruitment for controls. Although investigators recognize that there may be a long latent period in cancer development, they have also noted that reporting of past diet is influenced by current diet. It has been assumed that while total intake declines with age, the relative intake of different nutrients varies little in adult life (Willett, 1998d). However, increasing diversity in the foods available for consumption and the increasing consumption of convenience foods may mean that this assumption is no longer tenable in a number of countries (see Chapter 3).

Differences in the length of the reference period are a potential source of variability between studies in populations where availability of fruit and vegetables varies by season.

It is possible that early life exposure to fruit and vegetables is important in the etiology of cancer. The food frequency approach taken in cohort studies (of older individuals) to date provides little to no information on early-life exposure. To the extent that self-reported adult intake is a poor measure of early-life diet, additional exposure error is introduced into studies.

Differences in definition of exposure between types of study

Standard methods for classifying exposure to vegetables and fruit in epidemiological studies have not been established (Smith et al., 1995) (see Chapter 2). The instruments used in most studies have been designed to assess variation in nutrient intake, rather than variation in intake of fruit and vegetables per se. As an example of the lack of standardization, studies differ in whether fruit juice consumption is included in fruit consumption, vegetable juice intake with vegetable consumption, and whether potatoes or mature beans are included in vegetable intake (Slattery, 2001; Smith-Warner et al., 2001a).

The number of fruit and vegetable questions has varied considerably across studies, which may influence the specific fruit and vegetable groups examined and the intake estimates obtained. The contrast in intake estimates for the high versus low categories for relative risk estimation also has been highly variable across studies.

Differences in study instrument and its method of administration between types of study

The methods of dietary assessment used in epidemiological studies to estimate individual dietary exposure include FFQs, diet history interviews, 24-hour dietary recalls and food record methods (see Chapter 2). Most studies have used FFQs. Key factors that differ include the number and formulation of questions, inclusion of data on portion size and the method of administration. For example, in studies of colorectal cancer in which the number of items used to assess dietary intake was reported, this varied between 35 and 276 items for cohort studies, and 10 to 300 items for case–control studies (see below). Direct interviewing has been used in many case–control studies, whereas this is seldom used in cohort studies.

Measurement error

Issues in assessing evidence from different studies include (a) whether a validation study has been done; (b) if one has been done, its adequacy (see Chapter 2); and (c) whether information for the validation study was used in the analyses based on the primary study instrument. Little is known about the measurement error structure for reported fruit and vegetable intake in FFQs. Errors in the instrument being validated and in the reference method tend to be correlated (Plummer & Clayton, 1993; Goldbohm et al., 1995; Day et al., 2001; Kipnis et al., 2001), while the extent of error varies with characteristics of the subject (Prentice, 1996; Horner et al., 2002). In consequence, both the attenuation of the dietary effect and the loss of statistical power may be greater than previously estimated, making modest (but important) reductions in relative risk difficult to detect (Kipnis *et al.*, 2003). Potential solutions to this problem include the development and use of FFQs with far more detailed questions about fruit and vegetable intake; use of more intensive instruments (recalls, diaries) as the primary dietary assessment tool, and development of unbiased biomarkers of fruit and vegetable intake, analogous to urinary nitrogen as a biomarker of protein intake. At present, such fruit and vegetable biomarkers do not exist.

Adjustment for misclassification (calibration) may not deal with possible heterogeneity between studies because of differences in the design and administration of the primary study instrument.

End-points

In most studies, the primary end-point has been newly incident cancers. However, in some studies, mortality due to specific types of cancer has been the primary end-point and these would be biased if fruit or vegetable intake were associated with survival.

In randomized trials, and some observational studies, intermediate effect markers have been used as end-points. An intermediate effect biomarker is a detectable lesion or biological parameter with some of the histological or biological features of preneoplasia or neoplasia but without evidence of invasion, which is known either to be on the direct pathway from the initiation of the neoplastic process to the occurrence of invasive cancer, has a high probability of resulting in the development of cancer, or is a detectable biochemical abnormality which is highly correlated with the presence of such a lesion. Thus intermediate effect markers include (*a*) detectable precancerous changes in an organ (confirmed by histology), (*b*) alteration of a gene that is considered to play a causative role, (*c*) DNA damage, (*d*) other indicators of carcinogenesis, such as the expression of a marker of an exposure known to be a cause of a cancer (e.g., positivity for human papillomavirus (HPV) DNA), and (*e*) effects on metabolic factors thought to be involved in etiology, e.g., effects on phase I and phase II enzymes, antioxidant pathways and steroid hormone metabolism. Causation is not a requirement for inclusion in this group, but the expectation is that the relevant biomarkers can eventually be connected in a biologically mechanistic manner to the cancer (Miller *et al.*, 2001).

There is likely to be a hierarchy of intermediate biomarkers. Those that are known to be on the causal pathway to cancer are at the top and can be truly called intermediate effect markers. Then there are markers where present knowledge indicates only a probability of cancer association, but it is uncertain as to whether they are on the causal pathway – they can only be called intermediate markers. A subset of intermediate effect markers, which can be modulated, have been called surrogate end-point biomarkers (Kelloff *et al.*, 2000).

It has not been convincingly shown that the use of fruits and vegetables, or derivatives from them, in men and women with any type of preneoplastic lesion can substantially reduce the subsequent development of truly invasive cancer (see subsequent sections of this chapter). In general, not enough is known on the natural history of precancerous lesions to identify those that will progress to invasive cancer if allowed to do so, nor to define the time point in the natural history of progression of intermediate end-points to cancer where an intervention will prevent the development of the cancer. If an intervention, such as fruit and vegetables, acts at the later stages of carcinogenesis, a randomized trial with an intermediate end-point will fail to demonstrate any effect. It would only be if the intervention was administered after the occurrence of the intermediate end-point, and was shown not to prevent the development of subsequent cancer, that a benefit from the intervention could be excluded. Such studies are, however, likely to be precluded for ethical reasons, and therefore it may be impossible to use randomized trials to evaluate the effect of inhibition of the later stages of carcinogenesis.

Confounding

An association between intake of fruit and vegetables and cancer could be due to confounding. This may be because a high intake of fruit and vegetables is associated with other behaviours related to health (Serdula *et al.*, 1996; Williams *et al.*, 2000). In particular, smokers consume lower quantities of vegetables and fruit than non-smokers; some studies (Serdula *et al.*, 1996, Agudo *et al.*, 1999; Voorrips *et al.*, 2000a; Sauvaget *et al.*, 2003) but not all (Nuttens *et al.*, 1992; McPhillips *et al.*, 1994; Wallstrom *et al.*, 2000) have shown that differences in consumption are greater for fruit than for vegetables. Mean intake of fruit and vegetables of past smokers may be higher than those of current smokers (Miller *et al.*, 2003).

In most studies, data on smoking behaviour have been self-reported and the accuracy of these data may vary between studies (e.g., Lindqvist *et al.*, 2002). In some studies, higher levels of alcohol consumption have been associated with lower intake of fruit and vegetables (Serdula *et al.*, 1996; Wallstrom *et al.*, 2000). In addition, high intakes of fruit and vegetables are associated with reduced intake of potentially harmful foods such as red meat. Thus intervention studies aimed at increasing intake of vegetables and fruit may also result in reduced fat intake (Smith-Warner *et al.*, 2000). Physical inactivity is a consistent risk factor for colon and breast cancer and may be associated with other types of cancer (e.g., endometrium, prostate) (IARC, 2002) and fruit and vegetable consumption is likely to be correlated with physical activity. Even though many studies adjust for physical activity, this characteristic is not measured with great accuracy and residual confounding remains a possibility. In addition, consumption of fruit and vegetables varies by age, gender, socioeconomic status and ethnicity. In most countries where the relationship between fruit and vegetable intake and measures of socioeconomic status has been investigated, the general pattern has been that intake was higher among people of higher socioeconomic status (Subar et al., 1990; Murphy et al., 1992; Potter, 1997) (see Chapter 3).

When confounders are measured inaccurately, it follows that the analysis cannot properly control for confounding. If both the primary exposure of interest and the confounder are measured inaccurately, it is possible that the two sets of errors may be interrelated, so the apparent relationship between exposure and confounder may be quite different from that between the underlying variables (Clayton & Hills, 1993).

Due to the association between intake of fruit and vegetables and important risk factors for cancer like smoking and cancer on one side, and the possible errors in measuring these factors on the other side (e.g., Marshall et al., 1996; Lindqvist et al., 2002; Stram et al., 2002), it is difficult to exclude residual confounding completely. For example, Stram et al. (2002) illustrated with a simulation that even a modest correlation between smoking and serum β-carotene, combined with errors in smoking assessment, might plausibly explain the observed inverse association of serum β-carotene levels with lung cancer risk in terms of residual confounding.

Effect modification
Components of fruit and vegetables can interact with biological targets by modifying the risk associated with carcinogenic exposures. For example, DNA damage related to tobacco smoking could be inhibited by fruit and vegetable components. Such effect modification needs to be clearly distinguished from confounding, because it represents a genuine protective effect that occurs only in those exposed to the carcinogens. For this reason, it is important to analyse epidemiological data not only with an approach based on adjustment for potential confounders (e.g., smoking), but also stratifying by carcinogenic exposures (e.g., never-smokers, ex-smokers, current smokers).

If fruit and vegetable intake is protective only for persons with a specific genetically determined metabolic profile, the incorporation of appropriate genetic information into epidemiological studies could 'sharpen' the relative risks observed in the 'susceptible' group. Work on such nutrition–gene interactions presents considerable difficulties, however, given that there are many bioactive constituents of fruits and vegetables and many enzymes involved in their absorption and metabolism, with functionally important allelic variants for at least some of these enzymes.

Statistical analysis
Categorization of exposure
An issue in statistical analysis is whether to consider reported dietary intake as a continuous or a categorical variable. When the objective of dietary assessments is to rank subjects according to their intake rather than to provide a precise quantitative measure of absolute intake, analysis by ordered categories such as tertiles, quartiles or quintiles is less sensitive to the effects of outliers than analysis of continuous variables (Willett, 1998e). The measure of the effect of the nutrient on disease can be interpreted as the effect of changing intake between quantiles of intake, e.g. from the lowest to the highest. Categorization by quantiles can be based on the distribution of (*a*) cases, (*b*) non-cases and (*c*) all subjects. These three methods have been found to give the same statistical power to detect a trend across quantiles over a wide range of study situations (Hsieh et al., 1991). The choice of method may be influenced by consideration of how the quantiles relate to the source population and by ease of implementation.

Adjustment for energy intake
Total energy intake requires attention in the analysis and interpretation of nutritional epidemiology studies for several reasons. (1) It may be a primary cause of disease. Low energy intakes have reduced the incidence of tumours in experimental animals. Thus, adjustment for energy intake may be performed in human observational studies to mimic the isocaloric conditions in animal experiments. (2) It may be associated with disease in a non-causal manner and, since reported intakes of many specific food groups or nutrients tend to be correlated with total reported intake, total energy intake may confound associations with many food groups or nutrients. (3) Factors such as physical activity, body size and metabolic variation influence energy intake and may influence the risk of disease; variation in nutrient intake secondary to the influence of these factors on total energy intake is extraneous when investigating the effect of variation in nutrient intake on disease (Willett, 1990).

Methods of adjustment have been discussed by Willett (1990) and Kushi et al. (1992). More recently, it has been noted that the impact of measurement error on energy-adjustment models is uncertain (Kipnis et al., 1997), and there is renewed debate about energy adjustment (Block, 2001; Day et al., 2001; Day, 2002; Willett, 2001a, b, c). There is some doubt as to whether energy adjustment is required for assessment of fruit and vegetable intake. Fruits and vegetables are sources of non-fat energy. It has been suggested that adjustment for body weight may be a better approach to adjust for the overall effects of energy (Day & Ferrari, 2002).

Low intake or missing values
Treatment of data from subjects reporting very low total intake or with a high proportion of missing values can lead to (a) selection bias from excluding such subjects or (b) misclassification introduced by imputation of values to avoid this (Vach & Blettner, 1991; Greenland & Finkle, 1995; Demissie et al., 2003; Lyles & Allen, 2003). It is important to consider what method has been used, and whether the investigators reported any impact on the study results from different methods of dealing with this problem.

Study context
Heterogeneity between studies could arise from differences in many aspects of study context, including the types of fruit and vegetables available for consumption, their growing conditions, typical methods of preparation (storage, cooking), variability of exposure in the study population and of genetic background.

In cohort studies, few participants consume more than 4–5 servings of vegetables (or fruits) per day. This simply reflects the ranges of fruit and vegetable intake common in the USA and Europe, where these studies were conducted. The cohort studies to date could not evaluate whether substantial cancer protection is associated with higher levels of intake.

Integration of evidence
In reviewing the evidence in the rest of this chapter, the Working Group used inclusion criteria. Case reports were not considered, and ecological studies were not used in the evaluation. Cohort and case–control studies were always considered unless in the judgement of the Working Group they were inadequate in conception, design, conduct or analysis.

There have been several instances of sequential or multiple publications of analyses of the same or overlapping data-sets. When the reports clearly related to the same or overlapping data-sets, only data from the largest or most recent publication were included.

Meta-analyses and pooled analyses that were available are described at the end of the relevant section.

The data considered are presented in detail in the tables. In general, the tables include only data for total fruit, total vegetables, and total fruit and vegetables combined, unless for a specific study, the subgroups for which data were presented appeared to comprise a substantial proportion of fruit or vegetable intake, e.g. fresh fruits for fruits, or raw and cooked vegetables for vegetables. However, the data on sub-groups do not contribute to the evaluations, and no data are presented on cruciferous vegetables, as they will be the subject of a future evaluation. The odds ratios (ORs) or relative risks (RRs) presented are always those reported relating the highest quantile of consumption (of total fruit or total vegetables) to the lowest. Confidence intervals for these ORs are included when reported by the authors. When the authors reported ORs for the lowest to the highest consumption, the Working Group computed the inverse, and the result of these computations (and of the inverse of the confidence intervals if available) appears in square brackets in the tables.

The data used in the evaluations also appear as plots (Figures 16–51). Only those studies on total fruit or vegetables which reported confidence intervals and adjusted for the main confounders for the relevant sites are included in the plots. Meta-analyses and pooled analyses reported in the tables or discussed in the text have not been included in the plots. An estimate of the overall effect across all the evaluable studies, calculated as explained below, is presented, taking the size of the study (as reflected in the confidence interval) into account when weighting the individual study findings. The result of applying a test for heterogeneity is given with each plot. The reader is cautioned that these summary estimates do not constitute the result of a formal meta-analysis, and they should not be interpreted as such.

The summary estimates in the plots were calculated as follows. Using the log of the relative risks for the highest versus lowest exposure categories in the individual studies, designated as β_i, the pooled estimate (summary value, β_ρ) was obtained, separately for cohort and case–control studies, as

$$\beta_\rho = [\Sigma_i\ \beta_i/\text{var}(\beta_i)]/[\Sigma_i\ 1/\text{var}(\beta_i)]$$

with estimated standard error

$$\text{SE}(\beta_\rho) = [\Sigma_i\ 1/\text{var}(\beta_i)]^{-1/2}$$

The χ^2 for heterogeneity was calculated as

$$\chi^2 = \Sigma_i\ (\beta_i - \beta_\rho)^2/\text{var}(\beta_i)$$

with (N–1) degrees of freedom, where N is the total number of studies.

The analyses and generation of the plots were performed using the R software (Ihaka & Gentleman, 1996). Individual studies are presented in the plot in chronological order, with the 'box size' proportional to the inverse of their variance.

For some studies, results are reported for subcategories of the population under study, for example, males and females, pre- and post-menopausal women, colon and rectal cancer. In the calculation of the overall effect and in the final plot, the subgroups counted as individual studies; however, when counting the number of evaluable studies for different cancer sites, subgroups were considered as coming from a single study.

In reviewing the evidence on each cancer site, the Working Group considered the following criteria:
- Overall quality of design
- Comparability of source population of cases and controls
- Adequacy of control for potential confounding
- Evidence of dose–response effect
- Evidence of effect modification
- Evidence for difference in effect by age, gender and subsite of cancer
- Evidence of publication bias
- Evidence of heterogeneity of effect between studies

Effects by site

The tables summarizing epidemiological studies and their results by site (Tables 10–112 are grouped on pages 103–245).

Grouped sites of the upper gastrointestinal tract

The most important factors responsible for the occurrence of cancers of the upper gastrointestinal tract (oral, pharyngeal and oesophageal cancers), as well as cancer of the larynx, are tobacco smoking and alcohol drinking, which interact in a multiplicative way (WCRF/AICR, 1997). There are therefore serious risks of residual confounding in observational studies of cancers at all these sites.

Combined fruit and vegetables
Cohort studies
Three cohort studies have reported upon fruit and vegetable consumption in relation to grouped sites of the upper gastrointestinal tract, two conducted in Europe and one in the USA. One included all incident cancers from mouth to oesophagus (Boeing, 2002); another also included larynx (Kjaerheim et al., 1998) and a third additionally included nasopharynx and stomach (Kasum et al., 2002). Boeing (2002) reported a significantly decreased risk associated with consumption of fruit and vegetables combined; the other studies reported data only on subcategories (Table 10).

Oral cavity and pharynx
Fruit
Cohort studies
No cohort study on fruit consumption and risk of oral or oropharyngeal cancer was identified by the Working Group.

Case–control studies
Five studies in the USA and Australia have been reported (Table 11). Wynder et al. (1957) used a hospital-based case–control design and included 543 males and 116 females with cancer in their analysis. Neither vegetable nor fruit consumption was significantly different in males, but women with tongue cancer ($n = 57$) had lower citrus fruit consumption than controls (the findings are not tabulated). One study, which included deceased subjects, found an inverse association (Winn et al., 1984). Three analyses of data from a large study in the USA (McLaughlin et al., 1988; Gridley et al., 1990; Day et al., 1993) found inverse associations for fruit consumption except among blacks in total and black females.

In four South American hospital-based studies, inverse associations for fruit or citrus fruit consumption were significant in three.

In Europe, most of the case–control studies were conducted in northern Italy and nearby areas. Case recruitment was hospital-based and controls were hospital patients. In addition to reports from single study centres (Franceschi et al., 1991a; La Vecchia et al., 1991), combined analyses have been conducted using the various data sources in different combinations (Bosetti et al., 2000b). The publications of Negri et al. (1991) and La Vecchia et al. (1991) seem to have used overlapping data-sets. The results of Negri et al. (1991) were used for the Working Group's evaluation because of the larger number of subjects reported. Except for the first, the studies revealed inverse associations, one of which was non-significant. A sub-analysis for never-smokers showed a non-significant risk reduction in those having more than a low intake of fresh fruit (Fioretti et al., 1999). Franceschi et al. (1999) reported on a multicentre study conducted between 1992 and 1997, using an expanded validated questionnaire. More recent studies elsewhere in Europe have shown a consistent inverse relationship with fruit consumption.

Fruit consumption was inversely related to oropharyngeal cancer in one of the two older studies in southern Asia. However, this study reported only raw data without adjustment. A recent hospital-based case–control study in India showed a protective effect of fruit consumption in the whole study population, as well as among male smokers and non-smokers and alcohol drinkers and non-drinkers (Rajkumar et al., 2003b).

In most studies that addressed the issue (Winn et al., 1984; Oreggia et al., 1991; Tavani et al., 2001; Sánchez et al., 2003), an inverse association with fruit consumption was found across all strata of smoking and alcohol-drinking status.

Vegetables
Cohort studies
In the large cohort study of Hirayama (1990) in Japan, the frequency of intake of green-yellow vegetables was

inversely associated with risk of oropharyngeal cancer non-significantly in men and significantly in women.

Case–control studies
Three analyses of data from a large study in the USA (McLaughlin *et al.*, 1988; Gridley *et al.*, 1990, Day *et al.*, 1993) found a significantly reduced risk associated with vegetable consumption only in black men (Table 12).

In four studies in South or Central America, there was no significant effect of vegetable consumption except for a study in Uruguay involving 57 cases of squamous-cell carcinoma of the tongue.

The European case–control studies on diet and risk of oral and oropharyngeal cancer used hospital-based case recruitment and hospital patients as controls. The studies in northern Italy, except that of Franceschi *et al.* (1991a), show a consistent significant inverse relationship between vegetable intake and risk of oral and pharyngeal cancer. A sub-analysis on never-smokers revealed no protection by vegetables (Fioretti *et al.* 1999).

In a recent study in southern India, vegetable intake was inversely related to risk (Rajkumar *et al.*, 2003b). This was true for current smokers and non-smokers as well as for alcohol drinkers and non-drinkers. Neither of two studies from northern Asia presented data on total vegetable consumption.

Most other studies that addressed the issue suggest that the inverse association with vegetable consumption persists across all strata of smoking and alcohol-drinking status.

Combined fruit and vegetables
Results on total fruit and vegetable consumption from three case–control studies in North America have been reported. Graham *et al.* (1977) reported no difference between 584 cases of oral cavity cancer and 1222 hospital controls in intake of various fruit and vegetables, but no numerical data were presented. Gridley *et al.* (1992) reported that fruit and vegetable intake was associated with reduced risk (presented as a point estimate) for oral and pharyngeal cancer, independent of supplement use (Table 13). Winn *et al.* (1984) also reported a significant inverse relationship for combined fruit and vegetable consumption.

Precancerous lesions
Three case–control studies investigated precancerous lesions with respect to fruit and vegetables (Table 14). In two studies of submucous fibrosis and leukoplakia in male tobacco users in different states of India, cases and controls were selected by medical examination of household members. Only in the study of Gupta *et al.* (1999) was total fruit and vegetable consumption evaluated, and no inverse association was reported. Similarly, the study of Morse *et al.* (2000) did not show a significant inverse association with fruit and vegetable consumption.

Salivary gland
Zheng *et al.* (1996) (Table 15) did not find an association of either fruit or vegetable consumption with salivary gland cancer.

Nasopharynx
In the two case–control studies (Table 16), significant inverse associations were reported only for orange and tangerine consumption.

Discussion
The data available for evaluation are almost entirely from case–control studies, of varying design. Fruit consumption was evaluable in 10 studies: the mean odds ratio (OR) was 0.45 (95% confidence interval (CI), 0.38–0.53), range 0.10–0.70 (Figure 16). Vegetable consumption was evaluable in seven studies: mean OR = 0.49 (95% CI 0.39–0.62), range 0.19–0.80 (Figure 17).

Most of these studies adjusted for the potential confounding effects of tobacco and alcohol consumption, though many, especially the earlier studies, did so rather crudely. Therefore it is not possible to exclude an effect of residual confounding. Further, many of the case–control studies were hospital-based, and even in those that were population-based, full comparability of the data from cases and controls may not have been achieved, nor can the inherent biases associated with this design be eliminated.

Only three case–control studies considered the effect of fruit and vegetable consumption on presumed precursor lesions of the mouth. No significant inverse association was found. Similarly, no effect of these exposures on salivary gland cancer (one study) was found, while for nasopharyngeal cancer (two studies), only subcategories of exposure were considered.

Oesophagus
Fruit
Cohort study
Only one cohort study considered total fruit consumption (Table 17). This was conducted in the Life Span Study in Japan that included 120 321 atomic bombing survivors and non-exposed controls. A borderline significant inverse association was found (Sauvaget *et al.*, 2003).

Case–control studies
Three of the five studies in the USA found significant inverse associations for fruit consumption (Table 18). Four out of six studies in South America also found significant inverse associations, while two that did not report an effect were on citrus and non-citrus fruit, and not all fruits combined. The findings from four studies in South America were also included in a

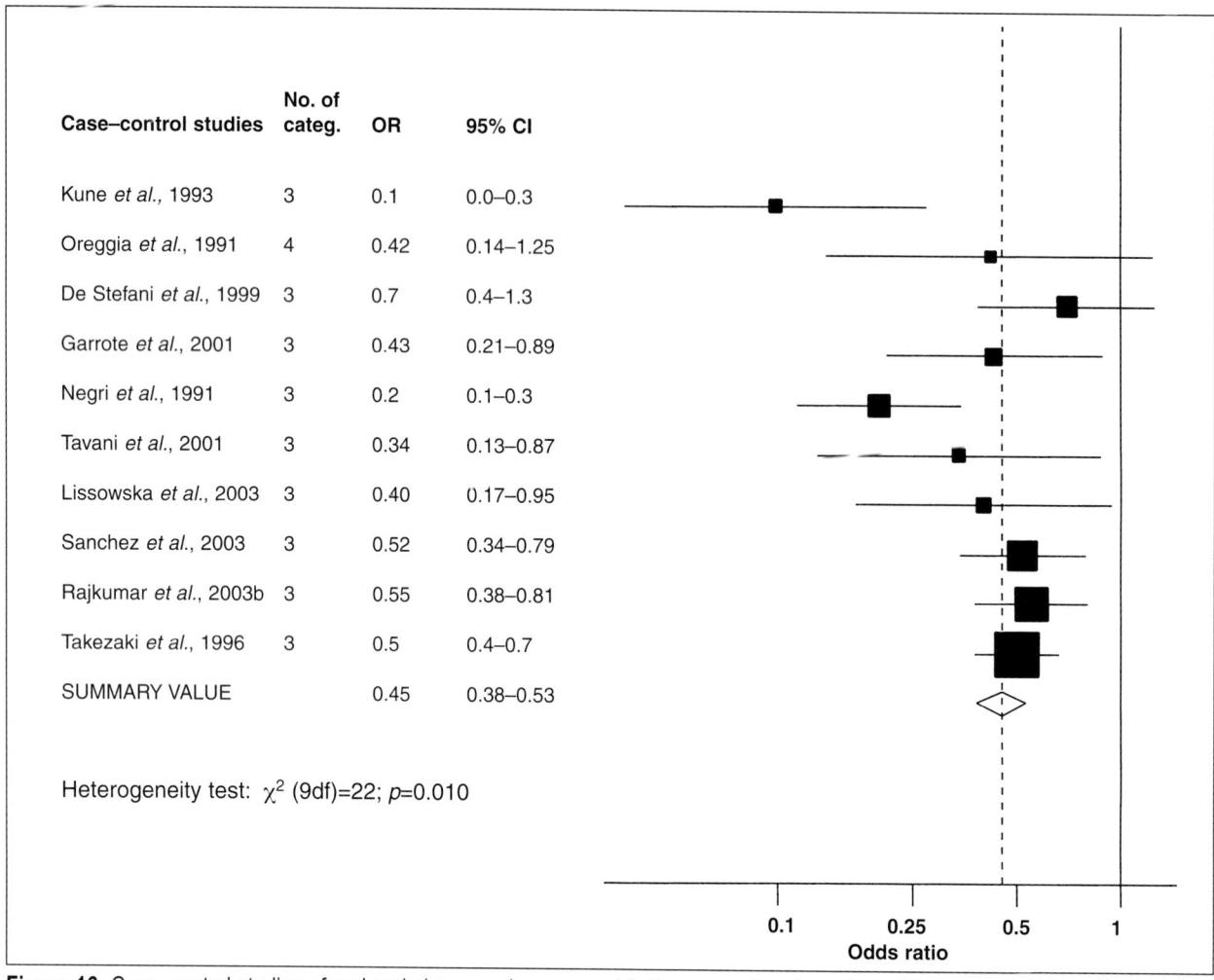

Case–control studies	No. of categ.	OR	95% CI
Kune et al., 1993	3	0.1	0.0–0.3
Oreggia et al., 1991	4	0.42	0.14–1.25
De Stefani et al., 1999	3	0.7	0.4–1.3
Garrote et al., 2001	3	0.43	0.21–0.89
Negri et al., 1991	3	0.2	0.1–0.3
Tavani et al., 2001	3	0.34	0.13–0.87
Lissowska et al., 2003	3	0.40	0.17–0.95
Sanchez et al., 2003	3	0.52	0.34–0.79
Rajkumar et al., 2003b	3	0.55	0.38–0.81
Takezaki et al., 1996	3	0.5	0.4–0.7
SUMMARY VALUE		0.45	0.38–0.53

Heterogeneity test: χ^2 (9df)=22; p=0.010

Figure 16 Case–control studies of oral and pharyngeal cancer and fruit consumption (see Table 11)

pooled analysis (Castellsague et al., 2000) which found a significant inverse association.

The studies in Europe also generally found fruit consumption to be inversely related to risk, except for a small study in Greece. The large study of Tuyns et al. (1987) evaluated citrus fruit and other fresh fruit but not total fruit. Many hospital-based case–control studies were conducted in northern Italy. Following an early report (Decarli et al., 1987), Negri et al. (1991) (294 cases in June 1990) summarized the results of the studies so far conducted. The reports of Tavani et al. (1993) for women, Tavani et al. (1994) for non-smokers and Tavani et al. (1996) for non-drinkers were based on the same data-set extended to 316 cases until December 1992. Most of the cases were already covered by the report of Negri et al. (1991). Bosetti et al. (2000a) used an expanded validated questionnaire in a multi-centre study on citrus and other fruits conducted between 1992 and 1997. In nearly all these studies, significant inverse associations were found.

Several studies in southern Asia have been reported. Cook-Mozaffari et al. (1979) conducted a population-based study between 1974 and 1976 with 344 incident cancers of the oesophagus and twice the number of controls. When they considered recent diet, they found relative risk estimates below 1.0, most of them significant for nearly all fruit items considered, but they did not present relative risk estimates for total fruit. The hospital-based case–control study of Prasad et al. (1992) in Hyderabad, India, included only 35 cases and did not present relative risk estimates for food items. The hospital-based study of de Jong et al. (1974) among Singapore

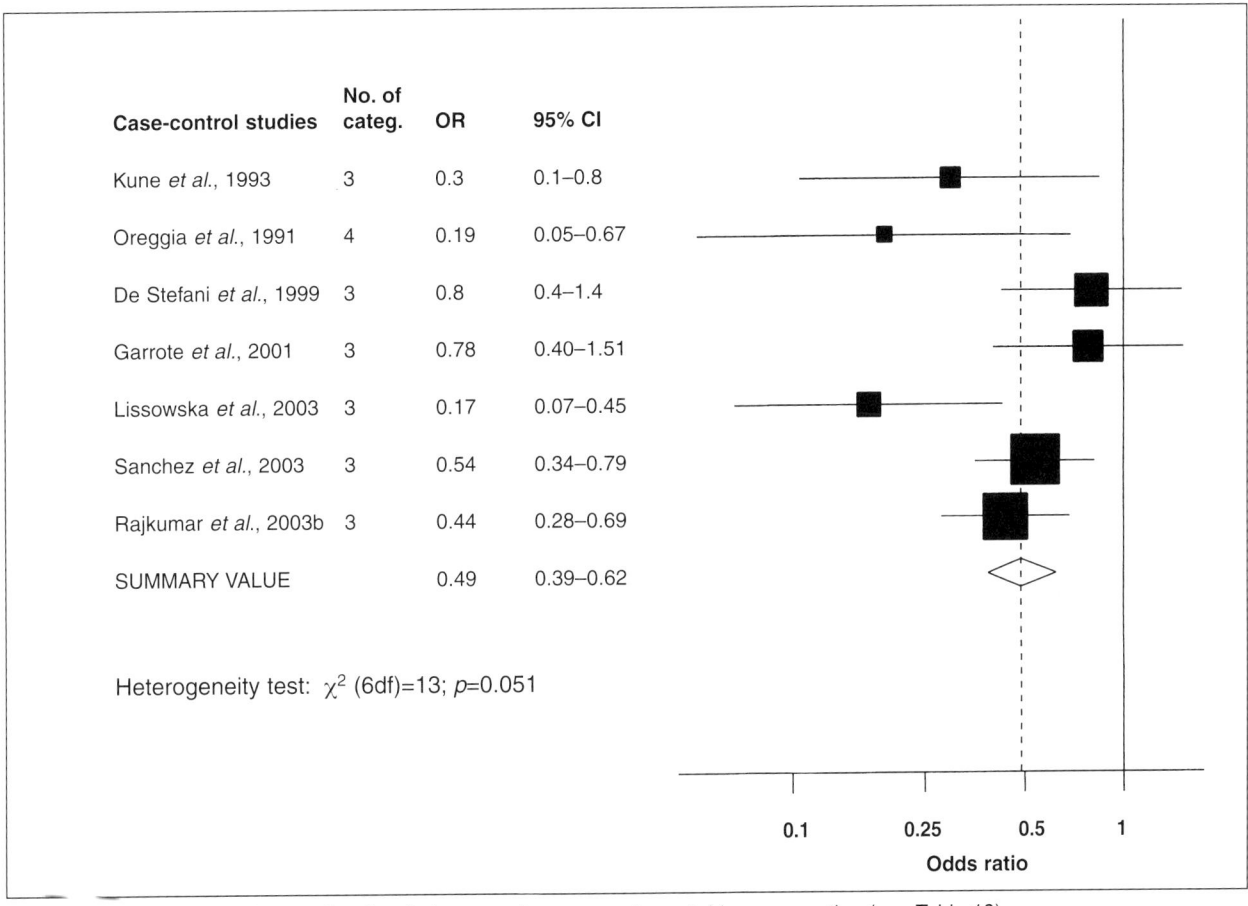

Case–control studies	No. of categ.	OR	95% CI
Kune et al., 1993	3	0.3	0.1–0.8
Oreggia et al., 1991	4	0.19	0.05–0.67
De Stefani et al., 1999	3	0.8	0.4–1.4
Garrote et al., 2001	3	0.78	0.40–1.51
Lissowska et al., 2003	3	0.17	0.07–0.45
Sanchez et al., 2003	3	0.54	0.34–0.79
Rajkumar et al., 2003b	3	0.44	0.28–0.69
SUMMARY VALUE		0.49	0.39–0.62

Heterogeneity test: χ^2 (6df)=13; p=0.051

Figure 17 Case–control studies of oral and pharyngeal cancer and vegetable consumption (see Table 12)

Chinese with 131 squamous-cell oesophageal cancer cases and 345 hospital controls also did not analyse total fruit, but only banana consumption. Of the four studies from India and Turkey included in Table 18, risk estimates were below 1.0 in one of the Indian studies and both in Turkey.

Of the nine studies in northern Asia included in Table 18, five considered total fruit, one finding a significant inverse association only for men. Of the remainder, one was based on oesophagitis diagnosed by oesophagoscopy in relatives in households.

Tavani et al. (1994, 1996) found that fruit intake was significantly inversely related to risk in the low-exposure groups of alcohol drinkers and smokers. Cheng et al. (1995) also reported that among never-smokers and non-drinkers, selected from a previously analysed study population, consumption of citrus fruit was inversely related to risk.

Vegetables
Cohort studies
All four cohort studies were conducted in China or Japan, but none considered the effect of total vegetable consumption (Table 19).

Case–control studies
All five studies in the USA showed an inverse association between vegetable consumption and risk of oesophageal cancer (Table 20). Wynder & Bross (1961) also reported lower intake of vegetables among 150 squamous-cell oesophageal cancer patients compared with 150 other tumour patients used as controls. Similarly, of the five studies in South America, all but one showed an inverse association between vegetable consumption and risk of oesophageal cancer. This was confirmed in the overview analysis of data from four of the studies (Castellsague et al., 2000). Further, except for squamous-cell carcinoma in one small study in Greece, all the studies in Europe showed inverse associations, though only four assessed total

vegetable intake. The studies conducted in northern Italy are best represented by the reports of Negri et al. (1991) and Bosetti et al. (2000a).

In the study in Iran by Cook-Mozaffari et al. (1979), relative risk estimates below 1.0, most of them not significant, were found for nearly all vegetable items, though total vegetable intake was not considered. The two studies in India and the two in Turkey all found inverse associations with vegetable consumption, although one of those in India did not assess total vegetable consumption.

Similarly, all but one of the nine cancer studies conducted in northern Asia found inverse associations between various groupings of vegetables and oesophageal cancer, though only one considered total vegetable consumption. This was supported for women but not men by the study of Chang-Claude et al. (1990) of oesophagitis among relatives.

The study of Tavani et al. (1994) in never-smokers revealed that vegetable consumption measured as total green vegetable consumption or carotene index is inversely related to risk of cancer of the oesophagus and in both low and high alcohol drinkers. Cheng et al. (1995) reported that among never-smokers and non-drinkers, selected from a previously analysed study population, consumption of green leafy vegetables was inversely related to risk.

Combined fruit and vegetables
Cohort studies
No studies were identified by the Working Group.

Case–control studies
The hospital-based case–control study by Mettlin et al. (1981) of male patients with 147 cases and 264 controls was one of the first to investigate fruit and vegetable consumption with respect to risk of oesophageal cancer. However, the only comparison was between case consumption and the consumption by the total study population. The findings indicated that fruit and vegetable consumption was significantly inversely related to case status.

All six studies with published estimates on combined fruit and vegetable intake found an inverse relationship with oesophageal cancer risk (Table 21).

Discussion
For oesophageal cancer, fruit consumption was evaluable in 16 case–control studies: the mean OR was 0.54 (95% CI 0.48–0.61), range 0.14–1.50 (Figure 18). Vegetable consumption was evaluable in 10 case–control studies, giving a mean OR = 0.64 (95% CI 0.57–0.72), range 0.10–0.97 (Figure 19).

The observation of an inverse association with fruit and vegetable intake in most of the studies was confirmed by a recent meta-analysis by Riboli & Norat (2003). For both dietary factors, the combined relative risk estimate was significantly below 1.0.

The data indicate that cancer cases have usually eaten less fruit and vegetables over their lifetime and that those eating more fruit and vegetables than the rest of the study population usually experience less oesophageal cancer. However, it remains uncertain whether this results from a true protective effect or is due to residual confounding by tobacco smoking, alcohol drinking and social factors. Studies that looked at effects of fruit and vegetables in particular subgroups of never-smokers and non-drinkers and those that looked at effects of these food items across strata of smoking habits and alcohol drinking indicate similar associations of fruit and vegetable consumption across all the subgroups considered, but the power of these studies was low.

Stomach
Despite reductions in incidence and mortality rates in most countries, stomach cancer is still one of the most common malignant neoplasms worldwide. The reasons for the decline and for geographical differences are not fully understood, but domestic refrigeration, increased year-round availability of fruits and vegetables, and reduced use of salt are believed to be relevant factors.

Fruit
Cohort studies
The association between intake of fruit and the risk of stomach cancer has been examined in 11 cohort studies (Table 22), most of which reported an inverse, although often non-significant, association.

Guo et al. (1994) found no association for either cardia or non-cardia cancer.

Case–control studies
Most of the 37 case–control studies of the association between intake of fruit and risk of stomach cancer included in Table 23 showed an OR below 1.0.

Two studies reported associations according to anatomical subsite; these showed significant inverse associations for both cardia and non-cardia cancer (Palli et al., 1992; Ekström et al., 2000). Six case–control studies reported upon the association according to histological subtype. In three, there was a significant inverse association for each histological type (Correa et al., 1985; Harrison et al., 1997; Ekström et al., 2000), in one a significant inverse association for the intestinal type in females only (Kato et al., 1990), in one a significant inverse association for the differentiated histological type (Ito et al., 2003) and in one no association for any subtype (Ward & Lopez-Carrillo, 1999).

Vegetables
Cohort studies
The association between intake of vegetables and risk of stomach cancer

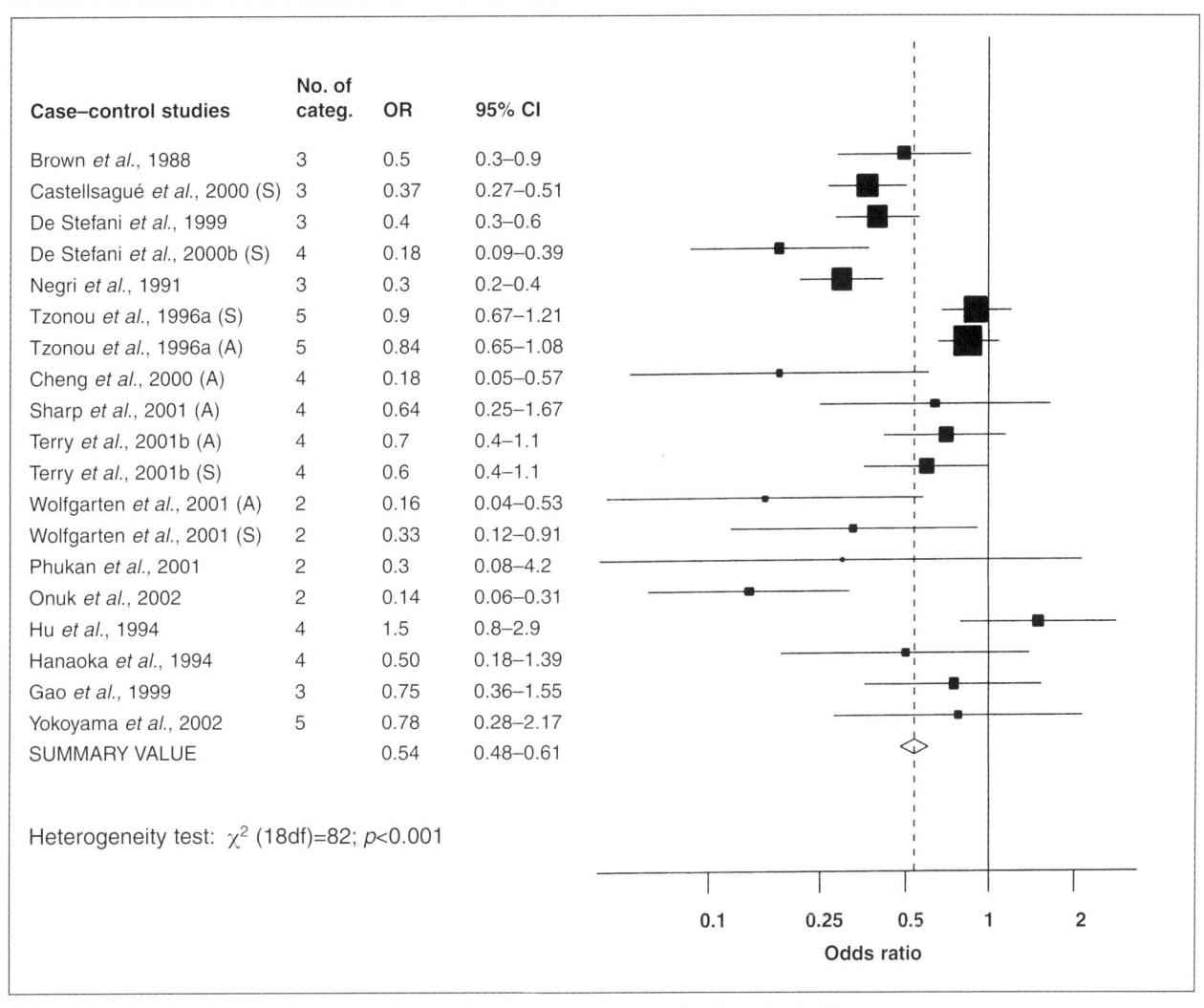

Case–control studies	No. of categ.	OR	95% CI
Brown et al., 1988	3	0.5	0.3–0.9
Castellsagué et al., 2000 (S)	3	0.37	0.27–0.51
De Stefani et al., 1999	3	0.4	0.3–0.6
De Stefani et al., 2000b (S)	4	0.18	0.09–0.39
Negri et al., 1991	3	0.3	0.2–0.4
Tzonou et al., 1996a (S)	5	0.9	0.67–1.21
Tzonou et al., 1996a (A)	5	0.84	0.65–1.08
Cheng et al., 2000 (A)	4	0.18	0.05–0.57
Sharp et al., 2001 (A)	4	0.64	0.25–1.67
Terry et al., 2001b (A)	4	0.7	0.4–1.1
Terry et al., 2001b (S)	4	0.6	0.4–1.1
Wolfgarten et al., 2001 (A)	2	0.16	0.04–0.53
Wolfgarten et al., 2001 (S)	2	0.33	0.12–0.91
Phukan et al., 2001	2	0.3	0.08–4.2
Onuk et al., 2002	2	0.14	0.06–0.31
Hu et al., 1994	4	1.5	0.8–2.9
Hanaoka et al., 1994	4	0.50	0.18–1.39
Gao et al., 1999	3	0.75	0.36–1.55
Yokoyama et al., 2002	5	0.78	0.28–2.17
SUMMARY VALUE		0.54	0.48–0.61

Heterogeneity test: χ^2 (18df)=82; $p<0.001$

Figure 18 Case-control studies of oesophageal cancer and fruit consumption (see Table 18)
S = squamous cell carcinoma, A = adenocarcinoma

was examined in 11 cohort studies (Table 24). Although all studies except two showed relative risks below 1.0, the association was generally not significant.

One study showed a significant inverse association for cases with differentiated histological type, but none for those with undifferentiated type (Kobayashi et al., 2002). In two studies, the association between total intake of vegetables and the risk of stomach cancer was examined according to anatomical subsite; in each there was no significant association for either cardia or non-cardia cancer (Inoue et al., 1994; Kobayashi et al., 2002).

Case–control studies
Most of 39 case–control studies reported in Table 25 showed an OR below 1.0.

In two studies, the association between intake of total vegetables and the risk of stomach cancer was examined according to anatomical subsite; in one there were significant inverse associations for both cardia and non-cardia cancer for raw vegetables (Palli et al., 1992), while in the other the association was not significant (Ekström et al., 2000). Five studies reported upon the association between intake of vegetables and the risk of stomach cancer according to histological subtype; in three there was a significant inverse association for both histological types (Ward & Lopez-Carrillo, 1999; Ekström et al., 2000;

Case–control studies	No. of categ.	OR	95% CI
Brown et al., 1988	3	0.7	0.4–1.3
Chen et al., 2002a (A)	4	0.45	0.2–1.0
De Stefani et al., 1999	3	0.7	0.5–0.9
Castellsagué et al., 2000	3	0.62	0.44–0.88
De Stefani et al., 2000b	4	0.64	0.34–1.20
Tzonou et al., 1996a (A)	5	0.62	0.48–0.80
Tzonou et al., 1996a (S)	5	0.97	0.74–1.28
Launoy et al., 1998	4	0.24	0.11–0.55
Cheng et al., 2000	4	0.58	0.22–1.55
Terry et al., 2001b (A)	4	0.5	0.3–0.8
Terry et al., 2001b (S)	4	0.6	0.4–1.0
Onuk et al., 2002	2	0.10	0.04–0.23
SUMMARY VALUE		0.64	0.57–0.72

Heterogeneity test: χ^2 (11df)=34; p=0.00033

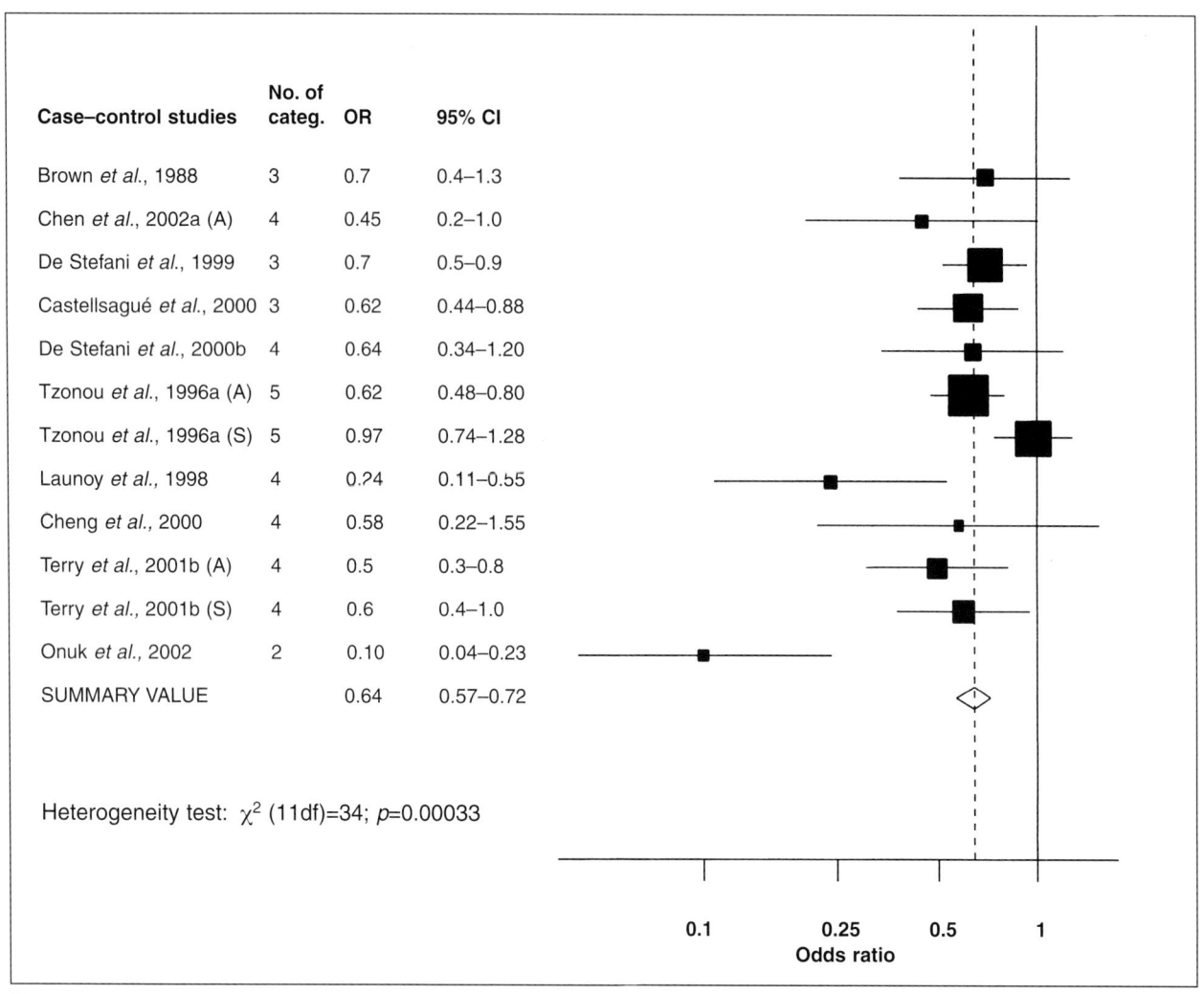

Figure 19 Case–control studies of oesophageal cancer and vegetable consumption (see Table 20)
A = adenocarcinoma; S = squamous-cell carcinoma

Ito et al., 2003), in one for the intestinal type only in males (Kato et al., 1990) and in one a non-significant inverse association (Harrison et al., 1997).

Combined fruit and vegetables
Cohort studies
Three cohort studies examined the association between combined intake of total fruit and vegetables and the risk of stomach cancer (Table 26). In two of these, there was a significant inverse association, although one study considered only fresh fruit and raw vegetables.

Case–control studies
In all three of the case–control studies that evaluated the combination of fruit and vegetables, there was a significant inverse association (Table 27).

Discussion
Fruit consumption was evaluable in 10 cohort studies of stomach cancer. The mean relative risk (RR) was 0.85 (95% CI 0.77–0.95), range 0.55–1.92 (Figure 20). In the 28 evaluable case–control studies, the mean OR was 0.63 (95% CI 0.58–0.69), range 0.31–1.39 (Figure 21).

Vegetable consumption was evaluable in five cohort studies. The mean RR was 0.94 (95% CI 0.84–1.06), range 0.70–1.25 (Figure 22). Twenty case–control studies were evaluable and the mean OR was 0.66 (95% CI 0.61–0.71), range 0.30–1.70 (Figure 23).

Cohort studies	No. of categ.	OR	95% CI
Chyou et al., 1990	4	0.8	0.4–1.3
Nomura et al., 1990	3	0.8	0.5–1.3
Kneller et al., 1991	4	1.5	0.75–2.93
Kato et al., 1992	3	1.92	1.03–3.59
Guo et al., 1994	2	0.9	0.8–1.1
Inoue et al., 1996	3	0.55	0.22–1.35
Botterweck et al., 1998	5	0.97	0.64–1.48
Galanis et al., 1998	2	0.6	0.4–0.9
Kobayashi et al., 2002	4	0.70	0.48–1.01
Sauvaget et al., 2003	3	0.80	0.65–0.98
SUMMARY VALUE		0.85	0.77–0.95

Heterogeneity test: χ^2 (9df)=15; p=0.083

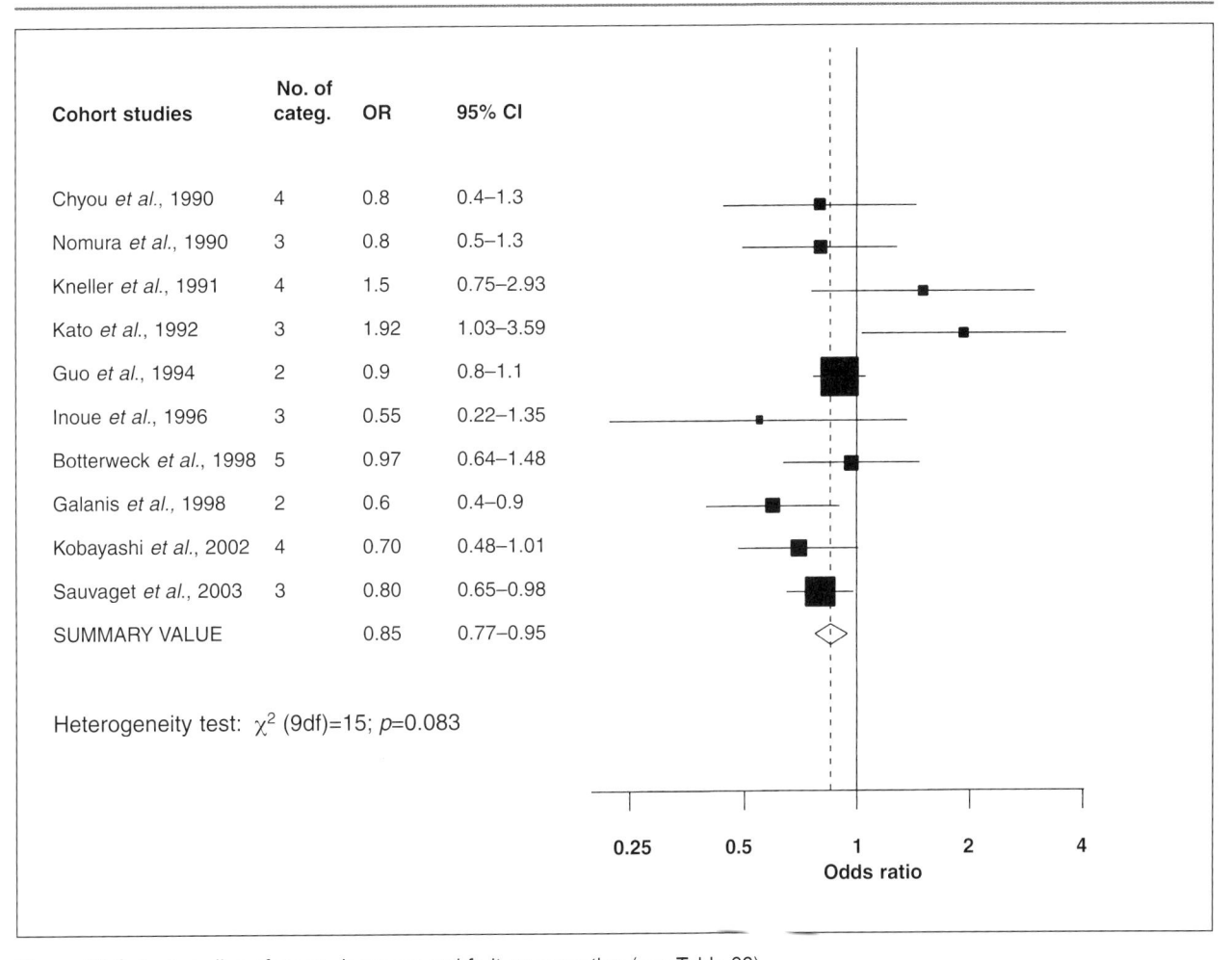

Figure 20 Cohort studies of stomach cancer and fruit consumption (see Table 22)

The results of the cohort studies are not consistent. Besides differences in population and the types of fruit and vegetables consumed, other factors that could explain the heterogeneity are the quality of design, food intake assessment, uncontrolled confounding and effect modification. In most cohort studies, there were inverse associations, but these were statistically significant in only two studies for fruit and one for vegetables. In two cohort studies, a positive association was reported between fruit intake and stomach cancer risk, one in a high-risk male American population and the second in Japanese. However, the numbers of cases in both studies were low. In all except two of the cohort studies, the dietary questionnaire was not validated and the numbers of total items in the questionnaire were low.

Stomach cancer is a disease of complex etiology involving multiple risk factors including dietary, infectious, occupational, genetic and preneoplastic factors. It is possible that unmeasured or unidentified risk factors may have affected some study results. While all the studies adjusted for sex and age, adjustment for *Helicobacter pylori* infection was rarely possible. Only three cohort studies adjusted for history of stomach disease and family history of stomach cancer. Two studies did not adjust for tobacco or alcohol intake and one of these reported a significant risk increase associated with high intake of fruit.

The relationship between stomach cancer risk and diet has been extensively investigated in case–control studies, mainly in European and Asian populations. The case–control studies showed more consistent and stronger effects of fruit and vegetables on stomach cancer risk than the cohort studies. Most of the case–control

Case–control studies	No. of categ.	OR	95% CI
Correa et al., 1985 (B)	4	0.33	0.16–0.66
Correa et al., 1985 (W)	4	0.47	0.24–0.92
Jedrychowski et al., 1986	3	0.31	0.15–0.64
Kono et al., 1988 (H)	2	0.7	0.4–1.0
Kono et al., 1988 (P)	2	0.5	0.3–0.8
De Stefani et al., 1990a	3	0.36	0.23–0.56
Kato et al., 1990 (M)	3	0.83	0.51–1.33
Kato et al., 1990 (F)	3	0.77	0.33–1.78
Wu-Williams et al., 1990	3	0.67	0.29–1.67
Boeing et al., 1991a	3	0.56	0.35–0.91
Yu & Hsieh, 1991	2	0.5	0.3–0.8
Hoshiyama & Sasaba, 1992	3	0.8	0.5–1.3
Jedrychowski et al., 1992	3	0.72	0.56–0.94
Sanchez-Diez et al., 1992	2	0.31	0.11–0.87
Ramon et al., 1993	4	0.85	0.21–1.11
Inoue et al., 1994	2	0.86	0.70–1.10
Cornée et al., 1995	3	0.50	0.25–1.03
Muñoz et al., 1997	3	0.47	0.21–1.05
Xu et al., 1996	4	0.5	0.4–0.8
Harrison et al., 1997 (I)	*	0.5	0.3–0.9
Harrison et al., 1997 (D)	*	0.5	0.2–1.0
La Vecchia et al., 1997	3	0.6	0.5–0.8
Gao et al., 1999	3	0.88	0.47–1.67
Ward & Lopez-Carrillo, 1999	4	1.0	0.5–2.2
Ekström et al., 2000 (C)	4	0.5	0.2–1.0
Ekström et al., 2000 (N)	4	0.6	0.4–0.8
Huang et al., 2000 (FH +)	*	1.39	0.69–2.82
Huang et al., 2000 (FH -)	*	1.11	0.74–1.67
Mathew et al., 2000	4	0.7	0.2–3.6
De Stefani et al., 2001	3	0.35	0.21–0.59
Hamada et al., 2002	2	0.4	0.2–0.9
Kim et al., 2002	3	0.67	0.33–1.39
Nishimoto et al., 2002	4	0.6	0.3–1.2
Ito et al., 2003	4	0.68	0.40–1.16
SUMMARY VALUE		0.63	0.58–0.69

Heterogeneity test: χ^2 (33df)=54.4; p=0.0108

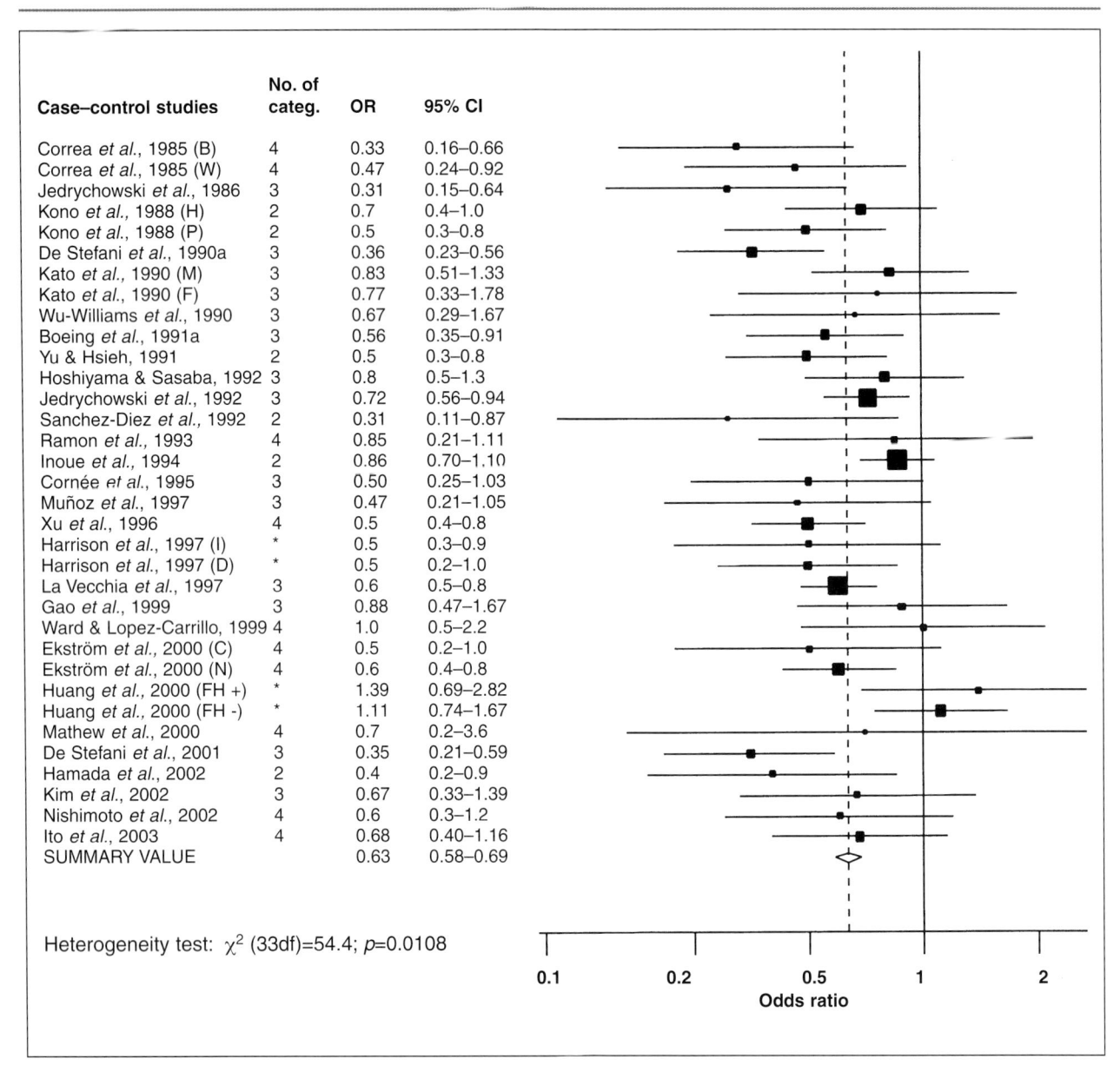

Figure 21 Case–control studies of stomach cancer and fruit consumption (see Table 23)
B = blacks; W = whites, H = hospital controls; P = population controls; M = males, F = females; I = intestinal type; D = diffuse type; C = cardia; N = non-cardia; FH+ = gastric cancer family history positive; FH– = gastric cancer family history negative; * = not applicable

Cancer-preventive effects

Cohort studies	No. of categ.	OR	95% CI
Chyou et al., 1990	4	0.7	0.4–1.1
Kneller et al., 1991	4	0.9	0.48–1.78
Botterweck et al., 1998	5	0.86	0.58–1.26
McCullough et al., 2001 (M)	3	0.89	0.76–1.05
McCullough et al., 2001 (F)	3	1.25	0.99–1.58
Kobayashi et al., 2002	5	0.75	0.54–1.04
SUMMARY VALUE		0.94	0.84–1.06

Heterogeneity test: χ^2 (5df)=9.5; p=0.09

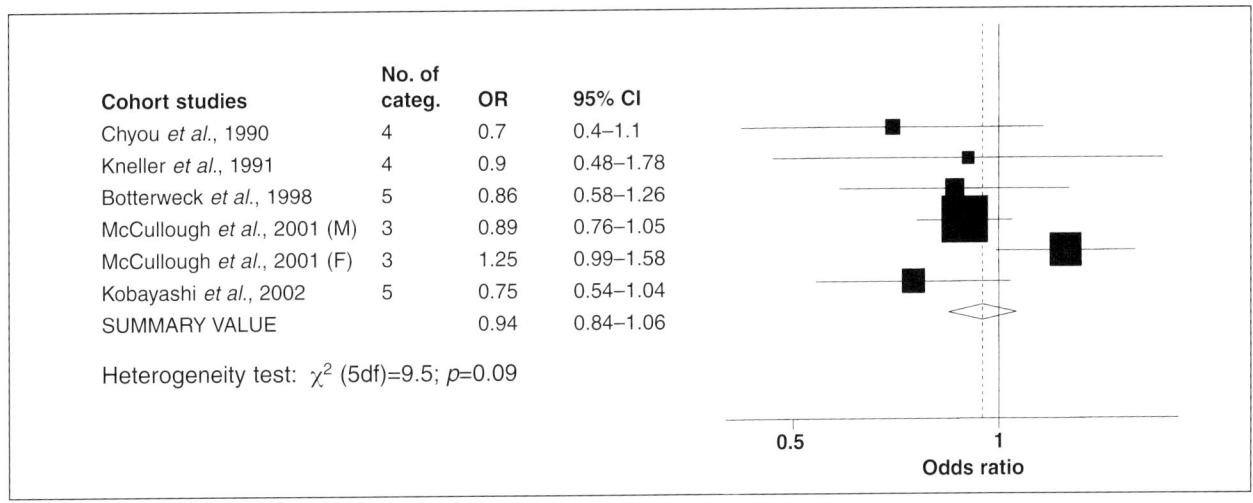

Figure 22 Cohort studies of stomach cancer and vegetable consumption (see Table 24)
M = males; F = females

Case–control studies	No. of categ.	OR	95% CI
Correa et al., 1985	4	0.50	0.25–1.00
Risch et al., 1985	*	0.84	0.72–0.96
Jedrychowski et al., 1986	3	0.61	0.25–1.49
De Stefani et al., 1990a	3	0.37	0.23–0.59
Boeing et al., 1991a	3	0.86	0.54–1.36
Jedrychowski et al., 1992	3	0.60	0.46–0.78
Memik et al., 1992	3	0.6	0.31–1.23
Sanchez-Diez et al., 1992	2	0.70	0.41–1.08
Hansson et al., 1993	4	0.50	0.32–0.78
Cornée et al., 1995	3	0.77	0.37–1.60
Xu et al., 1996	3	0.5	0.4–0.8
Harrison et al., 1997 (I)	*	0.8	0.5–1.3
Harrison et al., 1997 (D)	*	0.7	0.4–1.2
Muñoz et al., 1997	3	0.47	0.22–1.03
Ji et al., 1998 (M)	4	0.4	0.3–0.5
Ji et al., 1998 (F)	4	0.7	0.5–1.1
Ward & Lopez-Carrillo, 1999	4	0.3	0.1–0.6
Ekström et al., 2000 (C)	4	0.5	0.3–1.1
Ekström et al., 2000 (N)	4	0.7	0.5–1.0
Mathew et al., 2000	3	1.1	0.2–5.0
De Stefani et al., 2001	3	0.83	0.49–1.43
Chen et al., 2002	4	1.7	0.77–3.7
Kim et al., 2002	3	0.64	0.31–1.32
SUMMARY VALUE		0.66	0.61–0.71

Heterogeneity test: χ^2 (22df)=50; p=0.00059

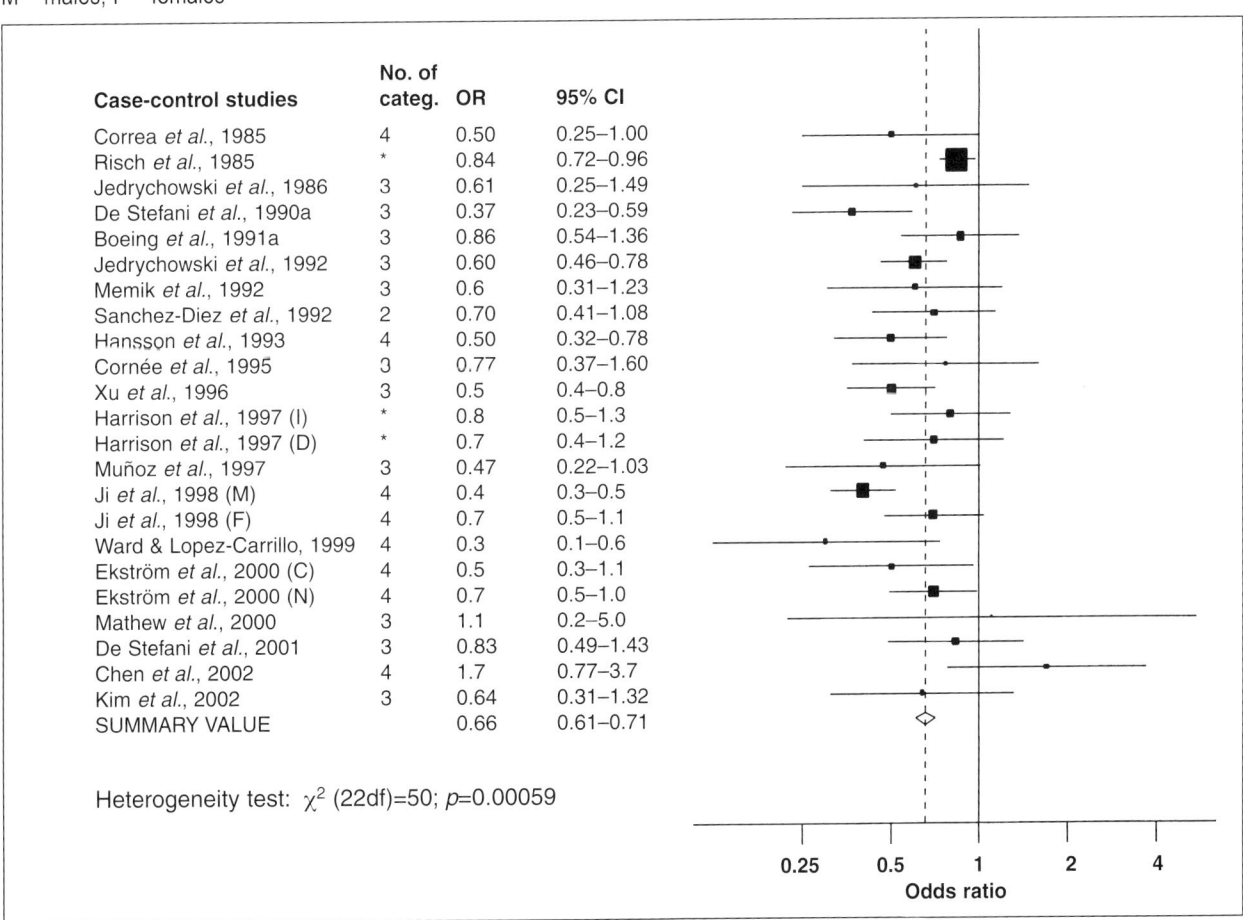

Figure 23 Case–control studies of stomach cancer and vegetable consumption (see Table 25)
I = intestinal type; D = diffuse type; M = males; F = females; C = cardia; N = non-cardia; * = not applicable

studies adjusted for more potential confounders than the cohort studies, particularly for other dietary factors, family antecedents of stomach cancer and socioeconomic status. The use of hospital-based or population-based controls was not a clear indicator of any difference in results. Only a few studies analysed the results by gender and there is very limited information about associations according to histology or tumour subsite.

The reason why case–control studies were more likely to show inverse associations is not clear. One explanation could be recall bias. Further, people with preclinical symptoms of stomach carcinoma or stomach disorders may change their dietary habits months or years before the diagnosis. In the Netherlands Cohort Study, analyses limited to cases occurring in the first year of follow-up revealed a strong inverse association with high combined fruit and vegetable consumption. With these cases excluded, the associations were much closer to the null value. Also stratified analyses (on stomach cancer and vegetable and fruit consumption combined) for subjects with and without stomach disorders revealed a stronger inverse association in subjects with stomach disorders (Botterweck et al., 1998).

Three cohort studies and three case–control studies evaluated combined intake of fruit and vegetables, and in all except one cohort study there were significant inverse associations. The absence of such estimates in other reports could be because the hypotheses were related to particular sub-groups of fruits and vegetables, or perhaps due to publication bias.

Colon and rectum

Because of potential end-point misclassification between specific colorectal subsites, this section focuses on colorectal cancer *in toto*. Where reports include separate risk estimates for colon and rectal cancer, these site-specific findings are noted in the accompanying tables.

Fruit
Cohort studies
Table 28 summarizes data from 12 cohort studies of fruit consumption and colorectal cancer. Results from these studies, conducted in Europe, in the USA and one in Japan, were published within the last ten years. In only one of these studies (Terry *et al.*, 2001a) is there evidence of a significant inverse association with fruit consumption.

A pooled analysis of data from 10 cohort studies (many included in Table 28) has so far been reported only in an abstract (Smith-Warner *et al.*, 2002a). The analysis included 4966 cases of colorectal cancer from a total of 533 753 men and women followed for 6–16 years. The pooled multivariate relative risks for the highest versus lowest quartile of intake of total fruit were 0.94 (95% CI 0.84–1.04) for colon and 0.96 (0.78–1.17) for rectal cancer.

Case–control studies
Table 29 presents data from 21 case–control studies of fruit consumption and colorectal cancer, some published nearly two decades ago. These investigations were nearly evenly split between population-based and hospital-based case–control studies. The geographical diversity is somewhat greater than for the cohort studies, some studies having been conducted in Asia, South America and Australia.

The findings are also diverse; only five studies reported significant inverse associations and then often for only one gender, five showed non-significant inverse associations and for the remainder, the ORs tended to centre around 1.0.

Vegetables
Cohort studies
Table 30 presents data from 13 cohort studies of vegetable consumption in relation to colorectal cancer. Again, these studies were conducted only within Europe and the USA. For none was a significant inverse association reported between vegetable consumption and colorectal cancer (or colon and rectum cancer separately).

A pooled analysis of data from 10 cohort studies (many included data in Table 30) has so far been reported only in an abstract (Smith-Warner *et al.*, 2002a). The analysis included 4966 cases of colorectal cancer from a total of 533 753 men and women followed for 6–16 years. The pooled multivariate relative risks for the highest versus lowest quartile of intake of total vegetables were 0.95 (95% CI 0.85–1.05) for colon and 0.93 (0.79–1.10) for rectal cancer.

Case–control studies
Data from 27 hospital-based and population-based case–control studies of colorectal cancer, published over the last 25 years, are summarized in Table 31. These studies were conducted in Asia, Australia and South America, as well as Europe and North America. Significant inverse associations for vegetable consumption were reported in 15 studies, though for some of these the associations were in only one gender, or for colon or rectal cancer. In addition non-significant inverse associations were noted in eight studies.

Combined fruit and vegetables
Cohort studies
Table 32 presents data from six cohort studies that considered combined fruit and vegetable consumption in relation to colorectal cancer, all conducted within Europe and the USA. In one there were significant inverse associations with colorectal cancer as a whole

and with rectal cancer (Terry et al., 2001a), in another with colon cancer in females (Shibata et al., 1992).

Case–control studies
Five case–control studies of colorectal cancer have evaluated total fruit and vegetable consumption (Table 33). One found a significant inverse association for females (Shannon et al., 1996) and another for both sexes combined (Deneo-Pellegrini et al., 2002).

Adenomatous polyps
Fruit
Cohort study. One cohort study has reported upon fruit consumption and the detection of polyps on endoscopy (Table 34). A significant inverse association was reported.

Case–control studies. Six case–control studies have considered adenomatous polyps (Table 35); three reported inverse associations with fruit intake. In one small study, there was a significant positive association with hospital controls, but not with population controls (Almendingen et al., 2001). [The Working Group was uncertain that the controls in this study were comparable to the cases, in view of the disparity between numbers of cases and controls and the much smaller number of controls.]

Vegetables
Cohort study. One cohort study reported no association between vegetable consumption and the detection of polyps on endoscopy (Table 36).

Case–control studies. Six case–control studies of adenomas have evaluated vegetable consumption (Table 37). There were inverse associations in males in one (Smith-Warner et al., 2002b) and in females in another (Sandler et al., 1993), but no clear association was noted in other studies that evaluated risk in both genders together. In a small study, there was a suggestion of an inverse association in comparison with hospital controls, but not with healthy controls (Almendingen et al., 2001).

Combined fruit and vegetables
Randomized trial. The Polyp Prevention Trial (PPT) was a randomized intervention study of the effect of a low-fat, high-fibre, high-fruit and vegetable diet on the recurrence of colorectal adenomatous polyps in individuals older than 35 years (Schatzkin et al., 2000). Intervention participants increased their intake of fruit and vegetables from 2.05 to 3.41 servings per 1000 kcal energy intake; control participants increased only from 2.00 to 2.23 servings per 1000 kcal. Intervention participants, compared with controls, lowered their fat intake by approximately one third and increased total fibre intake by about 75%. The primary trial result, however, was null: adenoma recurrence rates were virtually identical in the intervention and control groups over a four-year follow-up period (RR = 1.00; 0.90–1.12).

Cohort study. No cohort study has reported upon combined fruit and vegetable consumption and adenomas.

Case–control studies. One case–control study of adenomas reported non-significant inverse associations (Table 38).

Discussion
Colorectal cancer
The evidence for an inverse association between fruit intake and colorectal cancer is weaker in the cohort studies than in the case–control studies. The small reduction in risk observed in cohort studies is restricted to women. Over the 11 evaluable cohort studies, the mean RR was 1.00 (95% CI 0.96–1.05), range 0.50–1.60 (Figure 24) and for the nine evaluable case–control studies, the mean OR was 0.87 (95% CI 0.78–0.97), range 0.30–1.74 (Figure 25). A meta-analysis (Riboli & Norat, 2003) has shown a small statistically significant reduction in risk (per 100 gram increase in daily consumption) for the case–control studies (0.93; 95% CI 0.87–0.99) and a small non-significant reduction for cohort studies (0.96; 95% CI 0.90–1.01).

Similarly, the evidence for an inverse association between vegetable consumption and colorectal cancer is considerably weaker in the cohort studies than in the case–control studies. The mean RR for the 10 evaluable cohort studies was 0.9 (95% CI 0.85–1.05), range 0.72–1.78 (Figure 26) and for the 13 evaluable case–control studies the mean OR was 0.63 (95% CI 0.56–0.70), range 0.18–1.29 (Figure 27). The meta-analysis showed a substantial reduction in risk (per 100 grams) for the case–control studies (0.87; 95% CI 0.80–0.95) but only a small non-significant reduction in risk (0.96; 95% CI 0.90–1.05) for the cohort studies (Riboli & Norat, 2003). [If the relationship between vegetable consumption and colorectal cancer were linear, the OR of 0.87 per 100 grams of vegetable intake would translate into a risk reduction of approximately 40% for five servings versus one serving of vegetables daily.]

Adenomatous polyps
Adenomatous polyps are considered necessary precursor lesions for most large-bowel malignancies (Schatzkin et al., 1994). Both observational and experimental studies of adenomas can thus be informative with respect to etiological factors operating in the earlier stages of colorectal carcinogenesis.

The one randomized intervention trial showed no apparent protective effect from an intervention for adeno-

Cohort studies	No. of categ.	OR	95% CI
Shibata et al., 1992 (M)	3	1.12	0.69–1.81
Shibata et al., 1992 (F)	3	0.50	0.31–0.80
Steinmetz et al., 1994	4	0.86	0.58–1.29
Kato et al., 1997	4	1.49	0.82–2.70
Hsing et al., 1998a (CR)	4	1.6	0.9–2.8
Pietinen et al., 1999	4	1.1	0.8–1.7
Michels et al., 2000 (F,C)	5	0.96	0.89–1.03
Michels et al., 2000 (F,R)	5	0.96	0.83–1.11
Michels et al., 2000 (M,C)	5	1.08	1.00–1.16
Michels et al., 2000 (M,R)	5	1.09	0.94–1.26
Voorrips et al., 2000a (M,C)	5	1.33	0.90–1.97
Voorrips et al., 2000a (M,R)	5	0.85	0.55–1.32
Voorrips et al., 2000a (F,C)	5	0.73	0.48–1.11
Voorrips et al., 2000a (F,R)	5	0.67	0.34–1.33
Terry et al., 2001a (CR)	4	0.68	0.52–0.89
Flood et al., 2002	5	1.15	0.86–1.53
Sauvaget et al., 2003	3	0.97	0.73–1.29
McCullough et al., 2003 (M, C)	5	1.11	0.76–1.62
McCullough et al., 2003 (F, C)	5	0.74	0.47–1.16
SUMMARY VALUE		1.00	0.96–1.05

Heterogeneity test: χ^2 (18df) =37; p=0.0046

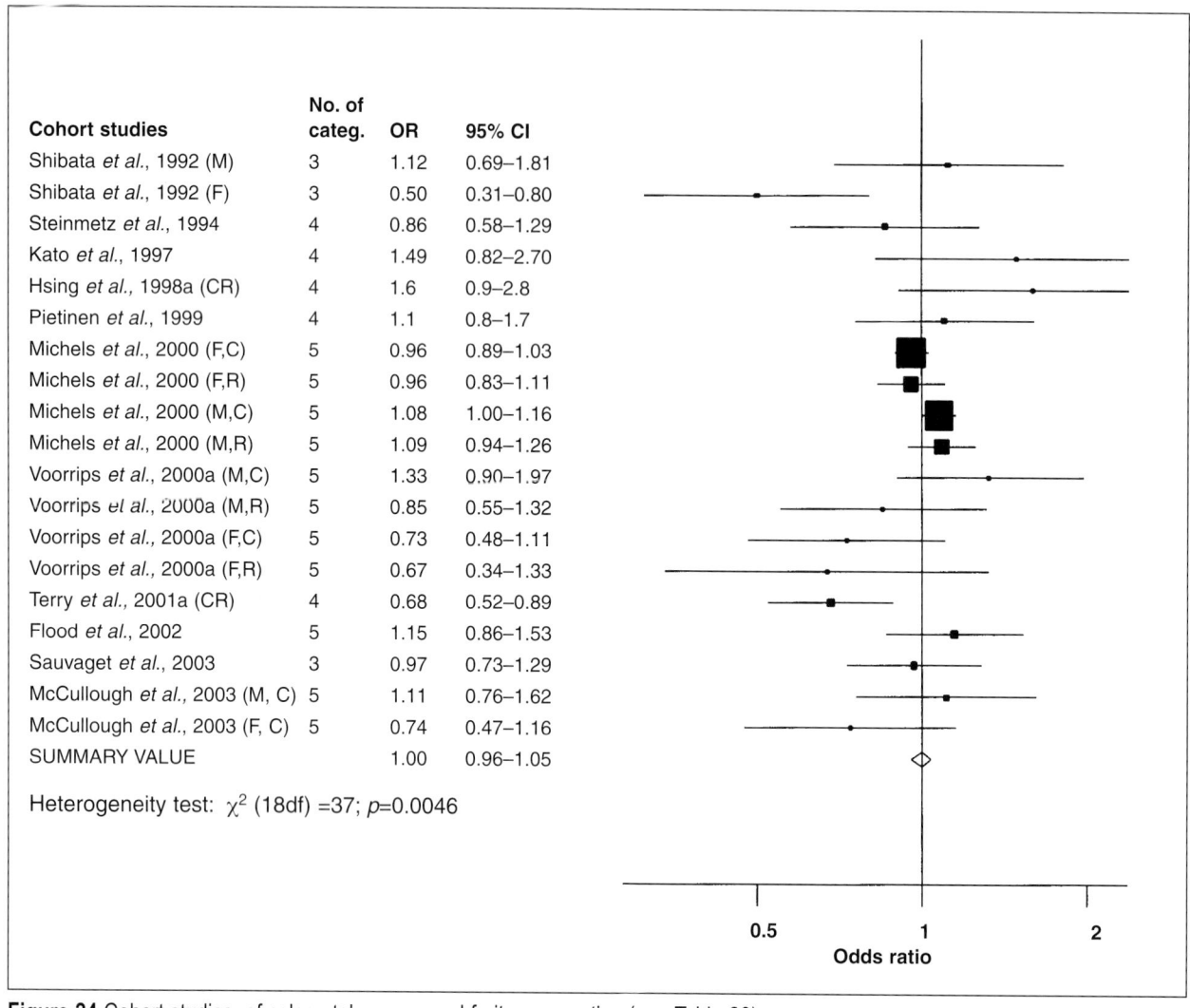

Figure 24 Cohort studies of colorectal cancer and fruit consumption (see Table 28)
M = males; F = females; CR = colorectal; C = colon; R = rectal

matous polyps (see above). However, this trial, in which most of the endpoints were small recurrent adenomas, could not rule out the possibility that fruit and vegetable intake operates to prevent the growth of small into large adenomas, or large adenomas into carcinomas. Thus, the null results of this trial do not definitively exclude a protective role for fruit and vegetables against malignant disease of the large bowel.

However, no clear pattern of protection by fruit or vegetables is evident from the case–control studies of colorectal adenomas. Nevertheless, in the one cohort study that has so far reported data, there was a statistically significant inverse association with fruit consumption.

Limitations of the data
The case–control studies of fruit and vegetables in relation to colorectal cancer have been carried out over more than two decades in several countries among both men and women. Although the aggregate risks from these studies suggest that total fruit and total vegetables confer protection against colorectal cancer, the case–control studies taken as a whole reflect considerable heterogeneity in association (Riboli & Norat, 2003).

The most serious problem with the case–control studies, however, is the possibility that recall and selection biases account for the observed asso-

Case-control studies	No. of categ.	OR	95% CI
Slattery et al., 1988 (M)	4	0.3	0.1–0.6
Slattery et al., 1988 (F)	4	0.6	0.3–1.3
Steinmetz & Potter 1993 (M)	4	1.74	0.88–3.46
Steinmetz & Potter 1993 (F)	4	0.90	0.38–2.11
Centonze et al., 1994 (CR)	3	1.02	0.53–1.95
Kampman et al., 1995 (M)	3	1.00	0.49–2.03
Kampman et al., 1995 (F)	3	0.54	0.23–1.23
Kotake et al., 1995 (C)	4	0.8	0.27–2.41
Kotake et al., 1995 (R)	4	0.7	0.21–2.08
Shannon et al., 1996 (M)	4	0.77	0.44–1.36
Shannon et al., 1996 (F)	4	0.44	0.24–0.82
Boutron-Ruault et al., 1999	4	1.0	0.6–1.6
Murata et al., 1999 (C)	4	0.94	0.78–1.13
Murata et al., 1999 (R)	4	0.98	0.79–1.22
Deneo-Pellegrini et al., 2002 (CR)	4	0.7	0.5–0.9
SUMMARY VALUE		0.87	0.78–0.97

Heterogeneity test: χ^2 (14df)=21; p=0.095

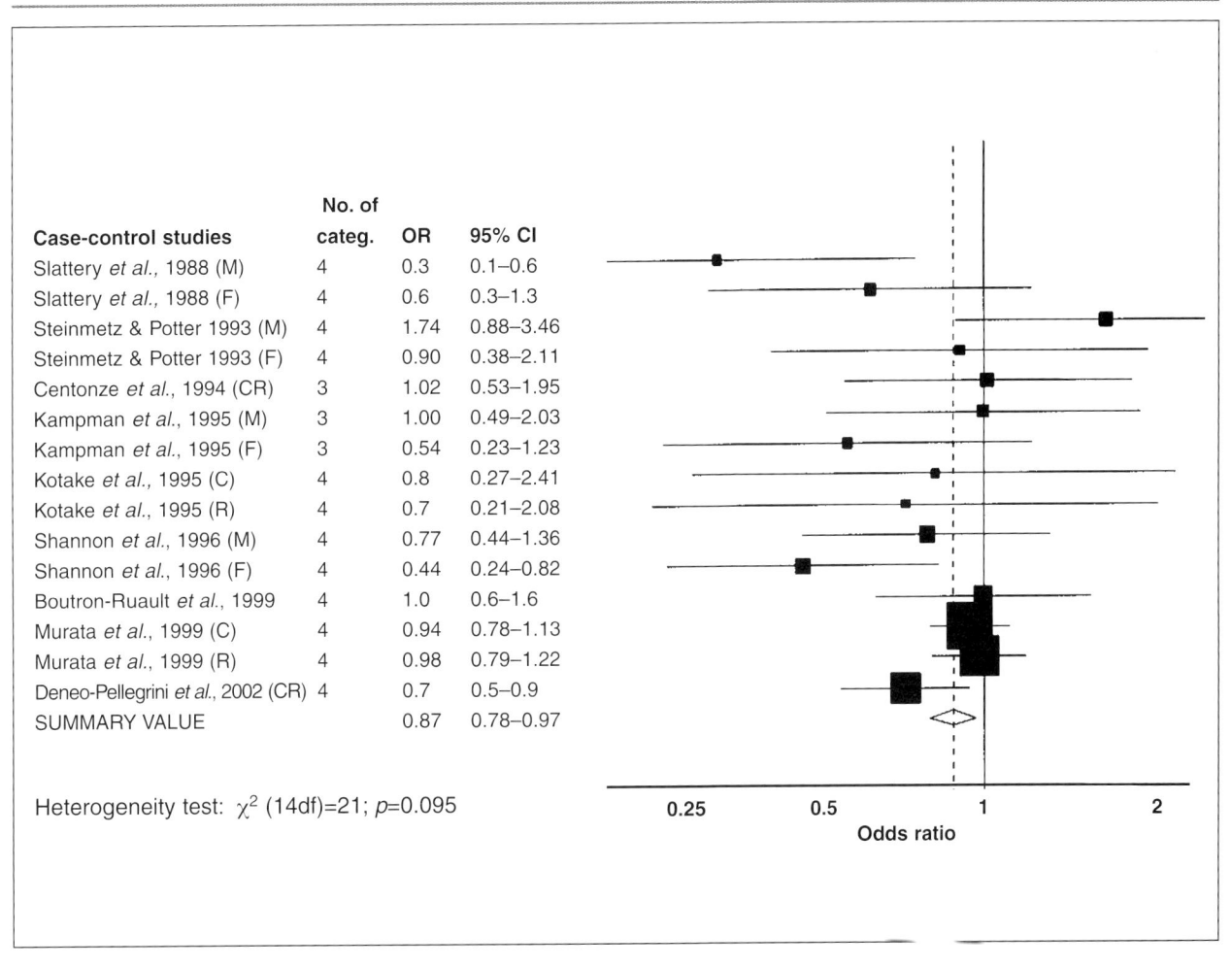

Figure 25 Case–control studies of colorectal cancer and fruit consumption (see Table 29)
M = males; F = females; CR = colorectal; C = colon; R = rectal; * = not applicable

ciations. This possibility is lent credence by the qualitatively different aggregate findings for the cohort studies of fruit and vegetables and colorectal cancer. Cohort studies are generally not susceptible to either recall or selection bias (though the cohort studies of this question also exhibit considerable heterogeneity of association). Case–control studies of adenomas avoid recall bias if dietary assessment is carried out before endoscopy—the adenomas are generally asymptomatic—but sigmoidoscopic screening (a frequent setting for such studies) can result in selection bias and allows study only of left-sided colorectal lesions.

In the report of one cohort study (Terry et al., 2001a), it was suggested that a threshold phenomenon exists, whereby extremely low intake of fruit and vegetables, relative to virtually all higher categories of consumption, is associated with increased risk. The overall data are currently too sparse to further evaluate this possibility.

There may be systematic bias (e.g., overreporting) at the individual level and this bias may be present—and correlated—in both the food frequency questionnaire and the reference instrument (24-hour recalls or dietary records) typically used to 'calibrate' a food frequency questionnaire in cohort studies. The existence of this correlated 'person-specific' bias may lead to considerably greater relative risk attenuation than has been previously appreciated (Kipnis et al., 2003).

Cohort studies	No. of categ.	OR	95% CI
Shibata et al., 1992 (M)	3	1.39	0.84–2.30
Shibata et al., 1992 (F)	3	0.72	0.45–1.16
Steinmetz et al., 1994	4	0.73	0.47–1.13
Kato et al., 1997	4	1.63	0.92–2.89
Hsing et al., 1998a (CR)	4	1.3	0.8–2.4
Pietinen et al., 1999	4	1.2	0.8–1.9
Michels et al., 2000 (C)	5	1.00	0.72–1.38
Michels et al., 2000 (R)	5	1.17	0.63–2.18
Voorrips et al., 2000a (M,C)	5	0.85	0.57–1.27
Voorrips et al., 2000a (M,R)	5	0.88	0.55–1.41
Voorrips et al., 2000a (F,C)	5	0.83	0.54–1.26
Voorrips et al., 2000a (F,R)	5	1.78	0.94–3.38
Terry et al., 2001a (CR)	4	0.84	0.65–1.09
Flood et al., 2002	5	0.95	0.71–1.26
McCullough et al., 2003 (M, C)	5	0.69	0.47–1.02
McCullough et al., 2003 (F, C)	5	0.91	0.56–1.48
SUMMARY VALUE		0.97	0.87–1.08

Heterogeneity test: χ^2 (15df)=19; p=0.21

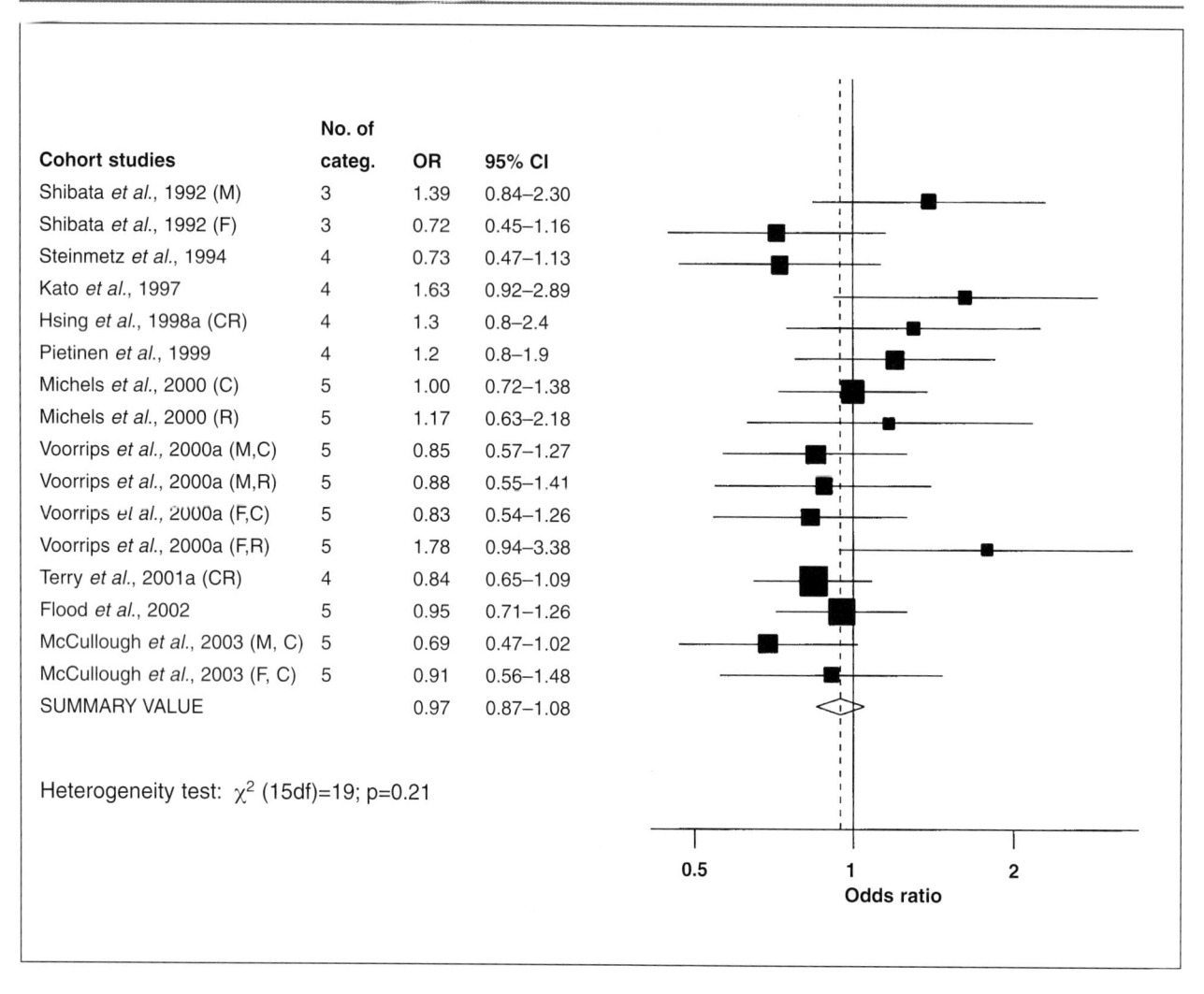

Figure 26 Cohort studies of colorectal cancer and vegetable consumption (see Table 30)
M = males; F = females; CR = colorectal; C = colon; R = rectal

Because the risk reductions for fruit and vegetables are so modest, it is virtually impossible to rule out confounding by unknown or unmeasured lifestyle and other factors associated with fruit and vegetable consumption as an explanation for the observed associations.

Liver
Fruit
Cohort study
One study of liver cancer showed no effect of fruit intake (Table 39).

Case–control studies
Many of the case–control studies of liver cancer were conducted with principal objectives other than consideration of fruit and vegetables.

Frequently, therefore, the dietary instrument used was not very detailed. None of three studies of hepatocellular carcinoma found a significant inverse association with fruit consumption (Table 40). Hadziyannis et al. (1995) reported that "for fruits ... the association was essentially null". In the study of Parkin et al. (1991) related to cholangiocarcinoma, the significant association for fresh fruit was from a

Cancer-preventive effects

Case-control studies	No. of categ.	OR	95% CI
Slattery et al., 1988 (M)	4	0.6	0.3–1.3
Slattery et al., 1988 (F)	4	0.3	0.1–0.9
Young & Wolf, 1988	5	0.72	0.48–1.07
Lee et al., 1989 (CR)	3	0.69	0.45–1.05
Hu et al., 1991	3	0.18	0.05–0.61
Iscovich et al., 1992	4	0.075	0.02–0.30
Steinmetz & Potter, 1993 (M)	4	1.29	0.67–2.51
Steinmetz & Potter, 1993 (F)	4	1.11	0.50–2.45
Centonze et al., 1994 (CR)	3	0.51	0.25–1.04
Kampman et al., 1995 (C)	4	0.40	0.23–0.69
Kotake et al., 1995 (C)	4	1.01	0.24–4.22
Kotake et al., 1995 (R)	4	0.5	0.12–1.96
Shannon et al., 1996 (M)	4	0.78	0.45–1.35
Shannon et al., 1996 (F)	4	0.51	0.28–0.93
Boutron-Ruault et al., 1999	4	0.7	0.4–1.3
La Vecchia et al., 1999 (M)	3	0.74	0.59–0.91
La Vecchia et al., 1999 (F)	3	0.43	0.32–0.56
Deneo-Pellegrini et al., 2002 (CR)	4	0.7	0.5–0.9
SUMMARY VALUE		0.63	0.56–0.70

Heterogeneity test: χ^2 (17df)=37; p=0.0038

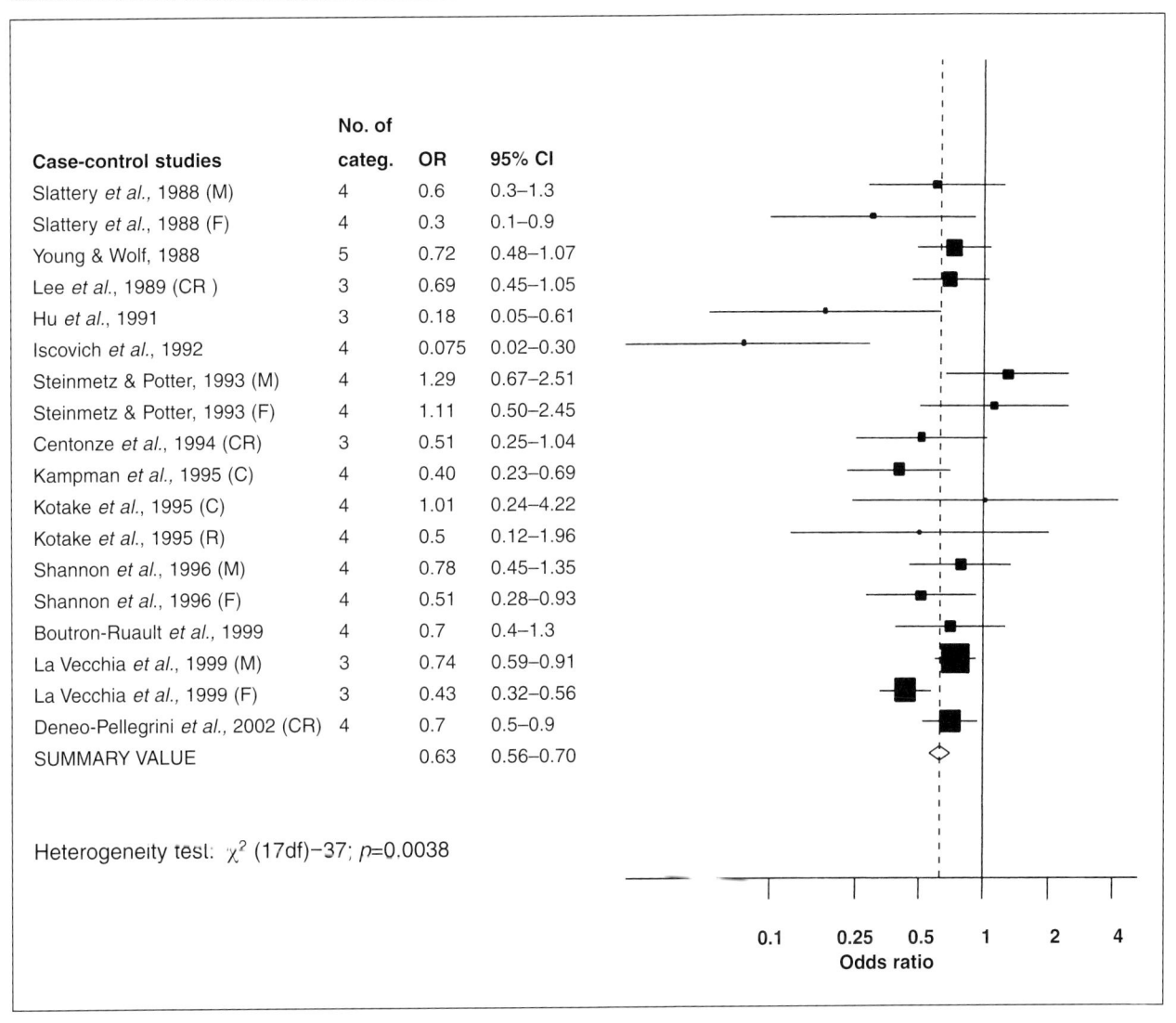

Figure 27 Case–control studies of colorectal cancer and vegetable consumption (see Table 31)
M = males; F = females; CR = colorectal cancer; C = colon; R = rectal

univariate analysis; when included in a multivariate model with all other food items, the association was no longer significant.

Vegetables
Cohort studies
The largest of the three cohort studies (Table 41), that of Hirayama (1990), included only limited information on diet, and for the class of vegetables, only frequency of consumption of green-yellow vegetables. Death from liver cancer was the end-point. [The Working Group noted that it is not clear whether all of these were from hepatocellular carcinoma].

The study of Yu et al. (1995) was a full cohort analysis of vegetable consumption, previously reported as a nested case–control study by Yu et al. (1993). Yu et al. (1995) noted that the inverse association for vegetable consumption appeared to be restricted to carriers of hepatitis B surface antigen (HBsAg) [RR 0.21, 0.09–0.50] and cigarette smokers [0.26, 0.12–0.59].

In the study of Sauvaget et al. (2003), green-yellow vegetable consumption was associated with a significant reduction in liver cancer mortality.

Case–control studies
Six case–control studies have reported data, two with significant inverse associations for vegetable consumption (Table 42). No numerical data were reported in the study of Fukuda *et al.* (1993), which was primarily designed to evaluate viral risk factors for hepatocellular carcinoma. However, the authors appear to have considered only mean consumption levels of fresh and green-yellow vegetables, and these were said to be similar for cases and controls. Similarly, Hadziyannis *et al.* (1995) reported that "for ... vegetables, the association was essentially null."

Combined fruit and vegetables
Cohort studies
No studies were identified by the Working Group.

Case–control studies
Only one study assessed the combination of fruit and vegetables, with an inverse association reported in both males and females (Table 43).

Discussion
Consumption of total fruit was not significantly associated with liver cancer, in either cohort or case–control studies. Consumption of total vegetables was significantly inversely associated with liver cancer only in one cohort study.

Biliary tract
Fruit
Cohort study
One cohort study has reported that there was no significant association between fruit consumption and gallbladder cancer (Table 44).

Case–control studies
No studies were identified by the Working Group.

Vegetables
Cohort studies
Hirayama (1990) tabulated gallbladder cancer as one of the end-points, but in the table in the section devoted to dietary factors, it is linked to bile-duct cancer. It is unclear whether the numbers of cases cited in Table 45 include bile-duct cancer. Comparison of daily with less frequent consumption of vegetables revealed no association. The study of Sauvaget *et al.* (2003) did not show any significant association.

Case–control studies
No studies were identified by the Working Group.

Combined fruit and vegetables
Case–control study
One case–control study has been reported of fruit and vegetable consumption and biliary tract cancer. The results were presented separately for gallbladder and bile duct cancer, and data for gallbladder cancer are summarized in Table 48. For bile-duct cancer, there were inverse associations for fruits, lettuce/cabbage, green-yellow vegetables and other vegetables in the univariate analysis, but these did not persist in the multivariate analysis.

Discussion
The available studies of biliary tract cancer in relation to fruit and vegetable consumption are too few to allow any conclusion to be drawn.

Pancreas
Fruit
Cohort studies
Of six cohort studies on diet and pancreas cancer, four used death from pancreas cancer as end-point and none found a significant inverse association with fruit consumption (Table 47). That of Mills *et al.* (1988) did not evaluate fruit consumption *per se*, but did report a protective effect of high consumption of vegetarian protein products, including raisins, dates and dry fruit. Zheng *et al.* (1993) provided no numerical data on risks for fruit consumption but reported that fruit consumption showed no clear association with pancreatic cancer risk.

Case–control studies
Many of the studies reported used proxy interviews for dead cases. For the few that used only direct interviews (with consequent exclusion of many cases who died within a short period), this is indicated in the comments section of Table 48. Eight of the 13 studies reported inverse associations for estimated fruit intake, one also for citrus fruit.

Farrow & Davis (1990), however, while reporting no numerical data, indicated that cases and controls did not differ with respect to total intake of all fruit or citrus fruit. Howe *et al.* (1990) also reported negative findings for associations with fruit consumption, on the basis of a model that included fibre, but they reported a significant protective effect of estimated intake of fibre (RR = 0.38 for 28 g/d of fibre from fruit). This study had been designed to obtain estimates of effects of nutrients, rather than of food groups.

The studies of Howe *et al.* (1990), Baghurst *et al.* (1991) and Bueno de Mesquita *et al.* (1991) were part of the IARC multi-country SEARCH programme, designed to evaluate associations using similar protocols in several different countries, also including studies in Montreal, Canada and Poland, that did not report specifically on fruit and vegetable intake. Howe *et al.* (1992) reported a combined analysis of these studies, with a total of 802 cases and 1669 controls. Like the study of Howe *et al.* (1990), the analysis was primarily related to nutrients. However, the authors comment that the results provide "strong evidence" of an inverse association of pancreas cancer with markers of fruit intake, particularly dietary fibre and vitamin C. The RR for the highest versus lowest quintile of vitamin C intake was 0.55 (95% CI 0.39–0.78) in a model that included all nutrient variables and lifetime cigarette consumption.

Vegetables
Cohort studies
Of the six cohort studies with data on vegetable consumption and pancreas cancer, none found a significant inverse association (Table 49). Mills *et al.* (1988) did not evaluate vegetable consumption *per se*, but did report a protective effect of high consumption of vegetarian protein products (beans, lentils or peas). Zheng *et al.* (1993) provided no numerical data on risks for vegetable consumption but reported that consumption of vegetables showed "no clear association" with pancreatic cancer risk.

Case–control studies
Many of the studies have used proxy interviews for dead cases. For the few that used only direct interviews (with consequent exclusion of many cases who died within a short period), this is indicated in the comments section of Table 50.

Seven of the 13 studies found protective effects for estimated intake of vegetables. Some found significant associations only for cruciferous vegetables or carrots. Farrow & Davis (1990), however, while reporting no numerical data, indicated that apart from a non-significant higher consumption of green and yellow vegetables by cases, cases and controls did not differ with respect to their total intake of all vegetables and raw vegetables. Howe *et al.* (1990) also reported negative findings for associations with vegetable consumption, on the basis of a model that included fibre, and they reported a significant protective effect of estimated intake of fibre (RR = 0.56 for 28 g/d of fibre from vegetables). This study had been designed to obtain estimates of effects of nutrients, rather than of food groups.

Baghurst *et al.* (1991) reported no numerical estimates of associations for vegetables, but indicated that cases consumed significantly less of a number of vegetables than controls.

The studies of Howe *et al.* (1990), Baghurst *et al.* (1991) and Bueno de Mesquita *et al.* (1991) were part of the IARC multi-country SEARCH programme, designed to evaluate associations using similar protocols in several different countries, also including studies in Montreal, Canada and Poland, that did not report specifically on fruit and vegetable intake. Howe *et al.* (1992) reported a combined analysis of these studies, with a total of 802 cases and 1669 controls. Like the study of Howe *et al.* (1990), the analysis was primarily related to nutrients. However, the authors comment that the results provide "strong evidence" of an inverse association of pancreas cancer with several markers of vegetable intake, particularly dietary fibre. The RR for the highest versus lowest quintile of dietary fibre intake was 0.50 (0.34–0.72) in a model that included all nutrient variables and lifetime cigarette consumption.

Combined fruit and vegetables
Case–control studies
Two case–control studies have been reported with estimates of risk for combined fruit and vegetable consumption (Table 51). Both showed inverse associations.

Discussion
Six case–control studies on fruit consumption and pancreas cancer were evaluable. The mean OR was 0.72 (95% CI 0.63–0.83), range 0.07–0.92 (Figure 28). The mean OR for the five evaluable case–control studies of vegetable consumption was 0.80 (95% CI 0.69–0.93), range 0.32–1.03 (Figure 29).

Although inverse associations for fruit or vegetable consumption were seen in many case–control studies, these have largely not been replicated in the cohort studies. There has to be some concern over the mainly inverse associations with fruit and or vegetables found in many of the case–control studies when the response rates for controls were low. It is possible that responders are more likely to be health-conscious than non-responders and thus tend to eat more fruit and vegetables. Selection bias is also possible if the case series was restricted to those subjects still alive at the time of interview. In the two largest individual case–control studies, only living cases were interviewed. This involved many more exclusions in the study of Silverman *et al.* (1998) conducted in the USA than in that of Ji *et al.* (1995) conducted in China. Whether this accounts for the difference between the largely negative findings of Silverman *et al.* (1998) and the significant association in men for fruit in the study of Ji *et al.* (1995) is uncertain.

Larynx
Fruit
Cohort studies
No studies were identified by the Working Group.

Case–control studies
The ten case–control studies on total fruit intake in relation to larynx cancer risk (Table 52) all included men and some also included women. The majority of the studies were hospital-based.

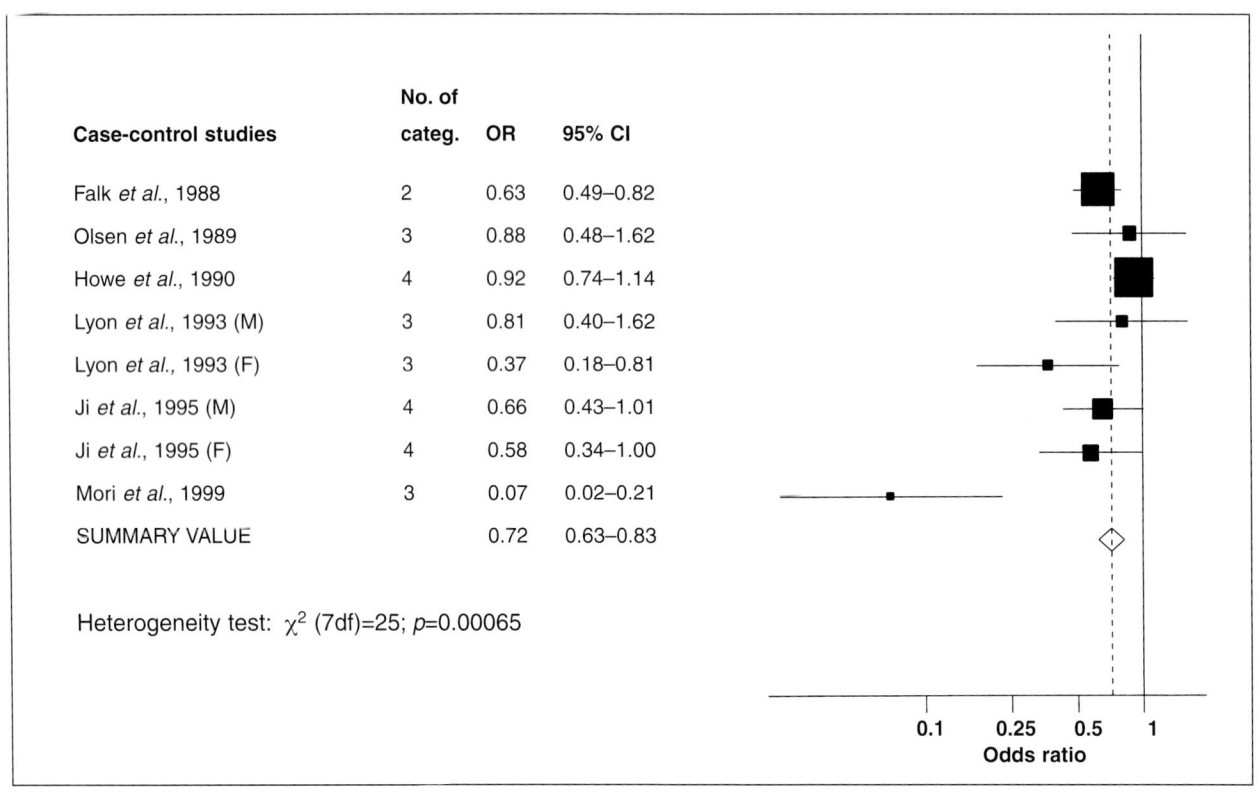

Case-control studies	No. of categ.	OR	95% CI
Falk et al., 1988	2	0.63	0.49–0.82
Olsen et al., 1989	3	0.88	0.48–1.62
Howe et al., 1990	4	0.92	0.74–1.14
Lyon et al., 1993 (M)	3	0.81	0.40–1.62
Lyon et al., 1993 (F)	3	0.37	0.18–0.81
Ji et al., 1995 (M)	4	0.66	0.43–1.01
Ji et al., 1995 (F)	4	0.58	0.34–1.00
Mori et al., 1999	3	0.07	0.02–0.21
SUMMARY VALUE		0.72	0.63–0.83

Heterogeneity test: χ^2 (7df)=25; p=0.00065

Figure 28 Case–control studies of pancreas cancer and fruit consumption (see Table 48)
M = males; F = females

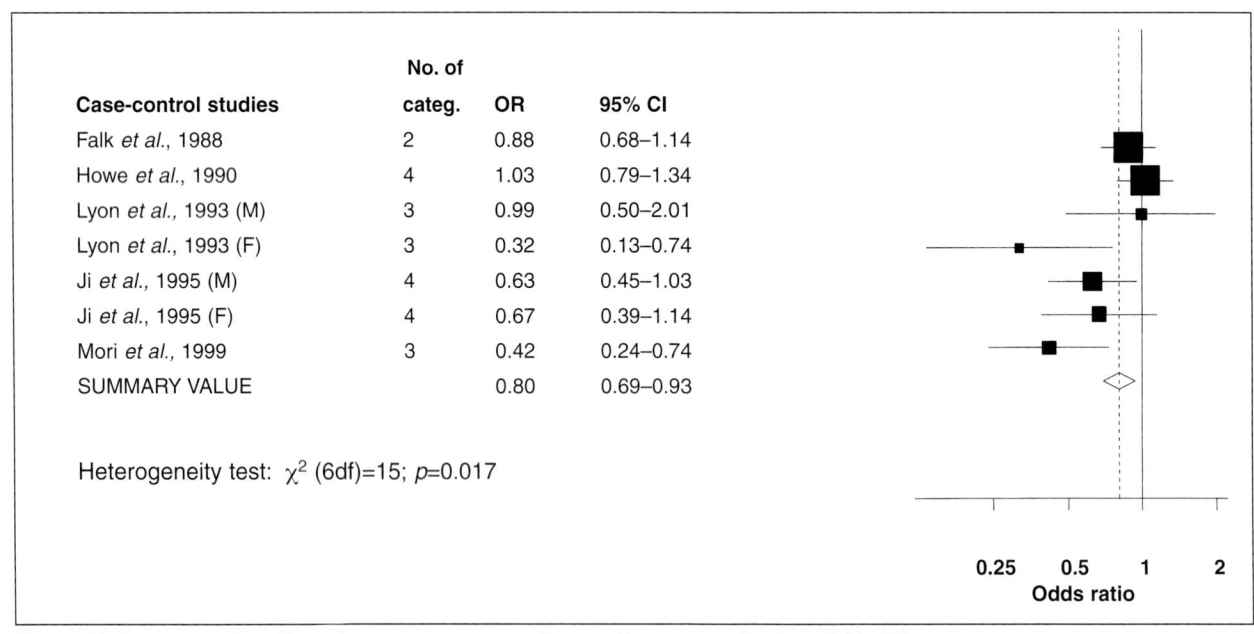

Case-control studies	No. of categ.	OR	95% CI
Falk et al., 1988	2	0.88	0.68–1.14
Howe et al., 1990	4	1.03	0.79–1.34
Lyon et al., 1993 (M)	3	0.99	0.50–2.01
Lyon et al., 1993 (F)	3	0.32	0.13–0.74
Ji et al., 1995 (M)	4	0.63	0.45–1.03
Ji et al., 1995 (F)	4	0.67	0.39–1.14
Mori et al., 1999	3	0.42	0.24–0.74
SUMMARY VALUE		0.80	0.69–0.93

Heterogeneity test: χ^2 (6df)=15; p=0.017

Figure 29 Case–control studies of pancreas cancer and vegetable consumption (see Table 50)
M = males; F = females

Most studies used a food frequency questionnaire to measure dietary intake, while one study used a diet history interview. The total number of measured food items varied widely between studies, as did the number of fruit items. This implies that very different numbers of fruits may be included in the category labelled 'total fruit'. Several reports do not state what is included under '(total) fruit'.

Almost all studies controlled for confounding by smoking (in different ways and detail) and alcohol, except three (De Stefani et al., 1987; Zheng et al., 1992b; Guo et al., 1995).

The (extreme) contrasts in intake of fruits considered were most often high versus low intake, based on tertiles or quartiles of intake.

All case–control studies showed inverse associations between intake of total fruit and risk of larynx cancer, with ORs for high versus low intake varying between 0.3 and 0.8. Although some studies did not show significant associations, the overall pattern of the case–control studies is of a consistent inverse association between total intake of fruit and risk of larynx cancer.

Only one study investigated these associations within subgroups of smoking, age and alcohol, or of supraglottis versus epiglottis and other subsites (Bosetti et al., 2002a). The observed ORs were weaker in the subgroups.

Vegetables
Cohort studies
No studies were identified by the Working Group.

Case–control studies
Nine case–control studies have reported on intake of (total) vegetables in relation to larynx cancer risk (Table 53). These studies all included men, and some also included women. The majority of the studies were hospital-based.

Most studies used a food frequency questionnaire to measure dietary intake, while one study used a diet history interview. The total number of measured food items varied widely between studies, as did the number of vegetable items. Not all studies reported the number of items but for the ones that did, the number of vegetable items varied up to 26. This implies that very different numbers of vegetables may be included in the category labelled 'total vegetables'.

Almost all studies controlled for confounding by smoking (in different ways and detail) and alcohol, except three (De Stefani et al., 1987; Zheng et al., 1992b; Guo et al., 1995).

All except one of the studies found inverse associations between intake of total vegetables and risk of larynx cancer, with ORs for high versus low intake varying between 0.17 and 0.9. Although most of the studies did not show significant associations, the overall pattern of the case–control studies is of a consistent inverse association between total intake of vegetables and risk of larynx cancer.

Only one study investigated these associations within subgroups of smoking, age and alcohol, or supraglottis versus epiglottis and other subsites (Bosetti et al., 2002a). No different ORs were found, however.

Combined fruit and vegetables
Cohort study
In one cohort study in the USA on upper aerodigestive tract cancer (Kasum et al., 2002), a non-significant inverse association of larynx cancer with intake of vegetables and fruits was mentioned, but no data were shown.

Case–control studies
In two case–control studies, there were significant inverse associations between combined fruit and vegetable intake and larynx cancer risk (Table 54).

Discussion
Only case–control studies on larynx cancer were available for evaluation. These studies were conducted in Europe, Asia and South America. For four evaluable case–control studies with total fruit, the mean OR was 0.63 (95% CI 0.52–0.77), range 0.38–0.80 (Figure 30). For four evaluable studies with vegetable consumption, the mean OR was 0.49 (95% CI 0.40–0.61), range 0.17–1.1 (Figure 31).

Control for smoking was rather crude and incomplete in the early studies; more recent studies have used more elaborate models and still observed inverse associations with fruit and vegetable intake. Only one study addressed associations between fruit and vegetables and larynx cancer in subgroups of smoking and alcohol intake. ORs for fruit became weaker in these subgroups, which might indicate residual confounding by smoking and alcohol. The possibility of recall and selection bias in the case–control studies cannot be excluded.

Lung
Fruit
Cohort studies
A total of 16 cohort studies have been reported on fruit intake and risk of lung cancer and in addition, results are available from a pooled analysis of primary data from eight cohort studies (Table 55).

Six studies used mortality from lung cancer as the end-point. Follow-up times ranged from 4 to 25 years. All but two studies used a self-administered food frequency questionnaire to measure dietary intake. The number of fruit items varied up to 23. The considered contrasts in fruit intake also varied considerably between studies. All but one study (Wang & Hammond, 1985) corrected for possible confounding by smoking (often in more detail than in the case–control studies), as well as

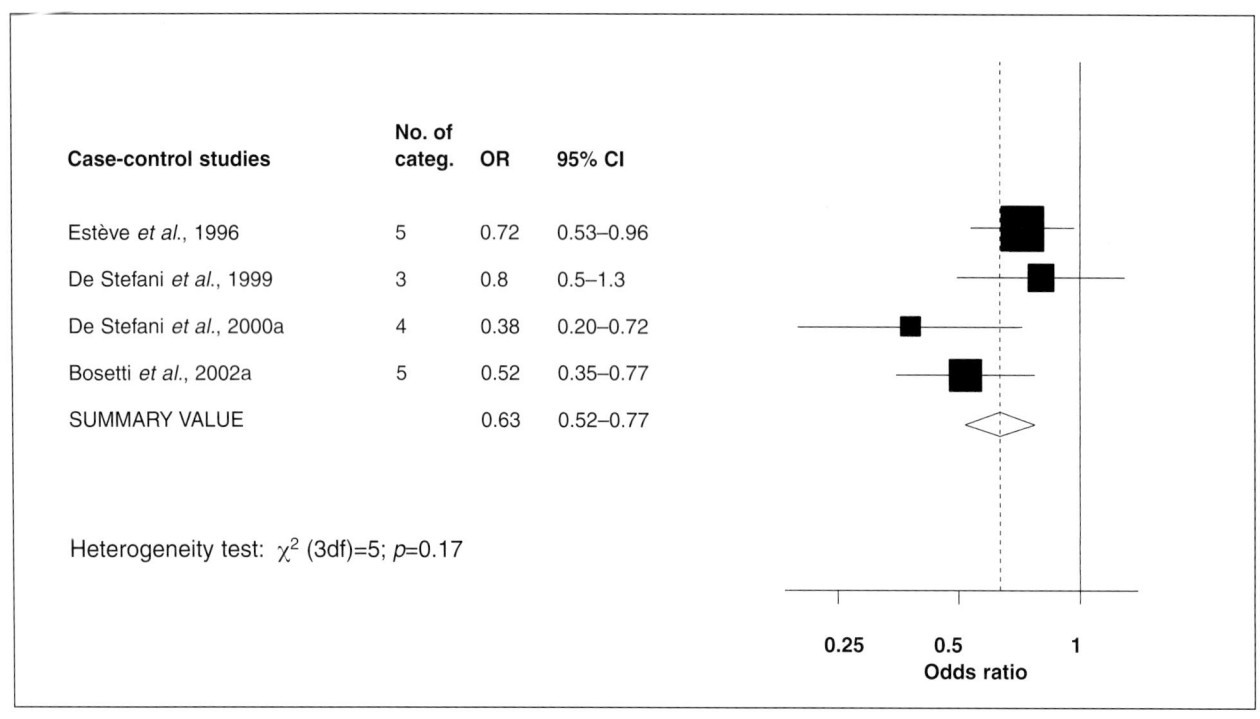

IARC Handbooks of Cancer Prevention Volume 8: Fruit and Vegetables

Case-control studies	No. of categ.	OR	95% CI
Estève et al., 1996	5	0.72	0.53–0.96
De Stefani et al., 1999	3	0.8	0.5–1.3
De Stefani et al., 2000a	4	0.38	0.20–0.72
Bosetti et al., 2002a	5	0.52	0.35–0.77
SUMMARY VALUE		0.63	0.52–0.77

Heterogeneity test: χ^2 (3df)=5; p=0.17

Figure 30 Case–control studies of larynx cancer and fruit consumption (see Table 52).

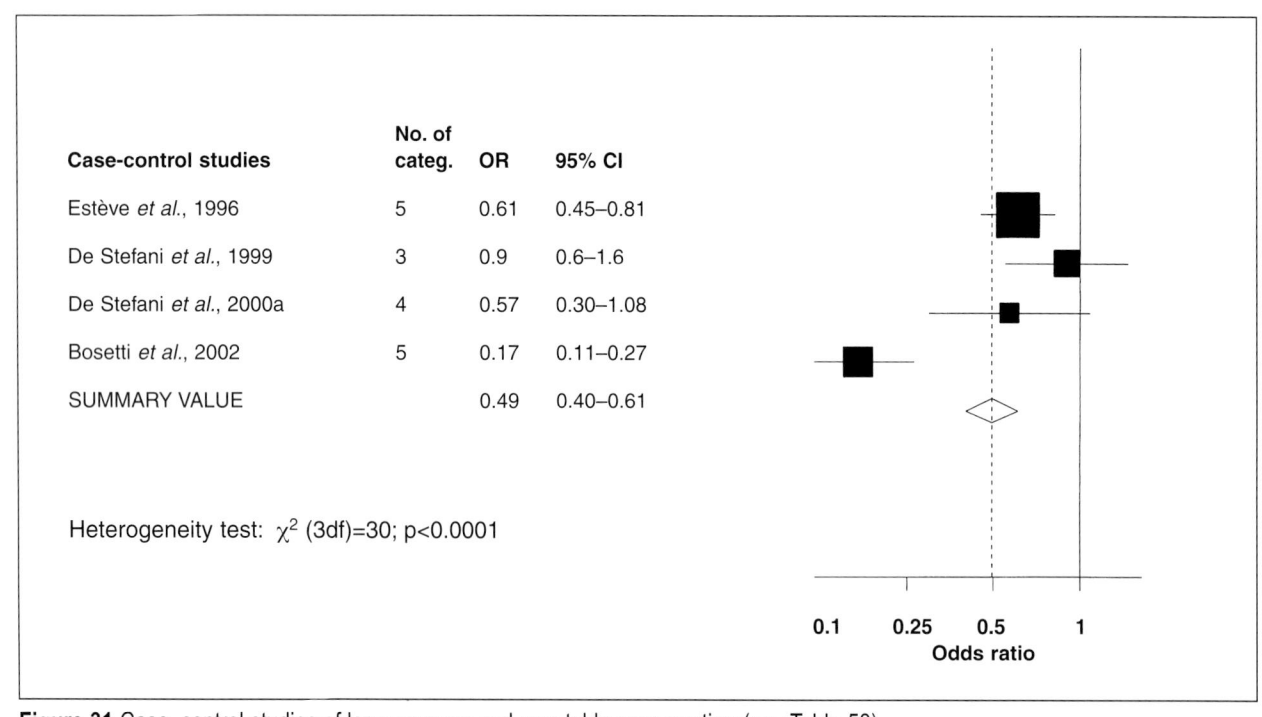

Case-control studies	No. of categ.	OR	95% CI
Estève et al., 1996	5	0.61	0.45–0.81
De Stefani et al., 1999	3	0.9	0.6–1.6
De Stefani et al., 2000a	4	0.57	0.30–1.08
Bosetti et al., 2002	5	0.17	0.11–0.27
SUMMARY VALUE		0.49	0.40–0.61

Heterogeneity test: χ^2 (3df)=30; $p<0.0001$

Figure 31 Case–control studies of larynx cancer and vegetable consumption (see Table 53)

age and several other confounders (e.g., education, occupation).

In most studies, there were inverse associations between fruit intake and lung cancer, although these were not always significant. The pooled analysis of cohort studies also showed a significant inverse association. The more recent cohort studies attempted more complete control for confounding by smoking (for example, incorporating duration and amount smoked as well as smoking status rather than pack-years in their final models) and similar associations were seen to those in the earlier studies.

Non-significant positive associations were observed in men in one study (Feskanich et al., 2000). Subgroup analyses in the studies did not clearly indicate that the inverse association was limited to particular morphological types of lung cancer. There is also no clear indication that a protective effect is seen only in (ex-)smokers. Several studies show inverse associations in never-smokers, including the pooled analysis of cohort studies; however, statistical significance was often not reached.

Case–control studies
30 case–control studies have reported on intake of (total) fruit and the association with lung cancer risk (Table 56). Ten were hospital-based, while the remainder used population controls. Almost all studies that included smokers controlled for confounding by age and smoking (smoking in different ways and detail), except two (Lei et al., 1996; Alavanja et al., 2001). Most studies also controlled for some measure of education or socioeconomic status. Other confounders considered have varied between studies. Eight studies were conducted among never- or non-current smokers, mostly in women.

The total number of measured food items varied widely between studies, as did the number of fruit items. Not all studies reported the number of items; for the ones that did, the number of fruit items varied up to 16. Several reports do not state what was included under '(total) fruit'.

In 22 of the studies, there were inverse associations between intake of fruit and risk of lung cancer; in 15 of these there were significant inverse associations, some only in sub-groups. Six studies, however, reported (non-significantly) increased odds ratios. Dorgan et al. (1993) reported inverse associations for white men or women and positive associations for black men or women.

Three studies showed separate results for men and women and in two of these, the inverse associations were somewhat stronger in women than men (Dorgan et al., 1993; Takezaki et al., 2001). Of the studies that evaluated effects in morphological subgroups, most reported somewhat stronger effects for squamous- and small-cell carcinoma than for other types. Effects were often stronger in ex- or current smokers. Among nine studies conducted among never- or non-smokers, four found significant inverse associations.

Vegetables
Cohort studies
Among a total of 15 cohort studies on intake of (total or specific) vegetables in relation to lung cancer risk (Table 57), 12 reported on total vegetable consumption. In addition, results from a pooled analysis of primary data from eight cohort studies, some also included in Table 57, are available (Smith-Warner et al., 2003).

Five studies used lung cancer mortality as the end-point. Follow-up times varied from 4 to 25 years. All but two studies used a self-administered food frequency questionnaire to measure dietary intake. The number of vegetable items mentioned varied considerably.

Many of the studies found inverse associations between vegetable intake and lung cancer risk, of which five were significant, at least in one gender. In the pooled analysis of eight cohort studies, inverse associations were seen in men and women, but were of only borderline significance in men (Smith-Warner et al., 2003). All studies corrected for possible confounding by smoking (often in more detail than in the case–control studies), as well as age and several other confounders (e.g., education, occupation).

Subgroup analyses in several studies indicated stronger inverse associations for squamous-cell, small- or large-cell carcinoma (sometimes aggregated as Kreyberg I) than for adenocarcinoma (Kreyberg II). Several studies showed stronger effects in ex-smokers.

Case–control studies
Of 25 case–control studies that have reported on intake of (total) vegetables in relation to lung cancer risk (Table 58), nine were hospital-based, while the remainder used population controls. Almost all studies that included smokers controlled for confounding effects of age and smoking (smoking in different ways and detail). Most studies also controlled for some measure of education or socioeconomic status. Seven studies were conducted among never- or non-current smokers, mostly in women.

Most studies used a food frequency questionnaire (or diet history) by interview to measure dietary intake. The total number of food items measured has varied widely between studies, as has the number of vegetable items. Not all studies reported the number of items, but in those that did, the number of vegetable items varied up to 28.

Regarding the associations between intake and lung cancer risk, the considered (extreme) contrasts in intake of vegetables were most often high versus low intake, based on tertiles, quartiles or quintiles of intake. Intake levels varied considerably between studies, as did the considered contrasts.

In most studies there were inverse associations between vegetable intake and risk of lung cancer and in 14 there were one or more significant inverse associations (sometimes for only one subgroup, e.g. females).

In the three studies that reported separate results for men and women, the inverse associations were somewhat stronger in women than men. Of the studies that evaluated effects by morphological subgroup, most reported somewhat stronger effects for squamous- and small-cell carcinoma than for other morphological types. Effects were often stronger in ex- or current smokers. Three of the seven studies conducted among never- or non-smokers reported significant inverse associations, one of them in females but not in males.

Combined fruit and vegetables
Cohort studies
Reports of six cohort studies included data on combined intake of fruit and vegetables in relation to lung cancer risk (Table 59). In all there were inverse associations, with RRs between 0.49 and 0.79 (mostly significant), two only in women. In the pooled analysis of eight cohort studies, there was a significant inverse association in both sexes combined (Smith-Warner et al., 2003).

Case–control studies
Reports of four case–control studies included data on intake of vegetables and fruits together in relation to risk of lung cancer (Table 60). All four showed inverse associations (mostly significant) when high versus low intake was compared, with odds ratios ranging from 0.40 to 0.77.

Discussion
The cohort studies considered for evaluation were conducted in North America, Europe or Japan, the case–control studies also in Australasia, other parts of Asia and South America. These studies mostly show an inverse association between intake of total fruit and/or vegetables and risk of lung cancer, although non-significant positive associations have also been observed. For fruit consumption, 13 cohort studies and 21 case–control stuides were evaluable. For cohort studies the mean RR was 0.77 (95% CI 0.71–0.84), range 0.26–1.22 (Figure 32), and for case–control studies the mean OR was 0.70 (95% CI 0.45–1.07), range 0.33–2.04 (Figure 33). For vegetable consumption, 11 cohort studies were evaluable. The mean RR was 0.80 (95% CI 0.73–0.88), range 0.47–1.37 (Figure 34). For the 18 evaluable case–control studies the mean OR was 0.69 (95% CI 0.63–0.76), range 0.30–1.49 (Figure 35).

The latest results from the cohort studies and a meta-analysis (Riboli & Norat, 2003) suggest a stronger inverse association for fruit than for vegetables. Studies vary considerably in terms of the number of items included in the fruit or vegetable group. There was no clear difference in results between men and women, between hospital- and population-based case–control studies or between morphological categories of lung cancer. The strength of the association was generally less for cohort studies than for case–control studies, leaving open the possibility of recall and/or selection bias in the case–control studies.

Because smoking is a strong risk factor for lung cancer, while smoking and fruit (and to a lesser extent, vegetable) consumption are inversely associated, appropriate control for confounding by smoking is crucial. Although the newer cohort studies have attempted to control for confounding by smoking much better than earlier ones, residual confounding by smoking cannot be excluded (Marshall & Hastrup, 1996; Stram et al., 2002), and cohort studies often fail to capture changes in smoking and diet after the baseline measurement. Subgroup analyses among categories of smoking also showed inverse associations in never-smokers (often non-significant) in the cohort studies. Case–control studies among never- or non-smokers were not entirely consistent in showing an inverse association with fruit or vegetables.

Breast
Studies of fruit and vegetable consumption in relation to breast cancer risk have been conducted over the past 40 years in North and South America, Australia, Asia and Europe. Most have focused on breast cancer in women; studies of breast cancer risk in men are discussed separately. The usual end-point has been breast cancer incidence, but some studies have examined associations with mortality. Cohort studies generally have measured recent diet at baseline, although diets during follow-up and during childhood also have been measured. Most case–control studies measured dietary intake during the 1–5 years preceding diagnosis, although some assessed dietary intake during childhood, adolescence and young adulthood.

Fruit
Cohort studies
Among the seven cohort studies, no statistically significant inverse association with fruit consumption was observed, although the relative risk of breast cancer was often well below 1.0 (Table 61). Reported menopausal status did not modify the association between fruit consumption and risk of breast cancer.

Cohort studies	No. of categ.	OR	95% CI
Fraser et al., 1991	3	0.26	0.10–0.70
Chow et al., 1992	4	0.7	0.4–1.3
Shibata et al., 1992 (M)	3	0.99	0.59–1.66
Shibata et al., 1992 (F)	3	0.68	0.37–1.24
Steinmetz et al., 1993	4	0.75	0.44–1.23
Ocké et al., 1997a	2	0.40	0.18–0.87
Breslow et al., 2000	4	0.9	0.5–1.6
Feskanich et al., 2000 (M)	5	1.22	0.80–1.87
Feskanich et al., 2000 (F)	5	0.76	0.56–1.02
Voorrips et al., 2000b	5	0.8	0.6–1.1
Jansen et al., 2001	3	0.69	0.46–1.02
Holick et al., 2002	5	0.87	0.74–1.02
Sauvaget et al., 2003	3	0.80	0.65–0.98
Miller et al., 2003	5	0.60	0.46–0.78
Neuhouser et al., 2003 (I)	5	0.79	0.57–1.11
Neuhouser et al., 2003 (P)	5	0.56	0.39–0.81
SUMMARY VALUES		0.77	0.71–0.84

Heterogeneity test: χ^2 (15df)=22; p=0.096

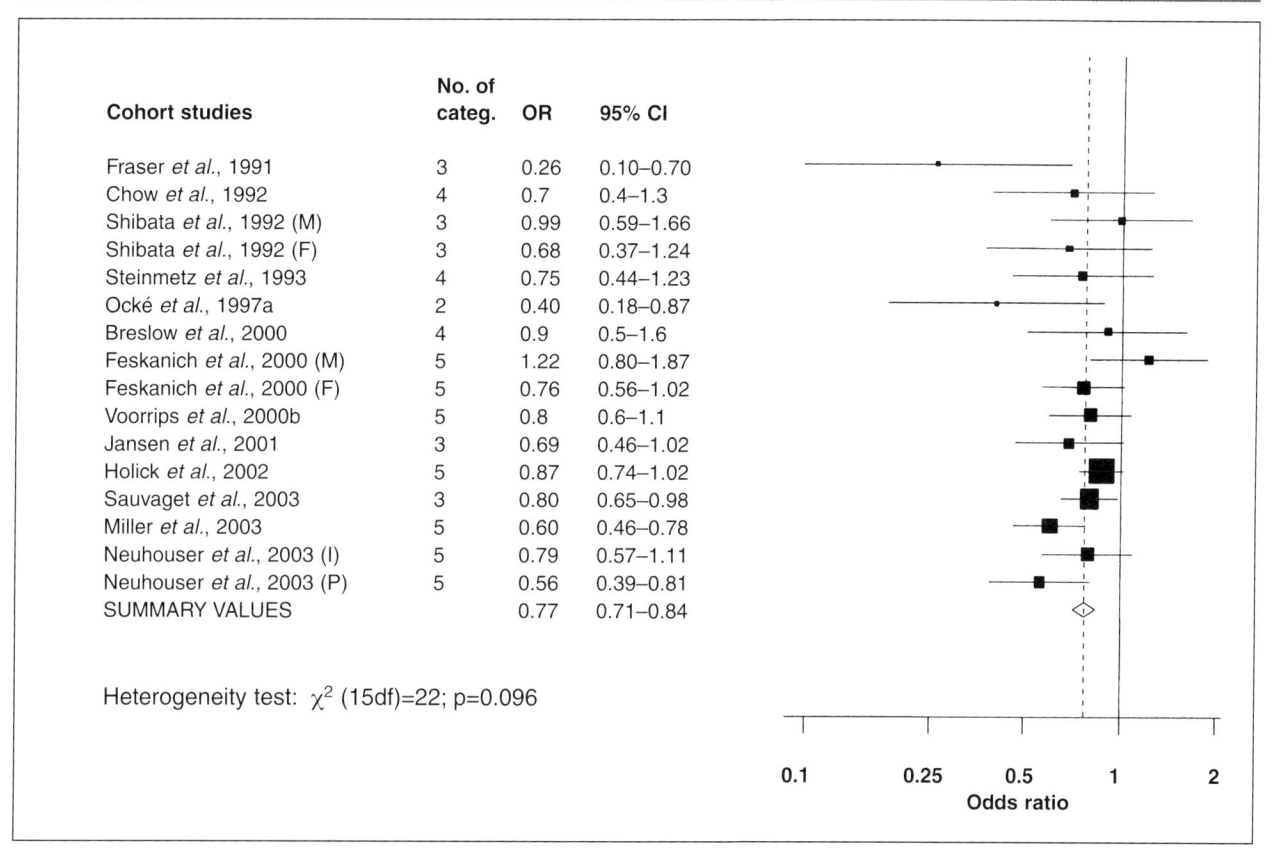

Figure 32 Cohort studies of lung cancer and fruit consumption (see Table 55)
M = males; F = females; I = intervention arm; P = placebo arm

In a meta-analysis of 10 case–control and two cohort studies including 9429 cases (Gandini et al., 2000), there was no association of breast cancer risk with fruit consumption when comparing high and low fruit intake (Table 61). However, when the analysis was restricted to the 11 studies for which dose–response information could be obtained, there was a 17% reduction in the risk of breast cancer for comparisons of six portions of fruit versus one per week (RR = 0.83, 95% CI 0.79–0.87). In this meta-analysis, for both comparisons, there was statistically significant between-study heterogeneity in the summary estimate ($p < 0.001$). This heterogeneity could have arisen because study-specific estimates were combined for total fruit, citrus fruit, other fruit and fruit rich in β-carotene for different comparison categories from studies using different study designs. In contrast, a more recent meta-analysis of eight case–control and ten cohort studies found no statistically significant association with fruit intake among cohort studies or case–control studies when considered separately or when combined (Riboli & Norat, 2003). However, there was significant heterogeneity across studies when the case–control studies were considered separately. Studies included in this meta-analysis were limited to those that considered total fruit, all fruit, fruit or fresh fruit and the study-specific relative risks were re-expressed based on an increase of 100 g per day of fruit consumption.

In a pooled analysis of the primary data from eight cohort studies (some of which were discussed above) using standardized criteria (Table 61), fruit consumption was not associated with breast cancer risk overall ($n = 7377$ cases) or when stratified by menopausal status (Smith-Warner et al., 2001).

Case–control studies
An inverse association with fruit consumption seen in about half of the 20 case–control studies was statistically significant in five (Table 62). The strongest association was observed in a small case–control study in Spain (Landa et al., 1994). In other case–

Case–control studies	No. of categ.	OR	95% CI
Fontham et al., 1988	3	0.66	0.54–0.82
Kalandidi et al., 1990	4	0.33	0.13–0.68
Candelora et al., 1992	4	0.6	0.3–1.1
Forman et al., 1992	4	1.10	0.57–2.08
Dorgan et al., 1993 (WM)	3	0.95	0.70–1.30
Dorgan et al., 1993 (WF)	3	0.56	0.40–0.79
Dorgan et al., 1993 (BM)	3	2.04	1.11–3.70
Dorgan et al., 1993 (BF)	3	1.30	0.44–3.85
Gao et al., 1993	3	0.45	0.30–0.67
Suzuki et al., 1994	3	1.2	0.4–3.1
Axelsson et al., 1996	3	0.73	0.43–1.23
Xu et al., 1996	4	0.6	0.5–0.9
Hu et al., 1997	4	0.7	0.4–1.2
Ko et al., 1997	2	1.0	0.5–1.7
Pawlega et al., 1997	3	0.42	0.23–0.77
Pillow et al., 1997	*	0.56	0.31–0.99
Nyberg et al., 1998	3	0.67	0.33–1.36
Brennan et al., 2000	3	1.09	0.6–1.5
Takezaki et al., 2001 (M,A)	4	0.98	0.61–1.58
Takezaki et al., 2001 (M,S)	4	0.61	0.40–0.95
Takezaki et al., 2001 (F,A)	4	0.68	0.27–1.70
Takezaki et al., 2001 (F,S)	4	0.49	0.11–2.13
De Stefani et al., 2002	4	0.84	0.62–1.13
Kreuzer et al., 2002	3	0.66	0.37–1.19
Marchand et al., 2002 (M)	3	0.7	0.4–1.5
Rachtan, 2002a	2	0.49	0.32–0.74
Seow et al., 2002 (Sm)	3	0.63	0.28–1.44
Seow et al., 2002 (NonSm)	3	0.60	0.39–0.93
SUMMARY VALUE		0.70	0.45–1.07

Heterogeneity test: χ^2 (27df)=45; p=0.015

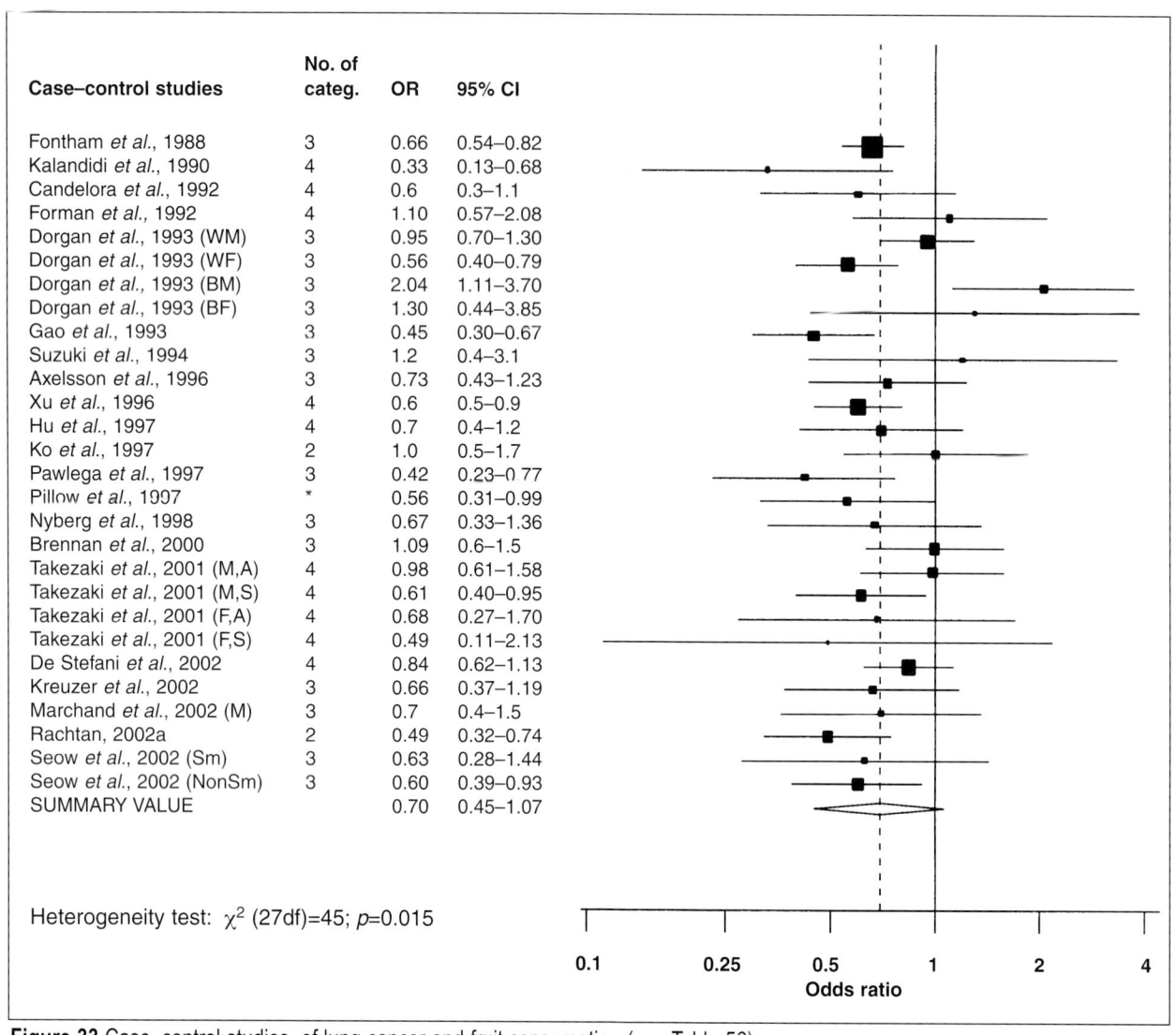

Figure 33 Case–control studies of lung cancer and fruit consumption (see Table 56)
W = white; B = black; M = males, F = females; A = adenocarcinoma; S = squamous and small cell carcinoma; Sm = smokers; NonSm = non smokers; * = not applicable

control studies, the relative risks have shown no more than a 10% increase or decrease in the risk of breast cancer for comparisons of high versus low consumption. A few studies have reported in the text that fruit consumption was not associated with the risk of breast cancer. In a Swedish case–control study, the OR was elevated in women over 50 years of age but not associated with breast cancer risk in women 50 years and younger (Holmberg et al., 1994). The test for effect modification by age group was not statistically significant. A similar pattern was observed in a Russian case–control study (Zaridze et al., 1991).

Vegetables
Cohort studies
Among the seven cohort studies (Table 63), a statistically significant inverse association with vegetable consumption was observed only in the Nurses' Health Study when the analysis was limited to premenopausal breast cancer (Zhang et al., 1999). When only postmenopausal women who were

Cohort studies	No. of categ.	OR	95% CI
Chow et al., 1992	4	1.2	0.6–2.3
Shibata et al., 1992 (M)	3	1.37	0.74–2.25
Shibata et al., 1992 (F)	3	0.58	0.32–1.05
Steinmetz et al., 1993	4	0.50	0.29–0.87
Ocké et al., 1997	2	0.47	0.21–1.03
Breslow et al., 2000	4	0.9	0.5–1.5
Feskanich et al., 2000 (M)	5	1.04	0.69–1.57
Feskanich et al., 2000 (F)	5	0.68	0.51–0.90
Voorips et al., 2000b	5	0.7	0.5–1.0
Jansen et al., 2001	3	0.90	0.61–1.33
Holick et al., 2002	5	0.75	0.63–0.88
Miller et al., 2003	5	1.00	0.76–1.30
Neuhouser et al., 2003 (I)	5	0.81	0.65–1.21
Neuhouser et al., 2003 (P)	5	0.82	0.59–1.14
SUMMARY VALUE		0.80	0.73–0.88

Heterogeneity test: χ^2 (13df)=18; p=0.16

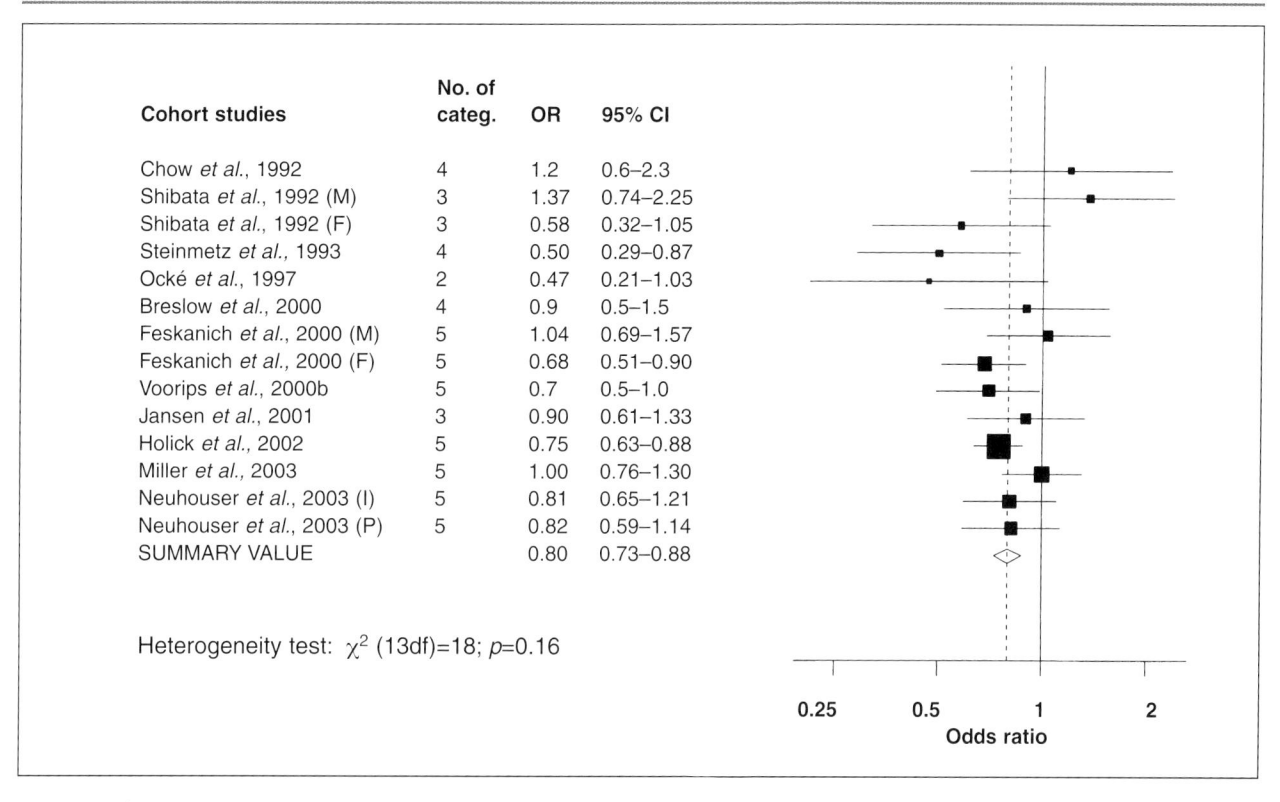

Figure 34 Cohort studies of lung cancer and vegetable consumption (see Table 57)
M = males; F = females; I = intervention arm; P = placebo arm

current users of hormone replacement therapy were examined, there was a suggestion of an inverse association. In three other cohort studies, a reduction of less than 15% in the risk of breast cancer was observed for higher versus lower vegetable consumption.

In a meta-analysis of 10 case–control and 10 cohort studies, breast cancer risk was decreased by 4% for an increment of 100 grams of vegetables per day (Riboli & Norat, 2003). When the two study designs were examined separately, an inverse association was suggested only in the case–control studies, but there was statistically significant heterogeneity in the results across the studies. Studies included in this meta-analysis were limited to those that considered total fruit, all fruit, fruits or fresh fruits and the study-specific relative risks were re-expressed based on an increase of 100 g per day of fruit consumption.

In a pooled analysis of eight cohort studies including 7377 breast cancer cases, total vegetable consumption was not associated with the risk of breast cancer (Table 63) (Smith-Warner et al., 2001). There was also no evidence of effect modification by family history, history of benign breast disease, hormone replacement therapy use, body mass index, fat consumption, alcohol consumption and several reproductive factors.

Case–control studies
In most of the 24 case–control studies, inverse associations with vegetable consumption have been found (Table 66). The strongest association observed was in a small case–control study in Greece (Katsouyanni et al., 1986). In the 13 case–control studies that found a statistically significant inverse association, the risk of breast cancer was generally 40–60% lower for comparison of the highest versus lowest intakes of total vegetables. In one study in Russia, the risk of breast cancer was reported to be lower among women who had increased their vegetable consumption during the past 10 years compared with those who had decreased consumption (Zaridze et al., 1991). In none of the case–control studies showing an odds ratio of at least 1.2 with higher vegetable consumption was the association statistically significant.

Some case–control studies of premenopausal women have suggested that higher vegetable consumption is

Case–control studies	No. of categ.	OR	95% CI
MacLennan et al., 1977	2	0.45	0.30–0.67
Fontham et al., 1988	3	0.90	0.74–1.11
Le Marchand et al., 1989 (M)	4	0.31	0.17–0.56
Le Marchand et al., 1989 (F)	4	0.18	0.06–0.53
Jain et al., 1990	4	0.60	0.40–0.88
Kalandidi et al., 1990	4	1.09	0.44–2.68
Candelora et al., 1992	4	0.3	0.1–0.5
Forman et al., 1992	4	0.60	0.30–1.18
Dorgan et al., 1993 (WM)	3	0.80	0.58–1.10
Dorgan et al., 1993 (WF)	3	0.59	0.42–0.82
Dorgan et al., 1993 (BM)	3	1.10	0.59–2.04
Dorgan et al., 1993 (BF)	3	0.67	0.23–1.96
Sankaranarayanan et al., 1994	4	0.32	0.13–0.78
Axelsson et al., 1996	3	0.37	0.23–0.61
Agudo et al., 1997	3	0.65	0.32–1.31
Ko et al., 1997	2	0.4	0.2–0.8
Pillow et al., 1997	*	1.49	0.84–2.63
Nyberg et al., 1998	3	0.57	0.29–1.13
Kubik et al., 2001	4	0.84	0.6–1.3
De Stefani et al., 2002	4	0.72	0.54–0.97
Marchand et al., 2002 (M)	3	1.4	0.7–2.9
Seow et al., 2002 (Sm)	3	0.48	0.23–1.00
Seow et al., 2002 (NonSm)	3	0.78	0.51–1.20
SUMMARY VALUE		0.69	0.63–0.76

Heterogeneity test: χ^2 (22df)=58; p<0.0001

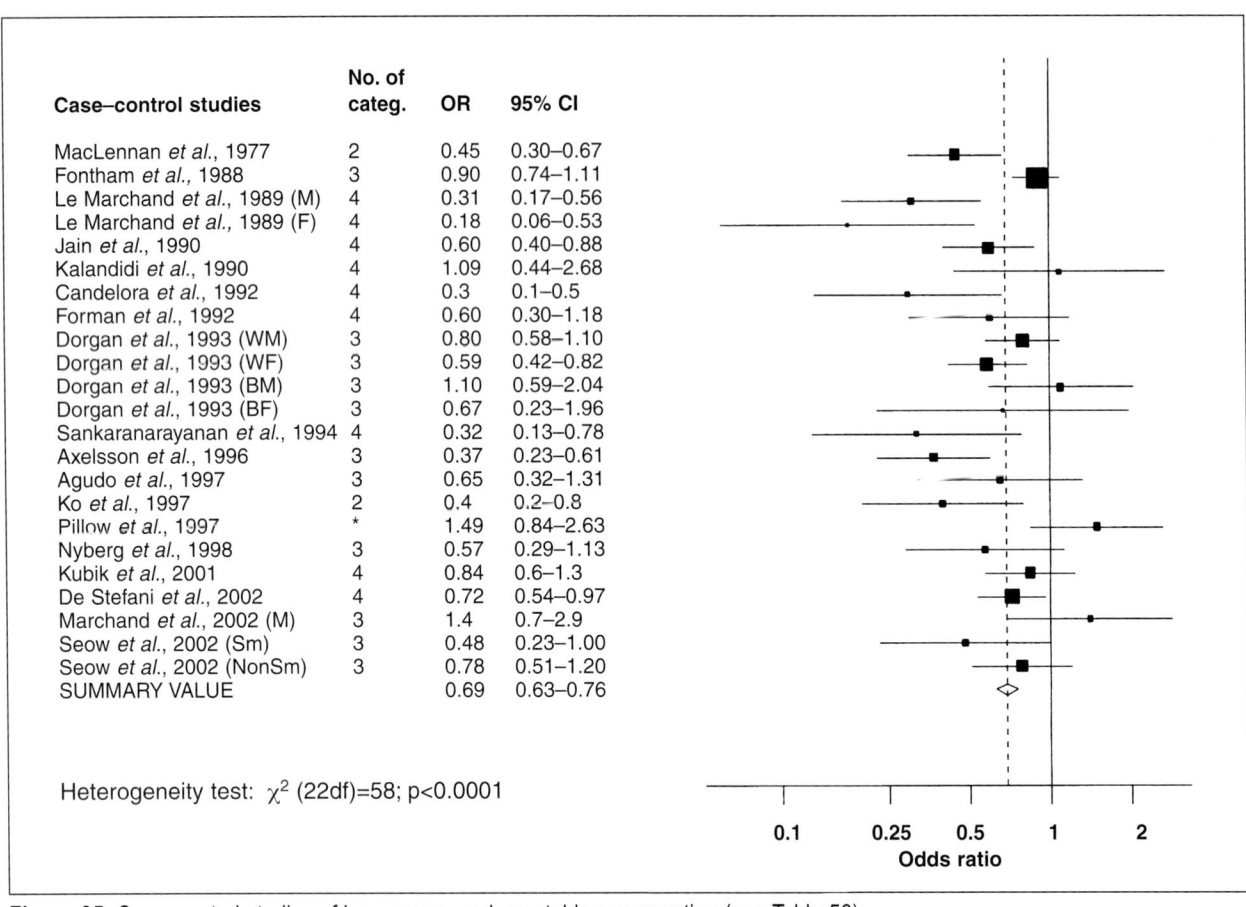

Figure 35. Case–control studies of lung cancer and vegetable consumption (see Table 58)
M = males; F = females; W = white; B = black; Sm = smokers; NonSm = non-smokers.

associated with reduced risk of breast cancer. However, relatively few studies have examined whether the association between vegetable consumption and breast cancer risk is modified by menopausal status. In those studies that have examined both pre-menopausal and postmenopausal breast cancer, no effect modification by menopausal status or by age group was generally observed. However, in a large Italian case–control study, raw vegetable consumption was inversely associated with the risk of pre-menopausal, but not postmenopausal, breast cancer (p-value for interaction = 0.01) (Franceschi et al., 1995; Braga et al., 1997b). Educational level also has not been found to modify the association between vegetable consumption and the risk of breast cancer.

In a meta-analysis of 14 case–control studies and three cohort studies of 16 052 cases (Gandini et al., 2000), a summary estimate for vegetables was generated by combining study-specific risk estimates for vegetables, cooked vegetables, raw vegetables, green vegetables and other vegetables (Table 63). Overall, there was a 25% reduction in the relative risk of breast cancer for comparison of the highest versus lowest categories of vegetable intake; however, there was statistically significant between-study heterogeneity ($p < 0.001$). When the analysis was restricted to the 16 studies with dose–response information, reductions in the risk of breast cancer were observed for intakes as low as three portions compared to one per week (RR = 0.91, 95% CI 0.89–0.93). A 20% reduction in risk was observed for eating six portions versus one per week (RR = 0.79, 95% CI 0.77–0.80). Again, there was statistically significant between-study heterogeneity for these summary estimates ($p < 0.001$). The results for vegetable consumption were suggestive of weaker associations among studies using a validated questionnaire (RR = 0.85, 95% CI 0.71–1.01 for high versus low consumption) than with a non-validated one (RR = 0.66, 95% CI 0.55–0.81; *p* for interaction = 0.13), among studies reporting univariate (RR = 0.86, 95% CI 0.77–0.97) versus multivariate relative risks (RR = 0.68, 95% CI 0.56–0.83; *p* for interaction = 0.22), and among non-Mediterranean (RR = 0.77, 95% CI 0.66–0.92) compared with Mediterranean countries (RR = 0.67, 95% CI 0.54–0.87; *p* for interaction = 0.48). Other sources of heterogeneity are that relative risks for different categories of intake for different vegetable groups were combined into a summary estimate.

Combined fruit and vegetables
Cohort studies
Total fruit and vegetable consumption was not significantly associated with breast cancer risk in two out of three cohort studies (Table 65). In the Nurses' Health Study, there was an inverse association with total fruit and vegetable consumption among premenopausal women (Zhang *et al.*, 1999). The association was stronger among premenopausal women with a family history of breast cancer or who drank at least 15 grams of alcohol per day. In this study, fruit and vegetable consumption was not associated with breast cancer risk among postmenopausal women, but an inverse association was suggested among postmenopausal women who were current users of hormone replacement therapy.

In a pooled analysis of eight prospective studies (including the Nurses' Health Study mentioned above), total fruit and vegetable consumption was not associated with breast cancer risk overall or for premenopausal or postmenopausal breast cancer (*p* for interaction by menopausal status = 0.57) (Smith-Warner *et al.*, 2001).

Case–control studies
Among the four case–control studies that considered combined fruit and vegetable consumption, a significant inverse association was found in only one (Ronco *et al.*, 1999) (Table 66).

Breast cancer in men
In three case–control studies of the association between fruit and vegetable consumption and risk of breast cancer in men (Table 67), the results are inconsistent and the evidence is too limited to allow any conclusion to be drawn.

Discussion
About 30 studies have evaluated the categories of total fruit or total vegetables in relation to risk of breast cancer. Total fruit consumption generally has not been significantly associated with risk in either a protective or harmful direction, the relative risks being mostly between 0.8 and 1.2 for comparisons of high versus low fruit intake. For the six evaluable cohort studies, the mean RR was 0.82 (95% CI 0.71–0.95), range 0.74–1.08 (Figure 36) and for the 12 case–control studies the mean OR was 0.99 (95% CI 0.92–1.07), range 0.57–1.82 (Figure 37). For total vegetable consumption, case–control studies have been more suggestive of an inverse association than the cohort studies, but they are more susceptible to recall and selection bias than cohort studies. For the five evaluable cohort studies, the mean RR was 0.94 (95% CI 0.83–1.07), range 0.64–1.43 (Figure 38) and for the 12 case–control studies the mean OR was 0.66 (95% CI 0.57–0.75), range 0.09–1.40 (Figure 39). There was little suggestion that associations between fruit and vegetable consumption and breast cancer risk differ by menopausal status. The Working Group could not exclude the possibility that fruit and vegetable consumption is associated with a slight decrease in the risk of breast cancer. Errors in the measurement of fruit and vegetable consumption may have attenuated the results, so it is possible that stronger inverse associations could be observed if more accurate dietary assessment methods were used to estimate fruit and vegetable intake. There are inadequate data on effects of diet during early life on subsequent risk of developing breast cancer. Few studies have examined effect modification.

Cervix
Fruit
Cohort studies
No studies were identified by the Working Group.

Case–control studies
In five studies that addressed the association of intake of fruit with invasive cervix cancer, most point estimates were below 1.0, although confidence intervals generally included the null (Table 68). The exception with a significant inverse association reported was a hospital-based study in Japan (Hirose *et al.*, 1996).

Vegetables
Cohort studies
No studies were identified by the Working Group.

Case–control studies
There is evidence of an inverse association, but confidence intervals often included the null (Table 69).

Combined fruit and vegetables
Two studies have examined total fruit and vegetable intake with regard to risk of cancer of the cervix (Table 70), one showing evidence of an inverse association and the other no significant effect.

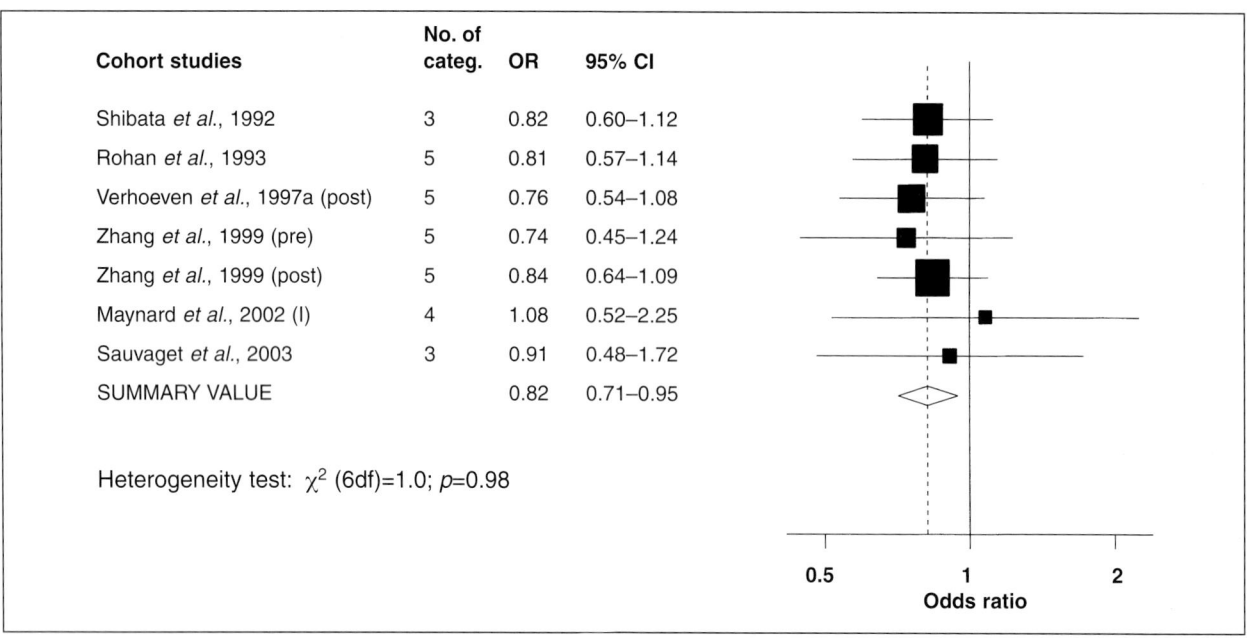

Cohort studies	No. of categ.	OR	95% CI
Shibata et al., 1992	3	0.82	0.60–1.12
Rohan et al., 1993	5	0.81	0.57–1.14
Verhoeven et al., 1997a (post)	5	0.76	0.54–1.08
Zhang et al., 1999 (pre)	5	0.74	0.45–1.24
Zhang et al., 1999 (post)	5	0.84	0.64–1.09
Maynard et al., 2002 (I)	4	1.08	0.52–2.25
Sauvaget et al., 2003	3	0.91	0.48–1.72
SUMMARY VALUE		0.82	0.71–0.95

Heterogeneity test: χ^2 (6df)=1.0; p=0.98

Figure 36 Cohort studies of breast cancer in women and fruit consumption (see Table 61)
Pre = premenopausal; post = postmenopausal; I = incidence

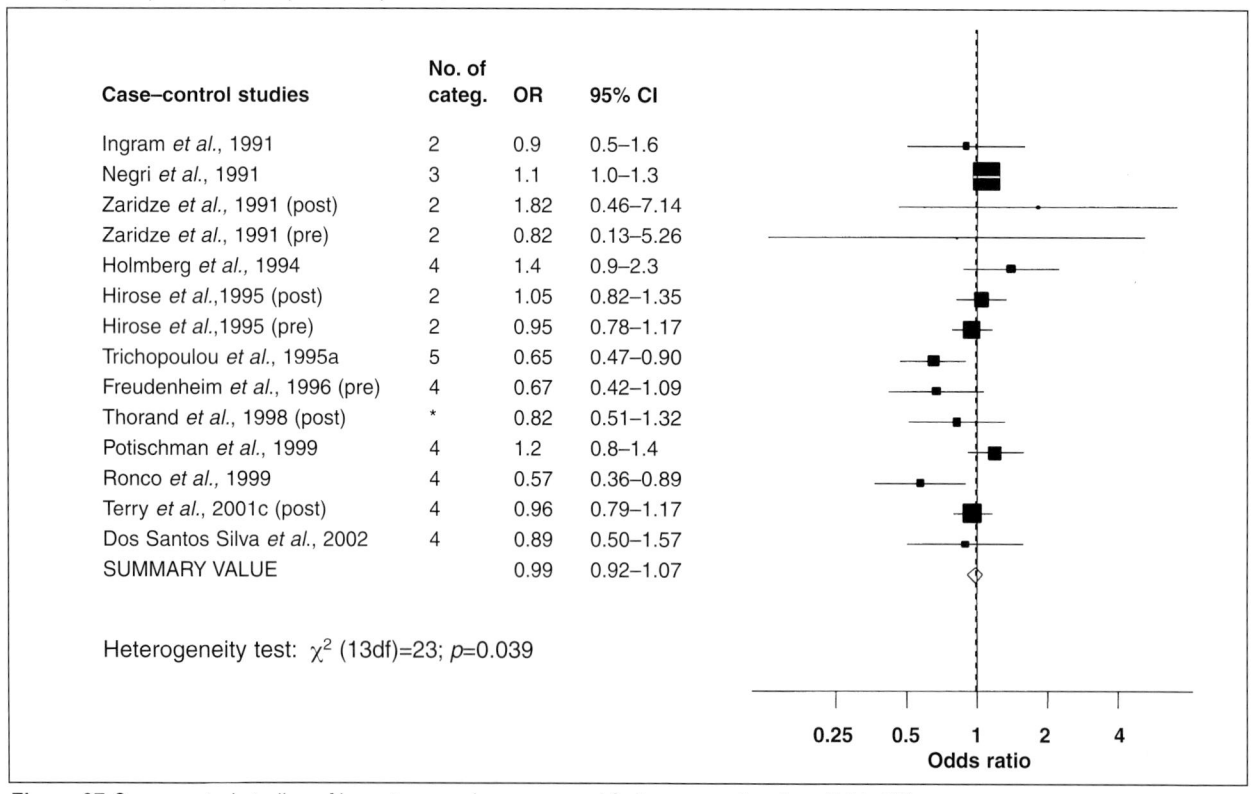

Case–control studies	No. of categ.	OR	95% CI
Ingram et al., 1991	2	0.9	0.5–1.6
Negri et al., 1991	3	1.1	1.0–1.3
Zaridze et al., 1991 (post)	2	1.82	0.46–7.14
Zaridze et al., 1991 (pre)	2	0.82	0.13–5.26
Holmberg et al., 1994	4	1.4	0.9–2.3
Hirose et al.,1995 (post)	2	1.05	0.82–1.35
Hirose et al.,1995 (pre)	2	0.95	0.78–1.17
Trichopoulou et al., 1995a	5	0.65	0.47–0.90
Freudenheim et al., 1996 (pre)	4	0.67	0.42–1.09
Thorand et al., 1998 (post)	*	0.82	0.51–1.32
Potischman et al., 1999	4	1.2	0.8–1.4
Ronco et al., 1999	4	0.57	0.36–0.89
Terry et al., 2001c (post)	4	0.96	0.79–1.17
Dos Santos Silva et al., 2002	4	0.89	0.50–1.57
SUMMARY VALUE		0.99	0.92–1.07

Heterogeneity test: χ^2 (13df)=23; p=0.039

Figure 37 Case–control studies of breast cancer in women and fruit consumption (see Table 62)
Pre = premenopausal; post = postmenopausal; * = not applicable

Cancer-preventive effects

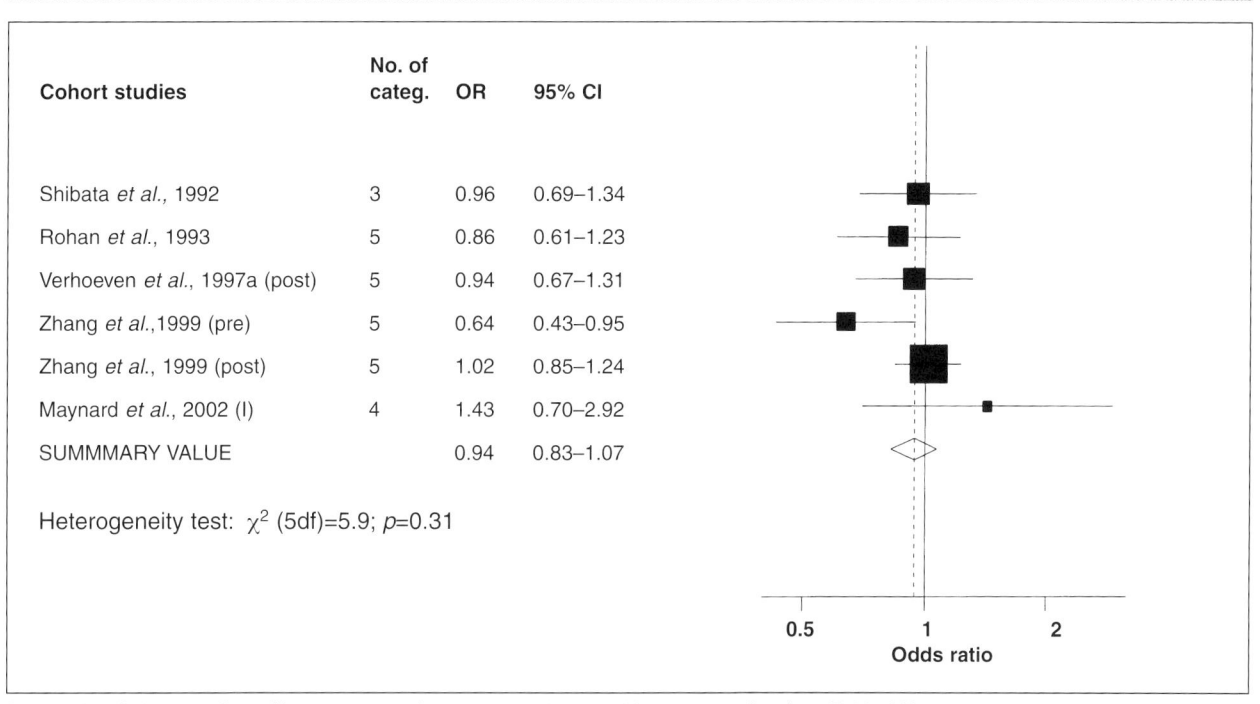

Cohort studies	No. of categ.	OR	95% CI
Shibata et al., 1992	3	0.96	0.69–1.34
Rohan et al., 1993	5	0.86	0.61–1.23
Verhoeven et al., 1997a (post)	5	0.94	0.67–1.31
Zhang et al.,1999 (pre)	5	0.64	0.43–0.95
Zhang et al., 1999 (post)	5	1.02	0.85–1.24
Maynard et al., 2002 (I)	4	1.43	0.70–2.92
SUMMMARY VALUE		0.94	0.83–1.07

Heterogeneity test: χ^2 (5df)=5.9; p=0.31

Figure 38 Cohort studies of breast cancer in women and vegetable consumption (see Table 63)
Pre = premenopausal; post = postmenopausal; I = incidence

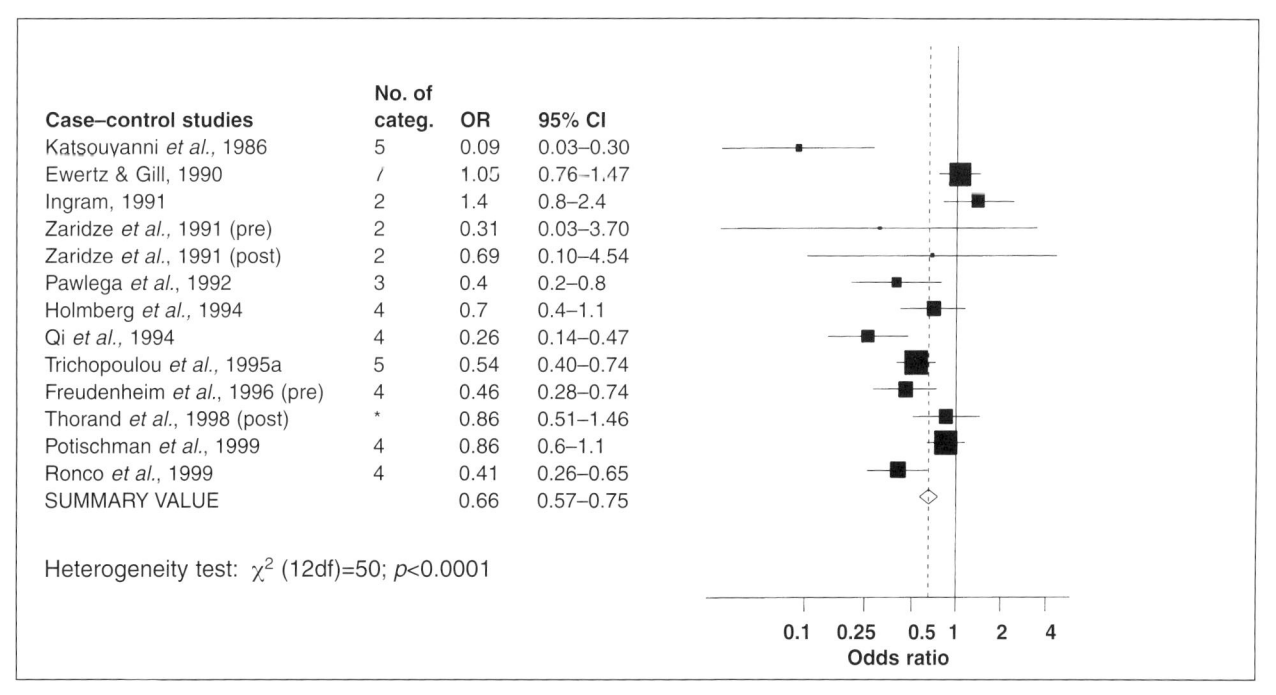

Case–control studies	No. of categ.	OR	95% CI
Katsouyanni et al., 1986	5	0.09	0.03–0.30
Ewertz & Gill, 1990	7	1.05	0.76–1.47
Ingram, 1991	2	1.4	0.8–2.4
Zaridze et al., 1991 (pre)	2	0.31	0.03–3.70
Zaridze et al., 1991 (post)	2	0.69	0.10–4.54
Pawlega et al., 1992	3	0.4	0.2–0.8
Holmberg et al., 1994	4	0.7	0.4–1.1
Qi et al., 1994	4	0.26	0.14–0.47
Trichopoulou et al., 1995a	5	0.54	0.40–0.74
Freudenheim et al., 1996 (pre)	4	0.46	0.28–0.74
Thorand et al., 1998 (post)	*	0.86	0.51–1.46
Potischman et al., 1999	4	0.86	0.6–1.1
Ronco et al., 1999	4	0.41	0.26–0.65
SUMMARY VALUE		0.66	0.57–0.75

Heterogeneity test: χ^2 (12df)=50; p<0.0001

Figure 39 Case–control studies of breast cancer in women and vegetable consumption (see Table 64)
pre = premenopausal; post = postmenopausal; * = not applicable

In situ cervical cancer

The association of fruit and vegetable intake with risk of *in situ* cervical cancer has been examined in only one case–control study (Table 71); there was an inverse association with fruit intake but not with vegetables.

Cervical dysplasia

One case–control study examining risk for cervical dysplasia in relation to intake of fruit and vegetables has been reported (Table 72). Cervical dysplasia is difficult to study because of problems with case ascertainment. In this study, there is some concern about the comparability of the study base for the cases and controls. Fruit intake appeared to be associated with reduced risk. There was no analysis of total vegetable intake.

Discussion

In all, nine case–control studies have addressed associations between fruit and vegetable intake and either invasive cancer or precancerous lesions of the cervix. The findings are not completely consistent and there is little evidence for a strong effect of intake of these foods on risk.

In considering these findings, several limitations need to be kept in mind. The lack of evidence from cohort studies makes it hard to evaluate the effect of recall and selection bias on the results. Further, there are concerns with measurement error. As in all observational studies, confounding is possible. Of particular concern for cervical cancer is the role of diet in a pathway that includes human papillomavirus (HPV). If fruit and vegetable intake is important in a causal pathway that includes HPV, it would be important to determine the HPV status of controls. Alternatively, HPV may operate as a confounder if both diet and HPV status are related to social status. However, in a study conducted in India where HPV was measured in both cases and controls, there was little difference between the OR measured for the full control group and that for the group of controls who were HPV-positive (Rajkumar *et al.*, 2003a).

Endometrium
Fruit
Cohort studies
No studies were identified by the Working Group.

Case–control studies
Eleven studies have examined the association between intake of fruit and risk of endometrial cancer (Table 73). In many of these, ORs were close to one and confidence intervals included the null. For the four studies where there was a significant inverse association, ORs were in the range 0.45–0.7.

Vegetables
Cohort studies
No studies were identified by the Working Group.

Case–control studies
Of 11 case–control studies that evaluated intake of vegetables, inverse associations were reported in eight, six being statistically significant (Table 74). In one study in Japan, a significant increase in risk was associated with consumption of raw but not green vegetables (Hirose *et al.*, 1996).

Combined fruit and vegetables
Cohort studies
In one cohort study, an inverse association between risk of endometrium cancer and combined fruit and vegetable intake was reported, but the confidence interval was wide and included the null (Table 75).

Case–control studies
In all three studies, total intake of fruit and vegetables was inversely associated with risk of endometrium cancer; in one the trend was significant (Table 76).

Discussion

Fruit consumption was evaluable in seven case–control studies, resulting in a mean OR of 1.03 (95% CI 0.90–1.17), range 0.67–1.97 (Figure 40). For the five evaluable studies on vegetable consumption, the mean OR was 0.75 (95% CI 0.64–0.89), range 0.65–1.00 (Figure 41). It is difficult to make comparisons among these studies because of differences in the composition of the diet in different regions and because of considerable differences in dietary assessment. There appears to be inconsistent evidence of an inverse association with these foods.

An important confounder to consider in the study of endometrial cancer is body mass index; most but not all of the studies included control for this.

Overall these results provide weak evidence at best for an effect of fruit and vegetable intake on risk of endometrial cancer.

Ovary
Fruit
Cohort studies
Neither of two cohort studies of fruit intake and ovary cancer risk found an association (Table 77).

Case–control studies
Among four case–control studies of total fruit intake in relation to risk of ovary cancer (Table 78), one found a significant inverse association, but in another fruit intake was positively associated with risk.

Vegetables
Cohort studies
In the two available studies, the association of vegetable intake with risk was inverse, but for both, the confi-

Cancer-preventive effects

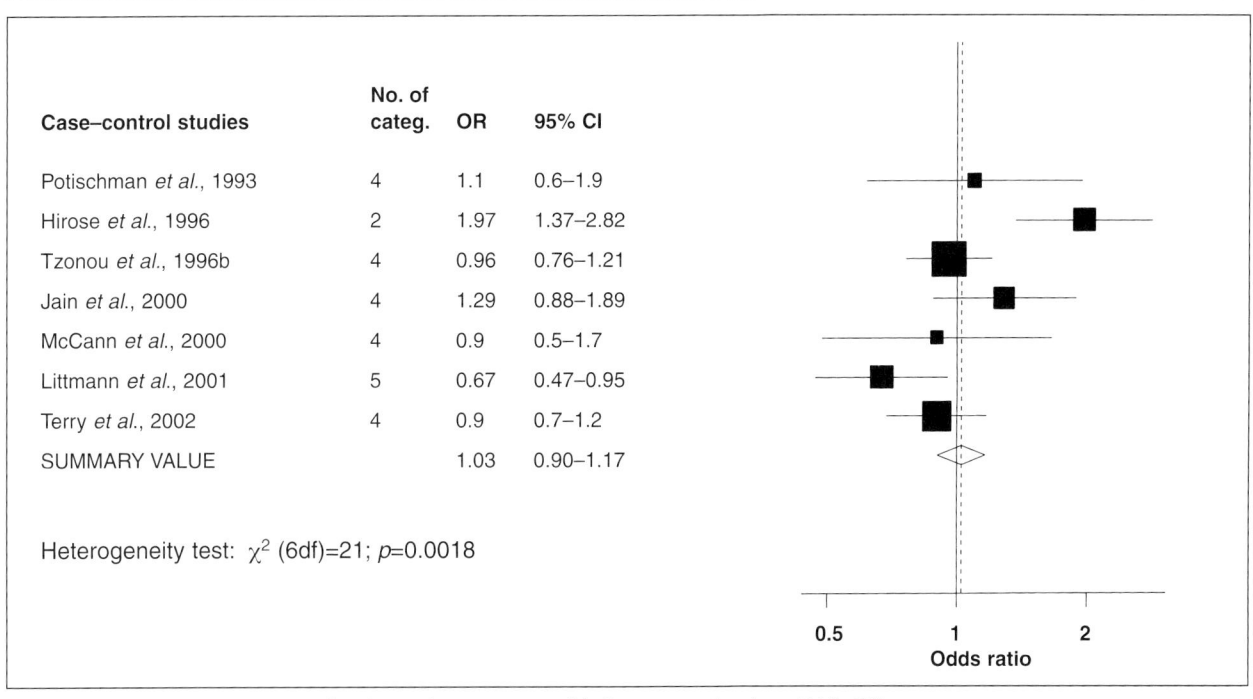

Case–control studies	No. of categ.	OR	95% CI
Potischman et al., 1993	4	1.1	0.6–1.9
Hirose et al., 1996	2	1.97	1.37–2.82
Tzonou et al., 1996b	4	0.96	0.76–1.21
Jain et al., 2000	4	1.29	0.88–1.89
McCann et al., 2000	4	0.9	0.5–1.7
Littmann et al., 2001	5	0.67	0.47–0.95
Terry et al., 2002	4	0.9	0.7–1.2
SUMMARY VALUE		1.03	0.90–1.17

Heterogeneity test: χ^2 (6df)=21; p=0.0018

Figure 40 Case–control studies of endometrium cancer and fruit consumption (see Table 73)

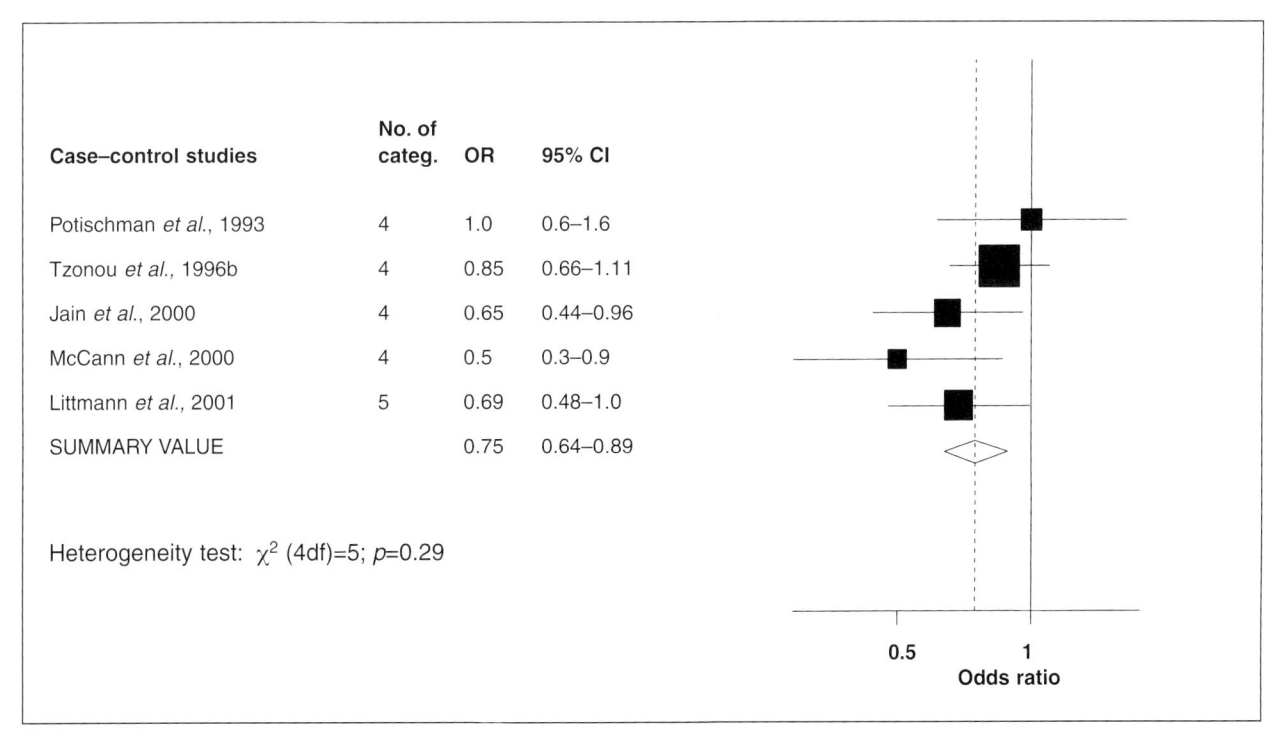

Case–control studies	No. of categ.	OR	95% CI
Potischman et al., 1993	4	1.0	0.6–1.6
Tzonou et al., 1996b	4	0.85	0.66–1.11
Jain et al., 2000	4	0.65	0.44–0.96
McCann et al., 2000	4	0.5	0.3–0.9
Littmann et al., 2001	5	0.69	0.48–1.0
SUMMARY VALUE		0.75	0.64–0.89

Heterogeneity test: χ^2 (4df)=5; p=0.29

Figure 41 Case-control studies of endometrium cancer and vegetable consumption (see Table 74)

dence intervals included the null (Table 79).

Case–control studies
Among six case–control studies of vegetable intake, a significant inverse association was seen in three (Table 80).

Combined fruit and vegetables
Cohort study
In one study, although adult intake was not associated with risk (Table 81), the reported intake of six fruits and vegetables during adolescence was associated with decreased risk (OR 0.54, 95% CI 0.29–1.03, *p* for trend 0.04) (Falrfield *et al.*, 2001).

Case–control study
In one hospital-based study, there was an inverse association with intake of combined fruit and vegetable intake (Table 82).

Discussion
In general, the limited number of cohort and case–control studies that considered fruit intake found little indication of an inverse association. Findings from two cohort studies indicated an approximately 25% reduction in risk with increased intake of vegetables; of the six case–control studies that addressed vegetable intake, five yielded point estimates below 1.0, although many of the confidence intervals included the null.

Wide confidence intervals may be the result of relatively small numbers of cases, especially in the cohort studies. The inverse association in one study with fruit and vegetable intake in adolescence is suggestive that early dietary exposures may be of importance.

Overall, these studies suggest that there may be a protective effect for ovary cancer associated with vegetable intake. The association with fruit intake is less consistent.

Prostate
The etiology of prostate cancer is very poorly understood and there are no established risk factors other than male sex, age, family history and ethnic group. The international variation in prostate cancer rates, together with ecological analyses, has suggested that dietary factors including fruit and vegetables may be associated with risk.

The surgical procedure trans-urethral resection of the prostate (TURP), employed for the treatment of urinary obstruction due to non-malignant enlargement of the peri-urethral zone of the prostate, became common in many countries in the late 1980s and led to increased diagnosis of small prostate cancers when the material removed was examined histologically. In the 1990s, the use of measurements of serum concentrations of prostate-specific antigen (PSA) became common both as part of the investigation of urinary symptoms and for testing asymptomatic men for prostate cancer. As a result, an increasing proportion of the prostate cancers diagnosed in the last 15 years have been small tumours which may behave non-aggressively, whereas in studies conducted in the 1970s and early 1980s most were diagnosed clinically. Thus the end-point in epidemiological studies has changed somewhat and this could potentially affect any associations of prostate cancer risk with dietary factors.

Some recent studies have suggested that tomatoes have a specific protective effect against prostate cancer. No attempt was made by the Working Group to evaluate this hypothesis. Lycopene (a constituent of tomatoes) was evaluated previously (IARC, 1998).

Fruit
Cohort studies
Results from ten cohort studies on the association of total fruit intake with prostate cancer risk have been published (Table 83). In three, non-significant inverse associations were found, but in six the relative risks for high fruit consumption were greater than 1.0.

Case–control studies
Eleven case–control studies with results on the association of total fruit intake with prostate cancer risk have been published (Table 84). In only one was a significant inverse association found, while in eight the relative risks for high fruit consumption were greater than 1.0

Vegetables
Cohort studies
Eight cohort studies with results on the association of total vegetable intake with prostate cancer risk have been published (Table 85). In four, relative risks for high vegetable consumption were less than 1.0, but none significantly so.

Case–control studies
Thirteen case–control studies with results on the association of total vegetable intake with prostate cancer risk have been published (Table 86). In nine, relative risks for high fruit consumption were less than 1.0, and significant reductions in risk were observed in four studies.

Combined fruit and vegetables
Cohort studies
In the two studies that considered combined fruit and vegetable consumption, there was no evidence of an inverse association (Table 87).

Case–control study
In one case–control study, there was evidence of an association between combined fruit and vegetable consumption and prostate cancer risk (Table 88).

Discussion

There is little evidence to support a protective effect of fruit intake on prostate cancer risk. For fruit consumption, eight evaluable cohort studies gave a mean RR of 1.11 (95% CI 0.98–1.26), range 0.84–1.57 (Figure 42) and nine evaluble case–control studies gave a mean OR of 1.08 (95% CI 0.98–1.18), range 0.40–1.70 (Figure 43). Vegetable consumption was evaluable in six cohort studies; mean RR 0.95 (95% CI 0.84–1.08), range 0.7–1.04 (Figure 44) and nine case–control studies, mean OR 0.90 (95% CI 0.82–1.00), range 0.6–1.39 (Figure 45).

Testis

Testicular cancer accounts for less than 2% of malignant neoplasms in men, but is the most common malignancy in young adult men aged 15–44 years in most developed countries, and its incidence has been increasing in developed countries throughout the world. An ecological association with consumption of fat, energy intake and dairy products was identified (Armstrong & Doll, 1975), but only two case–control studies (Table 89) have investigated the influence of total fruit and vegetable consumption on testicular cancer risk. In neither were there significant inverse associations with fruit or vegetable consumption.

An additional case–control study conducted in East Anglia, UK, aiming to test the hypothesis that milk and dairy products are risk factors for testicular cancer collected data on fresh fruit and vegetable consumption in adolescence (Davies et al., 1996). Although cases tended to have eaten fewer oranges, apples and fruit salads than the population controls, the difference was not statistically significant, while the reverse was the case for vegetable salads.

Discussion

The information available is too sparse to allow any conclusion on the association of fruit and vegetables with testis cancer to be drawn.

Bladder

The Working Group adopted the usual convention of including studies of all urothelial cancers among the general group of bladder cancers.

Fruit
Cohort studies
Of five cohort studies (Table 90), two show a statistically significant inverse association with fruit consumption. However, in the study by Zeegers et al. (2001), the trend is inconsistent and varies between different categories of smokers. In this study, stratified ORs by smoking habits indicated a non-significant inverse association among current smokers and in ex-smokers who smoked more than 15 cigarettes per day.

Case–control studies
Among the four case–control studies identified (Table 91), inverse associations were seen in three for total fruit intake, two of which were statistically significant.

Meta-analyses
Results of two formal meta-analyses considering fruit consumption and bladder cancer risk have been reported. Steinmaus et al. (2000) included nine studies with data on fruit (four cohort and five case–control). The OR for high versus low consumption was [0.71 (95% CI adjusted for heterogeneity statistic 0.55–0.92)]. There was little variation by study type. Riboli & Norat (2003) included eight studies in their meta-analysis (three cohort and five case–control); the OR for an increase in consumption of 100 g of fruit per day was 0.81 (0.73–0.91). Again there was little variation by study type.

Vegetables
Cohort studies
None of the four cohort studies reporting information on vegetables (Table 92) reported a statistically significant inverse association with the consumption of vegetables. Two reported non-significant inverse associations, but one was with green-yellow vegetables.

Case–control studies
Out of four case–control studies identified, only three reported information on total vegetables and one on green-yellow and other vegetables separately (Table 93). Two studies found inverse associations with vegetable consumption, but neither was statistically significant. In the study by Zeegers et al. (2001), stratified ORs by smoking habits indicated a non-significant inverse association only among current heavy smokers.

Meta-analyses
Results of two formal meta-analyses considering vegetable consumption and bladder cancer risk have been reported. Steinmaus et al. (2000) included 10 studies with data on vegetables (three cohort and seven case–control). The OR for high versus low consumption was [0.86 (95% CI adjusted for heterogeneity statistic 0.75–0.99)]. There was little variation by study type. Riboli & Norat (2003) included six studies in their meta-analysis (two cohort and four case–control); the OR for an increase in consumption of 100 g of vegetables per day was 0.91 (95% CI 0.82–1.00). Again there was little variation by study type.

Combined fruit and vegetables
Cohort studies
In two cohort studies, no association of combined fruit and vegetable intake with bladder cancer risk was seen (Table 94).

IARC Handbooks of Cancer Prevention Volume 8: Fruit and Vegetables

Cohort studies	No. of categ.	OR	95% CI
Mills et al., 1989	3	1.07	0.72–1.58
Severson et al., 1989	3	1.57	0.95–2.61
Hsing et al., 1990	4	0.9	0.6–1.4
Shibata et al., 1992	3	1.04	0.74–1.46
Giovannucci et al., 1995	*	0.84	0.59–1.84
Schuurman et al., 1998	5	1.31	0.96–1.79
Chan et al., 2000	5	1.3	0.8–2.2
Key et al., 2003	5	1.06	0.84–1.34
SUMMARY VALUE		1.11	0.98–1.26

Heterogeneity test: χ^2 (7df)=5.5; p=0.6

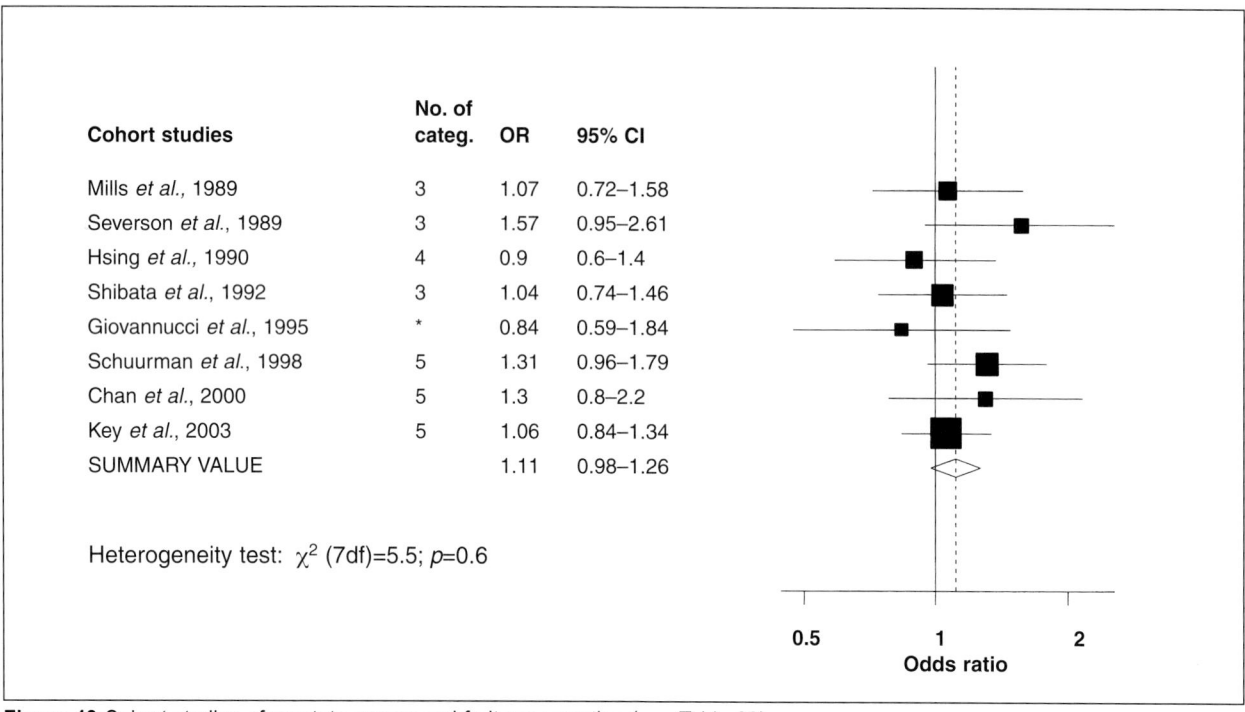

Figure 42 Cohort studies of prostate cancer and fruit consumption (see Table 83)
*Not applicable

Case–control studies	No. of categ.	OR	95% CI
Negri et al., 1991	3	0.4	0.3–0.8
De Stefani et al., 1995	3	1.7	1.1–2.8
Deneo-Pellegrini et al., 1999	4	0.8	0.4–1.4
Jain et al., 1999	4	1.51	1.14–2.01
Sung et al., 1999	2	1.16	0.57–2.35
Tzonou et al., 1999	5	0.98	0.86–1.13
Villeneuve et al., 1999	4	1.5	1.1–1.9
Cohen et al., 2000	4	1.07	0.72–1.60
Kolonel et al., 2000	5	1.01	0.79–1.28
SUMMARY VALUE		1.08	0.98–1.18

Heterogeneity test: χ^2 (8df)=33; p<0.0001

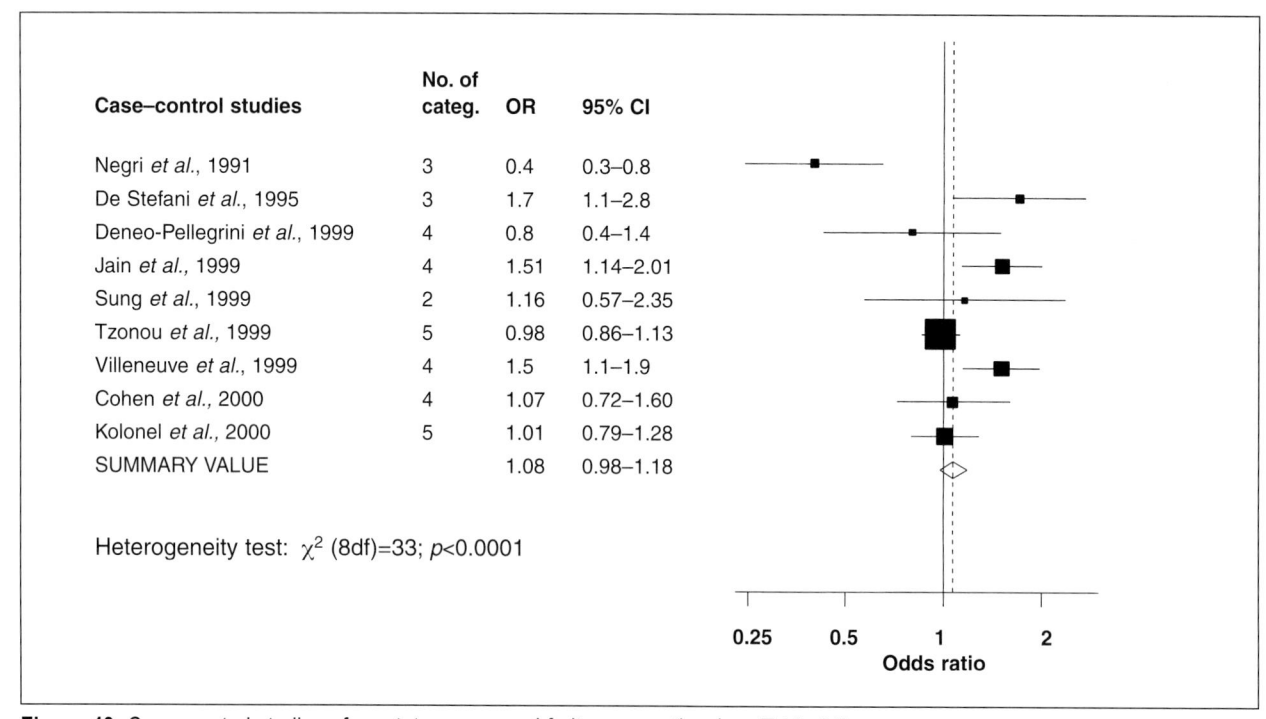

Figure 43 Case–control studies of prostate cancer and fruit consumption (see Table 84)

Cancer-preventive effects

Cohort studies	No. of categ.	OR	95% CI
Hsing et al., 1990	4	0.7	0.4–1.2
Shibata et al., 1992	3	1.04	0.74–1.46
Giovannucci et al., 1995	*	1.04	0.81–1.34
Schuurman et al., 1998	5	0.80	0.57–1.12
Chan et al., 2000	5	0.8	0.5–1.3
Key et al., 2003	5	1.00	0.81–1.23
SUMMARY VALUE		0.95	0.84–1.08

Heterogeneity test: χ^2 (5df)=3.7; p=0.6

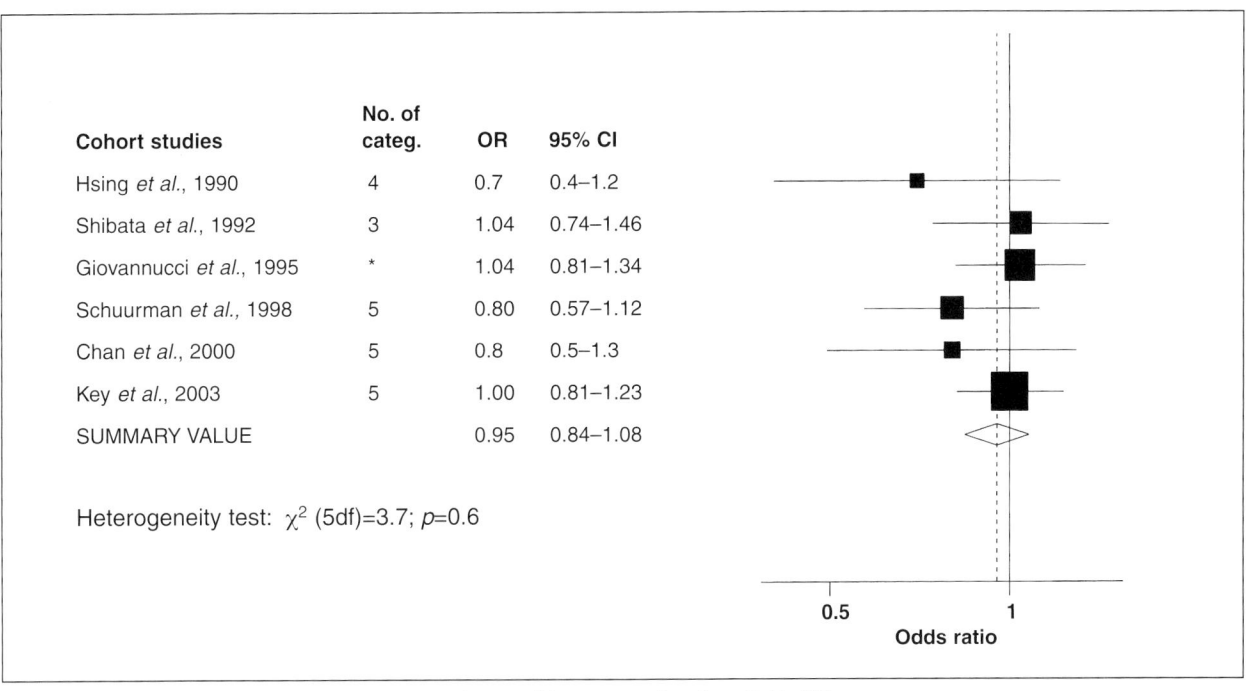

Figure 44 Cohort studies of prostate cancer and vegetable consumption (see Table 85)
*Not applicable

Case–control studies	No. of categ.	OR	95% CI
Oishi et al., 1988	3	0.07	0.43 1.76
Talamini et al., 1992	3	1.39	0.88–2.17
De Stefani et al., 1995	3	1.1	0.6–1.9
Deneo-Pellegrini et al., 1999	4	0.6	0.3–1.1
Jain et al., 1999	4	0.95	0.68–1.33
Tzonou et al., 1999	5	0.94	0.81–1.10
Villeneuve et al., 1999	4	1.0	0.8–1.3
Cohen et al., 2000	4	0.65	0.45–0.94
Kolonel et al., 2000	5	0.74	0.58–0.96
SUMMARY VALUE		0.90	0.82–1.00

Heterogeneity test: χ^2 (8df)=12; p=0.15

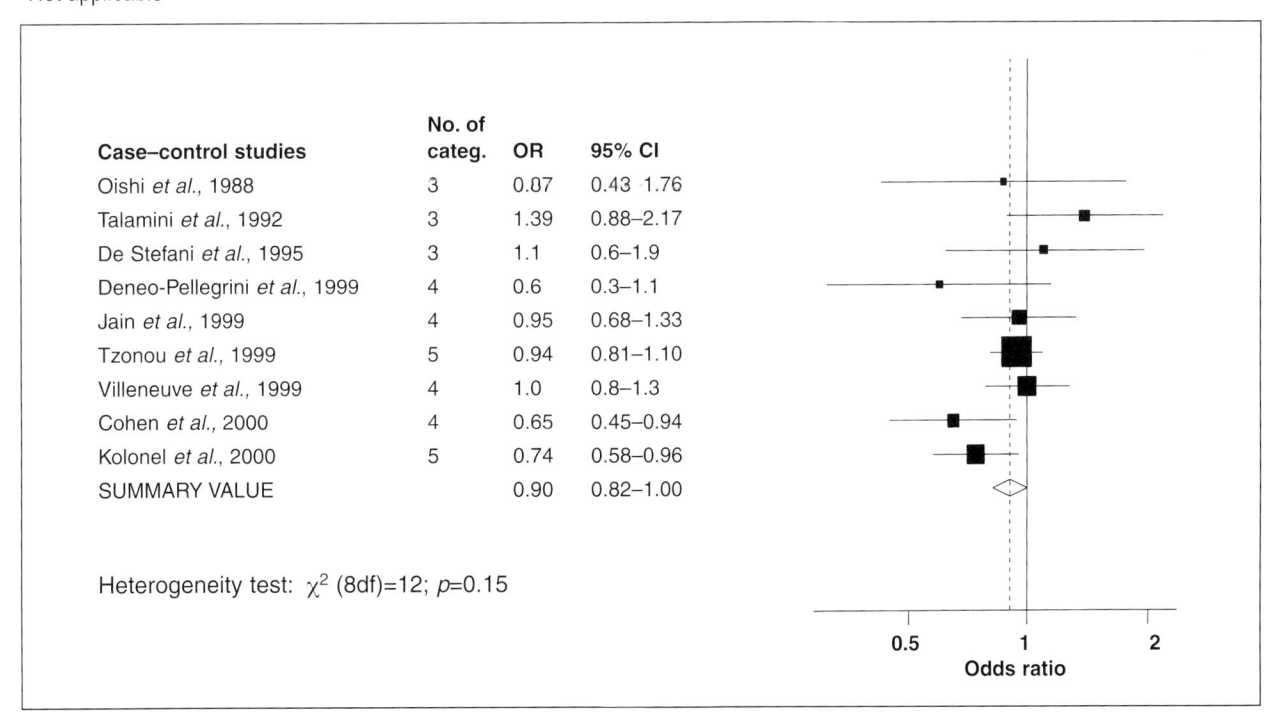

Figure 45 Case–control studies of prostate cancer and vegetable consumption (see Table 86)

Case–control studies
Inverse associations were noted in two out of three case–control studies in which combined fruit and vegetable intake was considered, but the association was significant only for males in one (Table 95).

Discussion
Cohort studies of the relationship between fruit and vegetable consumption and bladder cancer risk were generally set up to investigate diet, with the exception of that of Nagano *et al.* (2000), whose main goal was to study survivors of the atomic bombings. Most case–control studies had a hospital-based design; this design has limitations related to the recruitment of subjects with diet-associated diseases in the control group. Virtually all studies used food frequency questionnaires and adjusted for relevant confounders (gender, age, smoking and energy intake). The case–control studies more often found inverse associations than the cohort studies, but the findings were not consistent. For the five evaluable cohort studies on fruit consumption, the mean RR was 0.87 (95% CI 0.72–1.04), range 0.63–1.12 (Figure 46); for the four evaluable case–control studies, the mean OR was 0.74 (95% CI 0.59–0.92), range 0.53–0.95 (Figure 47). For vegetable consumption, the mean OR for the three evaluable cohort studies was 0.94 (95% CI 0.76–1.16), range 0.72–1.16 (Figure 48), and the mean OR for the three evaluable case–control studies was 0.89 (95%CI 0.69–1.14), range 0.66–1.04 (Figure 49).

Although both formal meta-analyses suggest protective effects of fruit and vegetables, the criteria for inclusion of studies varied, and in particular, that of Steinmaus *et al.* (2000) included studies that used surrogate estimates of fruit or vegetable consumption that were not considered by the Working Group.

Therefore, although the evidence of protective effects for fruit and vegetables and bladder cancer is suggestive, especially from the case–control studies, the Working Group felt it was not possible to exclude bias as accounting for the findings.

Kidney
In adults, cancer of the kidney encompasses two major histopathological entities, namely renal-cell (parenchymal) cancer and renal pelvis cancer. The epidemiology of renal pelvis cancer resembles that of bladder cancer more than that of renal-cell cancer and in some studies is included in the grouping urothelial cancer; it would thus have been covered in the previous section. The present review is therefore restricted to renal-cell cancer, which accounts for 80–90% of kidney cancers.

Fruit
Cohort studies
Of two cohort studies of renal-cell cancer reporting data on total fruit consumption (Table 96), only the one with the smaller numbers of cases found an inverse, but non-significant, association.

Case–control studies
The association between total fruit consumption and renal-cell cancer has been considered in seven case–control studies covering populations in North America, northern, central and southern Europe, Asia and Australia (Table 97). Significant inverse associations with fruit consumption were noted in four, but in one study only in males and in another only in non-smokers.

Data from three of these case–control studies (Chow *et al.*, 1994; Mellemgaard *et al.*, 1996; Lindblad *et al.*, 1997) as well as from an Australian study (McCredie & Stewart, 1992) were included in a multicentre analysis of 1185 renal-cell cancer cases and 1526 control subjects (Wolk *et al.*, 1996). In this analysis, there was a suggestion of an inverse association with total fruit consumption, but the association was not significant. In an analysis stratified by smoking status, the inverse association was confined to non-smokers. In the multicentre analysis, only a subset of 260 cases from the US study (Chow *et al.*, 1994) with direct interviews was included.

In a recent large case–control study among non-Asians of Los Angeles, California, which did not present results for total fruit, a strong significant inverse association was observed for citrus fruit (*p* for trend = 0.003) (Yuan *et al.*, 1998).

Vegetables
Cohort studies
In the one cohort study, there was no significant association with vegetable consumption (Table 98).

Case–control studies
Among five case–control studies with information on vegetable consumption, four found inverse associations, but they were significant only in men in one, and in another that considered dark green and yellow-orange vegetables separately (Table 99). In the multicentre study (Wolk *et al.*, 1996), there was a weak non-significant inverse association.

Combined fruit and vegetables
Cohort study
No significant association was observed in the one cohort study that considered combined intake of fruit and vegetables (Table 100).

Case–control studies
In one case–control study, a non-significant inverse association with combined intake of fruit and vegetables was noted in women, but not in men (Table 101).

Cancer-preventive effects

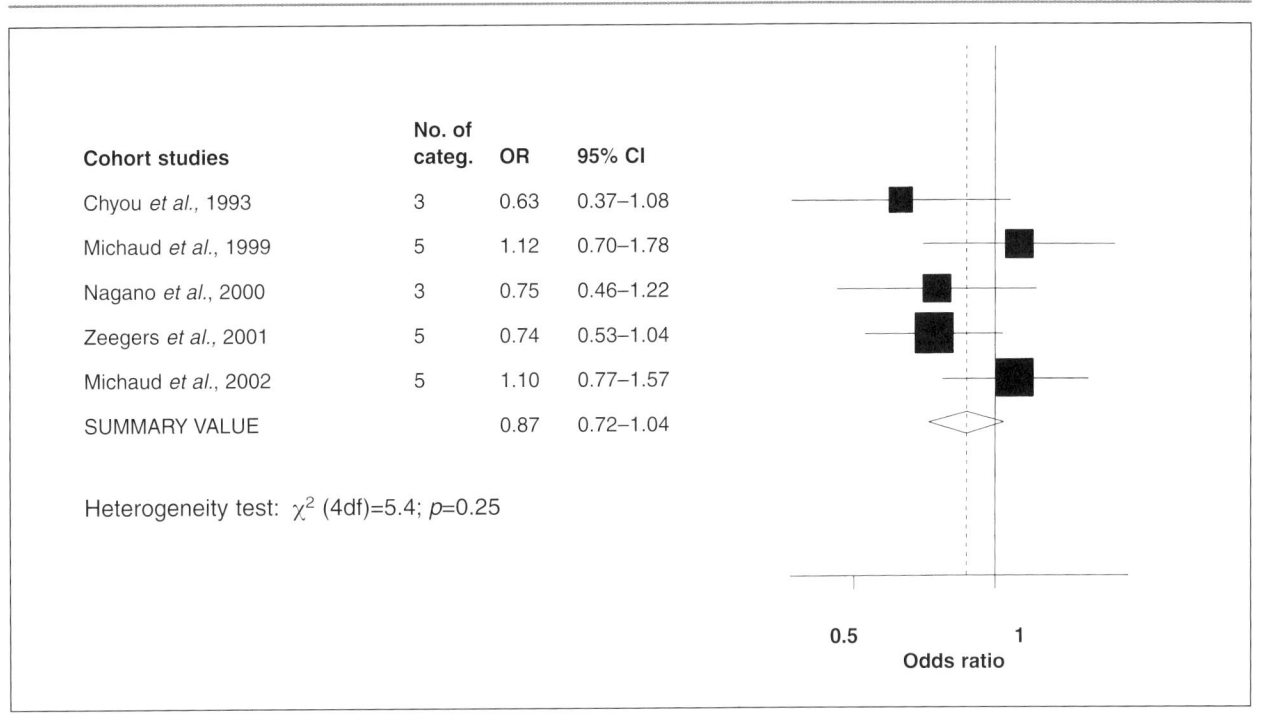

Cohort studies	No. of categ.	OR	95% CI
Chyou et al., 1993	3	0.63	0.37–1.08
Michaud et al., 1999	5	1.12	0.70–1.78
Nagano et al., 2000	3	0.75	0.46–1.22
Zeegers et al., 2001	5	0.74	0.53–1.04
Michaud et al., 2002	5	1.10	0.77–1.57
SUMMARY VALUE		0.87	0.72–1.04

Heterogeneity test: χ^2 (4df)=5.4; p=0.25

Figure 46 Cohort studies of bladder cancer and fruit consumption (see Table 90)

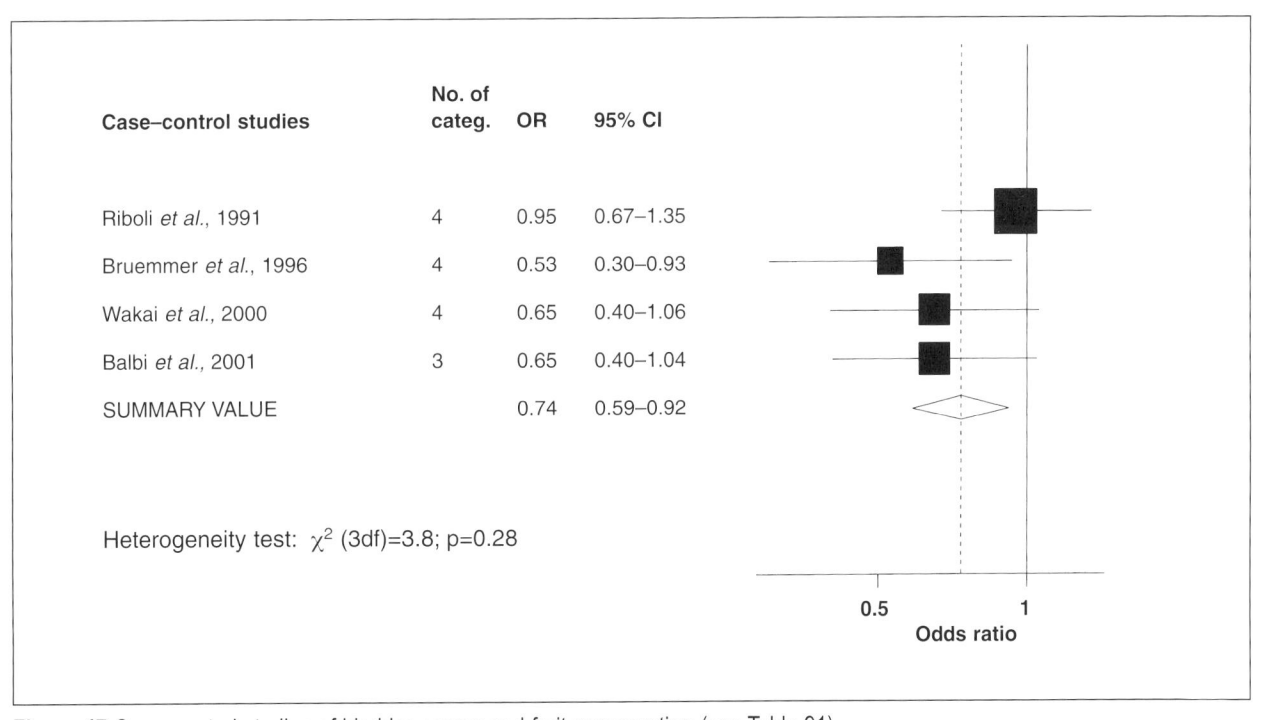

Case–control studies	No. of categ.	OR	95% CI
Riboli et al., 1991	4	0.95	0.67–1.35
Bruemmer et al., 1996	4	0.53	0.30–0.93
Wakai et al., 2000	4	0.65	0.40–1.06
Balbi et al., 2001	3	0.65	0.40–1.04
SUMMARY VALUE		0.74	0.59–0.92

Heterogeneity test: χ^2 (3df)=3.8; p=0.28

Figure 47 Case–control studies of bladder cancer and fruit consumption (see Table 91)

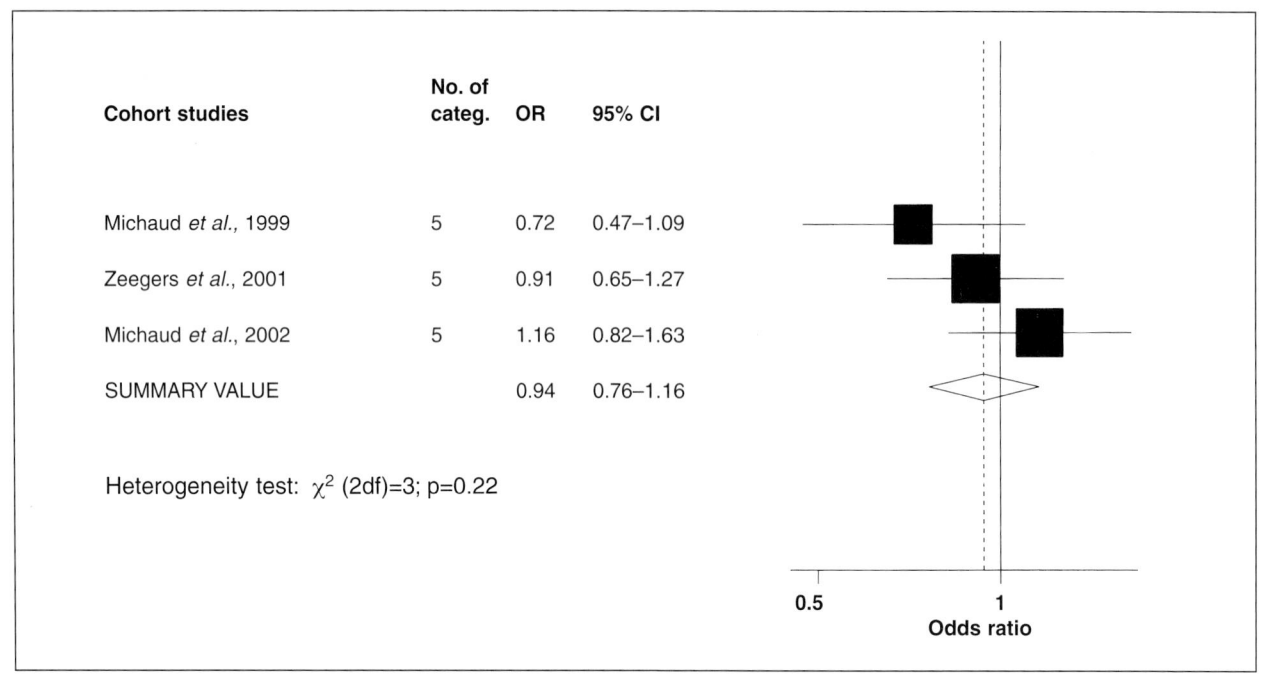

IARC Handbooks of Cancer Prevention Volume 8: Fruit and Vegetables

Cohort studies	No. of categ.	OR	95% CI
Michaud et al., 1999	5	0.72	0.47–1.09
Zeegers et al., 2001	5	0.91	0.65–1.27
Michaud et al., 2002	5	1.16	0.82–1.63
SUMMARY VALUE		0.94	0.76–1.16

Heterogeneity test: χ^2 (2df)=3; p=0.22

Figure 48 Cohort studies of bladder cancer and vegetable consumption (see Table 92)

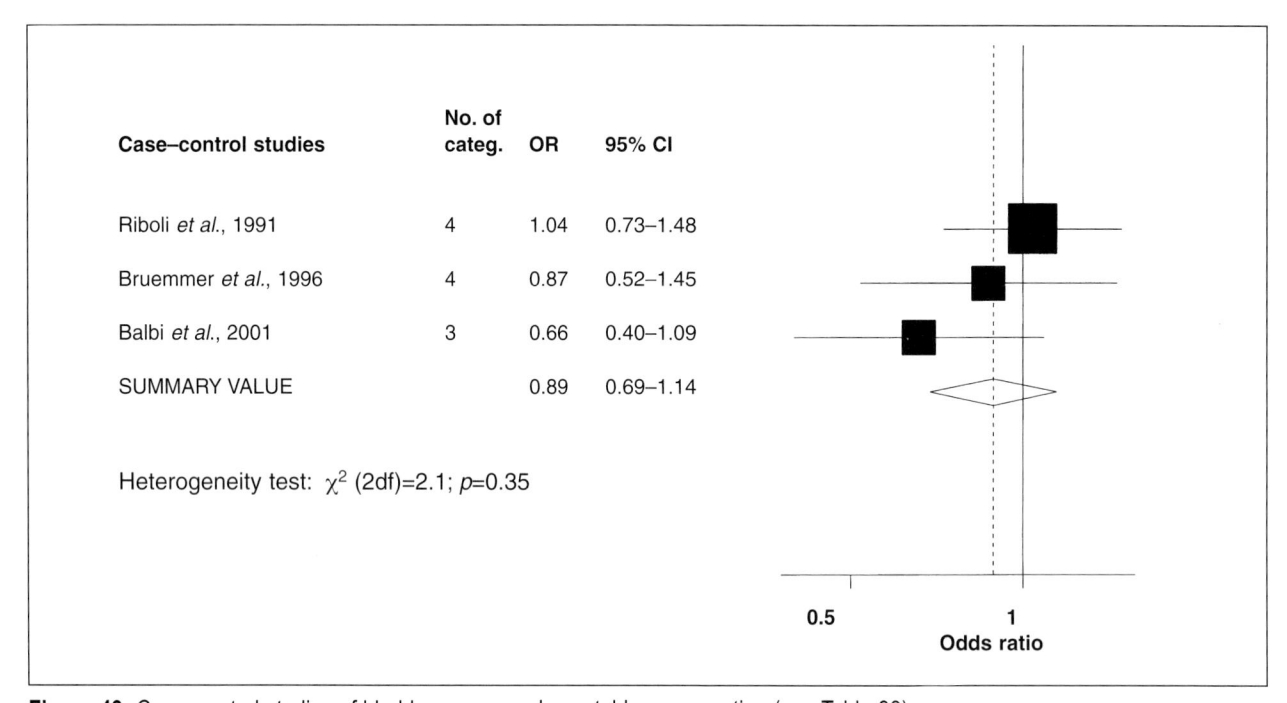

Case–control studies	No. of categ.	OR	95% CI
Riboli et al., 1991	4	1.04	0.73–1.48
Bruemmer et al., 1996	4	0.87	0.52–1.45
Balbi et al., 2001	3	0.66	0.40–1.09
SUMMARY VALUE		0.89	0.69–1.14

Heterogeneity test: χ^2 (2df)=2.1; p=0.35

Figure 49 Case–control studies of bladder cancer and vegetable consumption (see Table 93)

Discussion

A number of studies have examined fruit and vegetable consumption in relation to kidney cancer risk. There were only two cohort studies with small numbers of cases and nine case–control studies of which three were also analysed together with another as a multicentre study (Wolk *et al.*, 1996). The studies were performed in Australia, China, Europe and the USA and all renal-cell cancer cases were histologically confirmed. Most studies used population-based controls. Response rates were relatively high in most studies and adjustment was made for potential confounding by body mass index and smoking. However, recall bias cannot be excluded in the case–control studies.

The results are not consistent. For the seven evaluable case–control studies on fruit consumption, the mean OR was 0.76 (95% CI 0.63–0.91), range 0.20–1.20 (Figure 50) and for the four evaluable case–control studies on vegetable consumption, the mean OR was 0.86 (95% CI 0.67–1.09), range 0.30–1.60 (Figure 51).

Because smoking increases oxidative stress, it is of interest to examine the association with fruit and vegetables in subgroups of smokers and non-smokers. However, only two case–control studies took smoking status into account when analysing associations of fruit and vegetables with risk of renal-cell cancer. The results from these two studies and from the multicentre analysis are not consistent; one showing a significant inverse association for cruciferous/dark green vegetables both in ever-smokers and non-smokers (Yuan *et al.*, 1998), whereas the other study (Lindblad *et al.*, 1997) and the multicentre analysis found this relationship only among non-smokers.

Brain

Adult brain cancer

Fruit

Cohort studies. No cohort studies on adult brain cancer were identified by the Working Group.

Case–control studies: In two reports on a case–control study in north-east China, a significant inverse association with fruit consumption and risk of adult brain cancer was found (Table 102). No association with citrus fruit consumption was found in a study in the USA (Chen *et al.*, 2002b).

Vegetables

Cohort studies. No cohort studies on adult brain cancer were identified by the Working Group.

Case–control studies. In one case–control study in the USA and in two reports (possibly not independent) on a case–control study in north-east China, inverse associations between vegetable consumption and risk of adult brain cancer were found (Table 103).

Childhood brain cancer

Fruit

Cohort studies. No cohort studies on childhood brain cancer were identified by the Working Group.

Case–control studies. Although there have been several studies of dietary variables and childhood cancer (especially brain tumours), few have considered fruit and vegetables *per se*.

Four case–control studies have considered fruit consumption, with contrasting results (Table 104). Two of the three studies that considered maternal diet during pregnancy found inverse associations. In the study in Australia that did not find an overall association, however, there was an inverse association for fruit consumption in the first year of life of the child.

Vegetables

Cohort studies. No cohort studies on childhood brain cancer were identified by the Working Group.

Case–control studies. Three case–control studies have considered vegetable consumption, with contrasting results (Table 105). The two that found inverse associations both considered the diet of the mother during pregnancy, while the third found no association either during gestation or in the first year of life.

Discussion

Information on adult and childhood brain cancer in relation to consumption of fruit and vegetables is sparse and comes entirely from case–control studies. Although inverse associations have been found, the number of studies was considered by the Working Group to be too few to permit evaluation.

Thyroid

Thyroid cancer is a rare disease, which occurs more frequently among females than males. The majority of thyroid malignancies are well differentiated, and survival is high. Papillary carcinoma comprises between 50 and 80% of thyroid cancers and follicular carcinoma between 10 and 40%. Anaplastic carcinoma is less common (5–10%), occurs in the sixth to seventh decade of life and is highly malignant. Medullary carcinoma arises from parafollicular or C-cells, and is even rarer. The majority of the information that follows refers to differentiated thyroid carcinoma.

Fruit

Cohort studies

No cohort studies were identified by the Working Group.

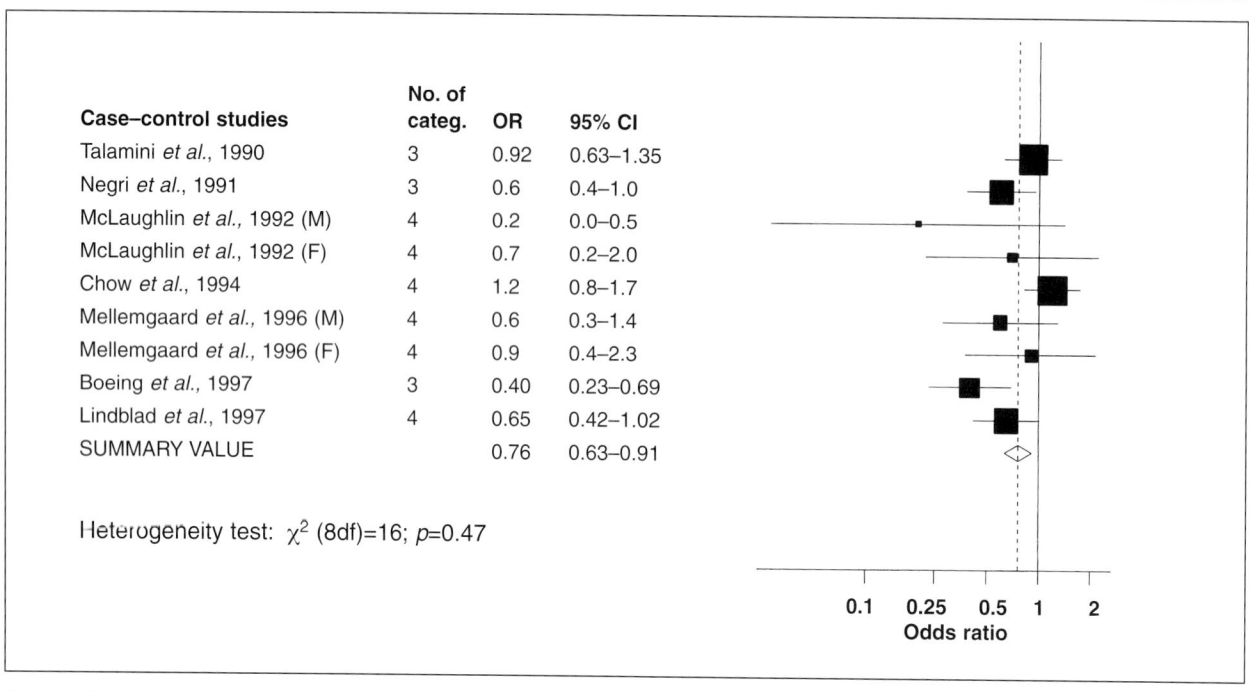

Case–control studies	No. of categ.	OR	95% CI
Talamini et al., 1990	3	0.92	0.63–1.35
Negri et al., 1991	3	0.6	0.4–1.0
McLaughlin et al., 1992 (M)	4	0.2	0.0–0.5
McLaughlin et al., 1992 (F)	4	0.7	0.2–2.0
Chow et al., 1994	4	1.2	0.8–1.7
Mellemgaard et al., 1996 (M)	4	0.6	0.3–1.4
Mellemgaard et al., 1996 (F)	4	0.9	0.4–2.3
Boeing et al., 1997	3	0.40	0.23–0.69
Lindblad et al., 1997	4	0.65	0.42–1.02
SUMMARY VALUE		0.76	0.63–0.91

Heterogeneity test: χ^2 (8df)=16; p=0.47

Figure 50 Case–control studies of renal-cell cancer and fruit consumption (see Table 97)
M = males; F = females

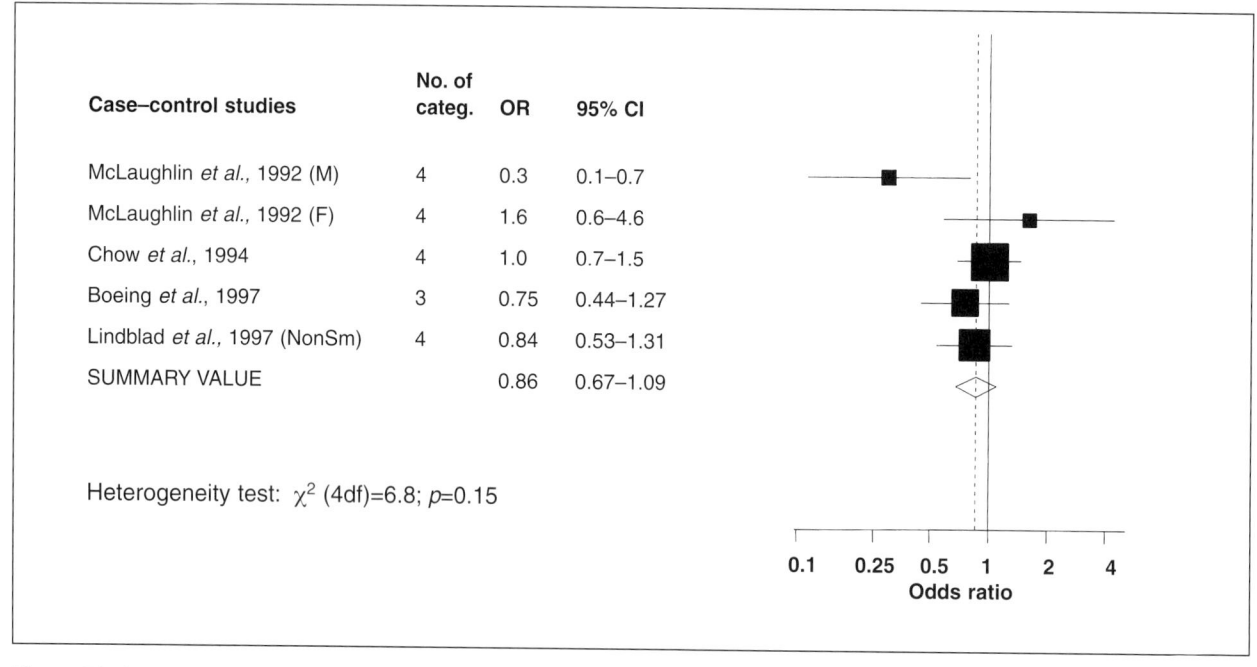

Case–control studies	No. of categ.	OR	95% CI
McLaughlin et al., 1992 (M)	4	0.3	0.1–0.7
McLaughlin et al., 1992 (F)	4	1.6	0.6–4.6
Chow et al., 1994	4	1.0	0.7–1.5
Boeing et al., 1997	3	0.75	0.44–1.27
Lindblad et al., 1997 (NonSm)	4	0.84	0.53–1.31
SUMMARY VALUE		0.86	0.67–1.09

Heterogeneity test: χ^2 (4df)=6.8; p=0.15

Figure 51 Case–control studies of renal-cell cancer and vegetable consumption (see Table 99)
M = males; F = females; NonSm = non-smokers

Case–control studies
Only two case–control studies have reported on the relationship between fruit consumption and thyroid cancer risk (Table 106). Neither reported a significant inverse association with total fruit consumption.

Vegetables
Cohort studies
No cohort studies were identified by the Working Group.

Case–control studies
Three case–control studies have reported on intake of either total or green/root vegetables and their association with thyroid cancer risk (Table 107). None reported a significant inverse association for vegetable consumption.

The association between cruciferous vegetables and other vegetable intake and thyroid cancer risk has been systematically re-analysed in a collaborative pooled analysis of 11 case–control studies (Bosetti et al., 2002b). A significant inverse association for intake of vegetables other than cruciferous was found (OR 0.82, 95% CI, 0.69–0.98).

Discussion
Information on thyroid cancer in relation to consumption of fruit and vegetables is sparse and comes entirely from case–control studies. Although an inverse association with consumption of vegetables other than cruciferous has been found in a collaborative re-analysis, the overall number of studies of total fruits or total vegetables was considered by the Working Group to be too low to permit evaluation.

Non-Hodgkin lymphoma
Fruit
Cohort studies
In two cohort studies, non-significant inverse associations between total fruit consumption and risk for non-Hodgkin lymphoma were found (Table 108).

Case–control studies
In the only case–control study of total fruit consumption and non-Hodgkin lymphoma identified (Table 109), there was no evidence of an inverse association.

Vegetables
Cohort studies
Three cohort studies of non-Hodgkin lymphoma include data on vegetable consumption. Hirayama (1990) mentioned malignant lymphoma as one of the end-points in relation to green-yellow vegetable consumption (Table 110), but gave no further details. In one study there was a significant inverse association for vegetable consumption, but there was no association in the other.

Case–control study
In the one case–control study of total vegetable consumption and non-Hodgkin lymphoma (Table 111), there was no evidence of an inverse association.

Discussion
Information on non-Hodgkin lymphoma in relation to consumption of fruit and vegetables is sparse and comes from two cohort and two case–control studies. Although inverse associations were found, the overall number of studies of total fruits or total vegetables was considered by the Working Group to be too low to permit evaluation.

Leukaemia
Fruit
No studies were identified by the Working Group.

Vegetables
Cohort study
Hirayama (1990) included leukaemia as one of the end-points in relation to green-yellow vegetable consumption (Table 112), but gave no further details.

Case–control studies
No studies were identified by the Working Group.

Table 10. Cohort study of combined fruit and vegetable consumption and risk of cancer at all sites of the upper gastrointestinal tract

Author, year, country	Cases/ cohort size, gender	Exposure assessment (no. of items)	Range contrasts (no. of categories)	Relative risk (95% CI)	Stat. sign.	Adjustment for confounding	Comments
Boeing, 2002, Europe	124/ 387 144, M,F	FFQ	> 456 g/d vs ≤ 287 g/d (3)	0.55 (0.32–0.95)		Follow-up time, sex, education, BMI, smoking, alcohol, energy	Incidence Preliminary results of EPIC

Table 11. Case–control studies of fruit consumption and risk of oral/pharyngeal cancer

Author, year, country	Cases/controls, gender	Exposure assessment (no. of items)	Range contrasts (no. of categories)	Relative risk (95% CI)	Stat. sign.*	Adjustment for confounding	Comments
North America/Australia							
Winn et al., 1984, USA	227 (156 incident/prevalent and 99 dead cases/405 (both hospital-based and dead), F	FFQ about usual adulthood diet (21), interviewed	Fresh fruit: ≥ 7.0 vs ≤ 1.0 times/wk (3)	0.6 (0.4–0.8)	$p = 0.001$	Respondent status, race, education, residence, cigarette smoking–snuff dipping, alcohol, relative weight, presence or absence of dentures, teeth missing, gum–tooth quality, regular or irregular use of mouthwash, number of meals/day, other food groups	Hospital-based
McLaughlin et al., 1988, USA	871 (oral and pharyngeal cancer)/979, M, F	FFQ about usual adulthood diet (61), interviewed	Highest vs lowest (4)	M 0.4 F 0.5	$p < 0.001$ $p = 0.01$	Smoking, alcohol	Population-based study on whites only In 22% of cases, closest next of kin was interviewed
Gridley et al., 1990, USA	190 (cancer of pharynx, tongue and other parts of oral cavity)/201, M, F	FFQ about usual adulthood diet (61), interviewed	Highest vs lowest (4)	M 0.2 F 0.6	$p = 0.006$ $p = 0.66$	Smoking, alcohol, energy	Population-based study among blacks
Day et al., 1993, USA	1065 (871 white, 194 black) (cancer of tongue, gums, other parts of the mouth, pharynx)/1182 (979 whites, 203 blacks), M, F	FFQ about usual adulthood diet(61), interviewed	Highest vs lowest (4)	Whites 0.3 Blacks 0.6 (95% CI includes 1)	$p < 0.001$ $p = 0.22$	Sex, age, study location, respondent status, smoking, drinking, energy	Population-based Response rate: 75–78%
Kune et al., 1993, Australia	41 (SCC of mouth and pharynx)/389, M	Dietary questionnaire, interviewed	Highest vs lowest (3)	0.1 (0.0–0.3)	$p < 0.001$	Age	Population-based
South America							
Franco et al., 1989, Brazil	232 (cancer of tongue, gum floor of the mouth, other parts of the oral cavity)/464, M, F	FFQ about average past consumption (20), interviewed	Citrus fruit: ≥ 4/wk vs < 1/mo (3)	0.5 (0.3–0.9)	$p = 0.03$	Matched by age, sex, study site, admission period. Adjusted for tobacco and alcohol consumption	Hospital-based Three hospitals covering 20, 100 and 100% of cases of the respective areas

Table 11 (contd)

Author, year, country	Cases/controls, gender	Exposure assessment (no. of items)	Range contrasts (no. of categories)	Relative risk (95% CI)	Stat. sign.*	Adjustment for confounding	Comments
Oreggia et al., 1991, Uruguay	57 (SCC of the tongue)/353, M	Short FFQ	≥ 5 vs < 1 times/wk (4)	[0.42 (0.14–1.25)]	p = 0.03	Age, county, type of tobacco, smoking intensity, total alcohol and other foods	Hospital-based
De Stefani et al., 1999, Uruguay	33 (oral and pharyngeal cancer)/-393, M, F	FFQ (64), interviewed	Highest vs lowest (3)	0.7 (0.4–1.3)		Age, sex, residence, urban/rural status, education, BMI, tobacco smoking (pack-years), alcohol, energy	Hospital-based; Controls for analysis of oral/pharyngeal, laryngeal and oesophageal cancer
Garrote et al., 2001, Cuba	200 (cancer of oral cavity, pharynx)/200, M, F	FFQ about lifetime dietary habits	> 13 vs < 7 servings/wk (3)	0.43 (0.21–0.89)	p < 0.05	Gender, age, area of residence, education, smoking and drinking habits and all four major foods (starchy foods, animal foods, vegetables)	Hospital-based
Europe Franceschi et al., 1991a, Italy	302 (cancer of oral cavity, and pharynx/699, M, F	FFQ about recent diet (40)	Fresh fruit: Highest vs lowest (3)	1.1	p = 0.75	Age, sex, occupation, smoking, drinking	Hospital-based No cancer registry – unknown number of cases in the area; no individual matching performed, but catchment areas of cases and controls were strictly comparable
Negri et al., 1991, Italy	119 (cancer of oral cavity and pharynx)/6147, M, F	FFQ (14–37, depending on cancer site)	Highest vs lowest (3)	0.2 (0.1–0.3)	p < 0.01	Age, area of residence, education, smoking, sex, vegetables	Hospital-based Data from a network of case–control studies
Levi et al., 1998, Switzerland	156 (oral and pharyngeal cancer)/284, M, F	FFQ about diet of recent 2 years (79), interviewed	Citrus fruit: > 3.5 vs ≤ 1.5 servings/wk (3) Other fruit: > 11 vs ≤ 5.2 servings/wk (3)	0.38 (0.20–0.73) 0.22 (0.11–0.44)	p < 0.01 p < 0.01	Age, sex, education, smoking, alcohol and non-alcohol energy intake	Hospital-based

Table 11 (contd)

Author, year, country	Cases/controls, gender	Exposure assessment (no. of items)	Range contrasts (no. of categories)	Relative risk (95% CI)	Stat. sign.*	Adjustment for confounding	Comments
Franceschi et al., 1999, Italy	598 (oral and pharyngeal cancer)/ 1491, M, F	FFQ about diet of recent two years (78), interviewed	Diversity of consumption: ≥ 6 vs < 4 servings/wk (3)	0.7 (0.4–1.2)	$p < 0.05$	Age, centre, sex, education, smoking habit, energy, alcohol, number of servings of all fruits and veg. consumed weekly	Hospital-based in specific areas
Tavani et al., 2001, Italy	132 (cancer of oral cavity, pharynx, tongue, mouth, oro-pharynx)/148, M, F	FFQ about recent year (25), interviewed	Total fruit: > 13 vs < 7 portions/wk (3)	0.34 (0.13–0.87)	$p < 0.05$	Age, sex, education, total number of portions, smoking, alcohol	Hospital-based
Lissowska et al., 2003, Poland	122 (cancers of oral cavity and pharynx)/124, M, F	FFQ (25), interviewed	≥ 7/wk vs < 3 wk (3)	0.40 (0.17–0.95)	$p < 0.01$	Gender, age, residence, smoking, alcohol	Hospital-based
Sanchez et al., 1984, USA	375 (cancer of oral and oropharynx)/ 375, M, F	FFQ (25)	≥ 11 vs ≤ 6 servings/wk (3)	0.52 (0.34–0.79)	$p < 0.001$	Gender, age, centre, years of schooling, smoking, alcohol	Hospital-based, three areas of Spain
Southern Asia							
Jafarey et al., 1977, Pakistan	1192 (carcinoma of oral cavity and oropharynx)/ 10 749 from an earlier study, M, F	FFQ	5–7 times/wk vs < 1/wk (4)	Males: [0.08 (0.06–0.12)] Females: [0.10 (0.07–0.15)]			Population-based Only frequencies of fruit and veg. consumption of males and females in five categories reported
Notani & Jayant, 1987, India	278 (cancer of oral cavity) plus 225 (pharyngeal cancer)/215 (hospital-based, H) and 177 (from population, P)	FFQ about usual diet before onset of the disease	At least once a week vs less than once a week (2)	Oral cavity: H: [1.15 (0.77–1.67)] P: [1.12 (0.71–2.0)] Pharynx: H: [1.16 (0.77–1.67)] P: [1.01 (0.63–1.67)]		Age, tobacco habits	Partly hospital-based, partly population-based
Rajkumar et al., 2003b, India	591 (cancers of oral cavity)/582, M, F	FFQ (21), interviewed	≥ 4 vs ≤ 2 servings/wk (3)	0.55 (0.38–0.81)	$p < 0.001$	Age, sex, centre, education, chewing, smoking, alcohol	Hospital-based

Table 11 (contd)

Author, year, country	Cases/controls, gender	Exposure assessment (no. of items)	Range contrasts (no. of categories)	Relative risk (95% CI)	Stat. sign.*	Adjustment for confounding	Comments
Northern Asia							
Zheng et al., 1992a, China	204 (oral and pharyngeal cancer) (115 M, 89 F)/414 (269 M, 145 F)	FFQ about usual diet of previous ten years (4, 30 fruits and veg.)	Oranges + tangerines: Highest vs lowest (3)	M 0.40 F 0.42	$p \leq 0.05$	Smoking, education	Population-based
			Other fruit: Highest vs lowest (3)	M 0.66 F 0.83	$p \leq 0.05$		
Takezaki et al., 1996, Japan	266 (oral cancers)/ 36 527, M, F	FFQ about diet before onset of symptoms	Highest vs lowest (3)	0.5 (0.4–0.7)	$p < 0.01$	Age, sex, smoking, drinking, year of visit	Hospital-based

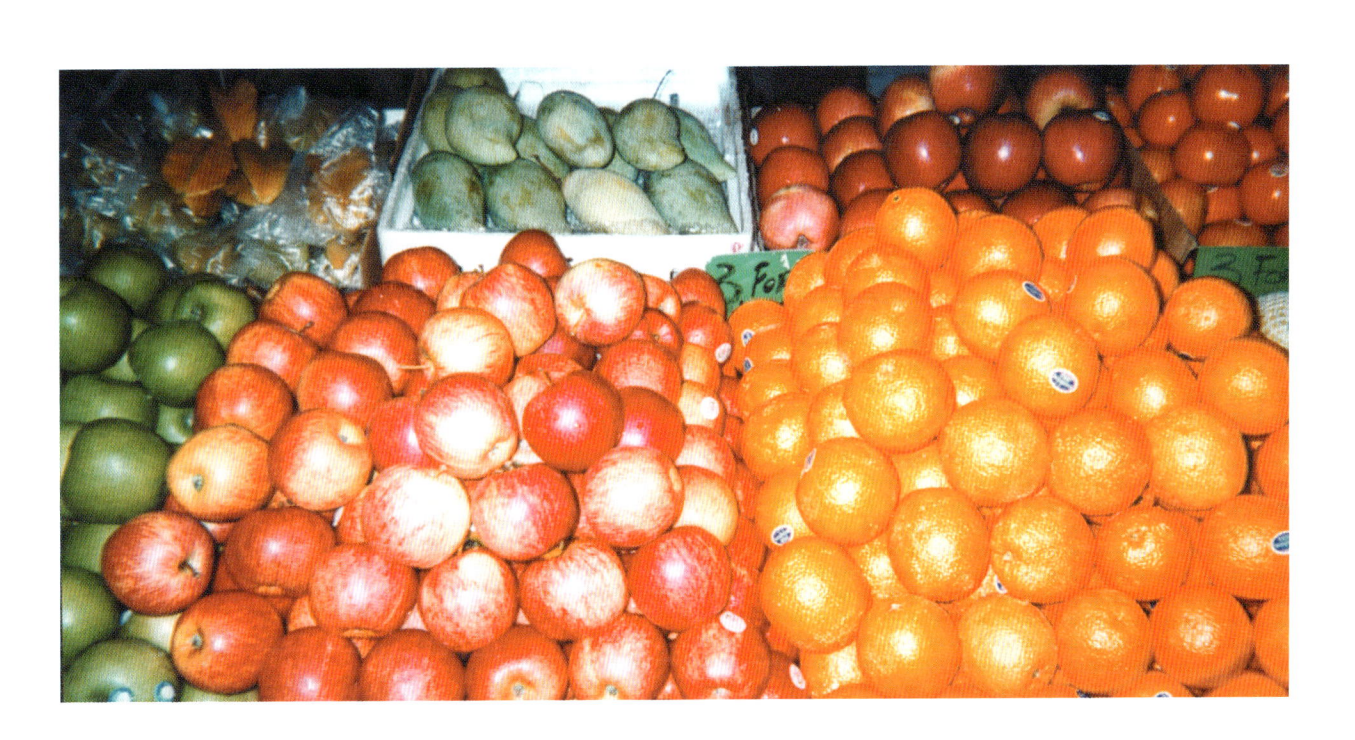

*p for trend when applicable

Table 12. Case-control studies of vegetable consumption and risk of oral/pharyngeal cancer

Author, year, country	Cases/controls, gender	Exposure assessment (no. of items)	Range contrasts (no. of categories)	Relative risk (95% CI)	Stat. sign.*	Adjustment for confounding	Comments
North America/Australia							
Winn et al., 1984, USA	227 (156 incident/prevalent cases and 99 dead cases)/405 (both hospital-based and dead), F	FFQ about usual adulthood diet (21), interviewed	Green leafy veg: ≥ 7.0 vs ≤ 2.0 times/wk (3)	0.7 (0.5–1.1)	$p = 0.06$	Respondent status, race, education, residence, cigarette smoking–snuff dipping, alcohol, relative weight, presence or absence of dentures, teeth missing, gum-tooth quality, regular or not regular use of mouthwash, number meals/day, other food groups	Hospital-based
			Other veg.: ≥ 7.1 vs ≤ 6.9 times/wk (3)	0.7 (0.4–1.3)	$p = 0.08$		
McLaughlin et al., 1988, USA	871 (oral and pharyngeal cancer)/979, M, F	FFQ about usual adulthood diet (61), interviewed	Highest vs lowest (4)	M 1.0 F 0.8	$p = 0.69$ $p = 0.20$	Smoking, alcohol	Population based study of Whites only. In 22% of cases closest next of kin was interviewed
Gridley et al., 1990, USA	190 (cancer of pharynx, tongue, and other parts of oral cavity)/201, M, F	FFQ about usual adulthood diet (61), interviewed	Highest vs lowest (4)	M 0.3 F 0.8	$p = 0.004$ $p = 0.92$	Smoking, alcohol, energy	Population-based study among Blacks
Day et al., 1993, USA	1065 (871 whites, 194 blacks) (cancer of tongue, gums, other parts of the mouth, pharynx)/1182 (979 whites, 203 blacks), M, F	FFQ about usual adulthood diet(61), interviewed	Highest vs lowest (4)	Whites 0.8 Blacks 0.5 (95% CI includes 1)	$p = 0.15$ $p = 0.07$	Sex, age, study location, respondent status, smoking, drinking, energy	Population-based
Kune et al., 1993, Australia	44 (SCC of mouth and pharynx)/398, M	Dietary questionnaire, interviewed	Highest vs lowest (3)	0.3 (0.1–0.8)	$p = 0.001$	Age	Population-based
South/Central America							
Franco et al., 1989, Brazil	232 (cancer of tongue, gum, floor of mouth, other parts of oral cavity)/464, M, F	FFQ about average past consumption (20), interviewed	Green veg.: ≥ 4/wk vs < 1/mo (3)	0.7 (0.4–1.4)		Matched by age, sex, study site, admission period. Adjusted for tobacco and alcohol consumption	Hospital-based. Three hospitals covering 20, 100 and 100% of cases of the respective areas

Table 12 (contd)

Author, year, country	Cases/controls, gender	Exposure assessment (no. of items)	Range contrasts (no. of categories)	Relative risk (95% CI)	Stat. sign.*	Adjustment for confounding	Comments
Oreggia et al., 1991, Uruguay	57 (SCC of tongue)/353, M	Short FFQ	≥ 5 vs < 1 times/wk (4)	[0.19 (0.05–0.67)]	p = 0.002	Age, county, type of tobacco, smoking intensity, alcohol, other foods	Hospital-based
De Stefani et al., 1999, Uruguay	33 (oral and pharyngeal cancer)/393, M, F	FFQ (64), interviewed	Highest vs lowest (3)	0.8 (0.4–1.4)		Age, sex, residence, urban/rural status, education, BMI, tobacco smoking (pack-years), alcohol, energy	Hospital-based Controls for analysis of oral/pharyngeal, laryngeal and oesophageal cancer
Garrote et al., 2001, Cuba	200 (cancer of oral cavity, pharynx)/200, M, F	FFQ about lifetime dietary habits	> 19 vs < 12 servings/wk (3)	0.78 (0.40–1.51)	p = 0.49	Gender, age, area of residence, education, smoking, alcohol, all major foods (starchy foods, animal foods, fruits)	Hospital-based
Europe Franceschi et al., 1991a, Italy	302 (cancer of oral cavity and pharynx)/699, M, F	FFQ about recent diet (40)	Highest vs lowest (3)	0.8	p = 0.34	Age, sex, occupation, smoking, alcohol	Hospital-based No cancer registry—unknown number of cases in the area No individual matching performed, but catchment areas of cases and controls were strictly comparable
Negri et al., 1991, Italy	119 (cancer of oral cavity and pharynx)/6147, M, F	FFQ (14–37, depending on cancer site)	Green veg.: Highest vs lowest (3)	0.3 (0.1–0.5)	p < 0.01	Age, area of residence, education, smoking, sex, veg.	Hospital-based Data from a network of case–control studies
Levi et al., 1998, Switzerland	156 (oral and pharyngeal cancer)/284, M, F	FFQ about diet of recent 2 y (79), interviewed	Raw veg.: > 8.5 vs ≤ 5 servings/wk (3) Cooked veg.: > 8.6 vs ≤ 5.2 servings/wk (3)	0.30 (0.16–0.58) 0.14 (0.07–0.19)	p < 0.01 p < 0.01	Age, sex, education, smoking, alcohol and non-alcohol total energy intake	Hospital-based

Table 12 (contd)

Author, year, country	Cases/controls, gender	Exposure assessment (no. of items)	Range contrasts (no. of categories)	Relative risk (95% CI)	Stat. sign.*	Adjustment for confounding	Comments
Franceschi et al., 1999, Italy	598 (oral and pharyngeal cancer)/1491, M, F	FFQ about diet of recent two years (78), interviewed	Diversity of consumption: ≥ 7 vs < 4 servings/wk (3)	0.6 (0.3–1.0)	NS	Age, centre, sex, education, smoking, energy, alcohol, number of servings of all fruits and veg. consumed weekly	Hospital-based in specific areas
Tavani et al., 2001, Italy	132 (cancer of oral cavity, pharynx, tongue, mouth/ 148, M, F	FFQ about recent year (25), interviewed	Total green veg.: > 13 vs < 7 portions/ wk (3)	0.37 (0.16–0.88)	$p < 0.01$	Age, sex, education, total number of portions, smoking, alcohol	Hospital-based
Lissowska et al., 2003, Poland	122 (oral cavity, and pharynx)/124, M, F	FFQ (25), interviewed	≥ 9/wk vs ≤ 6/wk (3)	0.17 (0.07–0.45)	$p < 0.01$	Gender, age, residence, smoking, alcohol	Hospital-based
Sanchez et al., 2003, Spain	375 (cancer of oral cavity and oropharynx)/375, M, F	FFQ (25)	≥ 8 vs < 3 servings/wk (3)	0.54 (0.34–0.79)	$p = 0.001$	Gender, age, centre, years of schooling, smoking, alcohol	Hospital-based, three areas in Spain
Southern Asia							
Jafarey et al., 1977, Pakistan	1192 (carcinoma of oral cavity and oropharynx)/ 10 749 from an earlier study, M, F	FFQ	5–7 times a week vs once a week or less (3)	M: [0.40 (0.29–0.56)] F: [0.47 (0.31–0.76)]			Population based Only frequencies of fruit and veg. consumption in 5 categories reported
Notani & Jayant, 1987, India	278 (cancer of oral cavity) plus 225 (pharyngeal cancer)/215 (hospital, H) and 177 (population, P), M	FFQ about usual diet before onset of the disease	Daily vs not daily (2)	Oral cavity H: [1.05 (0.71–1.67)] P: [0.42 (0.25–0.71)] Pharynx H: [1.03 (0.67–1.67)] P: [0.38 (0.22–0.63)]		Age, tobacco habits	Partly hospital-based, partly population-based
Rajkumar et al., 2003b, India	591 (cancers of oral cavity)/582, M, F	FFQ (21), interviewed	≥ 14 vs ≤ 7 servings/wk (3)	0.44 (0.28–0.69)	$p = 0.002$	Age, sex, centre, education, chewing, smoking, alcohol	Hospital-based

Table 12 (contd)

Author, year, country	Cases/controls, gender	Exposure assessment (no. of items)	Range contrasts (no. of categories)	Relative risk (95% CI)	Stat. sign.*	Adjustment for confounding	Comments
Northern Asia							
Zheng et al., 1992a, China	204 (oral and pharyngeal cancer), 115 M, 89 F)/414 (269 M, 145 F)	FFQ about usual diet of the previous ten years (41, 30 fruits and veg.)	Dark green veg.: Highest vs lowest (3)	M 1.37 F 1.22	NS NS	Smoking and education	Population-based
			Dark yellow veg.: Highest vs lowest (3)	M 0.32 F 0.78	$p < 0.05$ NS		
			Raw veg.: Highest vs lowest (3)	M 0.45 F 1.18	$p < 0.05$ NS		
Takezaki et al., 1996, Japan	266 (oral cancers)/36 527, M, F	FFQ about diet before onset of the symptoms	Green-yellow veg.: Highest vs lowest (3)	1.0 (0.7–1.3)	$p > 0.05$	Age, sex, smoking, drinking, year of visit	Hospital-based
			Raw veg: Highest vs lowest (3)	0.5 (0.4–0.7)	$p < 0.01$		

*p for trend when applicable

Table 13. Case–control studies on combined fruit and vegetable consumption and risk of oral and pharyngeal cancer

Author, year, country	Cases/controls, gender	Exposure assessment (no. of items)	Range contrasts (no. of categories)	Relative risk (95% CI)	Stat. sign.*	Adjustment for confounding	Comments
Winn et al., 1984, USA	227 (156 incident/-prevalent cases and 99 dead cases/405 (both hospital-based and dead)	FFQ about usual adult-hood diet (21), interviewed	> 21 vs 11 times/wk (3)	0.5 (0.3–0.8)	$p = 0.0002$	Respondent status, race, education, residence, cigarette smoking–snuff dipping, alcohol, relative weight, presence or absence of dentures, teeth missing, gum-tooth quality, regular or irregular use of mouthwash, number of meals/day, other food groups	Hospital-based
Gridley et al., 1992, USA	1103 (oral and pharyngeal cancers)/1262, M, F	FFQ, interviewed	Highest vs lowest (4)	No vitamin E supplement: 0.6 Vitamin E supplement: 0.2		Race, sex, tobacco and alcohol use	Population-based

*p for trend when applicable

Table 14. Case–control studies on fruit and vegetable consumption and oral/pharyngeal precancerous lesions

Author, year, country	Cases/controls, gender	Exposure assessment (no. of items)	Range contrasts (no. of categories)	Relative risk (95% CI)	Stat. sign.*	Adjustment for confounding	Comments
Gupta et al., 1998, India	318 (168 oral leukoplakia, 149 oral submucous fibrosis)/318, M	FFQ (92), interviewed	Fruit: Continuous variable Veg.: (pulses, roots and tubers excluded) Continuous variable	Submucous fibrosis 0.85 (0.70–1.04) Leukoplakia 0.78 (0.61–1.00)	$p = 0.1$ $p = 0.05$	Socioeconomic status, tobacco exposure, energy	Population-based study in state of Gujarat
Gupta et al., 1999, India	226 (oral leukoplakia, oral submucous fibrosis) 226, M	FFQ (81), interviewed	Fruit: Highest vs lowest (4) Veg.: Highest vs lowest (4)	1.01 (0.54–1.87) 0.83 (0.42–1.67)	NS	Tobacco, energy, economic status	Population-based study in state of Kerala Cases and controls all tobacco users
Morse et al., 2000, USA	105 (epithelial dysplasia)/103, M, F	FFQ (61)	Fruit: ≥ 2.9 vs < 1.8 servings/d Veg.: ≥ 3.6 vs < 2.25 servings/d Fruit and veg: ≥ 6.5 vs <4.6 servings/d	0.91 (0.33–2.5) 0.76 (0.28–2.1) 0.63 (0.21–1.9)	$p = 0.86$ $p = 0.70$ $p = 0.44$	Matched by age, gender, surgeon appointment date Adjusted for current smoking, number of drinks/week, education, season, energy	Hospital-based Only 87 case–control pairs utilized for this analysis

*p for trend when applicable

Table 15. Case–control study on fruit and vegetable consumption and risk of salivary gland cancer

Author, year, country	Cases/controls, gender	Exposure assessment (no. of items)	Range contrasts (no. of categories)	Relative risk (95% CI)	Stat. sign.*	Adjustment for confounding	Comments
Zheng et al., 1996	41/414, M, F	FFQ about usual frequency in the previous 10 years (41, 30 fruits and veg.)	Fruit: Daily vs never or occasionally (3) Veg: Daily vs never or occasionally (3)	1.3 (0.6–2.9) 0.9 (0.4–1.9)	$p > 0.10$ $p > 0.10$	Gender, age, income	Population-based

*p for trend when applicable

Table 16. Case–control studies on fruit and vegetable consumption and risk of cancer of nasopharynx

Author, year, country	Cases/controls, gender	Exposure assessment (no. of items)	Range contrasts (no. of categories)	Relative risk (95% CI)	Stat. sign.*	Adjustment for confounding	Comments
Armstrong et al., 1998, Malaysia	282/282, M, F	FFQ about diet five years before diagnosis and at age 10 y (55), interviewed	Oranges/tangerines: ≥ weekly vs < monthly (3) Chinese flowering cabbage: ≥ weekly vs < weekly (2) Other veg.: ≥ weekly vs < monthly (3)	0.52 (0.31–0.85)[1] 0.98 (0.51–1.86)[2] 0.64 (0.40–1.04)[1] 0.47 (0.29–0.77)[2] 0.50 (0.23–1.07)[1] 0.59 (0.33–1.06)[2] [1] diet of recent 5 y [2] diet at age 10	$p < 0.01$ $p < 0.1$		Population-based
Yu et al., 1989, China	306/306, M, F	FFQ as reported by mother: 110 mothers of cases/139 mothers of controls Diet of children aged 10 y (41) and aged 1–2 y (19)	Oranges/tangerines: Diet at age 10 y: daily vs rarely (4) Diet at age 1–2 y: weekly vs rarely (3) Other fresh fruit: Diet at age 10 y: daily vs rarely (4) Diet at age 1–2 y: weekly vs rarely (3) Fresh green veg.: children diet at age 10 y: daily vs less than daily (2) children diet at age 1–2 y: weekly vs rarely (3)	0.3 (0.1–0.9)[1] 0.0 (0.0–0.8)[2] 0.6 (0.3–1.2)[1] 0.3 (0.1–1.1)[2] [0.59 (0.20–1.67)][1] [0.77 (0.20–3.33)][2] [1] during ages 1–2 y [2] at age 10 y	$p < 0.05$ NS NS NS NS NS		Neighbourhood controls Analysis of subjects' diet as reported by mothers; Only 82 matched case–mother control–mother pairs

*p for trend when applicable

Table 17. Cohort studies of fruit consumption and risk of oesophageal cancer

Author, year, country	Cases/cohort size, gender (years follow-up)	Exposure assessment (no. of items)	Range contrasts (no. of categories)	Relative risk (95% CI)	Stat. sign.*	Adjustment for confounding	Comments
Yu et al., 1993, China	1162/12 693, M, F 15 y	Interview	Fresh fruit: regular or occasional vs never (2)	0.99 (0.85–1.15)	$p > 0.1$	Age, sex	Incidence Interviews performed in 1989 in subjects recruited in 1974 for screening
Guo et al., 1994, China	639/3200, M, F, 5 y	FFQ for diet during the past 12 months, interviewed	Fresh fruit: ≥ once vs none/mo (2)	0.9 (0.8–1.1)	NS	Years of smoking, cancer history in first-degree relatives	Incidence Nested case–control study in randomized control trial
Sauvaget et al., 2003, Japan	80/38 540, M, F 17 y	FFQ (22), self-administered	Daily vs once/wk or less (3)	0.57 (0.31–1.04)	$p = 0.07$	Sex, age, radiation dose, city, BMI, smoking status, alcohol, education level	Mortality Atomic bombing survivors

*p for trend when applicable

Table 18. Case–control studies of fruit consumption and risk of oesophageal cancer

Author, year, country	Cases/controls, gender	Exposure assessment (no. of items)	Range contrasts (no. of categories)	Relative risk (95% CI)	Stat. sign.*	Adjustment for confounding	Comments
North America							
Ziegler et al., 1981, USA	120/250, M, black	FFQ about subjects' usual adult diet before 1974 (31, 3 fruits), interviewed	Highest vs lowest (3)	[0.50]	$p < 0.05$	Alcohol	Population-based Deaths from oesophageal cancer (cases) or other causes (controls) Interviews with next of kin completed for 67% of cases and 71% of controls
Brown et al., 1988, USA	Incidence: 74/157, M Mortality: 143/285, M	FFQ about usual adult diet, interviewed	Highest vs lowest (3)	0.5 (0.3–0.9)	$p < 0.01$	Use of cigarettes and alcohol	Hospital- and population-based Incidence series

114

Table 18 (contd)

Author, year, country	Cases/controls, gender	Exposure assessment (no. of items)	Range contrasts (no. of categories)	Relative risk (95% CI)	Stat. sign.*	Adjustment for confounding	Comments
Brown et al., 1995, USA	174 ADC/750, M (white)	FFQ about usual adult diet (60), interviewed	Highest vs lowest (4)	0.7	p = 0.24	Age, area, smoking, liquor use, income, energy, BMI	Population-based
Brown et al., 1998, USA	333 SCC (114 white, 219 black)/ 1238 (681 whites, 557 black), M	FFQ about usual adult diet (60)	Highest vs lowest (4)	White: 0.5 Black: 0.4	p = 0.04 p = 0.001	Age, area, smoking, alcohol, energy	Population-based
Chen et al., 2002a, USA	124 (ADC)/449, M, F	Short FFQ about diet before 1985 (54), interviewed by telephone	Citrus fruit and juices: Highest vs lowest (4)	0.48 (0.21–1.1)	p = 0.03	Age, sex, energy, respondent type, BMI, alcohol, tobacco, education, family history, vitamin supplement use, age squared	Population-based For 76% of cases and for 61% of controls, interviews conducted with next of kin
South America							
Victora et al., 1987, Brazil	164 SCC/327, M, F	FFQ (9), interviewed	log days/mo +1	0.66 (90% CI 0.52–0.83)	p = 0.002	Cachaça drinking, residence, smoking status, fruit and meat consumption	Hospital-based
De Stefani et al., 1990b, Uruguay	261 SCC/ 522, M, F	FFQ of recent diet, interviewed	Daily vs < once/wk (4)	0.33 (0.2–0.5)		Age, residence, smoking duration, type of tobacco, alcohol	Hospital-based
Castelletto et al., 1994, Argentina	131 (SCC)/ 262, M, F	FFQ about recent diet and diet 10 y before admission (10), interviewed	Citrus fruit: > 3/wk vs < 1/wk (3) Non-citrus fruit: > 3/wk vs < 1/wk (3)	1.6 (0.8–3.1) 0.7 (0.3–1.5)		Age, sex, hospital, education, average number of cigarettes/day, alcohol, barbecued meat, potatoes, raw and cooked veg.	Hospital-based
Rolón et al., 1995, Paraguay	131/381, M, F	FFQ about current diet (50), interviewed	Citrus fruit: Highest vs lowest (4) Non-citrus fruit: Highest vs lowest (4)	0.8 (0.4–1.7) 0.9 (0.4–2.1)	p = 0.43 p = 0.98	Lifetime consumption of alcohol, cigarette smoking, age group, sex, hospital group, meats, fats, fish, milk	Hospital-based

Table 18 (contd)

Author, year, country	Cases/controls, gender	Exposure assessment (no. of items)	Range contrasts (no. of categories)	Relative risk (95% CI)	Stat. sign.*	Adjustment for confounding	Comments
Castellsagué et al., 2000, Argentina, Brazil, Paraguay, Uruguay	830 SCC/1779, M, F	FFQ about recent diet (50), interviewed	Almost daily/daily vs never/-rarely (3)	0.37 (0.27–0.51)	$p < 0.00001$	Sex, age group, hospital, residence, years of education, average number of cigarettes/day, alcohol	Hospital-based Pooled analysis from four main studies (Victora et al.,1987; De Stefani et al., 1990b; Castelletto et al., 1994; Rolón et al., 1995); together with additional subjects from Uruguay.
De Stefani et al., 1999, Uruguay	66/393, M, F	FFQ (64), interviewed	Highest vs lowest (3)	0.4 (0.3–0.6)		Age, sex, residence, urban/rural status, education, BMI, tobacco smoking (pack-years), alcohol, energy	Hospital-based Controls for analysis of oral/pharyngeal, laryngeal and oesophageal cancer
De Stefani et al., 2000b, Uruguay	111 SCC/444, M, F	FFQ (64), interviewed	≥ 216.8 vs ≤ 74.7 g/d (4)	0.18 (0.09–0.39)	$p < 0.001$	Age, gender, residence, urban/rural status, education, BMI, tobacco smoking, alcohol drinking, energy	Hospital-based
Europe Tuyns et al., 1987, France	331/1975, M, F	FFQ about usual diet (40), interviewed	Citrus fruit: Highest vs lowest (4) Other fresh fruit: Highest vs lowest (4)	0.33 0.72	$p = 0.004$ $p = 0.034$	Age, alcohol, smoking, urban or rural residence	Population-based

Table 18 (contd)

Author, year, country	Cases/controls, gender	Exposure assessment (no. of items)	Range contrasts (no. of categories)	Relative risk (95% CI)	Stat. sign.*	Adjustment for confounding	Comments
Franceschi et al., 1990, Italy	68/505, M	FFQ about diet of last year (40), interviewed	Fresh fruit: ≥ 13 vs ≤ 4 servings/wk (3)	[0.49]			Hospital-based No cancer registry, unknown number of cases in the area OR computed from distribution of intake
Negri et al., 1991, Italy	294/6147, M, F	FFQ (14–37, depending on cancer site)	Highest vs lowest (3)	0.3 (0.2–0.4)	p < 0.01	Age, area of residence, education, smoking, sex, veg.	Hospital-based Data from a network of case–control studies
Tzonou et al., 1996a, Greece	43 SCC plus 56 ADC/200, M, F	FFQ about diet 1 y before onset of the disease (115), interviewed	Highest vs lowest (5)	SCC: 0.90 (0.67–1.21) ADC: 0.84 (0.65–1.08)	p = 0.49 p = 0.17	Gender, age, birthplace, schooling, height, analgesics, coffee drinking, alcohol, smoking, energy	Hospital-based
Launoy et al., 1998, France	208 SCC/399, M	FFQ about diet of previous year (39), interviewed	Fresh fruit: > 180 vs < 60 g/d (4) Citrus fruit: > 60 vs < 20 g/d (4)	0.59 (0.35–1.00) 0.54 (0.33–0.89)	p < 0.05 p < 0.05	Age, interviewer, smoking, beer, aniseed aperitifs, hot Calvados, whisky, total alcohol, energy	Hospital-based
Bosetti et al., 2000a, Italy	304 (SCC)/743, M, F	FFQ about diet 2 y before diagnosis (78), interviewed	Citrus fruit (5) Other fruit (5)	0.42 (0.25–0.71) 0.52 (0.31–0.87)	p < 0.01 p < 0.05	Age, sex, area of residence, education, smoking, alcohol, non-alcohol energy	Hospital-based in specific areas
Levi et al., 2000, Switzerland	101 (SCC and ADC)/ 327, M, F	FFQ about diet of recent 2 y (79), interviewed	Citrus fruit: > 3.5 vs ≤ 1.5 servings/wk (3) Other fruit: > 3.5 vs ≤ 1.5 servings/wk (3)	0.22 (0.1–0.6) 0.20 (0.1–0.4)	p < 0.01 p < 0.01	Age, sex, education, smoking, alcohol and non-alcohol energy	Hospital-based

Table 18 (contd)

Author, year, country	Cases/controls, gender	Exposure assessment (no. of items)	Range contrasts (no. of categories)	Relative risk (95% CI)	Stat. sign.*	Adjustment for confounding	Comments
Cheng et al., 2000a, UK	74 ADC/74, F	FFQ about diet of previous 3 y, interviewed	≥ 25.73 vs ≤ 12 items/wk (4)	0.18 (0.05–0.57)	p = 0.003	None	Population-based
Sharp et al., 2001, UK	158 SCC/158, F	FQQ about diet of previous 3 y, interviewed	> 25.73 vs <12 times/wk (4)	0.64 (0.25–1.67)	p = 0.394	Slimming diet, breakfast, salad, years smoking, regular use of aspirin, centre, temperature of tea/coffee	Population-based
Terry et al., 2001b, Sweden	189 ADC plus 167 SCC/815, M, F	FFQ about diet 20 y before interview (63) Information on fruits contributing to 13.1% of total fruit consumed in Sweden was not obtained	2.0 vs 0.2 median servings/d (4)	ADC: 0.7 (0.4–1.1) SCC: 0.6 (0.4–1.1)	p = 0.08 p = 0.04	Age, gender, energy, BMI, gastro-oesophageal reflux symptoms, smoking	Population-based
Wolfgarten et al., 2001, Germany	85 (45 SCC, 40 ADC)/100, M, F	Interview about nutritional habits (1100)	≥ 101–180 g vs < 100 g/d (2)	SCC: [0.33 (0.12–0.91)] ADC: [0.16 (0.04–0.53)]	p < 0.001 p < 0.001		Population-based
Southern Asia and Turkey							
Notani & Jayant, 1987, India	236/215 (hospital-based) plus 177 (population-based), M	FFQ about usual diet before onset of the disease, interviewed	≥ once/wk vs < once/wk (2)	Hospital controls [1.01 (0.67–1.67)] Population controls [0.81 (0.5–1.25)]		Age, tobacco habits	Partly hospital-based, partly population-based
Memik et al., 1992a, Turkey	78/610, M, F	Interview	Fresh fruit: 5 times/wk vs 0–1/wk (3)	[0.30 (0.14–0.64)]	p < 0.001		Hospital based [OR computed based on reported distribution of intake]

Table 18 (contd)

Author, year, country	Cases/controls, gender	Exposure assessment (no. of items)	Range contrasts (no. of categories)	Relative risk (95% CI)	Stat. sign.*	Adjustment for confounding	Comments
Phukan et al., 2001, India	502/1004	Interview	Occasionally vs never (2)	0.3 (0.08–4.2)	$p < 0.01$		Hospital-based
Onuk et al., 2002, Turkey	44/100, M, F	Information on dietary habits	Highest vs lowest (2)	[0.14 (0.06–0.31)]	$p < 0.001$		Hospital-based
Northern Asia							
Chang-Claude et al., 1990, China	52 Subjects diagnosed with oesophagitis (42 M, 10 F)/486 (312 M, 174 F)	FFQ about diet in the past 5 y	Fresh fruit in summer: ≥ 1/wk vs < 1/wk (2)	0.31 (0.15–0.60)		Household status, age, gender, oesophagitis among siblings	Population-based All subjects underwent oesophagoscopy with biopsy. One third of subjects selected from a household with a case of oesophageal cancer
Li et al., 1989, China	1242 (SCC, ADC and unknown types of oesophageal cancer)/1311, M, F	FFQ of diet in the late 1970s (recent) (72), interviewed	Fresh fruit: > 35 vs 0 times/y (4)	1.0 (0.8–1.2)		Age, sex, smoking	Population-based
Cheng et al., 1992a, Hong Kong	400 (SCC, ADC and other)/1598, M, F	FFQ about recent diet (22), interviewed	Citrus fruit: Daily or more vs < once/y (6)	0.096 (0.036–0.26)	$p < 0.001$	Age, educational attainment, birthplace	Hospital-based Chinese population
			Other fruit: Daily or more vs < once/y (6)	0.15 (0.05–0.45)	$p < 0.001$		
Gao et al., 1994, China	902 (624 M, 278 F)/1552 (85 M, 701 F)	FFQ of diet 5 y before interview (81), interviewed	Highest vs lowest (4)	M 0.6 F 0.6	$p < 0.001$ $p = 0.11$	Age, education, birthplace, tea drinking, smoking and alcohol (only for men)	Population-based
Hu et al., 1994, China	196/392, M, F	FFQ about recent diet and diet in 1966 (32), (interviewed, no mention which data were used)	Highest vs lowest (4)	1.5 (0.8–2.9)	$p = 0.29$	Alcohol, smoking, income, occupation	Hospital-based

Table 18 (contd)

Author, year, country	Cases/controls, gender	Exposure assessment (no. of items)	Range contrasts (no. of categories)	Relative risk (95% CI)	Stat. sign.*	Adjustment for confounding	Comments
Hanaoka et al., 1994, Japan	139/136, M	FFQ of diet before onset of the disease	5–7 vs < 1/wk (4)	0.50 (0.18–1.39)	p = 0.19	Alcohol	Hospital-based
Cheng et al., 1995, Hong Kong	67 never-smokers and 53 never-drinkers/ 539 never-smokers, 407 never-drinkers, M, F	FFQ about recent diet (22), interviewed	Citrus fruit: Daily vs ≤ 3 times/wk (3)	Never smokers: 0.39 (0.16–0.98) Never drinkers: 0.59 (0.23–1.52)	p = 0.007 p = 0.183	Gender, age, educational attainment, place of birth, preference for hot drinks or soups, green leafy veg., pickled veg., alcohol, tobacco	Hospital-based Chinese population
Gao et al., 1999, China	81/234, M, F	FFQ, interviewed	≥ once/wk vs < once/mo (3)	0.75 (0.36–1.55)		Age, sex	Population-based
Yokoyama et al., 2002, Japan	234/634, M	FFQ (na)	Almost every day vs seldom (5)	[0.78 (0.28–2.17)]		Age	Hospital-based. Controls were attending for health check-ups

*p for trend when applicable. ADC, adenocarcinoma; SCC, squamous-cell carcinoma

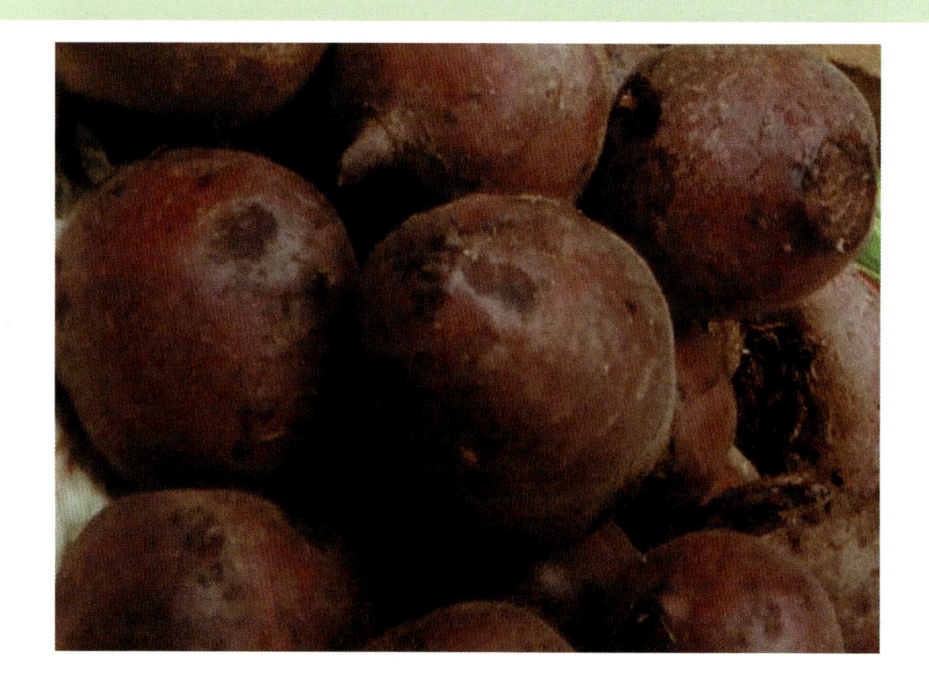

Table 19. Cohort studies of vegetable consumption and risk of oesophageal cancer

Author, year, country	Cases/cohort size, gender (years follow-up)	Exposure assessment (no. of items)	Range contrasts (no. of categories)	Relative risk (95% CI)	Stat. sign.*	Adjustment for confounding	Comments
Hirayama, 1990, Japan	585/265 118, M, F 17 y	FFQ (7)	Green-yellow veg.: Daily vs non-daily (2)	1.06 (90% CI, 0.91–1.24)		Age-adjusted rates	Mortality Census-based cohort in seven prefectures
Yu et al., 1993, China	1162/12 693. M, F 15 y	Interview about diet	Fresh veg.: Regular, occasionally vs never (2)	0.66 (0.44–0.99)	p = 0.044	Age, sex	Incidence Interviews performed in 1989 in subjects recruited in 1974 for screening
Guo et al., 1994, China	639/3200, M, F	FFQ for diet during the past 12 months	Fresh veg.: ≥ 60 vs ≤ 30 times/mo (3)	0.8 (0.6–1.0)	p = 0.08	Years of smoking, cancer history in first-degree relatives	Incidence Nested case–control study in randomized control trial
Sauvaget et al., 2003, Japan	80/38 540, M, F	FFQ (22) self-administered	Green-yellow veg.: Daily vs once/wk or less (3)	0.89 (0.48–1.63)	p = 0.63	Sex, age, radiation dose, city, BMI, smoking status, alcohol habits, education level	Mortality Atomic bombing survivors

*p for trend when applicable

Table 20. Case–control studies of vegetable consumption and risk of oesophageal cancer

Author, year, country	Cases/controls, gender	Exposure assessment (no. of items)	Range contrasts (no. of categories)	Relative risk (95% CI)	Stat. sign.*	Adjustment for confounding	Comments
North America							
Ziegler et al., 1981, USA	120/250, M, black	FFQ about subjects' usual adult diet before 1974 (31, 4 veg.), interviewed	Highest vs lowest (3)	[0.63]	$p < 0.10$	Alcohol	Study based on death from oesophageal cancer (cases) or other causes (controls) Interviews with next of kin completed for 67% of cases and 71% of controls
Brown et al., 1988, USA	Incidence 74/156, M Mortality 143/285, M	FFQ about usual adult diet, interviewed	Highest vs lowest (3)	0.7 (0.4–1.3)	NS	Smoking, alcohol	Hospital- and population-based Incidence and mortality series
Brown et al., 1995, USA	174 ADC/750, M white	FFQ about usual adult diet (60), interviewed	Highest vs lowest (4)	0.6	$p = 0.20$	Age, area, smoking, liquor use, income, energy, BMI	Population-based
Brown et al., 1998, USA	333 (114 white, 219 black) SCC/1238 (681 white, 557 black) M	FFQ about usual adult diet (60)	Highest vs lowest (4)	White: 0.4 Black: 1.0	$p = 0.06$ $p = 0.89$	Age, area, smoking, alcohol, energy	Population-based
Chen et al., 2002a, USA	124 ADC/449, M, F	Short FFQ about diet before 1985 (54), interviewed by telephone	Highest vs lowest (4)	0.45 (0.2–1.0)	$p = 0.04$	Age, sex, energy, respondent type, BMI, alcohol, education, family history, vitamin supplement use, age squared	Population-based
South America							
De Stefani et al., 1990b, Uruguay	261 SCC/522, M, F	FFQ of recent diet, interviewed	Daily vs < once/wk (4)	0.56 (0.3–1.0)		Age, residence, smoking duration, type of tobacco, alcohol	Hospital-based
Castelletto et al., 1994, Argentina	131 SCC/262, M, F	FFQ about recent diet and diet 10 y before admission (10), interviewed	> 3/wk vs < 1/wk (3)	Raw veg.: 0.9 (0.3–2.6) Cooked veg.: 0.7 (0.2–2.2)		Age, sex, hospital, education, average number of cigarettes/d, alcoho, barbecued meat, potatoes, raw or cooked veg.	

Table 20 (contd)

Author, year, country	Cases/controls, gender	Exposure assessment (no. of items)	Range contrasts (no. of categories)	Relative risk (95% CI)	Stat. sign.*	Adjustment for confounding	Comments
Rolón et al., 1995, Paraguay	131/381, M, F	FFQ about current diet (50), interviewed	Highest vs lowest (4)	0.8 (0.3–1.8)	p = 0.71	Lifetime consumption of alcohol, smoking, age group, sex, hospital group, meats, fats, fish, milk	Hospital-based
De Stefani et al., 1999, Uruguay	66/393, M, F	FFQ (64), interviewed	Highest vs lowest (3)	0.7 (0.5–0.9)		Age, sex, residence, urban/rural status, education, BMI, smoking (pack-years), alcohol, energy	Hospital-based Controls for analysis of oral/pharyngeal, laryngeal and oesophageal cancer
Castellsagué et al., 2000, Argentina, Brazil, Paraguay, Uruguay	830 SCC/1779, M, F	FFQ about recent diet (50) interviewed	Almost daily/daily vs never/rarely (3)	0.62 (0.44–0.88)	p = 0.08	Sex, age group, hospital residence, years of education, smoking, alcohol	Hospital-based Pooled analysis from four main studies (Victora et al.,1987; De Stefani et al., 1990b; Castelletto et al., 1994; Rolón et al., 1995); together with additional subjects from Uruguay
De Stefani et al., 2000b, Uruguay	111 SCC/444, M, F	FFQ (64), interviewed	≥ 127.7 vs ≤ 53.8 g/d (4)	0.64 (0.34–1.20)	p = 0.04	Age, gender, residence, urban/rural status, education, BMI, smoking, alcohol, energy	Hospital based
Europe Francheschi et al., 1990, Italy	68/505, M	FFQ about diet of last year (40), interviewed	≥ 14 vs < 7 servings/wk (3)	[0.37]			Hospital-based No cancer registry, unknown number of cases in the area OR computed based upon distribution of cases/controls

Table 20 (contd)

Author, year, country	Cases/controls gender	Exposure assessment (no. of items)	Range contrasts (no. of categories)	Relative risk (95% CI)	Stat. sign.*	Adjustment for confounding	Comments
Negri et al., 1991, Italy	294/6147, M, F	FFQ (14–37, depending on cancer site)	Green veg.: Highest vs lowest (3)	0.2 (0.1–0.3)	p < 0.01	Age, area of residence, education, smoking, sex, fruit consumption	Hospital-based Data from a network of case–control studies
Tuyns et al., 1987, France	331/1975, M, F	FFQ about usual diet (40), interviewed	Fresh veg.: Highest versus lowest (4)	0.58	p = 0.029	Age, alcohol, smoking, urban or rural residence	Population-based
Tzonou et al., 1996a, Greece	43 SCC plus 56 ADC/200, M, F	FFQ about diet one year before onset of disease (115), interviewed	(5)	SCC: 0.97 (0.74–1.28) ADC: 0.62 (0.48–0.80)	p = 0.83 p = 0.0003	Gender, age, birthplace, schooling, height, analgesics, coffee drinking, alcohol, smoking, energy	Hospital-based
Launoy et al.,1998, France	208 SCC/399, M	FFQ about diet of previous year (39), interviewed	> 400 vs < 200 g/d (4)	0.24 (0.11–0.55)	p < 0.001	Age, interviewer, smoking, beer, aniseed aperitifs, hot Calvados, whisky, total alcohol, energy, other significant food groups (butter, fresh fish, oil, veg.)	Hospital-based
Bosetti et al., 200a, Italy	304 SCC/743, M, F	FFQ about diet of 2 y before diagnosis (78), interviewed	Raw veg.: 12.6 vs < 3.9 servings/wk (5) Cooked veg: > 4.3 vs < 1.4 servings/wk (5)	0.32 (0.19–0.55) 0.79 (0.47–1.31)	p < 0.001 NS	Age, sex, area of residence, education, smoking, alcohol, non-alcohol energy	Hospital-based in specific areas
Cheng et al., 2000a, UK	74 ADC/74, F	FFQ about diet of previous 3 y, interviewed	≥ 25.90 vs ≤ 15.37 items/wk (4)	0.58 (0.22–1.55)	p = 0.371		Population-based

124

Table 20 (contd)

Author, year, country	Cases/controls, gender	Exposure assessment (no. of items)	Range contrasts (no. of categories)	Relative risk (95% CI)	Stat. sign.*	Adjustment for confounding	Comments
Levi et al., 2000, Switzerland	101 (SCC and ADC)/327, M, F	FFQ about diet of recent 2 y (79), interviewed	Raw veg.: > 9.5 vs ≤ 5.5 servings/wk (3) Cooked veg.: > 8.0 vs ≤ 5.3 servings/wk (3)	0.14 (0.1–0.4) 0.19 (0.1–0.3)	$p < 0.01$ $p < 0.01$	Age, sex, education, smoking, alcohol and non-alcohol total energy intake	Hospital-based
Terry et al., 2001b, Sweden	189 ADC plus 167 SCC/ 815, M, F	FFQ about diet 20 y before interview (63)	3.3 vs 1.1 median servings/d (4)	ADC: 0.5 (0.3–0.8) SCC: 0.6 (0.4–1.0)	$p = 0.001$ $p = 0.02$	Age, gender, energy, BMI, gastro-oesophageal reflux symptoms, smoking	Population-based Information on vegetables which contribute to 3.5% of total veg. consumed in Sweden were not obtained
Southern Asia and Turkey							
Notani & Jayant, 1987, India	236/215 (hospital-based)/177 (from population), M	FFQ about usual diet before onset of the disease, interviewed	Daily vs not daily (2)	Population controls [0.38 (0.23–0.67)] Hospital controls [1.08 (0.71–1.67)]		Age, tobacco habits	Partly hospital-based, partly population-based
Memik et al., 1992a, Turkey	78/610, M, F	Interview	≥ 5 vs 0–1 times/wk (3)	[0.34]			Hospital-based
Phukan et al., 2001, India	502/1004	Interview	Green leafy veg.: Daily vs never (4)	0.26 (0.01–2.9)	$p < 0.01$	NA	Hospital-based
Onuk et al., 2002, Turkey	44/100, M, F	Information on dietary habits	Highest vs lowest (2)	[0.10 (0.04–0.23)]	$p < 0.001$		Hospital-based
Northern Asia							
Chang-Claude et al., 1990, China	52 subjects with oesophagitis (42 M, 10 F)/486 (312 M, 174 F)	FFQ about diet in the past five years, interviewed	Green veg.: in winter: ≥ 1 vs < 1/wk (2) Raw veg.: ≥ 1 vs < 1/mo (2)	M 0.9 (0.4–2.1) F 0.3 (0.1–1.4) M 1.3 (0.6–2.6) F 0.2 (0.1–0.7)		Household status	All subjects underwent oesophagoscopy with biopsy One third of subjects selected from a household with a case of oesophageal cancer

Table 20 (contd)

Author, year, country	Cases/controls, gender	Exposure assessment (no. of items)	Range contrasts (no. of categories)	Relative risk (95% CI)	Stat. sign.*	Adjustment for confounding	Comments
Li et al., 1989, China	1243 (SCC, ADC and unknown types of cancer)/ 1314, M, F	FFQ of diet in the late 1970s (recent) (72), interviewed	Fresh veg.: > 973 vs < 483 times/y (4)	1.5 (1.2–1.9)		Age, sex, smoking	Population-based
Cheng et al., 1992a, Hong Kong	400 (SCC, ADC, other)/1598, M, F	FFQ about recent diet (22), interviewed	Green leafy veg.: Daily or more vs ≤ 3 times/wk (3)	0.39 (0.26–0.59)	p > 0.001	Age, educational attainment, birthplace	Hospital-based Chinese population
Gao et al.,1994, China	902 (624 M, 278 F)/ 1552 (851 M, 701 F)	FFQ of diet five years before interview (81), interviewed	Highest vs lowest (4)	M 0.8 F 0.9	p < 0.05 p = 0.25	Age, education, birthplace, tea drinking, smoking and alcohol (only for men)	Population-based
Cheng et al., 1995, Hong Kong	67 never-smokers, and 53 never-drinkers/539 never-smokers and 406 never-drinkers, M, F	FFQ about recent diet (22), interviewed	Green leafy veg.: Daily vs ≤ 3 times/wk (3)	Never-smokers: 0.33 (0.14–0.80) Never-drinkers: 0.65 (0.23–1.83)	p = 0.026 p = 0.231	Gender, age, educational attainment, place of birth, preference for hot drinks or soups, citrus fruits, pickled veg., smoking, alcohol	Hospital-based Chinese population
Hanaoka et al., 1994, Japan	139/136, M, F	FFQ of diet before onset of the disease	5–7 vs < 1/wk (4)	Green veg.: 0.82 (0.20–3.09) Yellow veg.: 2.32 (0.70–7.61)	p = 0.79 p = 0.16	Alcohol	Hospital-based
Hu et al., 1994, China	196/392, M, F	FFQ about recent diet and diet in 1966 (32), interviewed (no mention which data were used)	Total fresh veg.: highest vs lowest (4)	0.6 (0.3–1.06)	p = 0.05	Alcohol, smoking, income, occupation	Hospital-based
Gao et al., 1999, China	81/228, M, F	FFQ, interviewed	Raw veg.: Frequently vs never (3)	0.07 (0.03–0.19)		Age, sex	Population-based
Yokoyama et al., 2002, Japan	234/634, M	FFQ	Green-yellow veg.: Almost every day vs seldom (5)	[0.87 (0.10–7.14)]		Age	Hospital based Controls were attending for health check-ups

*p for trend when applicable; ADC, adenocarcinoma, SCC, squamous-cell carcinoma

Table 21. Case–control studies of fruit and vegetable consumption and risk of oesophageal cancer

Author, year, country	Cases/controls, gender	Exposure assessment (no. of items)	Range contrasts (no. of categories)	Relative risk (95% CI)	Stat. sign.*	Adjustment for confounding	Comments
Pottern et al., 1981, USA	120/250, M, black	FFQ about subjects' usual adult diet before 1974 (31), interviews with next of kin	Highest vs lowest (3)	[0.5]	$p < 0.05$	Alcohol	Study based on death from oesophageal cancer (cases) or other causes (controls) Interviews with next of kin completed for 67% of cases and 71% of controls
Ziegler et al., 1981, USA	120/250, M, black	FFQ about subjects' usual adult diet before 1974 (31, 3 fruits, 4 veg.), interviewed	Highest vs lowest (3)	[0.50]	$p < 0.05$	Alcohol	Population-based; deaths from oesophageal cancer (cases) or other causes (controls) Interviews with next of kin completed for 67% of cases and 71% of controls
Yu et al., 1988, USA	275/275, M, F	FFQ about usual consumption, interviewed	Fresh fruit or raw veg.: ≥ 5 vs ≤ 1 items/wk (3)	Directly interviewed: [0.40 (0.15–1.11)] All pairs: [0.43 (0.23–0.83)]	$p < 0.01$ $p < 0.001$		Neighbourhood controls. Only 129 cases directly interviewed, otherwise with next of kin
Brown et al., 2001, USA	347 (SCC)/1354, M	FFQ about usual adult diet (60)	Raw fruits and veg.: > 18.3 vs < 7.1 servings/wk (4)	White: [0.50 (0.26–0.91)] Black: [0.59 (0.32–1.00)]		Age, study area, years of cigarette smoking, alcohol, race	Population-based
Terry et al., 2001b, Sweden	189 ADC plus 167 SCC/815, M, F	FFQ about diet 20 y before interview (63)	4.8 vs 1.5 median servings/d (4)	ADC: 0.5 (0.3–0.8) SCC: 0.6 (0.4–1.0)	$p = 0.005$ $p = 0.01$	Age, gender, energy, BMI, gastro-oesophageal reflux symptoms, smoking	Population-based Information on fruits and veg. which contribute 3.5 % of total veg. and 13.1% of fruit consumed in Sweden was not obtained
De Stefani et al., 2000b, Uruguay	111/444, M, F	FFQ (64), interviewed	≥ 343 vs ≤ 155.7 g/d	0.22 (0.11–0.45)	$p < 0.001$	Age, gender, residence, urban/rural status, education, BMI, smoking, alcohol, energy	Hospital-based

*p for trend when applicable; ADC, adenocarcinoma, SCC, squamous-cell carcinoma

Table 22. Cohort studies of fruit consumption and risk of stomach cancer

Author, year, country	Cases/cohort size, gender (years follow-up)	Exposure assessment (no. of items)	Range contrasts (no. of categories)	Relative risk (95% CI)	Stat. sign.*	Adjustment for confounding	Comments
Chyou et al., 1990, Hawaii (Japanese)	111/361 (subcohort), M 18 y	24-h recall, interviewed (54)	≥ 301 vs 0 g/d (4)	0.8 (0.4–1.3)	p = 0.20	Age, smoking	Case–cohort Incidence All cohort: 8006
Nomura et al., 1990, Hawaii (Japanese)	149/7839, M 19 y	FFQ (20)	≥ 5 vs ≤ 1/wk (3)	0.8 (0.5–1.3)		Age	Incidence
Kneller et al., 1991, USA	75/17 633, M 20 y	FFQ (35), self-administered	Highest vs lowest (4)	1.5 (0.75–2.93)	NS	Age, cigarette smoking	Mortality
Kato et al., 1992, Japan	57/9753, M, F 6 y	FFQ (25), self-administered	Daily vs ≤ 1–2/wk (3)	1.92 (1.03–3.59)	p = 0.035	Age, sex	Mortality
Guo et al., 1994, China	538/2695, M, F 5 y	FFQ, interviewed	≥ once/mo vs none/mo (2)	0.9 (0.8–1.1)		Matched by age and sex. Adjusted for years of smoking and cancer history in first-degree relatives	Incidence Nested case–control in randomized controlled trial Similar finding for cardia/non-cardia cancer
Inoue et al., 1996, Japan	69/972, M, F 6 y	FFQ, self-administered	Daily vs rare (3)	Without atrophic gastritis: 0.55 (0.22–1.35)		Sex, age	Incidence Similar finding in subtypes with atrophic gastritis
Botterweck et al., 1998, Netherlands	281/3123 (subcohort), M, F 6.3 y	FFQ (150, 8 fruits)	≥ 325 vs ≤ 46 g/d (5)	0.97 (0.64–1.48)	p = 0.51	Age, sex, smoking, education, stomach disorders, family history of gastric cancer, veg.	Incidence Case–cohort analysis All cohort: 120 852
Galanis et al., 1998, Hawaii (Japanese)	108/11 907, M, F 14.8 y	FFQ (13), interviewed	≥ 7 vs < 7/wk (2)	0.6 (0.4–0.9)		Age, education, Japanese place of birth, gender (analyses among men: smoking, alcohol)	Incidence
McCullough et al., 2001, USA	910/436 654 M, 439/533 391 F 14 y	FFQ (32), self-administered	Citrus fruit: Highest vs lowest (3)	M: 0.88 (0.75–1.03) F: 0.97 (0.78–1.21)	p = 0.11 p = 0.79	Age, education, smoking, BMI, multivitamin and vitamin C use, aspirin use, race, family history	Mortality

Table 22 (contd)

Author, year, country	Cases/cohort size, gender (years follow-up)	Exposure assessment (no. of items)	Range contrasts (no. of categories)	Relative risk (95% CI)	Stat. sign.*	Adjustment for confounding	Comments
Kobayashi et al., 2002, Japan	404/39 993, M, F 10 y	FFQ (44), self-administered	Almost daily vs < 1 d/wk (4)	0.70 (0.48–1.01)	p = 0.25	Age, sex, area, education, smoking, BMI, alcohol, vitamin A, C, E supplement use, energy, salted food, history of peptic ulcer, family history of gastric cancer	Incidence, similar finding when cases in first 2 y excluded
Sauvaget et al., 2003, Japan	617/38 540, M, F 17 y	FFQ (22), self-administered	Daily vs 0–1 d/wk (3)	0.80 (0.65–0.98)	p = 0.03	Age, sex, radiation dose, city, BMI, smoking, alcohol, education	Mortality, atomic bombing survivors

*p for trend when applicable

Table 23. Case–control studies of fruit consumption and risk of stomach cancer

Author, year, country	Cases/controls, gender	Exposure assessment (no. of items)	Range contrasts (no. of categories)	Relative risk (95% CI)	Stat. sign.*	Adjustment for confounding	Comments
Correa et al., 1985, USA	Whites: 189/190, M, F Blacks 189/190, M, F	FFQ (59), interviewed	Highest vs lowest (4)	Whites: 0.47 (0.24–0.92) Blacks: 0.33 (0.16–0.66)	p < 0.005 p < 0.001	Matched by race, sex and age (within 5 y). Adjusted for sex, respondent status, income, duration of smoking	Hospital-based Similar finding by histological type
Jedrychowski et al., 1986, Poland	110/110, M, F	FFQ, interviewed	Daily or almost daily vs less frequently (3)	[0.31 (0.15–0.64)]		Matched by sex and age, adjusted for residence and smoking	Hospital-based
La Vecchia et al., 1987b, Italy	206/474, M, F	FFQ (29) interviewed	Fresh fruit: Highest vs lowest (3). Citrus fruit: Highest vs lowest (3)	0.73 0.63	NS p = 0.11	Age, sex, education, areas of residence, other dietary factors	Hospital-based
Kono et al., 1988, Japan	26/793 hospital, 91 population, M, F	FFQ, interviewed	Fruit, other than mandarin oranges: Daily vs less (2)	Hospital controls: 0.7 (0.4–1.0) Population controls: 0.5 (0.3–0.8)	p = 0.08 p = 0.008	Matched by age, sex and residence. Adjusted for smoking, mandarin orange, green tea	Hospital-based and population-based

Table 23 (contd)

Author, year, country	Cases/controls, gender	Exposure assessment (no. of items)	Range contrasts (no. of categories)	Relative risk (95% CI)	Stat. sign.*	Adjustment for confounding	Comments
You et al., 1988, China	564/1131, M, F	FFQ (85, 9 fruits), interviewed	Fresh fruit: > 30 vs < 5 kg/y (4)	0.6 (0.4–0.8)		Matched by age and sex. Adjusted for sex, age and family income	Population-based
Coggon et al., 1989, UK	94/185, M, F	FFQ (6), interviewed or self-administered	Fresh or frozen fruit: > 5 vs <1 time/wk (3)	0.6 (0.2–1.5)		Matched by age (2 y), sex. Adjusted for length of refrigerator use, salad veg. in winter, salt, smoked meat or fish (including bacon), socioeconomic status	Population-based
De Stefani et al., 1990a, Uruguay	210/630, M, F	FFQ, interviewed	5–7 vs 2 or less times/wk (3)	[0.36 (0.23–0.56)]	$p < 0.001$	Matched by age and sex. Adjusted for age, sex, residence, smoking duration, wine ingestion, meat, salted meat, veg. and 'mate'	Hospital-based
Kato et al., 1990, Japan	289/1247, M 198/1767, F	FFQ (10), self-administered	Almost daily vs ≤ once or twice per month (3)	M: 0.83 (0.51–1.33) F: 0.77 (0.33–1.78)		Age, residence	Hospital-based Significant reduction for intestinal type in females
Lee et al., 1990, Taiwan, China	210/810, M, F	FFQ, interviewed	≥ 6 vs ≤ 1/w Estimated at age ≤ 20 y Estimated at age 20–39 y	0.91 1.0		Matched by age, sex, hospital	Hospital-based
Wu-Williams et al., 1990, USA	130/135, M	FFQ, interviewed or self-administered	5 or more times/wk vs once or less/wk (3)	[0.67 (0.29–1.67)]		Matched by sex, age, race	Population-based
Boeing et al., 1991a, Germany	143/579, M, F	FFQ (74), interviewed	Highest vs lowest (3)	0.56 (0.35–0.91)	$p > 0.05$	Age, sex, hospital	Hospital-based
Gonzalez et al., 1991, Spain	354/354, M, F	Dietary history questionnaire (77), interviewed	Other [than citrus] fruit: Highest vs lowest (4)	0.7 (0.4–1.2)	$p = 0.08$	Matched by age, sex, and area of residence. Adjusted for energy intake	Hospital-based

Table 23 (contd)

Author, year, country	Cases/controls, gender	Exposure assessment (no. of items)	Range contrasts (no. of categories)	Relative risk (95% CI)	Stat. sign.*	Adjustment for confounding	Comments
Yu & Hsieh, 1991, China	52 M, 32 F	Questionnaire, interviewed or self-administered	Users vs non-users (2)	0.5 (0.3–0.8)		Age, sex, family income, family history of gastric cancer, family history of other cancer, history of tuberculosis, blood type, cigarette smoking, alcohol, strong tea, milk	Population-based
Hoshiyama & Sasaba, 1992, Japan	216/483, M	FFQ (24), interviewed	≥ 5 vs ≤ 1/wk (3)	0.8 (0.5–1.3)	$p = 0.34$	Age, smoking, other dietary variables	Population-based
Jedrychowski et al., 1992, Poland	741/741, M, F	FFQ, interviewed	Highest vs lowest (3)	0.72 (0.56–0.94)	$p = 0.015$	Matched by sex and age. Adjusted for age, sex, education, occupation of the index person and for residence, source of veg. and fruits, and status of the respondent (index person, other)	Hospital-based
Memik et al., 1992, Turkey	106/609, M, F	FFQ	≥ 5 vs ≤ 1/w (3)	[0.54]		Matched for age and sex	Population-based
Palli et al., 1992, Italy	923/1159, M, F	FFQ (146), interviewed	Citrus fruit: Highest vs lowest (3) Other fresh fruit: Highest vs lowest (3)	0.3 (0.2–0.6)[1] 0.6 (0.4–0.7)[2] 0.2 (0.1–0.5)[1] 0.4 (0.3–0.6)[2] [1]Gastric cardia [2]Other sites		Age, sex, area, place of residence, migration from the south, socioeconomic status, familial gastric cancer history, Quetelet index	Population-based
Sanchez-Diez et al., 1992, Spain	87/107, M, F	FFQ, interviewed	Daily vs no (2)	[0.31 (0.11–0.87)]	$p < 0.05$	Matched by age, sex, municipality of residence	Population-based
Tuyns et al., 1992, Belgium	449/3524, M, F	Dietary history questionnaire	Fresh fruit ≥ 1538 vs ≤ 300 g/w (4)	0.56	$p < 0.001$	Sex, age, province	Population-based
Ramon et al., 1993, Spain	117/234, M, F	FFQ (89), interviewed	≥ 461.4 vs ≤ 355.7 g/d (4)	0.85 (0.21–1.11)		Matched by sex, age, telephone ownership. Adjusted for sex, age, education, cigarettes, rice, cereals, pickled veg., salt intake	Population-based

Table 23 (contd)

Author, year, country	Cases/controls, gender	Exposure assessment (no. of items)	Range contrasts (no. of categories)	Relative risk (95% CI)	Stat. sign.*	Adjustment for confounding	Comments
Inoue et al., 1994, Japan	668/668, M, F	FFQ, self-administered	≥ 3 vs < 3/w (2)	0.86 (0.70–1.10)	p > 0.05	Matched by age, sex, time of hospital visit. Adjusted for sex	Hospital-based
Cornée et al., 1995, France	92/128, M, F	FFQ (30, 9 for fruits and veg.), interviewed	Highest vs lowest (3)	0.50 (0.25–1.03)	p = 0.02	Matched by age, sex (group matching). Adjusted for age, sex, occupation, energy	Hospital-based
Muñoz et al., 1997, Italy	88/103, M, F	FFQ (36), interviewed	≥ 11 vs < 5/w (3)	0.47 (0.21–1.05)	p < 0.05	Sex, age, area of residence, education	Hospital-based, subject with family history
Xu et al., 1996, China	293/959, M, F	FFQ, interviewed	≥ 55 vs 0 g/d (4)	0.5 (0.4–0.8)		Matched by sex, age. Adjusted for age, smoking, education, veg. consumption, stomach disease, family stomach cancer, veg. consumption	Iron and steel workers
Harrison et al., 1997, USA	91 (60 intestinal, 31 diffuse)/132, M, F	FFQ, self-administered	Increase in one standard deviation	Intestinal: 0.5 (0.3–0.9) Diffuse: 0.5 (0.2–1.0)	p < 0.05 p < 0.05	Energy, age, sex, race, education, smoking, alcohol, BMI	Hospital-based
La Vecchia et al., 1997, Italy	746/2053, M, F	FFQ, (29, 3 fruits), interviewed	≥ 3 different types of fruit/wk vs < 2/wk (3)	0.6 (0.5–0.8)	p < 0.001	Age, sex, area of residence, education, family history of gastric cancer, total number of serving, BMI, energy	Hospital-based
Ji et al., 1998, China	M: 770/819 F: 354/632	FFQ (74), interviewed	Fresh fruit: ≥ 18.1 vs ≤ 1.6 servings/mo (4)	M 0.4 (0.3–0.6) F: 0.5 (0.3–0.8)	p < 0.0001 p < 0.0006	Matched by age and sex. Adjusted for age, income, education, smoking, alcohol	Population-based
Gao et al., 1999, China	153/234, M, F	FFQ, interviewed	≥ 1 times/wk vs < 1 time/mo (3)	0.88 (0.47–1.67)		Matched by age, sex and neighbourhood. Adjusted for age and sex	Population-based

Table 23 (contd)

Author, year, country	Cases/controls, gender	Exposure assessment (no. of items)	Range contrasts (no. of categories)	Relative risk (95% CI)	Stat. sign.*	Adjustment for confounding	Comments
Ward & Lopez-Carrillo, 1999, Mexico	220/752, M, F	FFQ (70, 17 fruits), interviewed	≥ 5 times/d vs < 2 times/d (4)	1.0 (0.5–2.2)	p = 0.67	Matched by age. Adjusted for age, sex, energy, chili pepper consumption, added salt, history of peptic ulcer, cigarettes, socioeconomic status	Population-based Similar finding by histology
Ekström et al., 2000, Sweden	Cardia 73, non-cardia 404/1059, M, F	FFQ (45), dietary habits 20 years before interview	< 1/d vs ≤ 2/w (4)	Cardia: 0.5 (0.2–1.0) Non-cardia: 0.6 (0.4–0.8)	p = 0.03 p < 0.01	Matched by age, sex. Adjusted for age, sex, energy, smoking, BMI area, number of siblings, socioeconomic status, number of meals/day, multivitamin supplements, table salt use, urban environment	Population-based Similar finding by histology
Huang et al., 2000, Japan	1111/26 996, M, F	FFQ, self-administered	≥ 3 times/wk vs ≤ 3 times/mo	Gastric cancer family history (+): 1.39 (0.69–2.82) Gastric cancer family history (−): 1.11 (0.74–1.67)		Age, sex, smoking, drinking, pickled veg., fruit, raw veg., carrots, lettuce, pumpkin	Hospital-based
Mathew et al., 2000, India	194/305, M, F	FFQ, interviewed	> 9 vs ≤ 3/wk (4)	0.7 (0.2–3.6)	p = 0.99	Matched by age, sex, religion, residential area. Adjusted for age, sex, religion, income, smoking, alcohol	Hospital-based
De Stefani et al., 2001, Uruguay	160/320, M, F	FFQ (64, 9 fruits), interviewed	≥ 195.9 vs ≤ 99.3 g/d (3)	0.35 (0.21–0.59)	p < 0.001	Matched with sex, age, residence and urban/rural status. Adjusted for age, sex, residence, urban/rural status, education, BMI, energy, veg.	Hospital-based Tubers and legumes excluded
Hamada et al., 2002, Brazil	96/192, M, F	FFQ (30), interviewed	Daily vs ≤ 3–4 d/wk (2)	0.4 (0.2–0.9)		Matched by gender, age. Adjusted for country of birth, beef intake	Hospital-based and population-based, Japanese

Table 23 (contd)

Author, year, country	Cases/controls, gender	Exposure assessment (no. of items)	Range contrasts (no. of categories)	Relative risk (95% CI)	Stat. sign.*	Adjustment for confounding	Comments
Kim et al., 2002, Korea	136/136, M, F	FFQ (109) interviewed	Highest vs lowest (3)	0.67 (0.33–1.39)	$p = 0.56$	Matched by sex and age. Adjusted for sex, age, socioeconomic status, family history, refrigerator use	Hospital-based
Nishimoto et al., 2002, Brazil	236/236, M, F	FFQ (30), interviewed	Daily vs ≤ 1 d/wk (4)	0.6 (0.3–1.2)	$p = 0.08$	Matched by gender, age. Adjusted for race, education, smoking, other veg. intake	Hospital-based, non-Japanese
Ito et al., 2003, Japan	508 (156 differentiated, 352 non-differentiated)/ 36 490, F	FFQ, self-administered	Every day vs almost never (4) Differentiated Non-differentiated	0.68 (0.40–1.16) 0.31 (0.15–0.65) 1.16 (0.54–2.52)	$p < 0.001$ $p < 0.05$ $p < 0.05$	Age, year, season of visit, smoking, family history of gastric cancer	Hospital-based Cases restricted to those with histology subtype available (69%) Control response 90%

*p for trend when applicable

Table 24. Cohort studies of vegetable consumption and risk of stomach cancer

Author, year, country	Cases/cohort size, gender (years follow-up)	Exposure assessment (no. of items)	Range contrasts (no. of categories)	Relative risk (95% CI)	Stat. sign.*	Adjustment for confounding	Comments
Chyou et al., 1990, Hawaii (Japanese)	111/361 (sub-cohort), M, 18 y	24-h recall, interviewed (54)	≥ 80 g/d vs none (4)	0.7 (0.4–1.1)	$p = 0.001$	Age, smoking	Case–cohort, incidence All cohort: 8006
Kneller et al., 1991, USA	75/17 633, M 20 y	FFQ, self-administered (35)	Highest vs lowest (4)	0.9 (0.48–1.78)	NS	Age, cigarette smoking	Mortality
Kato et al., 1992, Japan	57/9753, M, F 6 y	FFQ, self-administered (25)	Green-yellow veg.: Daily vs < 1–2/wk (3) Other veg.: Daily vs < 1–2/wk (3)	1.54 (0.77–3.11) 1.15 (0.59–2.27)	$p = 0.23$ $p = 0.57$	Age, sex	Mortality Rural population

Table 24 (contd)

Author, year, country	Cases/cohort size, gender (years follow-up)	Exposure assessment (no. of items)	Range contrasts (no. of categories)	Relative risk (95% CI)	Stat. sign.*	Adjustment for confounding	Comments
Guo et al., 1994, China	538/2695, M, F 5 y	FFQ, interviewed	Fresh veg.: ≥ 60 vs ≤ 30 times/mo (3)	1.1 (0.8–1.4)		Matched by age and sex. Adjusted for years of smoking and cancer history in first-degree relatives	Incidence Nested case–control in randomized controlled trial
Inoue et al., 1996, Japan	69/972, M, F 6 y	FFQ, self-administered	Raw veg.: Daily vs rare (3) Green-yellow veg.: Daily vs rare (3)	0.67 (0.29–1.57) 0.74 (0.17–3.20)		Sex, age	Incidence Similar findings in subjects with atrophic gastritis
Botterweck et al., 1998, Netherlands	264/2953 (subcohort), M, F 6.3 y	FFQ (150, 17 veg.)	≥ 286 vs ≤ 103 g/d (5)	0.86 (0.58–1.26)	$p = 0.25$	Age, sex, smoking, education, stomach disorders, family history of gastric cancer, total fruit consumption	Incidence Case–cohort analysis. All cohort: 120 852
Galanis et al., 1998, Hawaii (Japanese)	108/11 907, M, F 14.8 y	FFQ (13), interviewed	Raw veg.: ≥ 7 vs < 7/wk (2)	0.8 (0.5–1.2)		Age, education, Japanese place of birth, gender (analyses among men; also smoking and alcohol)	Incidence
McCullough et al., 2001, USA	910/436 654, M 439/533 391, F 14 y	FFQ (32), self-administered	M: ≥ 13 vs < 8 d/wk (3) F: > 14 vs < 9 d/wk (3)	M: 0.89 (0.76–1.05) F: 1.25 (0.99–1.58)	$p = 0.17$ $p = 0.06$	Age, education, smoking, BMI, multivitamin and vitamin C use, aspirin use, race, family history	Mortality
Kasum et al., 2002, USA	56/34 351, F 14 y	FFQ (127), self-administered	Yellow/orange veg.: 3.5–106 vs 0–1 servings/wk (3)	0.63		Age, energy, alcohol, smoking	Incidence
Kobayashi et al., 2002, Japan	404/39 903, M, F 10 y	FFQ (44), self-administered	Highest vs lowest (5)	0.75 (0.54–1.04)	$p = 0.17$	Age, sex, area, education, smoking, BMI, alcohol, vitamin A, C, E supplement use, energy, salted food, history of peptic ulcer, family history of gastric cancer	Incidence Similar finding when first two years' cases excluded. Significant inverse association only for differentiated histology type
Sauvaget et al., 2003, Japan	617/38 540, M, F 17 y	FFQ (22), self-administered	Green-yellow veg.: Daily vs 0–1 d/wk (3)	0.91 (0.74–1.13)	$p = 0.35$	Age, sex, radiation dose, city, BMI, smoking alcohol, education	Mortality, atomic bombing survivors

*p for trend when applicable

Table 25. Case–control studies of vegetable consumption and risk of stomach cancer

Author, year, country	Cases/controls, gender	Exposure assessment (no. of items)	Range contrasts (no. of categories)	Relative risk (95% CI)	Stat. sign.*	Adjustment for confounding	Comments
Correa et al., 1985, USA	Blacks 186/190, M, F	FFQ (+food preparation, preservation methods) (59), interviewed	Highest vs lowest (4)	0.50 (0.25–1.00)	$p < 0.05$	Matched by race, sex, and age (within 5 y). Adjusted for age, sex, respondent status, income, duration of smoking	Hospital-based Study also included whites, but association with veg. not reported for them
Risch et al., 1985, Canada	246/246, M, F	Diet history (94), interviewed	Increase of 100 g/d	0.84 (0.72–0.96)	$p = 0.011$	Matched by sex, age, province of residence. Adjusted for total food intake, ethnicity, dietary fibre, nitrite, chocolate, carbohydrate, duration without refrigeration	Population-based
Jedrychowski et al., 1986, Poland	110/110, M, F	FFQ, interviewed	Daily or almost daily vs less frequently (3)	[0.61 (0.25–1.49)]		Matched by sex and age. Adjusted for residence and smoking	Hospital-based
La Vecchia et al., 1987b, Italy	206/474, M, F	FFQ (29), interviewed	Total green veg.: Highest vs lowest (3)	0.27	$p < 0.001$	Age, sex, education, areas of residence, other dietary factors	Hospital-based
Kono et al., 1988, Japan	77/1583, M, F	FFQ, interviewed	Raw veg.: > 1/d vs < 3/mo (3)	0.8	$p > 0.05$	Matched by age, sex and residence. Adjusted for occupational class	Hospital-based
			Green-yellow veg.: > 1/d vs < 3/mo (3)	1.3	$p > 0.05$		
You et al., 1988, China	564/113, M, F	FFQ (85, 36 veg.), interviewed	Total fresh veg.: ≥ 156 vs ≤ 73 kg/y (4)	0.4 (0.3–0.6)		Matched by age and sex. Adjusted for sex, age and family income	Population-based
Buiatti et al., 1989, Italy	1016/1159, M, F	FFQ (146), interviewed validated by pilot phase	Raw veg.: Highest vs lowest (3)	0.6	$p < 0.001$	Matched with age (5 y), sex, centre. Adjusted for sex, age, area, place of residence, migration from the south, socioeconomic status, familial gastric cancer history, Quetelet index	Population-based
			Cooked veg.: Highest vs lowest (3)	1.1	$p = 0.58$		

Table 25 (contd)

Author, year, country	Cases/controls, gender	Exposure assessment (no. of items)	Range contrasts (no. of categories)	Relative risk (95% CI)	Stat. sign.*	Adjustment for confounding	Comments
De Stefani et al., 1990a, Uruguay	210/630, M, F	FFQ, interviewed	5–7 vs 2 or less times/wk (3)	[0.37 (0.23–0.59)]	$p < 0.001$	Matched by age and sex. Adjusted for age, sex, residence, smoking duration, wine ingestion, meat, salted meat, fruits and 'mate'	Hospital-based
Graham et al., 1990, USA	186/181, M	FFQ, interviewed	Raw veg.: Highest monthly frequency vs less (2)	0.43 (0.23–0.78)		Matched by age, sex and neighbourhood. Adjusted for age, education	
Kato et al., 1990, Japan	289/1247, M 138/1767 F	FFQ (10), self-administered	Raw veg.: Almost daily vs ≤ once or twice/mo (3)	M: 0.59 (0.37–0.93) F: 0.84 (0.47–1.51)		Age and residence	Hospital-based Significant reduction for intestinal type in males
Boeing et al., 1991a, Germany	143/579, M, F	FFQ (74), interviewed	Highest vs lowest (3)	0.86 (0.54–1.36)	$p > 0.05$	Sex, age, hospital	Hospital-based
Gonzalez et al., 1991, Spain	354/354, M, F	Dietary history questionnaire (77), interviewed	Raw veg.: Highest vs lowest (4) Cooked veg.: Highest vs lowest (4)	0.8 0.6 (0.3–1.0)	$p = 0.25$ $p = 0.12$	Energy Energy and all groups of foods together	Hospital-based Matched by age, sex, and area of residence
Hoshiyama & Sasaba, 1992, Japan	216/483, M	FFQ (24), interviewed	Raw veg: ≥ 6 vs ≤ 1/wk (3) Green-yellow veg.: ≥ 8 vs ≤ 4/wk (3)	0.6 (0.3–1.0) 0.8 (0.4–1.4)	$p < 0.04$ $p = 0.30$	Age, smoking and other dietary variables	Population-based
Jedrychowski et al., 1992, Poland	741/741, M, F	FFQ, interviewed	Highest vs lowest (3)	0.60 (0.46–0.78)	$p < 0.001$	Matched by sex and age. Adjusted for age, sex, education, occupation of the index person and for residence, source of veg. and fruits, and status of the respondent (index person, other)	Hospital-based, multicentre Comparison based on dietary habits of case and control households

Table 25 (contd)

Author, year, country	Cases/controls, gender	Exposure assessment (no. of items)	Range contrasts (no. of categories)	Relative risk (95% CI)	Stat. sign.*	Adjustment for confounding	Comments
Memik et al., 1992, Turkey	117/609, M, F	FFQ	≥ 5 vs < 1/wk (3)	0.6 (0.31–1.23)	$p < 0.05$	Matched for age and sex	Population-based
Palli et al., 1992, Italy	923/1159, M, F	FFQ (146), interviewed	Raw veg.: Highest vs lowest (3) Cooked veg.: Highest vs lowest (3)	0.4 (0.2–0.8)[1] 0.6 (0.3–0.8)[2] 1.5 (0.8–2.8)[1] 1.1 (0.9–1.4)[2] [1]Gastric cardia [2]All others		Age, sex, area, place of residence, migration from the south, socio-economic status, familial gastric cancer history, Quetelet index (tertile categories of weight/ height squared)	Population-based
Sanchez-Diez et al., 1992, Spain	87/107, M, F	FFQ, interviewed	Daily vs none (2)	[0.70 (0.41–1.08)]		Matched by age, sex, municipality of residence	Population-based
Tuyns et al., 1992, Belgium	449/3524, M, F	Diet history questionnaire	Cooked veg.: ≥ 1150 vs ≤ 600 g/wk (4) Raw veg.: ≥ 268 vs ≤ 80 g/wk (4)	0.33 0.4	$p < 0.001$ $p < 0.001$	Sex, age, province	Population-based
Hansson et al., 1993, Sweden	338/669, M, F	FFQ (45), interviewed [1]Diet in adolescence [2]Diet consumed 20 years before interview	> 15 vs < 2.1 times/mo (4) Semi-continuous variables (effect per category)	[1]0.58 (0.37–0.89) [2]0.50 (0.32–0.78) [1]0.89 (0.77–1.03) [2]0.81 (0.70–0.94)	$p = 0.011$ $p = 0.005$	Age, gender, and socioeconomic status Age, gender, socio-economic status, consumption of a food item during adolescence and 20 years before interview	Population-based
Ramon et al., 1993, Spain	117/234, M, F	FFQ (89), interviewed	Highest vs lowest (4)	0.66	$p > 0.05$	Matched by sex, age, telephone possession. Adjusted for sex, age	Population-based
Inoue et al., 1994, Japan	668/668, M, F	FFQ, self-administered	Fresh veg.: ≥ 3 vs < 3/w (2)	0.70 (0.55–0.88)	$p < 0.05$	Matched by age, sex, time of hospital visit. Adjusted for sex	Hospital-based
Cornée et al., 1995, France	92/128, M, F	FFQ (30, 9 fruits and veg.), interviewed	Highest vs lowest (3)	0.77 (0.37–1.60)	$p = 0.68$	Matched by age, sex (group matching) Adjusted for age, sex, occupation, energy	Hospital-based Veg. comprise all types except dried veg. and potatoes

Table 25 (contd)

Author, year, country	Cases/controls, gender	Exposure assessment (no. of items)	Range contrasts (no. of categories)	Relative risk (95% CI)	Stat. sign.*	Adjustment for confounding	Comments
Lee et al., 1995, Korea	213/213, M, F	FFQ (64), interviewed	Fresh veg.: Highest vs lowest (3)	1.2 (0.8–1.9)	p > 0.01	Matched by age, sex. Adjusted for age, sex, education, economic status, residence	Hospital-based
Xu et al., 1996, China	293/959, M, F	FFQ, interviewed	≥ 7.4 vs ≤ 5.4 g/d (3)	0.5 (0.4–0.8)		Matched by sex, age. Adjusted for age, smoking, education, fruit consumption, stomach disease, family stomach cancer	Iron and steel workers
Harrison, et al., 1997, USA	91 (60 intestinal, 31 diffuse)/132, M, F	FFQ, self-administered	Increase in one standard deviation	Intestinal: 0.8 (0.5–1.3) Diffuse: 0.7 (0.4–1.2)		Energy, age, sex, race, education, smoking, alcohol, BMI	Hospital-based
La Vecchia et al., 1997, Italy	746/2053, M, F	FFQ (29, 7 veg.) interviewed	≥ 7 vs ≤ 5 different types of veg./wk (4)	0.5 (0.4–0.7)	p < 0.001	Age, sex, area of residence, education, family history of gastric cancer, total number of serving, BMI, energy	Hospital-based Data relate to diversity of types of veg. consumed, rather than number of all veg. items
Muñoz et al., 1997, Italy	88/103, M, F	FFQ (36), interviewed	≥ 8 vs ≤ 6/wk (3)	0.47 (0.22–1.03)	p > 0.05	Sex, age, area of residence, education	Hospital-based, subjects with family history. OR for subjects without family history 0.46
Ji et al., 1998, China	770/819, M 354/632, F	FFQ (74), interviewed	≥ 263.5 vs ≤ 158.9 servings/mo (4)	M: 0.4 (0.3–0.5) F: 0.7 (0.5–1.1)	p < 0.001 p > 0.05	Matched by age and sex. Adjusted for age, income, education, smoking, alcohol	Population-based
Gao et al., 1999, China	149/228, M, F	FFQ, interviewed	Raw veg.: Frequently vs almost never (3)	0.07 (0.04–0.13)		Matched by age, sex and neighbourhood. Adjusted for age and sex	Population-based
Ward & Lopez-Carrillo, 1999, Mexico	220/752, M, F	FFQ (70,13 veg.), interviewed	≥ 6 vs <4 times/d (4)	0.3 (0.1–0.6)	p = 0.001	Matched by age. Adjusted for age, sex, energy, chili pepper consumption, added salt, history of peptic ulcer, cigarettes, socioeconomic status	Population-based Similar findings by subtype

Table 25 (contd)

Author, year, country	Cases/controls, gender	Exposure assessment (no. of items)	Range contrasts (no. of categories)	Relative risk (95% CI)	Stat. sign.*	Adjustment for confounding	Comments
Ekström et al., 2000, Sweden	(Cardia; 69, non-cardia 395)/1061, M, F	FFQ (45), dietary habits 20 years before interview	≥ 2/d vs ≤ 5/w (4)	Cardia: 0.5 (0.3–1.1) Non-cardia: 0.7 (0.5–1.0)	$p = 0.05$ $p = 0.02$	Matched by age, sex. Adjusted for energy, smoking, BMI, area, number of siblings, socioeconomic status, number of meals/day, multi-vitamin supplements, table salt use, urban environment	Population-based Similar findings by histology
Huang et al., 2000, Japan	111/26 996, M, F	FFQ, self-administered	Raw veg.: ≥ 3 times/wk vs ≤ 3 times/mo	Gastric cancer family history (+): 0.52 (0.27–0.99) Gastric cancer family history (–): 0.95 (0.64–1.41)	$p < 0.05$ $p > 0.05$	Age, sex, smoking, drinking, pickled veg., fruit, raw veg., carrots, lettuce, pumpkin	Hospital-based
Mathew et al., 2000, India	194/305, M, F	FFQ, interviewed	> 9 vs ≤ 3/w (3)	1.1 (0.2–5.0)	$p = 0.08$	Matched by age, sex, religion, residential area. Adjusted for age, sex, religion, income, smoking, alcohol	Hospital-based
De Stefani et al., 2001, Uruguay	160/320, M, F	FFQ (64, 13 veg.), interviewed	≥ 128.8 g/d vs ≤ 71.6 g/d (3)	0.83 (0.49–1.43)	$p = 0.54$	Matched with sex, age, residence and urban/rural status. Adjusted for age, sex, residence, urban/rural status, education, BMI, energy, fruit	Hospital-based Tubers and legumes excluded
Chen et al., 2002a, USA	124/449, M, F	Short FFQ (54), interviewed, validated against full questionnaire	Highest vs lowest (4)	1.7 (0.77–3.7)	$p > 0.05$	Matched with age, sex and vital status. Adjusted for sex, age, energy, respondent type, BMI, alcohol, tobacco, education, family history, vitamin supplement use	Population-based

Table 25 (contd)

Author, year, country	Cases/controls, gender	Exposure assessment (no. of items)	Range contrasts (no. of categories)	Relative risk (95% CI)	Stat. sign.*	Adjustment for confounding	Comments
Kim et al., 2002, Korea	136/136, M, F	FFQ (109), interviewed	Highest vs lowest (3) Green veg.: Daily vs < 1d/wk (4)	0.64 (0.31–1.32) 0.9 (0.4–1.9)	p = 0.025 p = 0.73	Matched by sex and age. Adjusted for sex, age, socio-economic status, family history, refrigerator use	Hospital-based
Hamada et al., 2002, Brazil	96/192, M, F	FFQ (30), interviewed	Yellow veg.: Daily vs < 1d/wk(4) Other veg.: Daily vs < 1d/wk(4)	0.5 (0.1–1.5) 0.9 (0.3–3.0)	p = 0.47 p = 0.45	Matched by gender, age. Adjusted for country of birth	Hospital-based and population-based Japanese
Nishimoto et al., 2002, Brazil	236/236, M, F	FFQ (30), interviewed	Green veg.: Daily vs <1 d/wk (4) Yellow veg.: Daily vs <1 d/wk (4) Other veg.: Daily vs < 1 d/wk (4)	0.7 (0.4–1.3) 0.5 (0.6–0.99) 0.5 (0.3–0.97)	p = 0.33 p = 0.28 p = 0.02	Matched by gender, age. Adjusted for race, education, smoking, other veg./fruit intake	Hospital-based, non-Japanese
Ito et al., 2003 Japan	508/36 490, F	FFQ, self-administered	Raw veg.: Every day vs almost never (4)	0.50 (0.36–0.71)	p < 0.001	Age, year, season of visit, smoking, family history of gastric cancer	Hospital-based Similar findings for histological subtype

*p for trend when applicable

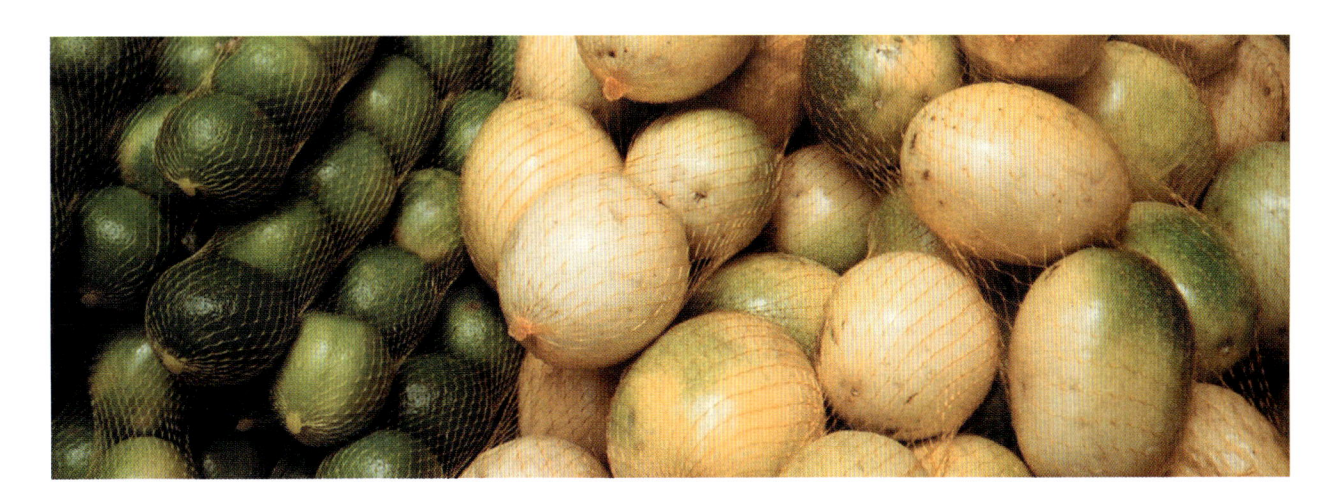

IARC Handbooks of Cancer Prevention Volume 8: Fruit and Vegetables

Table 26. Cohort studies of total fruit and vegetable consumption and risk of stomach cancer

Author, year, country	Cases/cohort size, gender (years follow-up)	Exposure assessment (no. of items)	Range contrasts (no. of categories)	Relative risk (95% CI)	Stat. sign.*	Adjustment for confounding	Comments
Botterweck et al., 1998, Netherlands	264/3123, M, F subcohorts 6.3 y	FFQ (150, 17 veg., 8 fruits)	≥ 544 vs ≤ 190 g/d (5)	0.72 (0.48–1.10)	$p = 0.14$	Age, sex, smoking, education, stomach disorders, family history of gastric cancer	Incidence Case–cohort analysis All cohort: 120 852
Galanis et al., 1998, Hawaii (Japanese)	108/11 907, M, F 14.8 y	FFQ (13), interviewed	Fresh fruit and raw veg.: ≥ 14 vs < 8/wk (3)	0.5 (0.3–0.8)	$p = 0.02$	Age, education, Japanese place of birth, gender (analyses among men; also smoking, alcohol)	Incidence
Terry et al., 1998, Sweden	116/11 546, M, F 25 y	FFQ (23), self-administered	High vs none/very little (4)	[0.18 (0.05–0.60)]	$p < 0.05$	Sex, age, smoking, BMI at 25 y, childhood socio-economic status, alcohol	Incidence Twin study

*p for trend when applicable

Table 27. Case-control studies of total fruit and vegetable consumption and risk of stomach cancer

Author, year, country	Cases/controls, gender	Exposure assessment (no. of items)	Range contrasts (no. of categories)	Relative risk (95% CI)	Stat. sign.*	Adjustment for confounding	Comments
Boeing et al., 1991b, Poland	741/741, M, F	FFQ (43, 8 fruits and 12 veg.), Fruit and veg. score	Highest vs lowest (5)	0.53 (0.37–0.75)	$p = 0.01$	Age, sex, occupation, education, residence	Hospital-based Similar results for intestinal and diffuse type
Hansson et al., 1993, Sweden	338/669, M, F	FFQ (45), interviewed	Highest vs lowest (4)	0.38 (0.21–0.67)		Age, gender, socio-economic status, consumption of a food item during adolescence and 20 years before interview	Population-based
De Stefani et al., 2001, Uruguay	160/320, M, F	FFQ (64, 22 fruits and veg.), interviewed	≥ 321.1 vs ≤ 192.1 g/d (3)	0.33 (0.19–0.56)	$p < 0.001$	Matched by sex, age, residence and urban/rural status. Adjusted for age, sex, residence, urban/rural status, education, BMI, energy, tubers, legumes	Hospital-based Tubers and legumes excluded

*p for trend when applicable

Table 28. Cohort studies of fruit consumption and risk of colorectal cancer

Author, year, country	Cases/cohort size, gender (years follow-up)	Exposure assessment (no. of items)	Range contrasts (no. of categories)	Relative risk (95% CI)	Stat. sign.*	Adjustment for confounding	Comments
Shibata et al., 1992, USA	105/11 580, F 9 y	FFQ (59, 23 fruits), self-administered	F ≥ 3.7 vs < 2.4 servings/day (3) M ≥ 3.5 vs < 2.2 servings/d (3)	Colon: 0.50 (0.31–0.80) 1.12 (0.69–1.81)	$p < 0.05$ NS	Age, smoking	Incidence Californian retirement community residents
Steinmetz et al., 1994, USA	212/ 41 837, F 5 y	FFQ (127) at baseline, self-administered	> 17.4 vs < 7.5 servings/wk (4)	Colon: 0.86 (0.58–1.29)	$p > 0.05$	Age, energy	Incidence Iowa Women's Health Study
Kato et al., 1997, USA	100/14 727, F average 7.1 y	FFQ at baseline, self-administered	Highest vs lowest (4)	Colorectum: 1.49 (0.82–2.70)	$p = 0.08$	Age, energy, enrolment site, education	Incidence NY University cohort
Hsing et al., 1998a, USA	120 colon, 25 rectum/17 633, M (white) 11.5 y	FFQ (35) at baseline, self-administered	> 67.0 vs < 29.3 times/mo (4)	Colorectum: 1.6 (0.9– 2.8) Colon: 1.6 (0.9–2.9)	$p = 0.04$ $p = 0.05$	Age, energy, smoking, alcohol	Mortality Lutheran Brotherhood cohort
Pietinen et al., 1999, Finland	185/26 926, M average 8 y	FFQ (276) at baseline, self-administered	216 vs 30 g/d (median values) (4)	Colorectum: 1.1 (0.8–1.7)	$p = 0.64$	Age, intervention group, years smoking, BMI, alcohol, education, physical activity, calcium	Incidence ATBC cohort, vitamin supplement trial
Michels et al., 2000, USA	569 colon, 155 rectum/88 764, F 16 y 368 colon, 89 rectum/47 325, M 10 y	FFQ (61, 6 fruits expanded to 15)	≥ 5 vs ≤ 1 servings/d (5)	F, Colon: 0.80 (RR for 1 additional serving/d: 0.96 (0.89–1.03)) Rectum: 0.66 (RR for 1 additional serving/d: 0.96 (0.83–1.11)) M, Colon: 1.35 (RR for 1 additional serving/d: 1.08 (1.00–1.16)) Rectum: 2.04 (RR for 1 additional serving/d: 1.09 (0.94–1.26))		Age, family history of colorectal cancer, sigmoidoscopy, height, BMI, smoking, alcohol, physical activity, aspirin, vitamin supplement use, energy (standard), red meat	Incidence Nurses' Health Study or Health Professional Study Pooled estimates for M and F not made because of heterogeneity

Table 28 (contd)

Author, year, country	Cases/cohort size, gender (years follow-up)	Exposure assessment (no. of items)	Range contrasts (no. of categories)	Relative risk (95% CI)	Stat. sign.*	Adjustment for confounding	Comments
Voorrips et al., 2000a, Netherlands	331 colon, 215 rectum/58 279, M 6.3 y 280 colon, 119 rectum/ 62 573, F 6.3 y	FFQ (150) at baseline, self-administered	M 286 vs 34 g/d (median values) (5) F: 343 vs 65 g/d (median values) (5)	Colon:1.33 (0.90–1.97) Rectum: 0.85 (0.55–1.32) Colon: 0.73 (0.48–1.11) Rectum: 0.67 (0.34–1.33)	0.22 0.29 0.12 0.44	Age, family history, alcohol	Incidence Netherlands cohort
Terry et al., 2001a, Sweden	291 colon, 259 rectum/ 61 463, F 9.6 y	FFQ (67) at baseline, self-administered	> 2 vs < 1 servings/d (4)	Colorectum: 0.68 (0.52–0.89) Colon: 0.76 (0.55–1.06) Rectum: 0.54 (0.33–0.89)	$p = 0.009$ $p = 0.23$ $p = 0.01$	Age, red meat, dairy food, energy	Incidence. Swedish mammography cohort
Bueno de Mesquita et al., 2002, Europe	773/405 667, M, F M: 3.3 y, F: 4.4 y	FFQs country specific. Interviewed or self-administered	Highest vs lowest (5)	Colorectum: 0.83 (CI includes 1.0)	$p = 0.88$	Stratified by age and centre. Adjusted for gender, weight, height, smoking, physical activity, energy, alcohol, veg.	Incidence EPIC cohort Excludes potatoes
Flood et al., 2002, USA	485/45 490, F Average 8.5 y	FFQ (62, 5 fruits) at baseline, self-administered	≥ 0.38 vs < 0.1 servings/day/ 1000 kJ (median values) (5)	Colorectum: 1.15 (0.86–1.53)		Age, energy (nutrient density), multivitamin supplement use, BMI, height, NSAIDs, smoking, education, physical activity, grains, red meat, calcium, vitamin D, alcohol, veg.	Incidence Breast Cancer Detection Demonstration Project cohort
Sauvaget et al., 2003, Japan	226/38 540, M 17 y	FFQ (22), self-administered	Daily vs 0–1 day/wk (3)	Colorectum: 0.97 (0.73–1.29)	$p = 0.81$	Age, sex, radiation dose, city, BMI, smoking, alcohol, education	Mortality, atomic bombing survivors
McCullough et al., 2003, USA	298/62 609, M 210/70 554, F 6 y	FFQ (68), self-administered	≥ 6.2 vs < 1.2 servings/ d (5) ≥ 6.0 vs < 1.2 servings/d (5)	Colon: 1.11 (0.76–1.62) Colon: 0.74 (0.47–1.16)	$p = 0.52$ $p = 0.47$	Age, education, exercise, aspirin, smoking, family history of colorectal cancer, BMI, energy, multivitamin use, total calcium, red meat, HRT use	Incidence Cancer Prevention Study II Nutrition Cohort

Cancer-preventive effects

Table 29. Case–control studies of fruit consumption and risk of colorectal cancer

Author, year, country	Cases/controls, gender	Exposure assessment (no. of items)	Range contrasts (no. of categories)	Relative risk (95% CI)	Stat. sign.*	Adjustment for confounding	Comments
Manousos et al., 1983, Greece	100/100, M, F	Dietary history (80), interviewed	Highest vs lowest (3)	Colorectum No difference in consumption between cases and controls		Age, sex	Hospital-based
Pickle et al., 1984, USA	Colon 58, rectum 28/176, M, F	Dietary history (57), interviewed	> 11.8 servings/wk versus less (2)	M: Colon: 1.12 Rectum: 0.97 F: Colon: 0.97 Rectum: 1.21		Age, sex, ethnic group, residence	Hospital-based Rural area
Macquart-Moulin et al., 1986, France	354/399, M, F	FFQ, interviewed	Highest vs lowest (4)	Colorectum: 0.74	NS	Age, sex, weight, energy	Hospital-based
Kune et al., 1987, Australia	Colon 392, rectum 323/727	Dietary history (> 300)	> 2440 vs < 610 g/wk (5)	M [0.74] F [0.61]	$p = 0.01$ in men	Age, sex	Population-based
La Vecchia et al., 1988c, Italy	Colon 339, rectum 236/778, M, F	FFQ (29)	Fresh fruit: Highest vs lowest (3)	Colon: 0.85 Rectum: 1.18	NS	Age, sex	Hospital-based
Slattery et al., 1988, USA	M, 112/185 F, 119/206	FFQ (99), interviewed	M: > 374 vs ≤ 158 g/d (4) F: > 431 vs ≤ 169 g/d (4)	Colon: M: 0.3 (0.1–0.6) F: 0.6 (0.3–1.3)		Age, BMI, religion, energy	Population-based
Tuyns et al., 1988, Belgium	Colon 453, rectum 365/2851, M, F	FFQ (extensive list), interviewed	Fresh fruit: > 1538 vs < 300 g/wk (4)	Colon: 0.91 Rectum: 0.87	$p = 0.19$ $p = 0.24$	Age, sex, province	Population-based
Benito et al., 1990, Spain	286/295, M, F	FFQ (99), interviewed	Fresh fruit: > 89 vs < 44 times/mo (4)	Colorectum: 1.09	NS	Age, sex, weight 10 years before	Population-based
Bidoli et al., 1992, Italy	Colon 123, rectum 125/699, M, F	FFQ, interviewed	Fresh fruit: Highest vs lowest (3)	Colon: 1.0 Rectum: 0.7	NS	Age, sex, social status	Hospital-based
Iscovich et al., 1992, Argentina	110/220	FFQ (140) interviewed		Colon: No association		Matched by age, sex, residence	Population-based, neigbour-hood controls
Peters et al., 1992, USA	746/746, M, F	Semi-quantitative FFQ (116), interviewed	Risk increase per 10 servings/mo	Colon: 1.00 (0.97–1.03)	NS	Age, sex, neighbourhood, fat, protein, carbohydrates, alcohol, calcium, family history, weight, physical activity, if female, pregnancy history	Population-based

145

Table 29 (contd)

Author, year, country	Cases/controls, gender	Exposure assessment (no. of items)	Range contrasts (no. of categories)	Relative risk (95% CI)	Stat. sign.*	Adjustment for confounding	Comments
Steinmetz & Potter, 1993, Australia	M 121/241 F 99/197	FFQ (141, 14 fruits), self-administered, previously validated	M: ≥ 28 vs ≤ 8 servings/wk (4) F: ≥ 34 vs ≤ 12 servings/wk (4)	Colon M: 1.74 (0.88–3.46) F: 0.90 (0.38–2.11)		Age, sex, occupation, Quetelet index, alcohol, protein intake, age at first live birth for women	Population-based
Centonze et al., 1994, Italy	Colorectal 119/119, M, F	FFQ (70), interviewed	≥ 480 vs ≤ 305 g/d (3)	Colorectum: 1.02 (0.53–1.95)	p = 0.96	Age, sex, smoking, education, changes in diet	Population-based
Kampman et al., 1995, Netherlands	M 130/136 F 102/123	FFQ (289), interviewed	M: > 269 vs < 100 g/d (3) F: > 327 vs < 143 g/d (3)	Colon: M: 1.00 (0.49–2.03) F: 0.54 (0.23–1.23)	p = 0.88 p = 0.13	Age, urbanization, energy, alcohol, cholecystectomy, family history	Population-based
Kotake et al., 1995, Japan	Colon 187, rectum 176/363 screening and hospital controls, M, F	FFQ (10)	Daily vs 1–2 times/wk (4)	Colon: 0.8 (0.27–2.41) Rectum: 0.7 (0.21–2.08)		Age, sex	Hospital-based
Shannon et al., 1990, USA	M 238/224 F 186/190	Semiquantitative FFQ (71), interviewed by telephone	M: > 17 vs ≤ 0.46 servings/d (4) F: > 2.1 vs ≤ 0.69 servings/d (4)	Colon: M: 0.77 (0.44–1.36) F: 0.44 (0.24–0.82)	p = 0.21 p = 0.007	Age, energy	Population-based
Franceschi et al., 1997, Italy	Colon 1225 Rectum 728/ 4154, M, F	FFQ (79), interviewed	Diversity of consumption: ≥ 6 vs ≤ 3 servings/wk (3)	Colon: 0.80 (0.63–1.01) Rectum: 0.94 (0.70–1.25)	NS p = 0.36	Age, sex, centre, education, energy, physical activity, veg., number of servings	Hospital-based
Boutron-Ruault et al., 1999, France	171/309, M, F	Dietary history, interviewed	M: > 273.2 vs < 130 g/d (4) F: > 286.4 vs < 137.4 g/d (4)	Colorectum: 1.0 (0.6–1.6)	p = 0.34	Age, sex, energy	Population-based
Levi et al., 1999, Switzerland	Colon 119, rectum 104/491, M, F	FFQ (79), interviewed	Citrus fruit: OR for an increase of one serving/d Other fruit: OR for an increase of one serving/d	Colorectum: 0.86 (0.78–0.96) Colorectum: 0.85 (0.75–0.96)		Age, sex, education, tobacco, alcohol, BMI, energy, physical activity	Hospital-based

Table 29 (contd)

Author, year, country	Cases/controls, gender	Exposure assessment (no. of items)	Range contrasts (no. of categories)	Relative risk (95% CI)	Stat. sign.*	Adjustment for confounding	Comments
Murata et al., 1999, Japan	Colon 265 Rectum 164/794, M, F	FFQ, self-administered	Daily vs rare (4)	Colon: 0.94 (0.78–1.13) Rectum: 0.98 (0.79–1.22)		Age, alcohol, tobacco, sex, eating attitude, other foods	Hospital-based
Deneo-Pellegrini et al., 2002, Uruguay	Colon: 260, Rectum: 224/ 1452	FFQ (64, 10 fruits), interviewed	Highest vs lowest (4)	Colorectum: 0.7 (0.5–0.9)	$p = 0.04$	Age, sex, residence, urban/rural status, education, family history of colon cancer, BMI, energy, red meat intake	Hospital-based

*p for trend when applicable

Table 30. Cohort studies of vegetable consumption and risk of colorectal cancer

Author, year, country	Cases/cohort size, gender (years follow-up)	Exposure assessment (no. of items)	Range contrasts (no. of categories)	Relative risk (95% CI)	Stat. sign.*	Adjustment for confounding	Comments
Shibata, et al., 1992, USA	105 F, 97 M/ 11 580 9 y	FFQ (59) at baseline, self-administered	F ≥ 4.8 vs < 3.2 servings/ d (3) M ≥ 4.5 vs < 3 servings/ d (3)	Colon: 0.72 (0.45–1.16) 1.39 (0.84–2.30)	NS NS	Age, smoking	Incidence California retirement community residents Includes potatoes
Thun et al., 1992, USA	539 F, 611, M/ 5746 6 y	FFQ (32) at baseline	Highest vs lowest (5)	Colon: F 0.66 M 0.80		Matched by age, race, sex	Mortality ACS Cancer Prevention II cohort: 426 838 F, 337 505 M Nested case–cohort design Inclusion of potatoes not specified
Steinmetz, et al., 1994, USA	212/41 837, F 5 y	FFQ (127) at baseline, self-administered	> 30.4 vs < 15.1 servings/wk (4)	Colon: 0.73 (0.47–1.13)	$p > 0.05$	Age, energy	Incidence Iowa Woman's Health Study Includes potatoes

Table 30 (contd)

Author, year, country	Cases/cohort size, gender (years follow-up)	Exposure assessment (no. of items)	Range contrasts (no. of categories)	Relative risk (95% CI)	Stat. sign.*	Adjustment for confounding	Comments
Kato, et al., 1997, USA	100/14 727, F Average 7.1 y	FFQ at baseline, self-administered	Highest vs lowest (4)	Colorectum: 1.63 (0.92–2.89)	$p = 0.40$	Age, energy, enrolment site, education	Incidence NY University cohort Excludes potatoes
Hsing, et al., 1998a, USA	125 colon, 25 rectum/17 633, M (white) 11.5 y	FFQ (35) at baseline, self-administered	> 4.5 vs < 1.2 times/mo	Colorectum: 1.3 (0.8–2.4) Colon: 1.5 (0.8–2.8)	$p = 0.3$ $p = 0.3$	Age, energy (standard), smoking, alcohol	Mortality Lutheran Brotherhood cohort Includes potatoes
Pietinen, et al., 1999, Finland	185/26 926, M Average 8 y	FFQ (276) at baseline, self-administered	191 vs 44 g/d (median values) (4)	Colorectum: 1.2 (0.8–1.9)	$p = 0.46$	Age, intervention group, years smoking BMI, alcohol, education, physical activity, calcium	Incidence ATBC cohort, vitamin supplement trial. All smokers Inclusion of potatoes not specified
Michels, et al., 2000, USA	368 colon, 89 rectum/47 325, M 569 colon; 155 rectum/88 764, F M 10 y, F 16 y	FFQ (61, 11 veg., expanded to 28)	≥ 5 vs ≤ 1 servings/d (5)	Colon: 1.00 (0.72–1.38) (RR for 1 additional serving/day: 1.03 (0.97–1.09)) Rectum: 1.17 (0.63–2.18) (RR for 1 additional serving/day: 1.02 (0.92–1.14))		Age, family history of colorectal cancer, sigmoidoscopy, height, BMI, smoking, alcohol, physical activity, menopausal status, hormone replacement therapy, aspirin, vitamin supplement use, energy, red meat	Incidence Nurses' Health Study or Health Professional Study Excludes potatoes Pooled estimates for M and F
Voorrips et al., 2000a, Netherlands	312 colon, 199 rectum/58 279, M 266 colon, 115 rectum/62 573, F 6.3 y	FFQ (150) at baseline, self-administered	M 285 vs 100 g/d (median values) (5) F 293 vs 107 g/d (median values) (5)	Colon: 0.85 (0.57–1.27) Rectum: 0.88 (0.55–1.41) Colon: 0.83 (0.54–1.26) Rectum: 1.78 (0.94–3.38)	$p = 0.45$ $p = 0.58$ $p = 0.31$ $p = 0.09$	Age, family history, alcohol	Incidence Netherlands cohort Excludes potatoes

148

Cancer-preventive effects

Table 30 (contd)

Author, year, country	Cases/cohort size, gender (years follow-up)	Exposure assessment (no. of items)	Range contrasts (no. of categories)	Relative risk (95% CI)	Stat. sign.*	Adjustment for confounding	Comments
Terry et al., 2001a, Sweden	291 colon, 159 rectum/61 463, F 9.6 y	FFQ (67) at baseline, self-administered	> 2 vs < 1 servings/d (4)	Colorectum: 0.84 (0.65–1.09) Colon: 0.90 (0.66–1.24) Rectum: 0.71 (0.45–1.12)	$p = 0.25$ $p = 0.43$ $p = 0.29$	Age, red meat, dairy food, energy	Incidence Swedish Mammography cohort Includes potatoes
Bueno de Mesquita et al., 2002, Europe	773/405 667, M, F M 3.3 y, F 4.4 y	FFQs country specific, interviewed or self-administered	Highest vs lowest (5)	Colorectum: 0.71 (CI does not include 1.0)	$p = 0.37$	Stratified by age and centre. Adjusted for gender, weight, height, smoking, physical activity, energy, alcohol, fruit	Incidence EPIC cohort Excludes potatoes
Flood et al., 2002, USA	485/45 490, F Average 8.5 y	FFQ (62, 5 fruits) at baseline, self-administered	≥ 0.79 vs < 0.33 servings/d 1000 kJ (5)	Colorectum: 0.95 (0.71–1.26)		Age, energy (nutrient density), multivitamin supplement use, BMI, height, NSAIDs, smoking, education, physical activity, grains, red meat, calcium, vitamin D, alcohol, fruits	Incidence Breast Cancer Detection Demonstration Project cohort Includes potatoes
Sauvaget et al., 2003, Japan	226/38,540, M, F 17 y	FFQ (22), self-administered	Green-yellow veg.: Daily vs 0–1 d/wk (3)	Colorectum: 1.10 (0.82–1.47)	$p = 0.52$	Age, sex, radiation dose, city, BMI, smoking, alcohol, education	Mortality, atomic bombing survivors
McCullough et al., 2003, USA	298/62 609, M 210/70 554 F 6 y	FFQ (68), self-administered	≥ 3.3 vs < 1.3 servings/d (5)	Colon: 0.69 (0.47–1.03) Colon: 0.91 (0.56–1.48)	$p = 0.10$ $p = 0.56$	Age, education, exercise, aspirin, smoking, family history of colorectal cancer, BMI, energy, multivitamin use, total calcium, red meat, HRT use	Incidence Cancer Prevention Study II Nutrition cohort Excludes potatoes

*p for trend when applicable

Table 31. Case–control studies of vegetable consumption and risk of colorectal cancer

Author, year, country	Cases/controls, gender	Exposure assessment (no. of items)	Range contrasts (no. of categories)	Relative risk (95% CI)	Stat. sign.*	Adjustment for confounding	Comments
Graham et al., 1978, USA	Colon 183/611 Rectum 243/492, M (white)	Interview (19 veg.)	> 61 vs ≤ 20 times/mo (4)	Colon: 1.76 Rectum: 1.60	p = 0.02 p = 0.012		Population-based
Manousos et al., 1983, Greece	100/100, M, F	Dietary histories (80), interviewed	Highest vs lowest (4)	Colorectum: cases less frequent consumption of veg. than controls	p < 0.05	Age, sex	Hospital-based
Miller et al., 1983, Canada	Colon 348 (171 M, 177 F), rectum 194 (114 M, 80 F)/ 535 hospital and 542 neighbourhood controls	FFQ (150), interviewed	M > 468 vs < 291 g/d (3) F > 395 vs < 251 g/d (3)	M, Colon: 0.8 Rectum: 1.1 F, Colon: 0.7 Rectum: 1.2	p = 0.19 p = 0.43 p = 0.06 p = 0.28	Age, sex, saturated fat, other foods	Hospital-based and population-based
Pickle et al., 1984, USA	Colon 58, rectum 28/17, M, F	Dietary history (57), interviewed	> 8.9 servings/wk vs less (2)	Colon: 1.77 Rectum: 1.43		Age, sex, ethnic group, residence	Hospital-based Rural area
Macquart-Moulin et al., 1986, France	399/399, M, F	FFQ, interviewed	Highest vs lowest (4)	Colorectum: Veg. with 1 g veg./100 g fibre: 0.42 Veg. with 2.8 g veg./100 g fibre: 0.58	p < 0.001 p = 0.004	Age, sex, energy, weight	Hospital-based
Kune et al., 1987, Australia	Colon 392, rectum 323/727, M, F	Dietary history (+300)	> 2370 vs < 1180 g/wk (4)	Colorectum: M [0.38] F [0.48]	p < 0.001 p < 0.001		Population-based
La Vecchia et al., 1988c, Italy	Colon 339, rectum 236/778, M, F	FFQ (29)	Green veg.: Highest vs lowest (3)	Colon: 0.50 Rectum : 0.51	p < 0.01 p < 0.01	Age, sex, education, area, other foods	Hospital-based
Slattery et al., 1988	M 112/185, F 119/206	FFQ (99), interviewed	M > 400.1 vs ≤ 220.5 g/d (4) F > 456 vs ≤ 231.2 g/d (4)	Colon: M 0.6 (0.3–1.3) F 0.3 (0.1–0.9)		Age, BMI, religion, energy	Population-based
Tuyns et al., 1988, Belgium	Colon 453, rectum 365/2851, M, F	FFQ (extensive list), interviewed	Cooked veg.: > 1375 vs < 800 g/wk (4) Raw veg.: > 268 vs < 80 g/wk (4)	Colon : 0.71 Rectum: 0.36 Colon: 0.37 Rectum: 0.49	p < 0.01 p < 0.013 p < 0.0001 p < 0.0001	Age, sex, province	Population-based

Table 31 (contd)

Author, year, country	Cases/controls, gender	Exposure assessment (no. of items)	Range contrasts (no. of categories)	Relative risk (95% CI)	Stat. sign.*	Adjustment for confounding	Comments
Young & Wolf, 1988, USA	353/618, M, F (white)	FFQ (25) Diet over age 35 y	Miscellaneous veg.: 20 times/mo vs 1/mo (5)	Colon: 0.72 (0.48–1.07)		Age, sex	Population-based
Lee et al., 1989, Singapore	Colon 131, Rectum 71/426, M, F	FFQ (116), interviewed	Highest vs lowest (3)	Colon: 0.79 (0.48–1.28) Rectum: 0.51 (0.27–0.98) Colorectum: 0.69 (0.45–1.05)	NS $p < 0.05$ NS	Age, sex, dialect, education, occupation	Hospital-based
Benito et al., 1990, Spain	265/267, M, F	FFQ (99), interviewed	> 117 vs < 64 times/mo (4)	Colorectum: 0.71	NS	Age, sex, weight 10 years prior	Population-based
Hu et al., 1991, China	Colon 111, rectum 225/336, M, F	FFQ (25)	> 193 vs < 75.5 kg/y (3)	[0.18 (0.05–0.61)]	$p = 0.003$	Age, sex, residence	Hospital-based
Bidoli et al., 1992, Italy	Colon 123, rectum 125/699, M, F	FFQ, interviewed	Highest vs lowest (3)	Colon: 0.7 Rectum : 0.6	NS	Age, sex, social status	Hospital-based
Iscovich et al., 1992, Argentina	110/220,	FFQ (140)	> 1281 vs < 483 times/y (4)	Colon: 0.075 (0.02–0.3)	$p < 0.001$	Age, sex, residence, other foods	Population-based, neighbourhood controls
Peters et al., 1992, USA	746/746, M, F	Semiquantitative FFQ (116), interviewed	Other non-cruciferous veg.: Risk increase per 10 servings/mo	1.01 (0.97–1.04)		Age, sex, neighbourhood, fat, protein, carbohydrates, alcohol, calcium, family history, weight, physical activity, if female, pregnancy history	Population-based
Steinmetz & Potter, 1993	M 121/241, F 99/197	FFQ (141, 48 veg.), self-administered, previously validated	M ≥ 32 vs < 15 servings/wk (4) F ≥ 38 vs < 19 servings/wk (4)	Colon: M 1.29 (0.67–2.51) F 1.11 (0.50–2.45)		Age, sex, occupation, Quetelet index, alcohol, protein intake, age at first live birth for women	Population-based

IARC Handbooks of Cancer Prevention Volume 8: Fruit and Vegetables

Table 31 (contd)

Author, year, country	Cases/controls, gender	Exposure assessment (no. of items)	Range contrasts (no. of categories)	Relative risk (95% CI)	Stat. sign.*	Adjustment for confounding	Comments
Centonze et al., 1994, Italy	119/119. M, F	FFQ (70), interviewed	> 329 vs ≤ 236 g/d (3)	Colorectum: 0.51 (0.25–1.04)	$p = 0.07$	Age, sex, smoking, education, changes in diet, cereals, dairy products, dried fruits, foods contained refined sugar, coffee, wine	Population-based
Kampman et al., 1995, Netherlands	232/259. M, F	FFQ (289), interviewed	> 247 vs < 142 g/d (4)	Colon: 0.40 (0.23–0.69)	$p = 0.0004$	Age, sex, urbanization, energy, alcohol, cholecystectomy, family history	Population-based
Kotake et al., 1995, Japan	Colon 187, rectum 176/363, screening and hospital controls	FFQ (10)	Daily vs 1–2 wk (4)	Colon: 1.01 (0.24–4.22) Rectum: 0.5 (0.12–1.96)		Age, sex	Hospital-based
Shannon et al., 1996, USA	M 238/224 F 186/190	Semiquantitative FFQ (71), interviewed by telephone	M: > 3.5 vs < 1.2 servings/d (4) F: > 3.9 vs < 1.5 servings/d (4)	Colon: M 0.78 (0.45–1.35) F 0.51 (0.28–0.93)	$p = 0.46$ $p = 0.02$	Age, energy	Population-based
Franceschi et al., 1997, Italy	Colon 1225, rectum 728/4154, M, F	FFQ (79), interviewed	Diversity of consumption: ≥ 8 vs ≤ 5 servings/wk (3)	Colon: 0.77 (0.62–0.95) Rectum: 0.85 (0.65–1.09)	$p < 0.05$ NS	Age, sex, centre, education, energy, physical activity, fruits, number of servings	Hospital-based
Boutron-Ruault et al., 1999, France	171/309, M, F	Dietary history, interviewed	M: > 251.8 vs < 130.8 g/d (4) F: > 243.4 vs < 120 g/d (4)	Colorectum: 0.7 (0.4–1.3)	$p = 0.19$	Age, sex, energy	Population-based
Levi et al., 1999, Switzerland	Colon 119, rectum 104/491, M, F	FFQ (79), interviewed	Raw veg.: OR for an increase of one serving per day Cooked veg.: OR for an increase of one serving	Colorectum: 0.85 (0.74–0.98) Colorectum: 0.69 (0.57–0.83)		Age sex, education, tobacco, alcohol, BMI, energy, physical activity	Hospital-based

Table 31 (contd)

Author, year, country	Cases/controls, gender	Exposure assessment (no. of items)	Range contrasts (no. of categories)	Relative risk (95% CI)	Stat. sign.*	Adjustment for confounding	Comments
La Vecchia et al., 1999, Italy	Colon 1225 (688 M, 537 F)/4154 (2073 M, 2081 F)	FFQ (78), validated	Highest vs lowest (3)	Colon: M [0.74 (0.59–0.91)] F [0.43 (0.32–0.56)]	NS $p < 0.01$	Age, sex, centre, education, physical activity, energy, meal frequency, family history	Hospital-based
Murata et al., 1999, Japan	Colon 265, rectum 164/794	FFQ, self-administered	Green veg,: Daily vs rare (4)	Colon: 0.87 (0.67–1.12) Rectum: 0.84 (0.62–1.14)		Age, alcohol, tobacco, sex, eating attitude, other foods	Hospital-based
Deneo-Pellegrini et al., 2002, Uruguay	Colon 260, rectum 224/1452 (882 M, 570 F)	FFQ (64, 18 veg.), interviewed	Highest vs lowest (4)	Colorectum: 0.7 (0.5–0.9)	$p = 0.04$	Age, sex, residence, urban/rural status, education, family history of colon cancer, BMI, energy, red meat	Hospital-based

*p for trend when applicable

Table 32. Cohort studies on fruit and vegetable consumption and risk of colorectal cancer

Author, year, country	Cases/cohort size, gender (years follow-up)	Exposure assessment (no. of items)	Range contrasts (no. of categories)	Relative risk (95% CI)	Stat. sign.*	Adjustment for confounding	Comments
Shibata et al., 1992, USA	905 F, 97 M/ 11 580 9 y	FFQ (52, 23 fruits and 21 veg.) at baseline, self-administered	F ≥ 8.3 vs < 5.9 servings/d (3) M ≥ 7.09 vs < 5.5 servings/d (3)	Colon: F 0.63 (0.40–1.00) M 1.50 (0.91–2.46)	$p < 0.05$ NS	Age, smoking	Incidence California retirement community residents Includes potatoes
Steinmetz et al., 1994, USA	212/41 837, F 5 y	FFQ (127) at baseline, self-administered	> 47 vs < 24.6 servings/wk (4)	Colon: 0.89 (0.57–1.40)	$p > 0.05$	Age, energy	Incidence Iowa Women's Health Study Includes potatoes

Table 32 (contd)

Author, year, country	Cases/cohort size, gender (years follow-up)	Exposure assessment (no. of items)	Range contrasts (no. of categories)	Relative risk (95% CI)	Stat. sign.*	Adjustment for confounding	Comments
Michels et al., 2000, USA	569 colon, 155 rectum/88 764, F 16 y 368 colon, 89 rectum/ 47 325, M 10 y	FFQ (61, 6 fruits and 11 veg. expanded to 15 fruits and 28 veg.)	≥ 6 vs ≤ 2 servings/d (5)	Colon: 1.08 (0.84–1.38) (RR for 1 additional serving/d: 1.02 (0.98–1.05)) Rectum: 0.99 (0.62–1.56) (RR for 1 additional serving/d: 1.02 (0.95–1.09))		Age, family history of colorectal cancer, sigmoidoscopy, height, BMI, smoking, alcohol, physical activity, aspirin, vitamin supplement use, energy (standard), red meat	Incidence Nurses' Health Study (F) and Health Professional Study (M) Pooled estimates for M and F
Voorrips et al., 2000a, Netherlands	312 colon, 199 rectum/ 58 279, M 266 colon, 115 rectum/ 62 573, F 6.3 y	FFQ (150) at baseline, self-administered	M 519 vs 177 g/d (median values) (5) F 578 vs 208 g/d (median values) (5)	Colon: 0.95 (0.64–1.41) Rectum: 0.88 (0.56–1.37) Colon: 0.66 (0.44–1.01) Rectum: 1.17 (0.63–2.17)	$p = 0.90$ $p = 0.90$ $p = 0.10$ $p = 0.84$	Age, family history, alcohol	Incidence Netherlands cohort Excludes potatoes
Terry et al., 2001a, Sweden	291 colon, 159 rectum/61 463, F 9.6 y	FFQ (67) at baseline, self-administered	> 5 vs < 2.5 servings/d (4)	Colorectum: 0.73 (0.56–0.96) Colon: 0.81 (0.59–1.13) Rectum: 0.60 (0.38–0.96)	$p = 0.03$ $p = 0.36$ $p = 0.02$	Age, red meat, dairy food, energy	Incidence Swedish mammography cohort
Bueno de Mesquita et al., 2002, Europe	773/405 667, M, F M 3.3 y F 4.4 y	FFQ country-specific, interviewed or self-administered	Highest vs lowest (5)	Colorectum: 0.74 (CI does not include 1)	$p = 0.45$	Stratified by age and centre. Adjusted for gender, weight, height, smoking, physical activity, energy, alcohol, veg.	Incidence EPIC cohort Excludes potatoes

*p for trend when applicable

Table 33. Case–control studies of total fruit and vegetable consumption and risk of colorectal cancer

Author, year, country	Cases/controls, gender	Exposure assessment (no. of items)	Range contrasts (no. of categories)	Relative risk (95% CI)	Stat. sign.*	Adjustment for confounding	Comments
Pickle et al., 1984, USA	58 colon, 28 rectum/176, M, F	Dietary history (57), interviewed	> 21.3 servings/wk vs less (2)	Colon 0.97 Rectum 1.21		Age, sex, ethnic group, residence	Hospital-based, rural area
Peters et al., 1989, USA	147/147 M white	Questionnaire, interviewed	Fresh fruit: or raw veg.: ≥ 5 vs ≤ 1 times/wk (3)	Colorectum: 0.6 (0.2–1.4)		Education, age	Population-based, neighbourhood controls
Steinmetz & Potter, 1993, Australia	M 121/141 F 99/197	FFQ (141, 14 fruits, 48 veg.), previously validated, self-administered	M: ≥ 59 vs ≤ 28 servings/wk (4) F: ≥ 70 vs ≤ 36 servings/wk (4)	Colon: M 1.39 (0.72–2.71) F 0.76 (0.33–1.76)		Age, sex, occcupation, Quetelet index, alcohol, protein intake, age at first live birth for women	Population-based
Shannon et al., 1996, USA	M 238/224 F 186/190	Semiquantitative FFQ (71), interviewed by telephone	M: > 5 vs 1.8 servings/d (4) F: > 5.7 vs < 2.4 servings/d (4)	0.93 (0.52–1.64) 0.48 (0.26–0.86)	$p = 0.61$ $p = 0.02$	Age, energy	Population-based
Deneo-Pellegrini et al., 2002, Uruguay	260 colon, 224 rectum/1452	FFQ (64, 10 fruits, 18 veg.), interviewed	Highest vs lowest (4)	Colorectum: 0.7 (0.5–0.9)	$p = 0.01$	Age, sex, residence, urban/rural status, education, family history of colon cancer, BMI, energy, red meat	Hospital-based

*p for trend when applicable

Table 34. Cohort study of fruit consumption and risk of adenomatous polyps

Author, year, country	Cases/cohort size gender (years follow-up)	Exposure assessment (no. of items)	Range contrasts (no. of categories)	Relative risk (95% CI)	Stat. sign.*	Adjustment for confounding	Comments
Platz et al., 1997, USA	690/16 448, M 9 y	FFQ (131)	> 8.4 vs < 1.3 g/d (5)	0.81 (0.59–1.11)	$p = 0.03$	Age, endoscopy before 1986, family history of colorectal cancer, BMI, pack-years smoking, physical activity, regular aspirin use, energy, alcohol, red meat, folate and methionine intake	Subjects who had endoscopy (left-sided adenomas)

*p for trend when applicable

Table 35. Case–control studies of fruit consumption and risk of adenomatous polyps

Author, year, country	Cases/controls, gender	Exposure assessment (no. of items)	Range contrasts (no. of categories)	Relative risk (95% CI)	Stat. sign.*	Adjustment for confounding	Comments
Macquart-Moulin et al., 1987, France	252/238	FFQ, interviewed	Highest vs lowest (4)	Colorectum: 0.70		Age, sex, energy, weight	Hospital-based
Sandler et al., 1993, USA	M 105/165 F 131/244	FFQ (>100), interviewed by telephone, previously validated	M > 19.9 vs < 6.3 servings/wk (5) F ≥ 22.3 vs < 8.4 servings/wk (5)	Colorectum: M 0.60 (0.24–1.52) F 0.44 (0.20–0.95)	$p = 0.50$ $p = 0.03$	Age, alcohol, BMI, energy	Hospital-based
Witte et al., 1996, USA	488/488, M, F	Semiquantitative FFQ (129), interviewed	≥ 25 vs < 2.5 servings/wk (5)	Colorectum: 0.92 (0.52–1.63)	$p = 0.99$	Race, BMI, physical activity, smoking, energy, saturated fat, fibre, folate, β-carotene, vitamin C	Asymptomatic screened controls
Lubin et al, 1997, Israel	196/196, M, F	FFQ (180), interviewed	Fruit/fresh juices > 478 vs < 283 g/d (3)	1.1 (0.6–1.9)	$p = 0.78$	Matched by age, sex, country of origin, follow-up. Adjusted for energy, physical activity	Asymptomatic screened controls
Almendinge et al., 2001, Norway	87/35 hospital and 35 healthy controls, M, F	Dietary record	Fruits and berries: > 321 vs < 110 g/d (3)	Hospital: 5.5 (1.3–23.1) Population: 2.9 (0.6–14.5)	$p = 0.01$ $p = 0.2$	Sex, age, BMI, history of colorectal cancer, energy, fat, fibre, smoking	Hospital-based and population-based
Smith-Warner et al., 2002b USA	564/535, M, F	Semi-quantitative FFQ (153, 59 fruits and veg.)	M > 27.9 vs < 2.1 servings/wk (5) F > 27.5 vs < 3.3 servings/wk (5)	Colorectum: M 0.75 (0.41–1.35) F 0.68 (0.32–1.43)	$p = 0.44$ $p = 0.29$	Age, energy, fat intake BMI, smoking, alcohol, use of NSAIDs, multivitamins, hormone replacement therapy	Population-based

*p for trend when applicable

Table 36. Cohort study of vegetable consumption and risk of adenomatous polyps

Author, year, country	Cases/cohort size, gender (years follow-up)	Exposure assessment (no. of items)	Range contrasts (no. of categories)	Relative risk (95% CI)	Stat. sign.*	Adjustment for confounding	Comments
Platz et al., 1997, USA	690/16 448, M 9 y	FFQ (131)	> 11.5 vs < 3.2 g/d (5)	0.93 (0.67–1.30)	$p = 0.33$	Age, endoscopy before 1986, family history of colorectal cancer, BMI, pack-years smoking, physical activity, regular aspirin use, energy, alcohol, red meat, folate and methionine intake	Subjects who had endoscopy (left-sided adenomas)

*p for trend when applicable

Table 37. Case–control studies of vegetable consumption and risk of adenomatous polyps

Author, year, country	Cases/controls, gender	Exposure assessment (no. of items)	Range contrasts (no. of categories)	Relative risk (95% CI)	Stat. sign.*	Adjustment for confounding	Comments
Macquart-Moulin et al., 1987, France	252/238, M, F	FFQ, interviewed	Veg. (low fibre): Highest vs lowest (4) Veg.: Highest vs lowest (4)	Colorectum: 0.78 1.24		Age, sex, energy, weight	Hospital-based
Witte et al., 1996, USA	488/488, M, F	Semiquantitative FFQ (129), interviewed	≥ 45.5 vs ≤ 9 servings/wk (5)	Colorectum: 0.90 (0.49–1.68)	$p = 0.27$	Race, BMI, physical activity, smoking, energy, saturated fat, fibre, folate, β-carotene, vitamin C	Asymptomatic screened controls
Lubin et al., 1997, Israel	196/196, M, F	FFQ (180), interviewed	> 460 vs < 290 g/d (3)	0.9 (0.6–1.6)	$p = 0.838$	Matched by age, sex, country of origin, follow-up. Adjusted for energy, physical activity	Asymptomatic screened controls
Sandler et al., 1993, USA	M 105/165 F 131/244	FFQ (> 100), interviewed by telephone, previously validated	M: ≥ 23.9 vs < 11.1 servings/wk (5) F: ≥ 24.8 vs < 11.2 servings/wk (5)	Colorectal adenomas: M 1.20 (0.49–2.93) F 0.74 (0.35–1.57)	$p = 0.72$ $p = 0.69$	Age, alcohol, BMI, energy	Hospital-based

IARC Handbooks of Cancer Prevention Volume 8: Fruit and Vegetables

Table 37 (contd)

Author, year, country	Cases/controls, gender	Exposure assessment (no. of items)	Range contrasts (no. of categories)	Relative risk (95% CI)	Stat. sign.*	Adjustment for confounding	Comments
Almendingen et al., 2001, Norway	87/35 hospital and 35 healthy controls, M, F	Dietary record	≥ 181 vs < 80 g/d (3)	Hospital: 0.4 (0.1–1.8) $p = 0.2$ Population: 1.1 (0.2–5.1) $p = 0.82$		Sex, age, BMI, history of colorectal cancer, energy, fat, fibre, smoking	Hospital-based and population-based
Smith-Warner et al., 2002b, USA	564/535, M, F	Semiquantitative FFQ (153, 59 fruits and veg.)	M ≥ 44.7 vs ≤ 8.8 servings/wk (5) F ≥ 51.4 vs ≤ 10.1 servings/wk (5)	Colorectal adenomas: M 0.55 (0.30–0.98) F 1.40 (0.67–2.92)	$p = 0.16$ $p = 0.24$	Age, energy, fat, BMI, smoking, alcohol, use of NSAIDs, multivitamins, hormone replacement therapy	Population-based

*p for trend when applicable

Table 38. Case–control studies of fruit and vegetable consumption and risk of adenomatous polyps

Author, year, country	Cases/controls, gender	Exposure assessment (no. of items)	Range contrasts (no. of categories)	Relative risk (95% CI)	Stat. sign.*	Adjustment for confounding	Comments
Smith-Warner et al., 2002b, USA	564/535, M, F	Semiquantitative FFQ (153, 59 fruits and veg.)	M: ≥ 75.9 vs ≤ 16.5 servings/wk (5) F: ≥ 82.8 vs ≤ 18.4 servings/wk	Colorectal adenoma: M 0.60 (0.32–1.12) F 0.76 (0.34–1.66)	$p = 0.20$ $p = 0.86$	Age, energy, fat, BMI, smoking, alcohol, use of NSAIDs, multivitamins, hormone replacement therapy	Population-based

*p for trend when applicable

Table 39. Cohort study of fruit consumption and risk of liver cancer

Author, year, country	Cases/ cohort size, gender (years follow-up)	Exposure assessment (no. of items)	Range contrasts (no. of categories)	Relative risk (95% CI)	Stat. sign.*	Adjustment for confounding	Comments
Sauvaget et al., 2003, Japan	555/38 540, M 17 y	FFQ (22), self-administered	Daily vs 0–1 d/wk (3)	0.96 (0.78–1.19)	p = 0.81	Age, sex, radiation dose, city, BMI, smoking, alcohol, education	Mortality, atomic bombing survivors

*p for trend when applicable

Table 40. Case–control studies of fruit consumption and risk of liver cancer

Author, year, country	Cases/controls, gender	Exposure assessment (no. of items)	Range contrasts (no. of categories)	Relative risk (95% CI)	Stat. sign.*	Adjustment for confounding	Comments
La Vecchia et al., 1988b, Italy	151 HCC/1051, M, F	FFQ	Fresh fruit: Highest vs lowest (3)	0.76	NS	Age, sex, area of residence, education, history of hepatitis, alcohol, smoking, other dietary factors	Hospital-based
Parkin et al., 1991, Thailand	93 cholangiocarcinoma/103 hospital or visitor, M, F	FFQ (54)	Fresh fruit: ≥ 3/month vs < 3/month (2)	0.5 (0.3–0.9)		Matched by sex, age, residence	Hospital-based
Hadziyannis et al., 1995, Greece	65 HCC/65 metastatic liver cancer, 65 hospital, M, F	Semiquantitative FFQ (115)		No association			Hospital-based Response rate for cases 89%, for metastatic liver cancer controls 90% and for hospital controls 93%
Kuper et al., 2000, Greece	97 HCC/128, M, F	Semiquantitative FFQ (~ 120)	One quintile increment	1.00 (0.71–1.41)	p = 0.99	Age, gender, schooling, HBV/HCV infection, alcohol, tobacco, energy, other food groups	Hospital-based

*p for trend when applicable

Table 41. Cohort studies of vegetable consumption and risk of liver cancer

Author, year, country	Cases/cohort size, gender, (years follow-up)	Exposure assessment (no. of items)	Range contrasts (no. of categories)	Relative risk (95% CI)	Stat. sign.*	Adjustment for confounding	Comments
Hirayama, 1990, Japan	1251/265 118, M, F 17 y	FFQ (7)	Green-yellow veg.: daily vs non-daily (2)	0.91 (90% CI 0.82–1.01)		Not reported	Mortality Census-based cohort in seven prefectures
Yu et al., 1995, Taiwan	50/8436, M 54 y	FFQ	≥ 6 veg-containing meals/wk vs < 6	[0.4 (0.2–0.8)]	$p = 0.006$	Age, HBsAg carrier status, cigarette smoking, habitual alcohol consumption, history of liver disease	Incidence Cohort recruited primarily for a study of biological markers of HCC
Sauvaget et al., 2003, Japan	555/38 540, M 17 y	FFQ (22), self-administered	Green-yellow veg.: Daily vs 0–1 d/wk (3)	0.75 (0.60–0.95)	$p = 0.009$	Age, sex, radiation dose, city, BMI, smoking, alcohol, education	Mortality, atomic bombing survivors

*p for trend when applicable

Table 42. Case–control studies of vegetable consumption and risk of liver cancer

Author, year, country	Cases/controls, gender	Exposure assessment (no. of items)	Range contrasts (no. of categories)	Relative risk (95% CI)	Stat. sign.*	Adjustment for confounding	Comments
Lam et al., 1982, Hong Kong	106/107, M, F	FFQ	Yellow veg.: weekly vs less Green veg.: daily vs less	0.6 1.0			Hospital-based Response rate for cases 72%
La Vecchia et al., 1988b, Italy	151/1051, M, F	FFQ	Green veg.: Highest vs lowest (3)	0.58	$p < 0.05$	Age, sex, area of residence, education, history of hepatitis, alcohol, smoking, other dietary factors	Hospital-based
Srivatanakul et al., 1991, Thailand	65/65 matched hospital or visitor, M, F	FFQ (54)	"Other" fresh veg.: ≤ twice a day vs less (2)	0.2 (0.04–1.0)	$p < 0.05$	HBsAg status, alcohol, betel-nut chewing, shrimp paste and powdered peanut consumption	Hospital-based. 'Other' fresh veg. consumption excludes cucumber and cabbage (Parkin et al., 1991)

Table 42 (contd)

Author, year, country	Cases/controls, gender	Exposure assessment (no. of items)	Range contrasts (no. of categories)	Relative risk (95% CI)	Stat. sign.*	Adjustment for confounding	Comments
Fukuda et al., 1993, Japan	368/485, M, F	FFQ (12)		No difference in consumption between cases and controls			Hospital-based Response rates high, only 7 cases not interviewed, and 3 controls excluded with incomplete information
Hadziyannis et al., 1995, Greece	65/65 controls with metastatic liver cancer, 65 hospital controls, M, F	Semiquantitative FFQ (115)		No association			Hospital-based Response rate for cases 89%, for metastatic liver cancer controls 90% and for hospital controls 93%
Kuper et al., 2000, Greece	97/128, M, F	Semiquantitative FFQ (~ 120)	One quintile increment	1.21 (0.80–1.82)	$p = 0.36$	Age, gender, schooling, HBV/HCV infection, alcohol, tobacco, energy, other food groups	Hospital-based

*p for trend when applicable

Table 43. Case–control study of fruit and vegetable consumption and risk of liver (hepatocellular) cancer

Author, year, country	Cases/controls, gender	Exposure assessment (no. of items)	Range contrasts (no. of categories)	Relative risk (95%)	Stat. sign.*	Adjustment for confounding	Comments
Braga et al., 1997a, Italy	320/1408, M, F	FFQ	Fresh fruit, green veg. and carrots combined: Highest vs lowest (3)	[0.46 (0.32–0.67)]		Age, sex, area of residence, smoking history, diabetes, liver cirrhosis	Hospital-based. This is an extension of La Vecchia et al. (1988b). Attributable risk estimated to be 40% (26–54%), 44% for males (28–60%) and 32% for females (4–60%)

*p for trend when applicable

Table 44. Cohort study of fruit consumption and risk of gallbladder cancer

Author, year, country	Cases/cohort size, gender (years follow-up)	Exposure assessment (no. of items)	Range contrasts (no. of categories)	Relative risk (95% CI)	Stat. sign.*	Adjustment for confounding	Comments
Sauvaget et al., 2003, Japan	157/38 540, M 17 y	FFQ (22), self-administered	Daily vs 0–1 d/wk (3)	0.85 (0.57–1.25)	$p = 0.53$	Age, sex, radiation dose, city, BMI, smoking, alcohol, education	Mortality, atomic bombing survivors

*p for trend when applicable

Table 45. Cohort study of vegetable consumption and risk of gallbladder cancer

Author, year, country	Cases/cohort size, gender (years follow-up)	Exposure assessment (no. of items)	Range contrasts (no. of categories)	Relative risk (95% CI)	Stat. sign.*	Adjustment for confounding	Comments
Hirayama, 1990, Japan	530/265 118, M, F 17 y	FFQ (7)	Green-yellow veg.: Daily vs non-daily (2)	1.06 (90% CI 0.90–1.24)		Not reported	Mortality Census-based cohort in seven prefectures
Sauvaget et al., 2003, Japan	157/38 540, M 17 y	FFQ (22), self-administered	Green-yellow veg.: Daily vs 0–1 d/wk (3)	1.09 (0.73–1.74)	$p = 0.73$	Age, sex, radiation dose, city, BMI, smoking, alcohol, education	Mortality, atomic bombing survivors

*p for trend when applicable

Table 46. Case–control study of fruit and vegetable consumption and risk of gallbladder cancer

Author, year, country	Cases/controls, gender	Exposure assessment (no. of items)	Range contrasts (no. of categories)	Relative risk (95% CI)	Stat. sign.*	Adjustment for confounding	Comments
Kato et al., 1989, Japan	109/218, M, F	FFQ (~ 46)	Daily vs less than daily (2)	0.26 (0.13–0.50)		Marital status, other food items	Population-based Response rates 84% for cases, virtually 100% for controls

*p for trend when applicable

Table 47. Cohort studies of fruit consumption and risk of pancreas cancer

Author, year, country	Cases/cohort size, gender (years follow-up)	Exposure assessment (no. of items)	Range contrasts (no. of categories)	Relative risk (95% CI)	Stat. sign.*	Adjustment for confounding	Comments
Mills et al., 1988, USA	40/34 000, M, F 7 y	FFQ		Protective, non-significant effect of fresh citrus fruits and fresh winter fruits			Mortality Cohort of Seventh-Day Adventists
Zheng et al., 1993, USA	57/17 633, M 20 y	FFQ (35), self-administered		No association			Mortality Cohort of insurance policy holders
Shibata et al., 1994, USA	65/13 979, M, F 9 y	FFQ (59, 23 fruits)	≥ 3.6 vs < 2.4 servings/d (3)	0.89 (0.49–1.62)	NS	Sex, age, cigarette smoking	Incidence Cohort of a retirement community
Appleby et al., 2002, UK	39/10 741, M, F 25 y	FFQ	Daily consumption of fresh fruit vs less than daily (2)	0.83 (0.38–1.80)	$p > 0.05$	Age, sex, smoking, other foods	Mortality Cohort of health-food shoppers
Stolzenberg-Solomon et al., 2002, Finland	163/27 111, M 13 y	FFQ (over 200), self-administered	Highest vs lowest (5)	0.85 (0.53–1.35)	$p = 0.52$	Age, years of smoking, energy	Incidence Cohort of smokers based on baseline data in a randomized trial
Sauvaget et al., 2003, Japan	177/38 540, M 17 y	FFQ (22), self-administered	Daily vs 0–1 d/wk (3)	0.81 (0.55–1.20)	$p = 0.23$	Age, sex, radiation dose, city, BMI, smoking, alcohol, education	Mortality, atomic bombing survivors

*p for trend when applicable

Table 48. Case–control studies of fruit consumption and risk of pancreas cancer

Author, year, country	Cases/controls, gender	Exposure assessment (no. of items)	Range contrasts (no. of categories)	Relative risk (95% CI)	Stat. sign.*	Adjustment for confounding	Comments
Norell et al, 1986, Sweden	99/163 hospital and 138 population controls, M, F	FFQ	Fruit juices: Almost daily vs seldom (3) Citrus fruit: Almost daily vs seldom (3)	0.6 (90% CI 0.3–1.2) 0.3 (90% CI 0.1–0.6)		Stratified by sex, age (two groups) and hospital	Hospital- and population-based Response rates 82% for cases Similar finding for population controls, and after adjustments for other risk factors
Voirol et al., 1987, Switzerland	88/336, M, F	Semiquantitative FFQ, interviewed	Average consumption: 88.6 g vs 40 g		Significant		Population-based Response rate 64% for controls
Falk et al., 1988, USA	363/1234, M, F	FFQ (59)	(2)	0.63 (0.49–0.82)	Significant	Sex, age, cigarette smoking, income, residence, Cajun ancestry, respondent type, history of diabetes	Hospital-based Similar finding when fruit juices were included When RR stratified for Cajun/non-Cajun ethnicity, associations were stronger for Cajuns for fruits and juices
Olsen et al., 1989, USA	212/220, M	FFQ	Fruit and juices: ≥ 53 vs ≤ 21 times/mo (3)	0.88 (0.48–1.62)		Age, education, history of diabetes, smoking, alcohol, meat	Population-based Data obtained on 81% of cases ascertained Similar finding for spouse interviews
Farrow & Davis, 1990, USA	148/188 (by random digit dialling), M	FFQ (135), interviewed by telephone		No significant difference in consumption between cases and controls			Population-based Interviews with case spouses

Table 48 (contd)

Author, year, country	Cases/controls, gender	Exposure assessment (no. of items)	Range contrasts (no. of	Relative risk (95% CI)	Stat. sign.*	Adjustment for confounding	Comments
Howe et al, 1990, Canada	249/505, M, F	Quantitative FFQ (over 200)	Highest vs lowest (4)	0.92 (0.74–1.14)		Fibre, energy, lifetime cigarette consumption	Population-based 547 cases ascertained 1636 potential controls approached 78% cases and 38% controls interviewed by proxy
La Vecchia et al., 1990a, Italy	247/1089, M, F	FFQ (14)	Fresh fruit: Highest vs lowest (3)	0.68 (0.41–0.98)	$p < 0.05$	Age, sex	Hospital-based
Baghurst et al., 1991, Australia	104/253, community controls, M, F	FFQ (179)		No difference in consumption between cases and controls			Population-based Response rate 62% for male and 63% for female cases, and 57% and 51% for controls, respectively
Bueno de Mesquita et al., 1991, Netherlands	164/480, M, F	Semi-quantitative FFQ (116)	Highest vs lowest (5)	1.09		Age, gender, response status (direct/proxy), smoking, energy	Population-based Overall response rate 72%. More than half of the cases directly interviewed
Lyon et al., 1993, USA	M 85/192 F 60/171	FFQ directed to period 20 y before interview (32)	Highest vs lowest (3)	M 0.81 (0.40–1.62) F 0.37 (0.18–0.81)	$p = 0.26$ $p < 0.05$	Age, cigarette smoking, coffee, alcohol	Population-based Response rate for cases 88%; for controls 77% All data derived from interviews of next of kin
Ji et al., 1995, China	451/1552, M, F	FFQ (86), interviewed	Highest vs lowest (4)	M 0.66 (0.43–1.01) F 0.58 (0.34–1.00)	$p = 0.02$ $p = 0.08$	Age, income, smoking, green tea drinks (females only) and response status	Population-based Deceased cases excluded (19%) Relatives assisted with interviews

Table 48. (contd)

Author, year, country	Cases/controls, gender	Exposure assessment (no. of items)	Range contrasts (no. of categories)	Relative risk (95% CI)	Stat. sign.*	Adjustment for confounding	Comments
Silverman et al., 1998, USA	436/2003, M, F	FFQ (60), interviewed	Highest vs lowest (4)	M: 0.9 F: 1.1		Age at diagnosis, race, study area, energy, diabetes mellitus, BMI, cholecystectomy, smoking, alcohol, income (men), marital status (women)	Population-based Multicentre study 1153 cases identified 78% ascertained potential controls interviewed
Mori et al., 1999, India	79 pancreatic ductal adenocarcinoma/146 visitor or friend control,	FFQ, interviewed	Every day vs seldom (3)	0.07 (0.02–0.21)	$p < 0.001$		Hospital-based 23 additional cases with chronic calcific pancreatitis and cancer showed no association with fruit consumption

*p for trend when applicable

Table 49. Cohort studies of vegetable consumption and risk of pancreas cancer

Author, year, country	Cases/cohort size, gender (years follow-up)	Exposure assessment (no. of items)	Range contrasts (no. of categories)	Relative risk (95% CI)	Stat. sign.*	Adjustment for confounding	Comments
Mills et al., 1988, USA	40/34 000, M, F 7 y	FFQ		Non-significant increase of risk for consumption of cooked green veg. and green salad			Mortality Cohort of Seventh-Day Adventists
Hirayama, 1990, Japan	679/265 118, M, F 17 y	FFQ (7)	Green-yellow veg.: daily vs non-daily (2)	1.11 (90% CI 0.96–1.29)		Not reported	Mortality Census-based cohort in seven prefectures
Zheng et al., 1993, USA	57/17 633, M 20 y	FFQ (35), self-administered		No association			Mortality Cohort of insurance policy holders
Shibata et al., 1994, USA	65/13 979, M, F 9 y	FFQ (59, 21 veg.), self-administered	≥ 4.7 vs < 3.2 servings/d (3)	0.82 (0.44–1.51)	NS	Sex, age, cigarette smoking	Mortality Cohort of members of a retirement community

Table 49 (contd)

Author, year, country	Cases/cohort size, gender (years follow-up)	Exposure assessment (no. of items)	Range contrasts (no. of categories)	Relative risk (95% CI)	Stat. sign.*	Adjustment for confounding	Comments
Stolzenberg-Solomon et al., 2002, Finland	163/27111, M 13 y	FFQ (over 200), self-administered	Highest vs lowest (5)	0.77 (0.47–1.27)	$p = 0.32$	Age, years of smoking, energy	Incidence Cohort based on baseline data in a randomized trial. Potatoes and legumes excluded
Sauvaget et al., 2003, Japan	177/38 540 M 17 y	FFQ (22), self-administered	Green-yellow veg.:daily vs 0–1 d/wk (3)	0.82 (0.54–1.24)	$p = 0.36$	Age, sex, radiation dose, city, BMI, smoking, alcohol, education	Mortality, atomic bombing survivors

*p for trend when applicable

Table 50. Case–control studies of vegetable consumption and risk of pancreas cancer

Author, year, country	Cases/controls, gender	Exposure assessment (no. of items)	Range contrasts (no. of categories)	Relative risk (95% CI)	Stat. sign.*	Adjustment for confounding	Comments
Norell et al., 1986, Sweden	99/163 hospital and 138 population controls, M, F	FFQ	Almost daily vs seldom (3)	0.5 (90% 0.3–1.1)		Stratified by sex, age (two groups) and hospital	Hospital- and population-based Response rates 82% for cases. Similar finding for population controls, for raw veg. and after adjustment for other risk factors.
Voirol et al., 1987, Switzerland	88/336, M, F	Semiquantitative FFQ, interviewed	Average consumption: 230 g vs 156.6 g	0.47	Significant		Population-based Response rate for controls 64%
Falk et al., 1988, USA	363/1234, M, F	FFQ (59)	(2)	0.88 (0.68–1.14)	NS	Sex, age, smoking, income, residence, Cajun ancestry, respondent type, history of diabetes	Hospital-based

Table 50 (contd)

Author, year, country	Cases/controls, gender	Exposure assessment (no. of items)	Range contrasts (no. of categories)	Relative risk (95% CI)	Stat. sign.*	Adjustment for confounding	Comments
Olsen et al., 1989, USA	212/220, M	FFQ	Non-cruciferous veg: ≥ 32 vs ≤16 times/mo (3)	0.95 (0.52–1.73)		Age, education, history of diabetes, smoking, alcohol, meat	Population-based. Data obtained on 81% of cases ascertained. Similar finding for spouse interviews.
Howe et al., 1990, Canada	249/505, M, F	Quantified FFQ (over 200)	Highest vs lowest (4)	1.03 (0.79–1.34)		Fibre, energy, lifetime cigarette consumption	Population-based. 547 cases ascertained. 1636 potential controls approached. 78% cases and 38% controls interviewed by proxy
Farrow & Davies, 1990, USA	148/188 (by random digit dialling), M	FFQ (135), interviewed by telephone		No significant difference in consumption between cases and controls			Population-based. Interviews with case spouses
La Vecchia et al., 1990a, Italy	247/1089, M, F	FFQ (14)	Green veg.: Highest vs lowest (3)	0.84 (0.58–1.22)		Age, sex	Hospital-based
Baghurst et al., 1991, Australia	104/253, M, F	FFQ (179)		No difference in consumption between cases and controls			Population-based. Response rate 62% for male and 63% for female cases, and 57% and 51% for controls, respectively
Bueno de Mesquita et al., 1991, Netherlands	164/480, M, F	Semi-quantitative FFQ (116)	Highest vs lowest (5)	0.34	$p < 0.05$	Age, gender, response status (direct/proxy), smoking, energy	Population-based. Overall response rate 72%. More than half of the cases directly interviewed

Table 50 (contd)

Author, year, country	Cases/controls, gender	Exposure assessment (no. of items)	Range contrasts (no. of categories)	Relative risk (95% CI)	Stat. sign.*	Adjustment for confounding	Comments
Lyon et al., 1993, USA	M 87/191, F 60/169	FFQ directed to period 20 y before interview (32)	Highest vs lowest (3)	M 0.99 (0.50–2.01) F 0.32 (0.13–0.74)	$p = 0.80$ $p = 0.01$	Age, cigarette smoking, alcohol, coffee consumption	Population-based Response rate 88% for cases and 77% for controls. All data derived from interviews of next of kin
Ji et al., 1995, China	451/1552, M, F	FFQ (86), interviewed	Highest vs lowest (4)	M 0.63 (0.45–1.03) F 0.67 (0.39–1.14)	$p = 0.03$ $p = 0.15$	Age, income, smoking, green tea drinks (females only), response status	Population-based Deceased cases excluded (19%) Relatives assisted with interviews.
Silverman et al., 1998, USA	436/2003, M, F	FFQ (60), interviewed	Highest vs lowest (4)	M 0.6 F 0.9	$p = 0.035$	Age at diagnosis, race, study area, energy, cholecystectomy, diabetes mellitus, BMI, cigarette smoking, alcohol, income (men), marital status (women)	Population-based. Multi-centre study. 1153 cases identified 78% ascertained potential controls interviewed
Mori et al., 1999, India	79 pancreatic ductal adenocarcinoma/146 visitor or friend control, M, F	FFQ, interviewed	Every day vs seldom or sometimes (3)	0.42 (0.24–0.74)	$p < 0.01$		Hospital-based 23 additional cases with chronic calcific pancreatitis and cancer showed similar, non-significant association with veg. consumption

*p for trend when applicable

IARC Handbooks of Cancer Prevention Volume 8: Fruit and Vegetables

Table 51. Case-control studies of fruit and vegetable consumption and risk of pancreas cancer

Author, year, country	Cases/controls, gender	Exposure assessment (no. of items)	Range contrasts (no. of categories)	Relative risk (95% CI)	Stat. sign.*	Adjustment for confounding	Comments
Gold et al., 1985, USA	201/201 hospital (H) and 201 population (P) controls, M, F	FFQ, interviewed	Raw fruits and veg.: ≥ 5 vs < 5 times/wk (2)	H: 0.58 (0.37–0.90) P: 0.55 (0.34–0.91)	p ≤ 0.02	Matched by age, race, sex	Hospital- and population-based Response rates for cases 70%, for hospital controls 54% and for population controls 50% (random digit dialling)
Mack et al., 1986, USA	326/363 neighbourhood controls, M, F	FFQ in broad groups, interviewed	Fresh fruit and veg.: ≥ 5 vs < 5 times/wk (2)	0.7 (0.5–0.9)		Matched by age, sex, race, neighbourhood	Population-based Response rate 66% for cases Direct interviews of 124 pairs, proxy interviews of the remainder

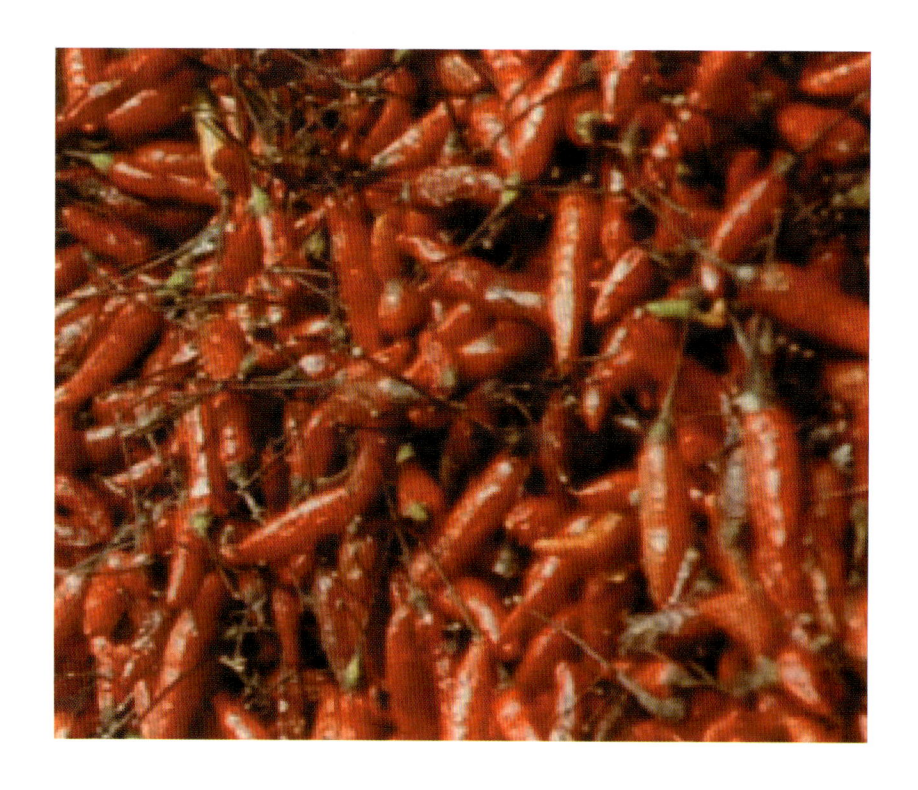

*p for trend when applicable

Table 52. Case–control studies of fruit consumption and risk of larynx cancer

Author, year, country	Cases/controls, gender	Exposure assessment (no. of items)	Range contrasts (no. of categories)	Relative risk (95% CI)	Stat. sign.*	Adjustment for confounding	Comments
De Stefani et al., 1987, Uruguay	107/290, M	FFQ, interviewed, frequency	Daily vs never (4)	[0.37 (0.19–0.77)]	p < 0.05	Age	Hospital-based No control for smoking and alcohol
Notani & Jayant, 1987, India	80/215 hospital controls, 177 population control, M	FFQ, interviewed, frequency	≥ once/wk vs < once/wk (2)	Hospital controls: [0.65 (0.33–1.25)] Population controls: [0.50 (0.24–1.0)]		Age, tobacco habits	Hospital-based and population-based
La Vecchia et al., 1990b, Italy	110/833, M	FFQ (17), interviewed, frequency	Fresh fruits: Highest vs lowest (3)	0.3	p < 0.01	Age, residence, education, smoking, intake of fish, green veg., alcohol	Hospital-based No interaction with tobacco or with alcohol
Zheng et al., 1992b, China	201/414, M, F	FFQ (41, 5 fruits), interviewed, frequency, portion size	Highest vs lowest (3)	M: 0.7 F: 0.5 (0.2–1.5)	M: p = 0.21	Age, education, smoking pack-years	Population-based No control for alcohol
Guo et al., 1995, China	100/100, M, F	FFQ, interviewed	Insufficient vs sufficient	0.44	p = 0.03	Age, number of cigarettes, mental factors, using firewood in winter, smoke in environment	Hospital-based No control for alcohol Unclear presentation
Estève et al., 1996, France, Switzerland, Spain, Italy	727 endolarynx/2736, M	Diet history, interviewed, frequency, portion size	> 250 vs ≤ 70 g/d (5)	[0.72 (0.53–0.96)]	p < 0.05	Age, study centre, smoking, alcohol, energy	Population-based Similar finding for epilarynx and hypopharynx
Maier & Tisch, 1997, Germany	164/656, M	FFQ, interviewed, frequency	Fresh fruit: ≥ once/wk vs less (2)	0.7 (0.4–1.1)	p = 0.08	Age, smoking, alcohol	Hospital-based Includes incident and prevalent cases
De Stefani et al., 1999, Uruguay	34/393, M, F	FFQ (64, 8 fruits), interviewed, frequency, portion size	Highest vs lowest (3)	0.8 (0.5–1.3)		Age, sex, residence, urban/rural, education, BMI, smoking pack-years, alcohol, energy	Hospital-based Part of larger case–control study on aerodigestive cancers

Table 52 (contd)

Author, year, country	Cases/controls, gender	Exposure assessment (no. of items)	Range contrasts (no. of categories)	Relative risk (95% CI)	Stat. sign.*	Adjustment for confounding	Comments
De Stefani et al., 2000a, Uruguay	148/444, M	FFQ (62, 8 fruits), interviewed, frequency, portion size	≥ 204 vs ≤ 69.8 g/d (4)	0.38 (0.20–0.72)	p = 0.001	Age, residence, urban/rural, education, BMI, smoking pack-years, alcohol, energy	Hospital-based
Bosetti et al., 2002a, Switzerland, Italy	527/1297, M, F	FFQ (78), interviewed, frequency, portion size	≥ 24.8 vs < 8.9 servings/wk (5)	0.52 (0.35–0.77)	p < 0.001	Age, sex, centre, education, smoking, alcohol and non-alcohol energy intake	Hospital-based OR weaker in subgroups of age, alcohol, smoking and for supraglottis, epiglottis or others

*p for trend when applicable

Table 53. Case–control studies of vegetable consumption and risk of larynx cancer

Author, year, country	Cases/controls, gender	Exposure assessment (no. of items)	Range contrasts (no. of categories)	Relative risk (95% CI)	Stat. sign.*	Adjustment for confounding	Comments
De Stefani et al., 1987, Uruguay	107/290, M	FFQ, interviewed, frequency	Daily vs infrequent (1–3 d/mo) (3)	[0.59 (0.34–1.11)]	NS	Age	Hospital-based No control for smoking and alcohol
Notani & Jayant, 1987, India	80/215 hospital controls, 177 population controls, M	FFQ, interviewed, frequency	Daily vs not daily (2)	Hospital controls:[0.78 (0.42–1.43)] Population controls: [0.36 (0.19–0.71)]		Age, tobacco habits	Hospital-based and population-based
La Vecchia et al., 1990b, Italy	110/833, M	FFQ (17), interviewed, frequency	Green veg.: Highest vs lowest (3)	0.4	NS	Age, residence, education, smoking, fish, fresh fruit, alcohol	Hospital-based No total veg.
Zheng et al., 1992b, China	201/414, M, F	FFQ (41, 26 veg.), interviewed, frequency, portion size	Highest vs lowest (3)	M: 1.2 F: 1.1 (0.4–3.2)	M: p = 0.61	Age, education, smoking pack-years	Population-based No control for alcohol

Table 53 (contd)

Author, year, country	Cases/controls, gender	Exposure assessment (no. of items)	Range contrasts (no. of categories)	Relative risk (95% CI)	Stat. sign.*	Adjustment for confounding	Comments
Guo et al., 1995, China	100/100, M, F	FFQ, interviewed	Sufficient vs insufficient	0.37	p = 0.03	Age	Hospital-based No control for alcohol
Estève et al., 1996, France, Italy, Spain, Switzerland	727 endolarynx/ 2736, M	Diet history, interviewed, frequency, portion size	> 350 vs ≤ 170 g/d (5)	[0.61 (0.45–0.81)]	p < 0.05	Age, study centre, smoking, alcohol, energy	Population-based Similar finding for epilarynx and hypopharynx
De Stefani et al., 1999, Uruguay	34/393, M, F	FFQ (64, 14 veg.), interviewed, frequency, portion size	Highest vs lowest (3)	0.9 (0.6–1.6)		Age, sex, residence, urban/rural, education, BMI, smoking pack-years, alcohol, energy	Hospital-based Part of larger case–control study on aerodigestive cancers
De Stefani et al., 2000a, Uruguay	148/444, M	FFQ (62, 11 veg.), interviewed, frequency, portion size	≥ 120.4 vs ≤ 54.1 g/d (4)	0.57 (0.30–1.08)	p = 0.18	Age, residence, urban/rural, education, BMI, smoking pack-years, alcohol, energy	Hospital-based
Bosetti et al., 2002a, Switzerland, Italy	527/1297, M, F	FFQ (78), interviewed, frequency, portion size	≥ 18.1 vs < 8.6 servings/wk (5)	0.17 (0.11–0.27)	p < 0.001	Age, sex, centre, education, smoking, alcohol and non-alcohol energy intake	Hospital-based OR similar for subgroups of age, alcohol, smoking and for supraglottis, epiglottis or others

Table 54. Case–control studies of fruit and vegetable consumption and risk of larynx cancer

Author, year, country	Cases/controls, gender	Exposure assessment (no. of items)	Range contrasts (no. of categories)	Relative risk (95% CI)	Stat. sign.*	Adjustment for confounding	Comments
Zatonski et al., 1991, Poland	249/965, M	FFQ (30), interviewed, frequency	Highest vs lowest (3)	0.34 (0.18–0.64)		Age, residence, education, smoking, alcohol	Population-based
De Stefani et al., 2000a, Uruguay	148/444, M	FFQ (62, 8 fruits and 11 veg.), interviewed, frequency, portion size	≥ 320.7 vs ≤ 143.0 g/d (4)	0.30 (0.15–0.59)	p < 0.001	Age, residence, urban/rural, education, BMI, smoking pack-years, alcohol, energy	Hospital-based

*p for trend when applicable

Table 55. Cohort studies of fruit consumption and risk of lung cancer

Author, year, country	Cases/cohort size, gender (years follow-up)	Exposure assessment (no. of items)	Range contrasts (no. of categories)	Relative risk (95 % CI)	Stat. sign.*	Adjustment for confounding	Comments
Kvale et al., 1983, Norway	168/13 785, M 11.5 y	FFQ (31, 9 fruits), self-administered, frequency	≥ 50 vs < 20 times/mo (4)	1.10	$p = 0.90$	Age, cigarette smoking, region, urban/rural residence	Incidence RR = 0.71 (NS) for squamous and small-cell carcinomas
Wang & Hammond 1985, USA	671/136 28, M 10 y	FFQ (16), self-administered, frequency	Fruit/fruit juice: 5–7 vs 0–2 d/wk (3)	[0.57]		Age	Mortality No control for smoking. RR = 0.52 in those taking vitamin pills; RR = 0.65 in heavy smokers
Fraser et al., 1991, USA	61/34 198, M, F 6 y	FFQ (51, 5 fruits), self-administered, frequency	≥ 2 times/d vs < 3 times/wk (3)	0.26 (0.10–0.70)	$p = 0.006$	Age, sex, smoking history	Incidence Seventh-Day Adventists RR = 0.28 in never-smokers, RR = 0.22 in ever-smokers. Similar finding for adenocarcinoma and tumours of other cell types
Chow et al., 1992, USA	219/17 633, M 20 y	FFQ (35), self-administered, frequency	> 90 vs < 31 times/mo (4)	0.7 (0.4–1.3)		Age, smoking status, occupation	Mortality Lutheran Brotherhood Significant association only for oranges
Shibata et al., 1992, USA	164 (94 M, 70 F)/11 580 9 y	FFQ (59, 23 fruits), self-administered, frequency	M: ≥ 3.5 vs < 2.2 servings/d (3) F: > 3.7 vs < 2.4 servings/d (3)	0.99 (0.59–1.66) 0.68 (0.37–1.24)	NS NS	Age, smoking	Incidence Retirement community
Steinmetz et al., 1993, USA	138/2814, F 4 y	FFQ (127, 15 fruits), self-administered, frequency, portion size; validated	≥ 18 vs ≤ 7 servings/wk (4)	0.75 (0.44–1.23)	$p = 0.08$	Age, pack-years of smoking, energy	Incidence Nested case–control; total cohort = 34 977 Strongest effect in large-cell carcinoma and in ex-smokers, but small numbers
Key et al., 1996, UK	59/10 771, M, F 17 y	FFQ (5), self-administered, frequency	Fresh fruit: Daily vs less than daily (2)	SMR: 0.59 (0.34–1.02)		Age, sex, smoking	Mortality Vegetarians and health-conscious people

Table 55 (contd)

Author, year, country	Cases/cohort size, gender (years follow-up)	Exposure assessment (no. of items)	Range contrasts (no. of categories)	Relative risk (95 % CI)	Stat. sign.*	Adjustment for confounding	Comments
Ocké et al., 1997a, Netherlands	54/561. M 20 y	Dietary history, spouse interview, frequency and portion size	> 33rd vs ≤ 33rd percentile (2)	0.40 (0.18–0.87)		Age, pack-years of cigarette smoking, energy	Incidence RR for stable dietary habits. Weaker RR for average habits
Breslow et al., 2000, USA	154/20 004, M, F 8.5 y	FFQ (59, 5 fruits), self-administered, frequency, portion size; validated	> 11.5 vs < 3 servings/wk (4)	0.9 (0.5–1.6)	$p < 0.489$	Age, sex, smoking duration, packs/day smoked	Mortality
Feskanich et al., 2000, USA	F 519/77 823 M 274/47 778 F: 12 y M: 10 y	FFQ (116, 15 fruits), self-administered, frequency, portion size; validated	F > 3.1 vs < 1.7 servings/d (5) M > 3.3 vs ≤ 1.7 servings/d (5)	0.76 (0.56–1.02) 1.22 (0.80–1.87)		Age, follow-up cycle, smoking status, years since quitting, cigarettes/day, age at start smoking, energy	Incidence In females, effect strongest in never-smokers; effect similar in Kreyberg I and II In males, protective effect only in never-smokers, and in Kreyberg I
Voorrips et al., 2000b, Netherlands	1010/2953 (subcohort), M, F 6.3 y	FFQ (150, 8 fruits), self-administered, frequency, portion size; validated	Highest (median 325 g/d) vs lowest (median 46 g/d) (5)	0.8 (0.6–1.1)	$p < 0.001$	Age, sex, family history of lung cancer, education, current smoker (y/n), years of smoking, cig./day	Incidence Total cohort = 120 852 Protective effect only in smokers (current and ex), and in all cell types
Jansen et al., 2001, Finland, Italy, Netherlands	149/1578, M, smokers 25 y	Dietary history, interviewed, frequency and portion size	Highest vs lowest (3)	0.69 (0.46–1.02)	$p = 0.05$	Age, cig./day, country, energy, veg.	Mortality. Protective effect only in heavy smokers (20+ cig/day) Effects less strong in Italy

Table 55 (contd)

Author, year, country	Cases/cohort size, gender (years follow-up)	Exposure assessment (no. of items)	Range contrasts (no. of categories)	Relative risk (95 % CI)	Stat. sign.*	Adjustment for confounding	Comments
Holick et al., 2002, Finland	1644/ 27 084, M, smokers 14 y	FFQ (276), self-administered, frequency, portion size; validated	> 188 vs < 45 g/d (5)	0.87 (0.74–1.02)	$p = 0.01$	Age, years smoked, cig./ day, intervention (α-tocopherol/β-carotene), previous supplement use (β-carotene and vitamin A), energy, cholesterol, fat	Incidence ATBC trial
Sauvaget et al. 2003, Japan	563/38 540, M, F 18 y	FFQ (22), self-administered, frequency; validated	Highest vs lowest (3)	0.80 (0.65–0.98)	$p = 0.035$	Age, sex, radiation dose, city, BMI, smoking status, alcohol, education	Mortality Atomic bombing survivors Strongest effect in never and current smokers No effect in women
Miller et al. 2003, 10 European countries	860/478 021, M, F 0–14 (mean 6 y)	FFQ (~300), self-administered or interviewed, frequency, portion size; calibration study	Highest vs lowest (5)	0.60 (0.46–0.78)	$p = 0.01$	Age, sex, weight, height, centre, smoking intensity and duration	Incidence Strongest effects in never- and current smokers
Neuhouser et al., 2003, USA	Intervention arm: 414/7072, M, F Placebo arm: 326/7048, M, F 12 y	FFQ, self-administered (45 items relating to fruit and veg.)	Intervention arm: Highest vs lowest (5) Placebo arm: Highest vs lowest (5)	0.79 (0.57–1.11) 0.56 (0.39–0.81)	$p = 0.13$ $p = 0.003$	Sex, age, smoking status, total pack-years of smoking, asbestos exposure, race/ ethnicity, enrolment centre	Follow-up of participants in CARET trial in smokers and asbestos workers
Smith-Warner et al., 2003, pooled analysis of 8 cohorts	3206/430 281 (8 cohorts), M, F 6–16 y	FFQ self-administered, frequency, portion size; validated	Highest vs lowest (5)	0.77 (0.67–0.87)	$p < 0.001$	Age, education, BMI, alcohol, energy, smoking status, duration, amount smoked	Incidence Effect strongest in never-smokers; significant effect only in current smokers; stronger effects in squamous-cell and adenocarcinoma than small-cell carcinoma Citrus fruit inversely associated

*p for trend when applicable

Table 56. Case–control studies of fruit consumption and risk of lung cancer

Author, year, country	Cases/controls, gender	Exposure assessment (no. of items)	Range contrasts (no. of categories)	Relative risk (95% CI)	Stat. sign.*	Adjustment for confounding	Comments
Ziegler et al., 1986, USA	763/900, M	FFQ (44, 12 fruits), interviewed, frequency	Highest vs lowest (4)	1.0	p = 0.35	Age, smoking	Population-based Small effect in current and recent smokers
Fontham et al., 1988, USA	1253/1274, M, F	FFQ (59), interviewed, frequency	Highest vs lowest (3)	0.66 (0.54–0.82)	Significant	Age, sex, race, pack-years cig., family income, ethnic group, respondent status, veg. intake	Hospital-based Somewhat stronger effect in squamous and small-cell than in adenocarcinoma
Koo, 1988, China	88/137, F, never-smokers (< 20 cig. in past)	FFQ, interviewed, frequency	Fresh fruit: Highest vs lowest (3)	[0.42 (0.19–0.92)]	p = 0.002	Age, no. of live births, schooling	Population-based RR = 0.65 in adenocarcinoma and large cell; RR = 0.43 in squamous and small-cell carcinoma
Jain et al., 1990, Canada	839/772, M, F	Diet history (81), interviewed, frequency, portion size; validated	> 378 vs < 110 g/d (4)	1.10	p = 0.76	Age, sex, residence, cumulative cig. smoking	Population-based
Kalandidi et al., 1990, Greece	91/120, F, never-smokers (lifelong)	FFQ (47), interviewed, frequency	Highest vs lowest (4)	0.33 (0.13–0.68)	p = 0.02	Age, years of education, interviewer, energy	Hospital-based ORs similar in adenocarcinoma and other types
Candelora et al., 1992, USA	124/263, F never-smokers (< 100 cig. in lifetime)	FFQ (60), interviewed, frequency, portion size	Highest vs lowest (4)	0.6 (0.3–1.1)	p = 0.04	Age, education, energy	Population-based
Forman et al., 1992, China	183/183, M tin miners	FFQ (27), interviewed, frequency	Highest vs lowest (4)	[1.10 (0.57–2.08)]		Age, cumulative tobacco intake (water pipe), pack-years cig., height, number of meals/day at home, socioeconomic status, radon and arsenic exposure	Population-based

Table 56 (contd)

Author, year, country	Cases/controls, gender	Exposure assessment (no. of items)	Range contrasts (no. of categories)	Relative risk (95% CI)	Stat. sign.*	Adjustment for confounding	Comments
Swanson et al., 1992, China	425/1007, M, tin mining community	FFQ (31), interviewed, frequency	Fresh fruit: > 3.9 vs < 1.1 times/mo (4)	0.94	p = 0.31	Age, respondent type, study site, smoking, family income, education, occupation	Population-based Associations for tin miners and mining community
Alavanja et al., 1993, USA	429/1021, F, not current smokers	FFQ (60, 16 fruits), self-administered, frequency, portion size	≥ 22.1 vs ≤ 9.2 servings/wk (5)	1.14	p = 0.99	Age, smoking history, previous lung disease, interview type, energy	Population-based
Dorgan et al., 1993, USA	1951 (355 blacks)/1238 (217 blacks), M, F	FFQ (44, 8 fruits), interviewed, frequency	≥ 37 vs ≤ 18 servings/mo (3)	WM: [0.95 (0.70–1.30)] WF: [0.56 (0.40–0.79)] BM: [2.04 (1.11–3.70)] BF: [1.30 (0.44–3.85)]	NS p < 0.01 p < 0.05 NS	Age, education, occupation, residence, smoking, passive smoking, study phase	Population-based Extension to females and blacks from Ziegler et al. (1986)
Gao et al., 1993, Japan	282/282, M, smokers	FFQ, interviewed, frequency	Daily vs sometimes (3)	0.45 (0.30–0.67)		Age, smoking status	Hospital-based Stronger effect in squamous and adenocarcinoma and in current smokers
Suzuki et al., 1994, Brazil	123/123, M, F	FFQ, interviewed, frequency	Daily vs < once/wk (3)	1.2 (0.4–3.1)	p = 0.57	Age, sex, race, pack-years, smoking, income	Hospital-based
Mayne et al., 1994, USA	413/413, M, F, not current smokers	FFQ (26), interviewed, frequency	Fresh fruit: Highest vs lowest (4)	0.44	p < 0.01	Age, sex, prior cig. use, religion, education, BMI, income	Population-based
Axelsson et al., 1996, Sweden	308/504, M	FFQ (80), interviewed, frequency	Fruit index: Almost daily vs < 1–2/mo (3)	0.73 (0.43–1.23)	p = 0.014	Age, cig./day, years smoked, marital status, socioeconomic job class	Population-based OR lower for 'other fruits and berries'. OR fruit = 1.02 when veg. index in model

Table 56 (contd)

Author, year, country	Cases/controls, gender	Exposure assessment (no. of items)	Range contrasts (no. of categories)	Relative risk (95% CI)	Stat. sign.*	Adjustment for confounding	Comments
Lei et al., 1996, China	792/792, M, F	FFQ, spouse interview, frequency	≥ almost daily vs never (3)	M: 0.79 (0.56–1.11) F: 0.87 (0.51–1.47)		Age	Population-based No control for smoking Deceased cases and controls; info. from spouses or cohabiting relatives
Xu et al., 1996, China	610/959, M iron and steel workers	FFQ, interviewed, frequency	≥ 55 vs 0 'jing'/y (4)	0.6 (0.5–0.9)		Age, smoking (pack-years), income, education, tea intake, pulmonary disease, family history of lung cancer	Population-based
Agudo et al., 1997, Spain	103/206, F	FFQ (33, 8 fruits), interviewed, frequency, portion size	Fresh fruit: Highest vs lowest (3)	1.20 (0.56–2.56)	$p = 0.66$	Age, residence, hospital, smoking status, pack-years	Hospital-based
Hu et al., 1997, China	227/227, M, F	FFQ (50, 4 fruits), interviewed, frequency	≥ 15 vs 0 kg/y (4)	0.7 (0.4–1.2)	$p = 0.10$	Age, sex, residence, cig./day, smoking, duration, income	Hospital-based OR = 0.9 in smokers, OR = 0.6 in non-smokers
Ko et al., 1997, Taiwan, China	105/105, F non-smokers	FFQ (12), interviewed, frequency, portion size	Daily vs 0–6/wk (2)	1.0 (0.5–1.7)		Age, date of interview, education, socioeconomic status, residential area	Hospital-based
Pawlega et al., 1997, Poland	176/341, M	FFQ, self-administered, frequency	>1 vs < 1 times/wk (3)	0.42 (0.23–0.77)	$p < 0.05$	Age, education, residence, pack-years smoking, occupational exposure	Population-based OR = 1.67 among drinkers of vodka above average
Pillow et al., 1997, USA, Sweden	137/187, M, F	FFQ (100), self-administered, frequency, portion size	Continuous variable	0.56 (0.31–0.99)	$p = 0.05$	Age, sex, ethnicity, pack-years smoking, energy	Population-based Increment is unclear

Table 56 (contd)

Author, year, country	Cases/controls, gender	Exposure assessment (no. of items)	Range contrasts (no. of categories)	Relative risk (95% CI)	Stat. sign.*	Adjustment for confounding	Comments
Nyberg et al., 1998, Sweden	124/235, M, F never-smokers	FFQ (19), interviewed, frequency	Fruit index: Highest vs lowest (3)	0.67 (0.33–1.36)		Age, sex, urban residence, occasional smoking, occupation, passive smoking, carrots	Population-based
Brennan et al., 2000, European centres	506/1045, M, F (never-smokers, < 400 cig. in life-time)	FFQ, interviewed, frequency	2–7/wk vs < 1/mo (3)	1.0 (0.6–1.5) SqCC 0.7 SmCC 0.9 ADC 0.9	$p = 0.81$	Age, sex, centre	Population-based Items differed per centre
Alavanja et al., 2001, USA	360/574, F	FFQ (70, 6 fruits), self-administered, frequency	Fruit and fruit juice: Highest vs lowest (5)	0.4 (0.3–0.6)	$p < 0.001$	Age, energy	Population-based No control for smoking
Takezaki et al., 2001, Japan	1045/4153, M, F	FFQ (24), self-administered, frequency	Daily vs almost never (4)	M, ADC: 0.98 (0.61–1.58) M, SqSC + SmCC: 0.61 (0.40–0.95) F, ADC: 0.68 (0.27–1.70) F, SqCC + SmCC: 0.49 (0.11–2.13)	$p = 0.383$ $p = 0.007$ $p = 0.536$ $p = 0.668$	Age, year of visit, occupation, prior lung diseases, smoking, meat, green veg.	Hospital-based
De Stefani et al., 2002, Uruguay	1032/1030, M, F	FFQ (11), interviewed, frequency, portion size	> 364 vs ≤ 52 servings/y (4)	0.84 (0.62–1.13)	$p = 0.14$	Age, sex, residence, urban/rural, education, year of diagnosis, smoking status, years since quitting, smoking intensity, age at start, energy	Hospital-based Strongest effects in large-cell carcinoma, in never- and current smokers

Table 56 (contd)

Author, year, country	Cases/controls, gender	Exposure assessment (no. of items)	Range contrasts (no. of categories)	Relative risk (95% CI)	Stat. sign.*	Adjustment for confounding	Comments
Kreuzer et al., 2002, Germany	234/535, F (never-smokers, < 400 cig. in lifetime)	FFQ (15) interviewed, frequency	Daily vs ≤ once/wk (3)	0.66 (0.37–1.19)	$p = 0.94$	Age, region	Population-based
Marchand et al., 2002, New Caledonia	134/295, M, F	FFQ (89), interviewed, frequency, portion size	Highest vs lowest (3)	M: 0.7 (0.4–1.5)	$p = 0.09$	Age, ethnicity, pack-years smoking	Population-based No significant association in women ('data not shown')
Rachtan, 2002a, Poland	242/352, F	FFQ (17), self-administered, frequency	Daily vs rarely (2)	0.49 (0.32–0.74)	$p = 0.001$	Age, pack-years	Population-based
Seow et al., 2002, Singapore	303/765, F	FFQ (39, 12 fruits), interviewed, frequency, portion size	≥ 9.7 vs < 3.8 servings/wk (3)	Smokers: 0.63 (0.28–1.44) Non-smokers: 0.60 (0.39–0.93)	$p = 0.4$ $p = 0.03$	Age, date of admission, place of birth, family history of cancer, (for smokers: duration, cig./day)	Hospital-based

*p for trend when applicable
ADC, adenocarcinoma; SqCC, squamous-cell carcinoma; SmCC, small-cell carcinoma

Table 57. Cohort studies of vegetable consumption and risk of lung cancer

Author, year, country	Cases/cohort size, gender (years follow-up)	Exposure assessment (no. of items)	Range contrasts (no. of categories)	Relative risk (95 % CI)	Stat. sign.*	Adjustment for confounding	Comments
Kvale et al., 1983, Norway	168/13 785, M 11.5 y	FFQ (31, 8 veg.), self-administered, frequency	Veg. index: ≥ 50 vs < 20 times/mo (4)	0.74	$p = 0.37$	Age, sex, cig. smoking, region, urban/rural residence	Incidence RR = 0.54 (NS) for squamous and small cell carcinomas
Fraser et al., 1991, USA	61/34 198, M, F 6 y	FFQ (51), self-administered, frequency	Cooked green veg.: ≥ 7 vs < 3 times/wk (3)	1.09 (0.41–2.87)	$p = 0.50$	Age, sex, cig. smoking status (never, ex, current)	Potatoes excluded Incidence Seventh-Day Adventists No information on total veg.
Chow et al., 1992, USA	219/17 633, M 20 y	FFQ (35), self-administered, frequency	> 160 vs < 46 times/mo (4)	1.2 (0.6–2.3)		Age, smoking status, occupation	Mortality Lutheran Brotherhood

Table 57 (contd)

Author, year, country	Cases/cohort size, gender (years follow-up)	Exposure assessment (no. of items)	Range contrasts (no. of categories)	Relative risk (95 % CI)	Stat. sign.*	Adjustment for confounding	Comments
Shibata et al., 1992, USA	164 (94 M 70 F)/11 580 9 y	FFQ (59, 21 veg.), self-administered, frequency	M: ≥ 4.5 vs < 3 servings/d (3) F: ≥ 4.8 vs < 3.2 servings/d (3)	1.37 (0.74–2.25) 0.58 (0.32–1.05)	NS NS	Age, smoking	Incidence Retirement community
Steinmetz et al., 1993, USA	138/2814, F 4 y	FFQ (127, 29 veg.), self-administered, frequency, portion size; validated	≥ 31 vs ≤ 14 servings/wk (4)	0.50 (0.29–0.87)	p = 0.01	Age, pack-years of smoking, energy	Incidence Nested case–control; total cohort 34 977 Strongest effect in large-cell carcinoma, and in ex-smokers, but small numbers
Ocké et al., 1997a, Netherlands	54/561, M 20 y	Dietary history, spouse interview; frequency and portion size	> 33rd vs ≤ 33rd percentile (2)	0.47 (0.21–1.03)		Age, pack-years of cig. smoking, energy	Incidence RR for stable dietary habits Weaker RR for average habits
Breslow et al., 2000, USA	158/20 004, M, F 8.5 y	FFQ (59, 12 veg.), self-administered, frequency, portion size; validated	> 13.6 vs < 5.2 servings/wk (4)	0.9 (0.5–1.5)	p < 0.786	Age, sex, smoking duration, packs/day smoked	Mortality
Feskanich et al., 2000, USA	519/77 823, F 274/47 778 M F 12 y M 10 y	FFQ (116, 23 veg.), self-administered, frequency, portion size; validated	F: > 4.3 vs ≤ 2.5 servings/d (5) M: > 4.1 vs ≤ 2.3 servings/d (5)	0.68 (0.51–0.90) 1.04 (0.69–1.57)		Age, follow-up cycle, smoking status, years since quitting, cig./day, age at start smoking, energy	Incidence Excludes beans and lentils, potatoes For females, effect strongest in current smokers, and in Kreyberg I For males protective effect only in never-smokers, and in Kreyberg I
Voorrips et al., 2000b, Netherlands	1010/2953 (sub-cohort), M, F 6.3 y	FFQ (150, 21 veg.), self-administered, frequency, portion size; validated	Highest (median 286 g/d) vs lowest (103 g/d) (5)	0.7 (0.5–1.0)	p = 0.001	Age, sex, family history of lung cancer, education, current smoker, years of smoking, cig./day	Incidence Total cohort = 120 852 Protective effect only in current and ex smokers, and in Kreyberg I (men)

Table 57 (contd)

Author, year, country	Cases/cohort size, gender (years follow-up)	Exposure assessment (no. of items)	Range contrasts (no. of categories)	Relative risk (95 % CI)	Stat. sign.*	Adjustment for confounding	Comments
Jansen et al., 2001, Italy, Netherlands	149/1578, M, smokers 25 y	Dietary history, interviewed, frequency and portion size	Highest vs lowest (3)	0.90 (0.61–1.33)	$p = 0.59$	Age, cig./day, country, energy, fruit	Mortality Protective effect only in heavy smokers (20+ cig./day), effects less strong in Italy
Ozasa et al., 2001, Japan	572/98 248, M, F 9 y	FFQ (32), self-administered, frequency	Green leafy veg.: Almost daily vs ≤ 1–2/wk (3)	M: 0.76 (0.59–0.98) F: 1.19 (0.75–1.90)	$p = 0.035$ $p = 0.45$	Age, family history of lung cancer, smoking status, cigts/day × duration, time since quitting	Mortality No information on total veg. Effects stronger in male ex-smokers and female non-smokers
Holick et al., 2002, Finland	1644/27 084, M, smokers 14 y	FFQ (276), self-administered, frequency, portion size; validated	> 156 vs < 52 g/d (5)	0.75 (0.63–0.88)	$p < 0.0001$	Age, years smoked, cig./day, intervention (α-tocopherol/β-carotene), previous supplement use (β-carotene and vitamin A), energy, cholesterol, fat	Incidence ATBC trial
Miller et al, 2003, 10 European countries	860/ 478,021, M, F (0–14 mean 6 y)	FFQ (300), self-administered or interviewed, frequency, portion size; calibration study	Highest vs lowest (5)	1.00 (0.76–1.30)	$p = 0.85$	Age, sex, weight, height, centre, smoking	Incidence No association in never-, current and ex-smokers
Neuhouser et al., 2003, USA	Intervention arm: 414/7072, M, F Placebo arm: 326/7048, M, F 12 y	FFQ, self-administered (45 items relating to fruit and veg.)	Intervention arm: Highest vs lowest (5) Placebo arm: Highest vs lowest (5)	0.81 (0.65–1.21) 0.82 (0.59–1.14)	$p = 0.46$ $p = 0.39$	Sex, age, smoking status, pack-years of smoking, asbestos exposure, race/ethnicity, enrolment centre	Follow up of participants in CARET trial in smokers and asbestos workers

Table 57 (contd)

Author, year, country	Cases/cohort size, gender (years follow-up)	Exposure assessment (no. of items)	Range contrasts (no. of categories)	Relative risk (95% CI)	Stat. sign.*	Adjustment for confounding	Comments
Sauvaget et al., 2003, Japan	563/38 540, M, F 18 y	FFQ (22), self-administered, frequency; validated	Green-yellow veg.: Highest vs lowest (3)	0.95 (0.76–1.19)	$p = 0.676$	Age, sex, radiation dose, city, BMI, smoking status, alcohol, education	Mortality Atomic bombing survivors No information on total veg. No association in smoking subgroups
Smith-Warner et al, 2003, pooled analysis	3206/430 281 (8 cohorts), M, F 6–16 y	FFQ, self-administered, frequency, portion size; validated	Highest vs lowest (5)	0.88 (0.78–1.00)	$p = 0.12$	Age, education, BMI, alcohol, energy, smoking status, duration, amount smoked	Incidence No difference between smoking status categories, or between morphological categories

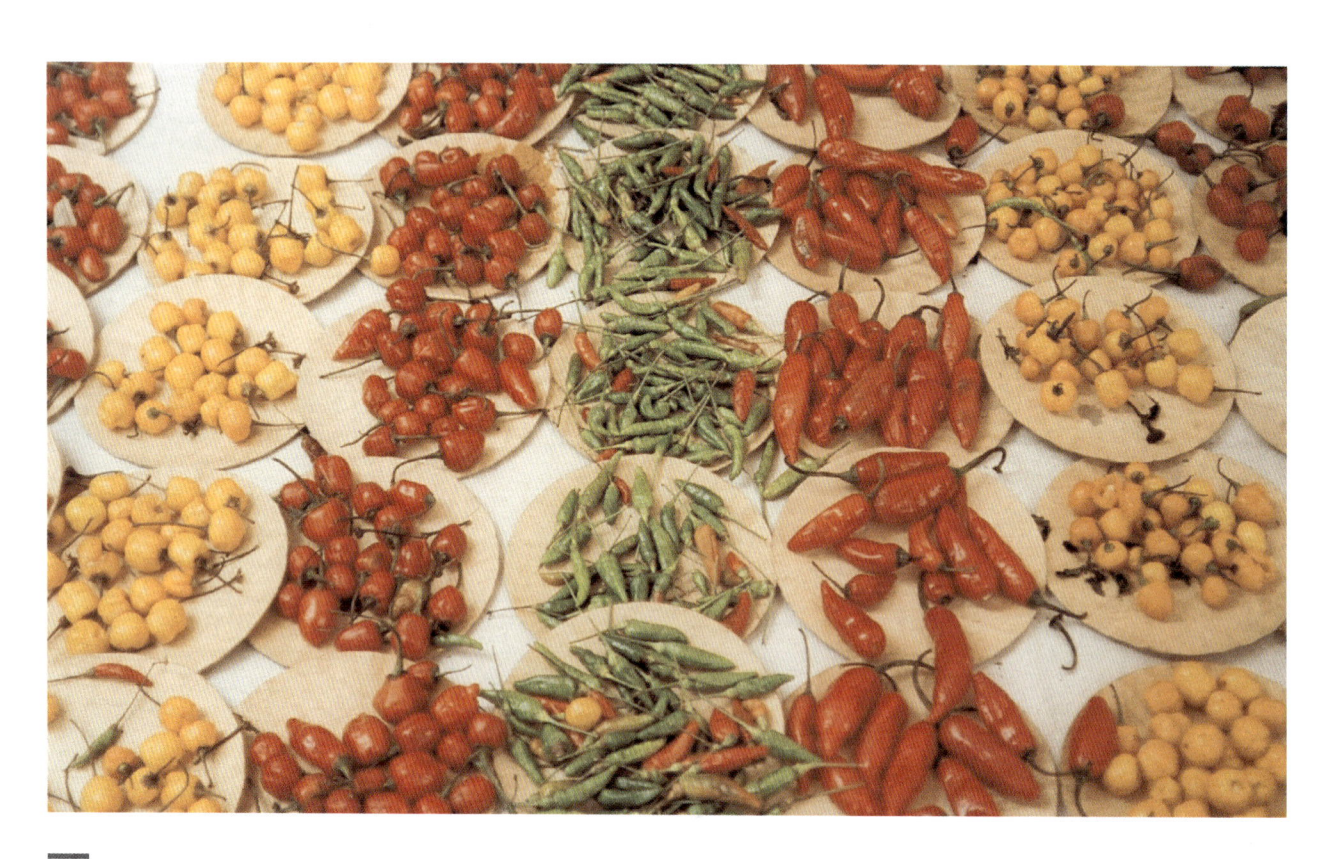

*p for trend when applicable

Table 58. Case–control studies of vegetable consumption and risk of lung cancer

Author, year, country	Cases/controls, gender	Exposure assessment (no. of items)	Range contrasts (no. of categories)	Relative risk (95% CI)	Stat. sign.*	Adjustment for confounding	Comments
MacLennan et al., 1977, Singapore	233/300, M, F	FFQ (8 veg.), interviewed, frequency	Veg. index: Highest vs lowest (2)	[0.45 (0.30–0.67)]		Age, sex, dialect, smoking, socio-economic status	Hospital-based
Ziegler et al., 1986, USA	763/900, M	FFQ (44, 16 veg.), interviewed, frequency	Highest vs lowest (4)	[0.71]	$p = 0.01$	Age, smoking	Population-based Strongest effect for squamous-cell carcinoma Effect limited to current and recent smokers
Fontham et al., 1988, USA	1253/1274, M, F	FFQ (59), interviewed, frequency	Highest vs lowest (3)	0.90 (0.74–1.11)	NS	Age, sex, race, pack-years cig., family income, ethnic group, respondent status, fruit intake	Hospital-based No difference between cell types
Le Marchand et al., 1989, USA	332/865, M, F	FFQ (>130, 22 veg.), interviewed, frequency, portion size; validated	Highest vs lowest (4)	M: [0.31 (0.17–0.56)] F: [0.18 (0.06–0.53)]	$p = 0.001$ $p = 0.001$	Age, ethnicity, smoking status, pack-years cig., cholesterol intake (M only), total vitamin C and folic acid intake	Population-based Effect most apparent in current and recent ex-smokers in M, and in never/ex-smokers in F Effect somewhat stronger for squamous- and small-cell in M
Jain et al., 1990, Canada	839/772, M, F	Diet history (81), interviewed, frequency, portion size; validated	> 308 vs < 129 g/d (4)	0.60 (0.40–0.88)	$p = 0.01$	Age, sex, residence, cumulative cig. smoking	Population-based
Kalandidi et al., 1990, Greece	91/120, F, never-smokers (lifelong)	FFQ (47), interviewed, frequency	Highest vs lowest (4)	1.09 (0.44–2.68)	$p = 0.86$	Age, years of education, interviewer, energy	Hospital-based
Candelora et al., 1992, USA	124/263, F (never-smokers, < 100 cig. in lifetime)	FFQ (60), interviewed, frequency, portion size	Highest vs lowest (4)	0.3 (0.1–0.5)	Significant	Age, education, energy, fruit consumption	Population-based ORs higher for self-reports than for next of kin interviews

Table 58 (contd)

Author, year, country	Cases/controls, gender	Exposure assessment (no. of items)	Range contrasts (no. of categories)	Relative risk (95% CI)	Stat. sign.*	Adjustment for confounding	Comments
Forman et al., 1992, China	183/183, M, tin miners	FFQ (27), interviewed, frequency	Highest vs lowest (4)	[0.60 (0.30–1.18)]		Age, cumulative tobacco intake (water pipe), pack-years cig. smoking, height, number of meals/day at home, socio-economic status, radon and arsenic exposure	Population-based Stronger protective effect for yellow-light green veg.
Alavanja et al., 1993, USA	429/1021, F, not current smokers	FFQ (60; 28 veg.), self-administered, frequency, portion size	≥ 25 vs ≤ 13 servings/wk (5)	0.99	p = 0.89	Age, smoking history, previous lung disease, interview type, energy	Population-based Includes potatoes
Dorgan et al., 1993, USA	1951 (355 blacks)/1238 (217 blacks), M, F	FFQ (44, 16 veg.), interviewed, frequency	≥ 66 vs ≤ 41 servings/mo (3)	WM: [0.80 (0.58–1.10)] WF: [0.59 (0.42–0.82)] BM: [1.10 (0.59–2.04)] BF: [0.67 (0.23–1.96)]	NS p < 0.01 NS NS	Age, education, occupation, residence, smoking, passive smoking, study phase	Population-based Extension to females and blacks from Ziegler et al. (1986) Effects stronger in squamous- and small-cell than adenocarcinoma Effect limited to current and ex cig. smokers
Sankaranarayanan et al., 1994, India	261/1190, M	FFQ (45, 12 veg.), interviewed, frequency	Highest vs lowest (4)	0.32 (0.13–0.78)	p = 0.02	Age, smoking, education, religion	Population-based Onions most protective (RR = 0.03)
Mayne et al., 1994, USA	413/413, M, F, not current smokers	FFQ (26), interviewed, frequency	Highest vs lowest (4)	M: 0.55 F: 0.47	NS p < 0.025	Age, prior cig. use, religion, education, BMI, income	Population-based

Table 58 (contd)

Author, year, country	Cases/controls, gender	Exposure assessment (no. of items)	Range contrasts (no. of categories)	Relative risk (95% CI)	Stat. sign.*	Adjustment for confounding	Comments
Axelsson et al., 1996, Sweden	308/504, M	FFQ (80), interviewed, frequency	Veg. index: Almost daily vs < 1–2/mo (3)	0.37 (0.23–0.61)	$p < 0.001$	Age, cig./day, years smoked, marital status, socio-economic job class	Population-based OR lower for cabbage, green pepper. OR=0.37 in current smokers; Lowest in 30+ y smokers Consistent low OR for all 4 hist. types
Agudo et al., 1997, Spain	103/206, F	FFQ (33, 11 veg.), interviewed, frequency, portion size	Highest vs lowest (3)	0.65 (0.32–1.31)	$p = 0.23$	Age, residence, hospital, smoking status, pack-years	Hospital-based Includes potatoes. Same OR in ADC and never smokers (only subgroups)
Hu et al., 1997, China	227/227, M, F	FFQ (50, 20 veg.), interviewed, frequency	Fresh veg.: > 138 vs < 77 kg/y (4)	0.8 (0.4–1.3)	$p = 0.65$	Age, sex, residence, cig./day, smoking duration, income	Hospital-based OR=1.0 in smokers, OR=0.6 in non-smokers
Ko et al., 1997, Taiwan	105/105, F, non-smokers	FFQ (12), interviewed, frequency, portion size	Daily vs 0–6 times/wk (2)	0.4 (0.2–0.8)		Age, date of interview, education, residential area	Hospital-based
Pawlega et al., 1997, Poland	176/341, M	FFQ, self-administered, frequency	Boiled veg: > 3 vs < 3 times/wk (3)	0.22 (0.11–0.43)	$p < 0.05$	Age, education, residence, pack-years smoking, occupational exposure	Population-based OR=0.08 among drinkers of vodka above average
Pillow et al., 1997, USA	137/187, M, F	FFQ (100), self-administered, frequency, portion size	Continuous variable	1.49 (0.84–2.63)	$p = 0.17$	Age, sex, ethnicity, pack-years smoking, energy	Population-based Increment is unclear

Table 58 (contd)

Author, year, country	Cases/controls, gender	Exposure assessment (no. of items)	Range contrasts (no. of categories)	Relative risk (95% CI)	Stat. sign.*	Adjustment for confounding	Comments
Nyberg et al., 1998, Sweden	124/235 M, F (never-smokers)	FFQ (19), interviewed, frequency	Veg. index: Highest vs lowest (3)	0.57 (0.29–1.13)	$p = 0.35$	Age, sex, urban residence, occasional smoking, occupation, passive smoking, non-citrus fruit	Population-based
Brennan et al., 2000, 8 European centres	506/1045, M, F (never smokers, < 400 cigs in lifetime)	FFQ, interviewed, frequency	Fresh veg.: 7/wk vs < 1/wk (3)	0.7 (0.5–1.0)	$p = 0.09$	Age, sex, centre	Population-based Items differed per centre. Effect only seen in adenocarcinoma
Kubik et al., 2001, Czech Republic	282/1120, F	FFQ (9), interviewed, frequency	> several times/wk vs. 'never' (4)	0.84 (0.6–1.3)		Age, residence, education, pack-years smoking	Hospital-based Effect only (OR=0.55) in squamous +small + large cell carcinoma
De Stefani et al., 2002, Uruguay	1032/1030, M, F	FFQ (11), interviewed, frequency, portion size	> 156 vs < 52 servings/y (4)	0.72 (0.54–0.97)	$p = 0.008$	Age, sex, residence, urban/rural, education, year of diagnosis, smoking status, years since quitting, smoking intensity, age at start, energy	Hospital-based Strongest effects in squamous-, small- cell carcinoma, in current and ex- smokers
Marchand et al., 2002, New Caledonia	134/295, M, F	FFQ (89), interviewed, frequency, portion size	Highest vs lowest (3)	M: 1.4 (0.7–2.9)	$p = 0.72$	Age, ethnicity, pack-years smoking	Population-based No significant association in women ('data not shown')

Table 58 (contd)

Author, year, country	Cases/controls, gender	Exposure assessment (no. of items)	Range contrasts (no. of categories)	Relative risk (95% CI)	Stat. sign.*	Adjustment for confounding	Comments
Rachtan, 2002b Poland	242/352, F	FFQ (17), self-administered, frequency	Veg. other than carrots: Daily vs. rarely (2)	0.24 (0.11–0.52)		Age, pack-years of smoking, passive smoking, consumption of beer and vodka, siblings with cancer, tuberculosis, place of residence, occupational exposures	Population-based
Seow et al., 2002, Singapore	303/765, F	FFQ (39, 19 veg.), interviewed, frequency, portion size	> 26.4 vs. < 14.3 servings/wk (3)	Smokers: 0.48 (0.23–1.00) Non-smokers: 0.78 (0.51–1.20)	$p = 0.04$ $p = 0.3$	Age, date of admission, place of birth, family history of cancer, (for smokers: duration, cig./day)	Hospital-based

*p for trend when applicable
ADC, adenocarcinoma, SqCC, squamous-cell carcinoma; SmCC, small-cell carcinoma

Table 59. Cohort studies of fruit and vegetable consumption and risk of lung cancer

Author, year, country	Cases/cohort size, gender (years follow-up)	Exposure assessment (no. of items)	Range contrasts (no. of categories)	Relative risk (95% CI)	Stat. sign.*	Adjustment for confounding	Comments
Shibata et al., 1992, USA	164 (94 M, 70 F)/ 11 580, 9 y	FFQ (59, 21 veg.), self-administered, frequency	M: ≥ 7.9 vs < 5.5 servings/d (3) F: ≥ 8.3 vs < 5.9 servings/d (3)	1.22 (0.72–2.07) 0.58 (0.32–1.04)	NS NS	Age, smoking	Incidence Retirement community
Steinmetz et al., 1993, USA	138/ 2814, F 4 y	FFQ (127, 15 fruits, 29 veg.), self-administered, frequency, portion size; validated	> 48 vs ≤ 24 servings/wk (4)	0.49 (0.28–0.86)	$p = 0.02$	Age, pack-years of smoking, energy	Incidence Nested case–control; total cohort 34 977 Strongest effect in large-cell carcinoma, and in ex-smokers, but small numbers

Table 59 (contd)

Author, year, country	Cases/ cohort size, gender (years follow-up)	Exposure assessment (no. of items)	Range contrasts (no. of categories)	Relative risk (95% CI)	Stat. sign.*	Adjustment for confounding	Comments
Feskanich et al., 2000, USA	F 519/77 823, 12 y M 274/ 47 778, 10 y	FFQ (116, 15 fruits, 23 veg.), self-administered, frequency, portion size; validated	F > 7.2 vs ≤ 4.5 servings/d (5) M > 7.2 vs ≤ 4.3 servings/d (5)	0.79 (0.59–1.06) 1.12 (0.74–1.69)		Age, follow-up cycle, smoking status, years since quitting, cig./day (current smokers), age at start smoking, energy	Incidence. Excludes beans and lentils, potatoes For females, effect strongest in never-smokers, and in Kreyberg I. For males, protective effect only in never-smokers, and in Kreyberg I
Voorrips et al., 2000b, Netherlands	1010/2953, (subcohort). M, F 6.3 y	FFQ (150, 8 fruits, 21 veg.), self-administered, frequency, portion size; validated	Highest (median 554 g/d) vs lowest (191 g/d) (5)	0.7 (0.5–1.0)	$p < 0.001$	Age, sex, family history of lung cancer, education, current smoker (yes/no), years of smoking, cig./day	Incidence Total cohort 120 852
Holick et al., 2002, Finland	1644/27 084, M, smokers 14 y	FFQ (276), self-administered, frequency, portion size; validated	> 332 vs < 116 g/d (5)	0.73 (0.62–0.86)	$p < 0.001$	Age, years smoked, cig./day, intervention (α-tocopherol/β-carotene), previous supplement use (β-carotene and vitamin A), energy, cholesterol, fat	Incidence ATBC trial
Neuhouser et al., 2003, USA	Intervention arm: 414/ 7072, M, F Placebo arm: 326/ 7048, M, F 12 y	FFQ, self-administered (45 items relating to fruits and veg.)	Intervention arm: Highest vs lowest (5) Placebo arm: Highest vs lowest (5)	0.76 (0.55–1.06) 0.73 (0.51–1.04)	$p = 0.13$ $p = 0.21$	Sex, age, smoking status, total pack-years of smoking, asbestos exposure, race/ethnicity, enrolment centre	Follow up of participants in CARET trial in smokers and asbestos workers
Smith-Warner et al., 2003, pooled analysis	3206/430 281 (8 cohorts), M, F 6–16 y	FFQ, self-administered, frequency, portion size; validated	Highest vs lowest (5)	0.79 (0.69–0.90)	$p = 0.001$	Age, education, BMI, alcohol, energy, smoking status, duration, amount smoked	Incidence. Effect strongest in never-smokers; significant effect only in current smokers; stronger effects in SqCC and ADC than SmCC

*p for trend when applicable
ADC, adenocarcinoma, SqCC, squamous-cell carcinoma; SmCC, small-cell carcinoma

Table 60. Case–control studies of fruit and vegetable consumption and risk of lung cancer

Author, year, country	Cases/controls, gender	Exposure assessment (no. of items)	Range contrasts (no. of categories)	Relative risk (95% CI)	Stat. sign.*	Adjustment for confounding	Comments
Ziegler et al., 1986, USA	763/900, M	FFQ (44, 12 fruits, 16 veg.), interviewed, frequency	Highest vs lowest (4)	[0.77]	p = 0.04	Age, smoking	Population-based
Fontham et al., 1988, USA	1253/1274, M, F	FFQ (59), interviewed, frequency	Highest vs lowest (3)	0.70 (0.55–0.91)	p = 0.004	Age, sex, race, pack-years cig., family income, ethnic group, respondent status	Hospital-based Somewhat stronger effect (RR = 0.65) for SqCC and SmCC; RR = 0.77 for ADC
Mayne et al., 1994, USA	413/413, M, F, not current smokers	FFQ (26), interviewed, frequency	Raw: Highest vs lowest (4) Processed: Highest vs lowest (4)	M: 0.41 F: 0.40 M: 1.02 F: 0.69	p < 0.005 p < 0.005 NS NS	Age, prior cig. use, religion, education, BMI, income	Population-based
De Stefani et al., 2002, Uruguay	1032/1030, M, F	FFQ (11), interviewed, frequency, portion size	> 494 vs ≤ 156 servings/y (4)	0.62 (0.45–0.84)	p = 0.002	Age, sex, residence, urban/rural, education, year of diagnosis, smoking status, years since quitting, intensity smoking, age at start, energy	Hospital-based Strongest effects for SqCC, in current and ex-smokers

*p for trend when applicable
SqCC, Squamous-cell carcinoma; SmCC, small-cell carcinoma

Table 61. Cohort studies of fruit consumption and risk of breast cancer in women

Author, year, country	Cases/cohort size (years follow-up)	Age, population subgroups	Exposure assessment (no. of items)	Range contrasts (no. of categories)	Relative risk (95% CI)	Stat. sign.*	Adjustment for confounding	Comments
Shibata et al., 1992, USA	219/11 580 9 y	Mean 74 y	FFQ (59, 23 fruits, self-administered, estimated frequency	≥ 3.7 vs < 2.4 servings/d (3)	0.82 (0.60–1.12)	NS	Age, smoking	Incidence Retirement community
Rohan et al., 1993, Canada	519/1182 6 y	40–59 y	Diet history (86), self-administered, estimated frequency and amount	≥ 491 vs < 189 g/d (5)	0.81 (0.57–1.14)	$p = 0.174$	Age, age at menarche, surgical menopause, age at first live birth, education, family history of breast cancer, history of benign breast disease, other contributors to total food intake	Incidence Nested in the Canadian Breast Screening Cohort (56 837 women) No statistically significant difference by menopausal status
Verhoeven et al., 1997a, Netherlands	519/ 62 573 4.3 y	55–69 y, only postmenopausal	Semi-quantitative FFQ, past year (150), self-administered, estimated frequency; validity assessed	Highest vs lowest (5) (median values 343.1 g/d vs 64.9 g.d)	0.76 (0.54–1.08)	$p = 0.10$	Age, energy, alcohol, history of benign breast disease, maternal breast cancer, breast cancer in sister(s), age at menarche, age at menopause, age at first birth, parity	Incidence
Zhang et al., 1999, USA	2697 (784 pre-menopausal, 1913 post-menopausal)/ 83 234 15 y	33–60 y	Semiquantitative FFQ, past year (61–126), estimated frequency; validity and reliability assessed	≥ 5.0 vs < 2 servings/d (5)	Premenopausal: 0.74 (0.45–1.24) Postmenopausal: 0.84 (0.64–1.09) Postmenopausal, current HRT user: 0.57 (0.33–1.00)	$p = 0.13$ $p = 0.10$	Age, length of follow-up, energy, parity, age at first birth, age at menarche, history of breast cancer in mother or sister, history of benign breast disease, alcohol, BMI at age 18, weight change from age 18, height, age at menopause, HRT use	Incidence Nurses' Health Study
Gandini et al., 2000	10 case-control; 2 cohort (n = 9429 cases) Studies publ. 1982–97			≥ 1 portion/d vs ≤ 3–4 portions/wk 6 vs 1 portion/wk	0.94 (0.79–1.11) 0.83 (0.79–0.87)			Meta-analysis of published literature p for heterogeneity < 0.001

Table 61 (contd)

Author, year, country	Cases/cohort size (years follow-up)	Age, population subgroups	Exposure assessment (no. of items)	Range contrasts (no of categories)	Relative risk (95% CI)	Stat. sign.*	Adjustment for confounding	Comments
Smith-Warner et al., 2001	7377 cases from eight cohort studies with total baseline population of 351 825 women Follow-up 1976–96			Highest vs lowest (4) Increment = 100 g/d	All: 0.93 (0.86–1.00) All: 0.99 (0.98–1.00). Premenopausal: 0.98 (0.94–1.02) Postmenopausal: 0.99 (0.98–1.01)	p = 0.8		Pooled analysis Study-specific RRs were calculated using the primary data and then combined using the random effects model Similar finding when fruit juices were excluded from total fruits p for heterogeneity: 0.89–0.94
Appleby et al., 2002, UK 25 y	90/6416 25 y	≥16 y	FFQ (5); estimated frequency	Fresh fruit Daily vs < daily (2)	0.66 (0.38–1.14)	NS	Age, smoking, other foods	Mortality Cohort of health food shoppers
Maynard et al., 2002, UK 64 y	82 incident, 36 fatal/1959 64 y	Mean 8 y	7-day household inventory	Highest (mean = 88.4 g/d) vs lowest (mean = 0.6 g/d) (4)	Incidence: 1.08 (0.52–2.25). Mortality: 1.25 (0.40–3.92)	p = 0.61 p = 0.73	Age, energy, food expenditure, Townsend score, season	Incidence and mortality Survey conducted at the household level 78% of the 4999 boys and girls originally identified were included in the cohort
Riboli & Norat, 2003	8 case–control, 10 cohort studies, publ. 1973–2001			Increment = 100 g/d	Cohort: 0.99 (0.98–1.00) Case–control: 0.92 (0.84–1.01) All: 0.99 (0.98–1.00)	p for heterogeneity = 0.99 p for heterogeneity < 0.01 p for heterogeneity = 0.88		Meta-analysis of published literature
Sauvaget et al., 2003, Japan	76/23 667 18 y	34–103 y	FFQ, past year (22), self-administered, estimated frequency	Daily vs ≤1/wk (3)	0.91 (0.48–1.72)	0.71	Age, radiation dose, city, BMI, smoking, alcohol, education	Mortality Atomic bombing survivors

*p for trend when applicable; HRT, hormone replacement therapy

Table 62. Case–control studies of fruit consumption and risk of breast cancer in women

Author, year, country	Cases/ controls	Age, population subgroups	Exposure assessment (no. of items)	Range contrasts (no. of categories)	Relative risk (95% CI)	Stat. sign.*	Adjustment for confounding	Comments
Katsouyanni et al., 1986, Greece	120/120	Mean 55 y for cases	FFQ, before onset of disease (120), interviewed, estimated frequency	Highest vs lowest (5)	[0.59]	$p = 0.10$	Age, interviewer, years of schooling	Hospital-based Response rate 92% for cases
Iscovich et al., 1989, Argentina	150/150 hospital controls, 150 neighbourhood controls	Mean = 56 y for cases	FFQ, 5 y up to 6 mo before interview (147, 13 fruits), interviewed, estimated frequency	Highest vs lowest (4)	Citrus fruit Hospital controls: 0.75 Neighbourhood controls: 0.58 Other than citrus: Hospital controls: 0.55 Neighbourhood controls: 0.41	NS $p < 0.05$ $p < 0.05$ $p < 0.05$	Age, education, husband's occupation, age at first pregnancy, parity, obesity index	Hospital-based and population-based Response rate 98% for cases
Toniolo et al., 1989, Italy	250 (70 premenopausal, 180 postmenopausal)/ 499	< 75 y	Interviewer-administered dietary history (70); estimated frequency and amount	Highest vs lowest (4)	1.1		Age, energy	Population-based Response rate 91% for cases, 79% for controls
Van't Veer et al., 1990, Netherlands	133/238	25–44, 55–64 y	Diet history, 12 mo before diagnosis (236), interviewed, estimated frequency and amount; validity and reliability assessed	Highest vs lowest (4)	0.55	$p = 0.35$	Age, history of benign breast disease, first and second degree of family history, number of cigarettes smoked daily, education, ever-use of oral contraceptives, age at menarche, age at first full-term pregnancy, BMI, energy, alcohol	Population-based Response rate 80% for cases, 53% for controls
Ingram et al., 1991, Australia	99/209	22–86 y	FFQ, current intake (179), self-administered	Highest vs lowest (2)	0.9 (0.5–1.6)	NS	Age, residence	Population-based Response rate 100% for cases

Cancer-preventive effects

Table 62 (contd)

Author, year, country	Cases/ controls	Age, population subgroups	Exposure assessment (no. of items)	Range contrasts (no. of categories)	Relative risk (95% CI)	Stat. sign.*	Adjustment for confounding	Comments
Negri et al., 1991, Italy	2860/3625	<75 y	FFQ (14–37 depending on cancer site)	Highest vs lowest (3)	1.1 (1.0–1.3)	$p < 0.01$	Age, area of residence, education, smoking, veg.	Hospital-based Data from a network of case–control studies Response rate >97%
Franceschi et al., 1995, Italy	2569/2588	20–74 y	FFQ, 2 y before diagnosis (79, 10 fruits), interviewed, estimated weekly frequency; validity assessed	Citrus fruit: > 7.3 vs < 1.3 servings/wk (5) Other fruit: > 20.5 vs < 7.6 (5)	1.06 (0.89–1.28) 0.89 (0.73–1.07)	NS NS	Age, study centre, education, parity, energy, alcohol	Hospital-based Response rate 96% No significant interaction by study centre, age group, menopausal status, education, parity and BMI
Zaridze et al., 1991, Russia	139 (58 premenopausal, 81 postmenopausal/ 139		FFQ, year before diagnosis (145), interviewed, estimated frequency	Increased vs decreased intake in last 10 years	Premenopausal: [0.82 (0.13–5.26)] Postmenopausal: [1.82 (0.46–7.14)]	NS NS	Age at menarche, age at first birth, education	Hospital-based Response rate 99% for cases, 94% for controls
Levi et al. 1993b, Switzerland	107/318	≤ 75 y	Questionnaire (50, 4 fruits), interviewed, estimated frequency	Fresh fruit: Highest vs lowest (3)	0.8		Age	Hospital-based Response rate > 85%
Holmberg et al., 1994, Sweden	265 (55 ≤ 50 y, 210 > 50 y)/432 screening controls	40–74 y	FFQ, past 6 mo (60), interviewed, estimated frequency	Highest vs lowest (4)	All: 1.4 (0.9–2.3) ≤ 50 years: 0.7 (0.3–2.1) > 50 years: 1.7 (1.0–3.0)		Age, county of residence, month of mammography	Population-based Response rate for cases 70%, for controls 82% Effect modification by age group non-significant
Landa et al., 1994, Spain	100/100	Mean 59 y	FFQ, before onset of disease (99), inteviewed, estimated frequency	Highest vs lowest (3)	[0.26]	$p < 0.05$	Age	Hospital-based

Table 62 (contd)

Author, year, country	Cases/ controls	Age, population subgroups	Exposure assessment (no. of items)	Range contrasts (no. of categories)	Relative risk (95% CI)	Stat. sign.*	Adjustment for confounding	Comments
Qi et al., 1994, China	244/244		Diet history starting from 1 y before diagnosis (40), interviewed, estimated frequency and amount		No association		Age, length of stay in Tianjin	Hospital-based
Hirose et al., 1995, Japan	1052 (607 premenopausal, 445 postmenopausal)/ 23 163	≥ 20 y	Questionnaire before symptoms, self-administered	Daily vs ≤ 3–4/wk (2)	Premenopausal 0.95 (0.78–1.17) Postmenopausal: 1.05 (0.82–1.35)	NS NS	Age, first-visit year, BMI, age at menarche, delivery, smoking, physical activity, type of breakfast, milk, dietary control, bean curd, green-yellow veg., carrots, potato/sweet potato, chicken, ham/sausage	Hospital-based Response rate 98%
Trichopoulou et al., 1995a, Greece	820 (270 premenopausal, 550 postmenopausal)/795 hospital controls, 753 visitor controls		Semi-quantitative FFQ, past year (115, 18 fruits, interviewed, estimated frequency, validated	Highest vs lowest (5) (Median 183 vs 42.5 times/mo)	0.65 (0.47–0.90)	$p = 0.004$	Age, place of birth, parity, age at first pregnancy, age at menarche, menopausal status, Quetelet index, energy	Hospital-based and population-based Response rate for cases 94%, for hospital controls 96%, for visitor controls 93% Confounding between fruits and veg. was limited Further adjustment for other food groups or fat did not change association No statistically significant effect modification by menopausal status ($p > 0.10$)

Table 62 (contd)

Author, year, country	Cases/ controls	Age, population subgroups	Exposure assessment (no. of items)	Range contrasts (no of categories)	Relative risk (95% CI)	Stat. sign.*	Adjustment for confounding	Comments
Freudenheim et al., 1996, USA	297/311	≥ 40 y Only premenopausal	FFQ, past year 2 y before interview (172, 21 fruits), interviewed, estimated frequency and amount; validity and reliability assessed	≥ 484 vs ≤ 204 g/d (4)	0.67 (0.42–1.09)	$p = 0.05$	Age, education, age at first birth, age at menarche, first-degree relative with breast cancer, previous benign breast disease, BMI, energy	Population-based Response rate 66% for cases, 62% for controls
Thorand et al., 1998, Germany	43/106	38–80 y All postmenopausal	Diet history, past year (201), interviewed, estimated frequency and amount; validity and reliability assessed; validated	Continuous variable, increment 206 g/d	0.82 (0.51–1.32)		Age, BMI, exogenous hormone use, age at menarche, nulliparity, smoking status, socio-economic status	Population-based Response rate 75% for cases, 45% for controls
Potischman et al., 1999, USA	568 in situ or invasive localized disease, did not report chemotherapy treatment/ 1451	20–44 y	FFQ, past year (100/25 fruits), self-administered, estimated frequency and amount; validated	Fruit and fruit juice: > 11.2 vs < 3.5 times/wk (4) Fruit: ≥ 8.3 vs < 2.1 times/wk (4)	1.08 (0.8–1.4) 1.2 (0.8–1.4)		Age at diagnosis, study site, ethnicity, education, age at first birth, alcohol, years of oral contraceptive use, smoking status	Population-based Response rate 84% for cases, 70% for controls Results were similar when limited to the 353 cases with localized disease or who were interviewed within three months of diagnosis
Ronco et al., 1999, Uruguay	400/405	20–89 y	FFQ (64, 9 fruits), interviewed; reliability assessed	> 7.9 vs < 3.5 servings/wk (4)	0.57 (0.36–0.89)	$p = 0.05$	Age, residence, urban/rural status, family history of breast cancer in a first-degree relative, BMI, age at menarche, parity, menopausal status, energy	Hospital-based. Response rate for cases 97%, for controls 94%. No effect modification by menopausal status

Table 62 (contd)

Author, year, country	Cases/ controls	Age, population subgroups	Exposure assessment (no. of items)	Range contrasts (no. of categories)	Relative risk (95% CI)	Stat. sign.*	Adjustment for confounding	Comments
Terry et al. 2001c, Sweden	2832/2650	50–74 y All postmenopausal	FFQ, past year (65, 19 fruits and veg.), self-administered, estimated frequency	Highest vs lowest (4)	0.96 (0.79–1.17)	$p = 0.81$	Age, height, BMI, current smoking, socio-economic status, alcohol, high-fibre grains and cereals, fatty fish, multivitamin use, parity, hormone replacement therapy, history of benign breast disease, family history of breast cancer, type of menopause, age at menopause, age at menarche, age at first birth	Population-based Response rate for cases 84%, for controls 82%
Dos Santos Silva et al., 2002, UK	240/477	< 75 y	FFQ, 2–3 y before (108, 23 fruits), interviewed, estimated frequency and amount; validity assessed	≥ 4 vs ≤ 1 servings/d (4)	0.89 (0.50–1.57)	$p = 0.45$	Age, general practitioner, energy, age at menarche, age at first birth, parous, parity, breastfeeding, family history of breast cancer, menopausal status, time since menopause, education	Population-based Population: women of South Asian ethnicity who had migrated to England Response rate 79% for cases, 76% for controls

*p for trend when applicable

Table 63. Cohort studies of vegetable consumption and risk of breast cancer in women

Author, year, country	Cases/cohort size (years follow-up)	Age, population subgroups	Exposure assessment (no. of items)	Range contrasts (no. of categories)	Relative risk (95% CI)	Stat. sign.*	Adjustment for confounding	Comments
Shibata et al., 1992, USA	219/11 580 9 y	Mean 74 y	FFQ (59, 21 veg.), self-administered, estimated frequency	> 4.8 vs < 3.2 servings/d (3)	0.96 (0.69–1.34)	NS	Age, smoking	Incidence Retirement community Includes potatoes
Rohan et al., 1993, Canada	519/1182 6 y	40–59 y	Diet history (86), self-administered, estimated frequency and amount	> 433 vs < 203 g/d (5)	0.86 (0.61–1.23)	p = 0.752	Age, age at menarche, surgical menopause, age at first live birth, education, family history of breast cancer, history of benign breast disease, and other contributors to total food intake	Incidence Nested in the Canadian Breast Cancer Screening Cohort (56 837 women) No statistically significant difference by menopausal status
Järvinen et al., 1997, Finland	88/4697 25 y	≥ 15 y	Diet history, interviewed, past year	Highest vs lowest (3)	No association		Age, BMI, parity, region, occupation, smoking	Incidence
Verhoeven et al., 1997a, Netherlands	519/62 573 4.3 y	55–69 y Only postmenopausal women	Semi-quantitative FFQ, past year (150), self-administered, estimated frequency; validity assessed	Highest vs lowest (5) (Median values: 303 vs 108 g/d)	0.94 (0.67–1.31)	p = 0.30	Age, energy, alcohol, history of benign breast disease, maternal breast cancer, breast cancer in sister(s), age at menarche, age at menopause, age at first birth, parity	Incidence
Zhang et al., 1999, USA	2697 (784 premenopausal, 1913 postmenopausal)/ 83 234 15 y	33–60 y	Semi-quantitative FFQ, past year (61–126), self-administered, estimated frequency, validity and reliability asssessed	> 5.0 vs < 2 servings/d (5)	Premenopausal: 0.64 (0.43–0.95) Postmenopausal: 1.02 (0.85–1.24) Postmenopausal, current HRT user: 0.87 (0.63–1.20)	p = 0.10 p = 0.61	Age, length of follow-up, energy, parity, age at first birth, age at menarche, history of breast cancer in mother or sister, history of benign breast disease, alcohol, BMI at age 18, weight change from age 18, height, age at menopause, HRT use	Incidence Nurses' Health Study

Table 63 (contd)

Author, year, country	Cases/cohort size (years follow-up)	Age, population subgroups	Exposure assessment (no. of items)	Range contrasts (no. of categories)	Relative risk (95% CI)	Stat. sign.*	Adjustment for confounding	Comments
Gandini et al., 2000	14 case-control, 3 cohort (n = 16 052 cases); Studies publ. 1982–97			≥ 1 portion/d vs ≤ 3–4 portion/wk 6 vs 1 portions/wk	0.75 (0.66–0.85) 0.79 (0.77–0.80)			Meta-analysis of published literature p for heterogeneity < 0.001
Smith-Warner et al., 2001	7377 cases from 8 cohort studies with total baseline population of 351 825 women Follow-up: 1976–1996			Highest vs lowest (4) Increment = 100 g/d	All: 0.96 (0.89–1.04) All: 1.00 (0.97–1.02) Premenopausal: 0.99 (0.93–1.06) Postmenopausal: 1.00 (0.97–1.02)	p = 0.54		Pooled analysis Study-specific RRs were calculated using the primary data and then were combined using the random effects model Excludes potatoes p for heterogeneity: 0.31–0.73
Maynard et al., 2002, UK	82 incident, 36 fatal/1959 64 y	Mean 8 y	7-day household inventory	Highest vs lowest (4) (mean = 115.2 vs 23.1 g/d) Increment = 100 g/d	Incidence: 1.43 (0.70–2.92) Mortality: 0.86 (0.30–2.47)	p = 0.59 p = 0.35	Age, energy, food expenditure, Townsend score, season	Incidence and mortality Survey conducted at the household level 78% of the 4999 boys and girls originally identified were included in the cohort
Riboli & Norat (2003)	10 case-control, 10 cohort studies publ. 1973–2001				Cohort: 1.00 (0.97–1.02) Case-control: 0.86 (0.78–0.94) All: 0.96 (0.94–0.98)	p for heterogeneity =0.99 p for heterogeneity <0.01 p for heterogeneity =0.89		Meta-analysis of published literature
Sauvaget et al., 2003, Japan	76/23 667 18 y	34–103 y	FFQ, past year (22), self-administered, estimated frequency	Green-yellow veg.: Daily vs ≤ 1/ wk (3)	1.28 (0.64–2.54)	0.54	Age, radiation dose, city, BMI, smoking, alcohol, education	Mortality Atomic bombing survivors

* p for trend when applicable; HRT, hormone replacement therapy

Table 64. Case–control studies of vegetable consumption and risk of breast cancer in women

Author, year, country	Cases/controls	Age, population subgroups	Exposure assessment (no. of items)	Range contrasts (no of categories)	Relative risk (95% CI)	Stat. sign.*	Adjustment for confounding	Comments
Zemla, 1984, Poland	328 (214 native upper Silesians, 114 migrants)/585	17–79 y	Questionnaire (5), interviewed	Raw veg. Rather regular vs none (3)	Upper Silesians 0.73 Migrants 1.57			Population-based, hospital visitor controls Response rate for cases 98%
Katsouyanni et al., 1986, Greece	120/120	Mean 55 y for cases	FFQ, before onset of disease (120), interviewed, estimated frequency	Highest vs lowest (5)	0.09 (0.03–0.30)	$p < 0.001$	Age, interviewer, years of schooling, parity, age at first birth, marital status, menopausal status, age at menopause, age at menarche, place of residence	Hospital-based Response rate for cases 92% No interaction with age, years of schooling, menopausal status
Iscovich et al., 1989, Argentina	150/150 hospital controls, 150 neighbourhood controls	Mean 56 y for cases	FFQ, 5 y up to 6 mo before interview (147, 12 veg., excluding potatoes, 4 pulses), interviewed, estimated frequency	Green leafy veg.: Highest vs lowest (4) All green veg.: Highest vs lowest (4)	Hospital controls: 0.32 Neighbourhood controls: 0.15 Hospital controls: 0.52 Neighbourhood controls: 0.40	$p < 0.05$ $p < 0.05$ $p < 0.05$ $p < 0.05$	Age, education, husband's occupation, age at first pregnancy, parity, obesity index	Hospital-based and population-based Response rate 98% for cases In multivariate analyses controlling for other food groups, the association with green vegetables remained
Toniolo et al., 1989, Italy	250 (70 premenopausal, 180 postmenopausal)/499	< 75 y	Diet history (70), interviewed, estimated frequency and amount	Highest vs lowest (4)	1.2		Age, energy	Population-based Response rate for cases 91%, for controls 79%
Ewertz & Gill, 1990, Denmark	1474/1322	< 70 y	Semi-quantitative FFQ, year before diagnosis (21), estimated frequency and amount; included summary question on veg.	7 vs < 2 (7) times/wk	[1.05 (0.76–1.47)]		Age, residence	Population-based Response rate for cases 88%, for controls 79% Questionnaire completed one year after diagnosis

Table 64 (contd)

Author, year, country	Cases/controls	Age, population subgroups	Exposure assessment (no. of items)	Range contrasts (no. of categories)	Relative risk (95% CI)	Stat. sign.*	Adjustment for confounding	Comments
Van't Veer et al., 1990, Netherlands	133/238	25–44, 55–64 y	Diet history, 12 mo before diagnosis (236), interviewed, estimated frequency and amount; validity and reliability assessed	Highest vs lowest (4)	0.86	$p = 0.66$	Age, history of benign breast disease, first- and second-degree of family history, number of cigarettes daily, education, ever-use of oral contraceptives, age at menarche, age at first full-term pregnancy, BMI, energy, alcohol	Population-based Response rate for cases 80%, for controls 53%
Ingram, 1991, Australia	99/209	22–86 y	FFQ, current intake (179), self-administered	Highest vs lowest (2)	1.4 (0.8–2.4)	NS	Age, residence	Population-based Response rate for cases 100%
Negri et al., 1991, Italy	2860/3625	< 75 y	FFQ; (14–37 depending on cancer site)	Green veg.: Highest vs lowest (3)	0.7 (0.6–0.8)	$p < 0.01$	Age, area of residence, education, smoking, fruit consumption	Hospital-based Data from a network of case–control studies Response rate > 97%
Richardson et al., 1991, France	409/515	28–66 y	Diet history (55), interviewed, estimated frequency and amount	Increased vs decreased intake in last 10 y	No difference in mean intake in cases (1092 g/wk) vs controls (1064 g/wk)		Age, menopausal status	Hospital-based Response rate > 98%
Zaridze et al., 1991, Russia	139 (58 premenopausal, 81 postmenopausal)/139		FFQ, year before diagnosis (145); interviewed, estimated frequency		Premenopausal: [0.31 (0.03–3.70)] Postmenopausal: [0.69 (0.10–4.54)]	NS NS	Age at menarche, age at first birth, education	Hospital-based Response rate for cases 99%, for controls 94%

202

Table 64 (contd)

Author, year, country	Cases/controls	Age, population subgroups	Exposure assessment (no. of items)	Range contrasts (no. of categories)	Relative risk (95% CI)	Stat. sign.*	Adjustment for confounding	Comments
Pawlega, 1992, Poland	127 (33 < 50 y, 94 ≥ 50 y)/250	≥ 35 y	Questionnaire, 20 y ago (44)	Boiled veg.: > 3 vs ≤ 1/wk (3)	≥ 50 years: 0.4 (0.2–0.8)	$p = 0.01$	Age, education, social class, marital status, number of persons in household, years of smoking, BMI, drinking of vodka 20 years earlier	Population-based Data on boiled veg. among women < 50 years were not accepted because of low reproducibility
Levi et al., 1993b, Switzerland	107/318	≤ 75 y	Questionnaire (50, 9 veg., 1 pulses, 1 potato), interviewed, estimated frequency	Green veg. Highest vs lowest (3)	0.4	$p < 0.01$	Age, education, energy	Hospital-based Response rate > 85%
Holmberg et al., 1994, Sweden	265 (55 ≤ 50 y, 210 > 50 y)/432 screening controls	40–74 y	FFQ, past 6 mo (60), interviewed, estimated frequency	Highest vs lowest (4)	All: 0.7 (0.4–1.1) < 50 years: 1.6 (0.5–4.7) > 50 years: 0.6 (0.3–1.0)		Age, county of residence, month of mammography	Population-based Response rate for cases 70%, for controls 82% Potatoes excluded Effect modification by age group non-significant
Landa et al., 1994, Spain	100/100	Mean 59 y	FFQ, before onset of disease (99), interviewed, estimated frequency	Highest vs lowest (3)	[0.52]	$p < 0.05$	Age	Hospital-based
Qi et al., 1994, China	244/244		Diet history, starting from one year before diagnosis (40), interviewed, estimated frequency and amount	≥ 600 vs < 400 g (4)	0.26 (0.14–0.47)		Age, length of stay in Tianjin, age at menarche, age at menopause, age at first birth	Hospital-based

Table 64 (contd)

Author, year, country	Cases/controls	Age, population subgroups	Exposure assessment (no. of items)	Range contrasts (no. of categories)	Relative risk (95% CI)	Stat. sign.*	Adjustment for confounding	Comments
Franceschi et al., 1995, Italy	2569/2588	20–74 y	FFQ, 2 y before diagnosis (79, 11 veg., 2 potatoes), interviewed, estimated weekly frequency; validity assessed	Raw veg.: > 12.5 vs < 4.9 servings/wk (5) Cooked veg: > 7.5 vs < 3.1 servings/wk (5)	0.73 (0.60–0.88) 0.96 (0.79–1.16)	$p < 0.01$	Age, study centre, education, parity, energy, alcohol	Hospital-based Response rate 96% Cooked vegetable group includes pulses
Hirose et al., 1995, Japan	1052 (607 premenopausal, 445 postmenopausal)/ 23 163	≥ 20 y	Questionnaire before symptoms, self-administered	Raw veg. Daily vs ≤ 3–4/wk (2)	Premenopausal: 1.00 (0.85–19) Postmenopausal: 0.99 (0.81–1.20)	NS NS	Age, first-visit year	Hospital-based Response rate 98%
Trichopoulou et al., 1995a, Greece	820, (270 premenopausal, 550 postmenopausal)/ 795 hospital controls, 753 visitor controls		Semi-quantitative FFQ, past year (115, 26 veg., 1 potato, 5 pulses), interviewed, estimated frequency; validated	Highest vs lowest (5) (median 142 vs 47 times/mo)	0.54 (0.40–0.74)	$p = 0.0001$	Age, place of birth, parity, age at first pregnancy, age at menarche, menopausal status, Quetelet index, energy	Hospital and population-based Response rate for cases 94%, for hospital controls 96%, for visitor controls 93%. Confounding between fruit and veg. was limited. Potatoes excluded. Further adjustment for other food groups or fat did not change association. No statistically significant effect modification by menopausal status ($p > 0.10$).
Freudenheim et al., 1996, USA	297/311	≥ 40 y, only premenopausal	FFQ, past year 2 y before interview (172, 31 veg.), interviewed, estimated frequency and amount; validity and reliability assessed	≥ 523 vs ≤ 276 g/d (4)	0.46 (0.28–0.74)	$p < 0.001$	Age, education, age at first birth, age at menarche, first-degree relative with breast cancer, previous benign breast disease, BMI, energy	Population-based. Response rate 66% for cases, 62% for controls. Potatoes excluded. Association attenuated after further adjustment for β-carotene (RR = 0.84, 0.43–1.63) and lutein/zeaxanthin (RR = 0.76, 0.41–1.44). No change in vegetable estimate after adjusting for vitamin C, α-tocopherol, folic acid, dietary fibre or α-carotene

Table 64 (contd)

Author, year, country	Cases/controls	Age, population subgroups	Exposure assessment (no. of items)	Range contrasts (no. of categories)	Relative risk (95% CI)	Stat. sign.*	Adjustment for confounding	Comments
Thorand et al., 1998, Germany	43/106	38–80 y, all postmenopausal	Diet history, past year (201), interviewed, estimated frequency and amount; validity and reliability assessed	Continuous variable, increment 260 g/d	0.86 (0.51–1.46)		Age, BMI, exogenous hormone use, age at menarche, nulliparity, smoking, status, socioeconomic status	Population-based Response rate 75% for cases, 45% for controls. Potatoes excluded. Similar finding when potatoes are included
Potischman et al., 1999, USA	568 in situ or invasive localized disease, did not report chemotherapy treatment/1451	20–44 y	FFQ, past year (100, 34 veg.), self-administered, estimated frequency and amount, validated	≥ 18.2 vs < 8.4 times/wk (4)	0.86 (0.6–1.1)		Age at diagnosis, study site, ethnicity, education, age at first birth, alcohol, years of oral contraceptive use, smoking status	Population-based Response rate 84% for cases, 70% for controls Vegetable group included potatoes, olives, avocado, garlic. Results not changed after further adjustment for cereals and grains. Results similar when limited to the 353 cases with localized disease or who were interviewed within three months of diagnosis
Ronco et al., 1999, Uruguay	400/405	20–89 y	FFQ (64, 15 veg.), interviewed, reliability assessed	> 16.3 vs< 9 servings/wk (4)	0.41 (0.26–0.65)	$p = 0.004$	Age, residence, urban/rural status, family history of breast cancer in a first-degree relative, BMI, age at menarche, parity, menopausal status, energy	Hospital-based Response rate for cases 97%, for controls 94% Vegetable group includes garlic and legumes, excludes potatoes. No effect modification by menopausal status. RR remained significant after further adjustment for other nutrient but became non-significant after further adjustment for lycopene

Cancer-preventive effects

Table 64 (contd)

Author, year, country	Cases/controls	Age, population subgroups	Exposure assessment (no. of items)	Range contrasts (no of categories)	Relative risk (95% CI)	Stat. sign.*	Adjustment for confounding	Comments
Tavani et al., 1999, Italy	579/668	22–39 y	FFQ (78); estimated weekly frequency; validated	Raw veg.: > 8 servings/wk vs less (2)	0.57 (0.33–0.98)		Study centre, year of recruitment, age, education, BMI, family history of breast cancer, parity, age at first birth	Hospital-based Subset of studies by Franceschi et al., 1995, Negri et al., 1991 Response rate generally > 96%
Dos Santos Silva et al., 2002, UK	240/477	< 75 y	FFQ, 2–3 y before (108, 40 veg, 21 pulses, lentils, dhals), interviewed, estimated frequency and amount; validity assessed	Veg. dishes: ≥ 4 vs ≤ 1 g/d (4)	0.48 (0.27–0.85)	p = 0.005	Age, general practitioner, energy, age at menarche, age at first birth, parous, parity, breast feeding, family history of breast cancer, menopausal status, time since menopause, education	Population-based Population: women of South Asian ethnicity who had migrated to England Response rate for cases 79%, for controls 76% Risk was attenuated after further adjustment for type of diet or meat consumption

* p for trend when applicable

Table 65. Cohort studies of total fruit and vegetable consumption and risk of breast cancer in women

Author, year, country	Cases/cohort size (years follow-up)	Age, population subgroups	Exposure assessment (no. of items)	Range contrasts (no. of categories)	Relative risk (95% CI)	Stat. sign.*	Adjustment for confounding	Comments
Shibata et al., 1992, USA	219/11 580 9 y	Mean 74 y	FFQ (59, 23 fruits, 21 veg.), self-administered, estimated frequency	≥ 8.3 vs < 5.9 servings/d (3)	0.87 (0.63–1.21)	NS	Age, smoking	Incidence Retirement community Veg. group includes potatoes
Byrne et al. 1996, USA	53/6156 4 y	32–86 y	FFQ (93), interviewed; estimated frequency	> 3 vs ≤ 3 servings/d (2)	0.7 (0.4–1.5)		Age	Incidence
Zhang et al. 1999, USA	2697 (784 premenopausal, 1913 postmenopausal)/ 83 234 15 y	33–60 y	Semi-quantitative FFQ, past year (61–126), self-administered, estimated frequency; validity and reliability assessed	≥ 5.0 vs < 2 servings/d (5)	Premenopausal: 0.77 (0.58–1.02) Premenopausal and positive family history: 0.29 (0.13–0.62) Premenopausal and drink ≥ 15 g/d of alcohol: 0.53 (0.27–1.04) Postmenopausal: 1.03 (0.81–1.31) Postmenopausal and current HRT user: 0.86 (0.54–1.39)	$p = 0.05$ $p = 0.003$ $p = 0.007$ $p = 0.73$	Age, length of follow-up, energy intake, parity, age at first birth, age at menarche, history of breast cancer in mother or sister, history of benign breast disease, alcohol, BMI at age 18, weight change from age 18, height, age at menopause, HRT use	Incidence Nurses' Health Study
Smith-Warner et al., 2001	7377 cases from 8 cohort studies with total baseline population of 351 825 women Follow-up: 1976–96			Highest vs lowest (4) Increment = 100 g/d	All: 0.93 (0.86–1.00) All: 0.99 (0.98–1.00) Premenopausal: 0.99 (0.96–1.02) Postmenopausal: 1.00 (0.98–1.01)	$p = 0.12$		Pooled analysis Study-specific RRs were calculated using the primary data and then were combined using the random effects model Veg. group excludes potatoes p for heterogeneity 0.78–0.99

*p for trend when applicable. HRT, hormone replacement therapy

Table 66. Case–control studies of total fruit and vegetable consumption and risk of breast cancer in women

Author, year, country	Cases/ controls	Age, population subgroups	Exposure assessment (no. of items)	Range contrasts (no. of categories)	Relative risk (95% CI)	Stat. sign.*	Adjustment for confounding	Comments
Potischman et al., 1998, USA	1647/1501	< 45 y	FFQ, 12–13 y of age (29, 2 fruits, 3 veg., 1 beans, 2 potatoes), interviewed, estimated frequency and amount; validity assessed	> 101 vs ≤ 54 times/mo (4)	0.89 (0.7–1.1)		Age, site, race, education, combination variable for age at first full-term birth and number of full-term births, oral contraceptive use, average lifetime exercise, exercise at ages 12–13 y, current alcohol consumption	Population-based Response rate for cases 86%, for controls 71% Veg. group includes potatoes, excludes beans Fruit group excludes juice. Results were similar when unreliable foods were removed from intake estimates. No effect modification by strata of adult fat or veg. intake
Potischman et al., 1999, USA	568 in situ or invasive localized disease/ 1451	20–44 y	FFQ, past year (100, 25 fruits, 34 veg.), self-administered, estimated frequency and amount; validated	≥ 29.4 vs < 14 times/wk (4)	0.94 (0.7–1.2)		Age at diagnosis, study site, ethnicity, education, age at first birth, alcohol, years of oral contraceptive use, smoking status	Population-based Response rate for cases 84%, for controls 70%. Results were similar when limited to the 353 cases with localized disease or interviewed < 3 months after diagnosis
Ronco et al., 1999, Uruguay	400/405	20–89 y	FFQ (64, 9 fruits, 15 veg.), interviewed, reliability assessed	Highest vs lowest (4)	0.42 (0.26–0.66)	p = 0.005	Age, residence, urban/ rural status, family history of breast cancer in a first-degree relative, BMI, age at menarche, parity, menopausal status, energy	Hospital-based Response rate for cases 97%, for controls 94% Veg. group includes garlic and legumes, excludes potatoes. No effect modification by menopausal status
Terry et al., 2001c, Sweden	2832/2650	50–74 y All post-menopausal	FFQ, past year (65, 19 fruits and veg.), self-administered, estimated frequency	Highest vs lowest (4)	0.97 (0.80–1.18)	p = 0.61	Age, height, BMI, current smoking, socioeconomic status, alcohol, high-fibre grains and cereals, fatty fish, multivitamin use, parity, HRT, history of benign breast disease, family history of breast cancer, type of menopause, age at menopause, age at menarche, age at first birth	Population-based Response rate for cases 84%, for controls 82%

* p for trend when applicable. HRT, hormone replacement therapy

Table 67. Case–control studies of fruit and vegetable consumption and risk of breast cancer in men

Author, year, country	Cases/ controls	Exposure assessment (no. of items)	Range contrasts (no. of categories)	Relative risk (95% CI)	Stat. sign.*	Adjustment for confounding	Comments
Hsing et al., 1998b, USA	178/512	Questionnaire, adult life (5), estimated frequency	Fruit: ≥ 7 vs < 1/wk (4) Veg.: ≥ 7 vs < 1/wk (4)	All respondents: 0.8 (0.4–1.3) Spouse respondents: 0.5 (0.2–1.2) All respondents: 0.5 (0.2–1.7) Spouse respondents: 0.3 (0.03–4.2)		Age at death, socioeconomic status	Mortality for cases and controls Questionnaire completed by next of kin
Rosenblatt et al., 1999, USA	220/291	FFQ (125), self-administered	Citrus fruit: Highest vs lowest (4) Other fruit: Highest vs lowest (4) Green veg.: Highest vs lowest (4) Yellow veg.: Highest vs lowest (4)	1.7 (1.0–2.8) 1.1 (0.7–1.9) 1.0 (0.6–1.7) 0.8 (0.4–1.3)	$p = 0.032$ $p = 0.85$ $p = 0.44$ $p = 0.35$	Age, study site, energy	Population-based Response rate for cases 75%, for controls 45%
Johnson et al., 2002, Canada	81/1905	FFQ (60), self-administered	Fruit and juice: ≥ 26 vs < 9.9 servings/wk (4) Fruit: ≥ 14.5 vs < 4.4 servings/wk (4) Veg.: ≥ 24 vs < 13 servings/wk (4) Veg. and veg. juice: ≥ 25 vs < 13.4 servings/wk (4)	2.26 (1.18–4.52) 1.15 (0.62–2.13) 0.70 (0.38–1.30) 0.75 (0.40–1.40)	$p = 0.02$ $p = 0.4$ $p = 0.33$ $p = 0.41$	Age, marriage status, coffee consumption, physical activity, BMI	Population-based Response rate for cases 68%, for controls 65%

*p for trend when applicable

Table 68. Case–control studies of fruit consumption and risk of invasive cervix cancer

Author, year, country	Cases/controls	Exposure assessment (no. of items)	Range contrasts (no. of categories)	Relative risk (95% CI)	Stat. sign.*	Adjustment for confounding	Comments
Verreault et al., 1989, USA	189/227	FFQ, (66) average frequency of use, assumed standard portion size, interviewed by telephone	≥ 10.7 vs ≤ 3.4 servings/wk (4)	1.3 (0.6–2.5)	$p = 0.68$	Age, education, smoking, frequency of Pap smears, oral and barrier contraceptive use, age at first intercourse, number of sexual partners, history of cervicovaginal infection	Population-based Response for cases 72%, for eligible controls 69% Interviews 2.8 years after diagnosis for cases
Ziegler et al., 1990, USA	271/502	FFQ (75, 15 fruits and fruit juices), interviewed, open-ended frequency categories	≥ 19 vs ≤ 7.3 servings/wk (4)	[0.74]	$p = 0.26$	Matched on age, race and telephone exchange. Adjusted for number of sexual partners, age at first intercourse, cigarettes per day, oral contraceptive use duration, history of non-specific genital infection, years since last Pap smear, age, study centre	Population-based Response for cases 73%, for eligible controls 74%
Herrero et al., 1991, four Latin American countries	748/1411	FFQ (58, 15 fruits), interviewed, frequency only, assumed average portion size	≥ 119 vs < 43 servings/mo (4)	0.86 (0.6–1.2)	$p = 0.44$	Age, study site, age at first intercourse, number of sexual partners, number of pregnancies, presence of HPV 16/18, time since last Pap smear, number of household facilities as measure of household socio-economic status	Hospital-based in two countries, hospital and community-based in other two countries Response for cases 99.1%, for controls 95.8% Controls with no sexual history excluded from analysis
Cuzick et al., 1996, UK	121/241	Diet assessment tool not clear, interviewed	≥ 8 vs 0 pieces/wk (4)	0.67 (0.19–2.35)	$p = 0.33$	Number of partners and age at first intercourse	Hospital-based
Hirose et al., 1996, Japan	556/26 751	Questionnaire on frequency of intake	Daily vs ≤ 3–4 servings/wk (2)	0.70 (0.59–0.83)	$p < 0.01$	Age and first visit year	Hospital-based 98% of first-visit patients completed questionnaire

*p for trend when applicable

Table 69. Case–control studies of vegetable consumption and risk of invasive cervical cancer

Author, year, country	Cases/controls	Exposure assessment (no. of items)	Range contrasts (no. of	Relative risk (95% CI)	Stat. sign.*	Adjustment for confounding	Comments
La Vecchia et al., 1988a, Italy	392/392	FFQ (5), frequency only	Green veg.: ≥ 14 vs < 7 servings/wk (3)	[0.21 (0.10–0.45)]	p < 0.001	Age, interviewer, marital status, education, parity, age at first intercourse, number of sexual partners, BMI, smoking, oral contraceptive use, other female hormone use	Hospital-based 98% response rate for cases and controls
Verreault et al., 1989, USA	189/227	FFQ (66), interviewed by telephone, average frequency of use, assumed standard portion size	Dark green and yellow veg.: ≥ 5.3 vs < 2 servings/wk (4)	0.6 (0.3–1.1)	p = 0.06	Age, education, smoking, frequency of Pap smears, oral and barrier contraceptive use, age at first intercourse, number of sexual partners, history of cervico-vaginal infection	Population-based Response rate for cases 72%, for eligible controls 69% Interviews 2.8 years after diagnosis for cases
			Light green veg.: ≥ 10.0 vs < 5.2 servings/wk (4)	0.9 (0.5–1.7)	p = 0.43		
Ziegler et al., 1990, USA	271/502	FFQ, (75, 20 veg.) interviewed, open-ended frequency categories	≥ 26 vs ≤ 11 servings/wk (4)	[0.86]	p = 0.43	Matched on age, race and telephone exchange. Adjusted for number of sexual partners, age at first intercourse, cigarettes per day, oral contraceptive use duration, history of non-specific genital infection, years since last Pap smear, age, study centre	Population-based Response rate for cases 73%, for eligible controls 74% Potatoes and legumes excluded
Herrero et al., 1991, four Latin American countries	748/1411	FFQ (58, 16 veg.), interviewed, frequency only, assumed average portion size	≥ 207 vs < 121 servings/mo (4)	0.97 (0.7–1.3)	p = 0.54	Age, study site, age at first intercourse, number of sexual partners, number of pregnancies, presence of HPV 16/18, time since last Pap smear, number of household facilities as measure of household socio-economic status	Hospital-based in two countries, hospital and community-based in two other countries Response for cases 99.1%, for controls 95.8%. Controls with no sexual history excluded from analysis

Table 69 (contd)

Author, year, country	Cases/controls	Exposure assessment (no. of items)	Range contrasts (no. of categories)	Relative risk (95% CI)	Stat. sign.*	Adjustment for confounding	Comments
Cuzick et al., 1996, UK	121/241	Diet assessment tool not clear, interviewed	≥ 7 vs ≤ 2 servings/wk (3)	Leafy veg.: 0.59 (0.24–1.48) Other veg.: 0.67 (0.23–1.98)	p = 0.11 p = 0.39	Number of partners, age at first intercourse	Hospital-based
Hirose et al., 1996, Japan	556/26 751	Questionnaire on frequency of intake	Raw veg.: Daily vs ≤ 3–4 servings/wk (2) Green veg.: ≥ 5 vs ≤ 2 servings/wk (3)	0.88 (0.74–1.04) 0.56 (0.45–0.71)	NS p < 0.01	Age and first-visit year	Hospital-based 98% of first visit patients completed questionnaire

*p for trend when applicable

Table 70. Case–control studies of fruit and vegetable consumption and risk of cervical cancer

Author, year, country	Cases/controls	Exposure assessment (no. of items)	Range contrasts (no. of categories)	Relative risk (95% CI)	Stat. sign.*	Adjustment for confounding	Comments
Ziegler et al., 1990, USA	271/502	FFQ (75, 15 fruits and fruit juices, 20 veg.), interviewed, open-ended frequency categories	≥ 44 vs ≤ 21 servings/wk (4)	[0.90]	p = 0.34	Matched on age, race and telephone exchange. Adjusted for number of sexual partners, age at first intercourse, cigarettes per day, oral contraceptive use duration, history of non-specific genital infection, years since last Pap smear, age, study centre	Population-based Response rate for cases 73%, for eligible controls 74%
Rajkumar et al., 2003a, India	205/213	FFQ (21), interviewed	≥ 7 vs < 6 servings/wk (3)	0.48 (0.24–0.98)	p = 0.04	Age, residence, occupation, marital status, age at first marriage, number of pregnancies, husband's extramarital affairs, BMI, chewing habits	Hospital-based Little difference when only HPV-positive controls were considered

*p for trend when applicable

Table 71. Case–control study of fruit and/or vegetable consumption and risk of *in situ* cervical cancer

Author, year, country	Cases/controls	Exposure assessment (no. of items)	Range contrasts (no. of categories)	Relative risk (95% CI)	Stat. sign.*	Adjustment for confounding	Comments
Ziegler et al., 1991, USA	229/502	FFQ, (75, 15 fruit and fruit juice, 20 veg.), interviewed, open-ended frequency categories	Fruit: ≥ 19 vs ≤ 7.3 servings/wk (4)	[0.61]	p = 0.09	Matched on age, race and telephone exchange. Adjusted for number of sexual partners, duration of cigarette use, oral contraceptive use duration, history of non-specific genital infection, years since last Pap smear, years of education, age, study centre	Population-based Limited to non-Hispanic whites Response for cases 78%, for eligible controls 74%
			Veg.: ≥ 26 vs ≤ 11 servings/wk (4)	[0.92]	p = 0.48		
			Fruit and veg.: ≥ 44 servings/wk vs ≤ 21 (4)	[0.74]	p = 0.43		

*p for trend when applicable

Table 72. Case–control study of fruit consumption and risk of cervical dysplasia

Author, year, country	Cases/controls	Exposure assessment (no. of items)	Range contrasts (no. of categories)	Relative risk (95% CI)	Stat. sign.*	Adjustment for confounding	Comments
De Vet et al., 1991, Netherlands	257/705	FFQ, self-administered, frequency of consumption and small, medium or large portion size	≥ 3 vs 0 servings/d (4)	0.29 (0.13–0.63)	p = 0.06	Demographic characteristics, season when questionnaire completed, marital status, education, smoking, parity, oral contraceptive use, age at first sexual intercourse, frequency of intercourse, number of sexual partners, frequency of Pap smears, consumption of other food groups	Population-based Cases were participants in a multi-centre trial; controls were drawn from population registries Response rate for cases 85%, for controls 67%

*p for trend when applicable

Table 73. Case–control studies of fruit consumption and risk of endometrium cancer

Author, year, country	Cases/controls	Exposure assessment (no. of items)	Range contrasts (no. of categories)	Relative risk (95% CI)	Stat. sign.*	Adjustment for confounding	Comments
La Vecchia et al., 1986, Italy	206/206	FFQ (10), frequency	Fresh fruit: ≥ 14 vs < 14 servings/wk (2)	0.57 (0.33–0.99)		Interviewer, age, marital status, years of education, BMI, parity, history of diabetes or hypertension, age at menarche, age at menopause, oral contraceptive use, other female hormone use	Hospital-based
Levi et al., 1993a, Switzerland, northern Italy	274/572	FFQ (50), interviewed, frequency	Total fresh fruit: Highest vs lowest (3)	0.45	$p = 0.01$	Age, study centre, energy	Hospital-based
Potischman et al., 1993, USA	399/296	FFQ (60, 7 fruits), interviewed, open-ended frequency of intake, one of three portion sizes	> 21.9 vs < 8.5 times/wk (4)	1.1 (0.6–1.9)		Age group, BMI, ever estrogen use, ever oral contraceptive use, number of births, current smoking, education, energy	Population-based Response rate among eligible cases 87%, among eligible controls 66%
Shu et al., 1993, China	268/268	FFQ (63, 5 fruits), interviewed, open-ended usual intake frequency, portion per unit time	Highest vs lowest (4)	0.7	$p = 0.25$	Age, number of pregnancies, BMI, energy	Population-based Response rate for cases 91%, for controls 96%
Hirose et al., 1996, Japan	145/26 751	Questionnaire, frequency of intake	Daily vs ≤ 3–4 servings/wk (2)	1.97 (1.37–2.82)	$p < 0.01$	Age and first-visit year	Hospital-based 98% of first-visit patients completed questionnaire
Tzonou et al., 1996b, Greece	145/298	Semi-quantitative FFQ, (115, 19 fruits), interviewed	Highest vs lowest (4)	0.96 (0.76–1.21)	$p = 0.73$	Age, education, age at menopause, age at menarche, parity, miscarriages, abortions, oral contraceptive use, hormone replacement therapy, smoking, alcohol, coffee, height, energy, BMI	Hospital-based Response rate for cases 83%, for controls 88%

Table 73 (contd)

Author, year, country	Cases/control	Exposure assessment (no. of items)	Range contrasts (no. of categories)	Relative risk (95% CI)	Stat. sign.*	Adjustment for confounding	Comments
Goodman et al., 1997, USA	332/511	FFQ (250), interviewed, open-ended usual intake frequency, portion size from pictures of three different portions	> 282 vs < 95 g/d (4)	0.5	p = 0.004	Pregnancy history, oral contraceptive usage, history of diabetes, BMI, energy	Population-based Response rate for cases 66%, for controls 73%
Jain et al., 2000, Canada	552/563	Diet history, interviewed, usual frequency, usual amount in relation to food models	> 555 vs < 229 g/d (4)	1.29 (0.88–1.89)	p = 0.41	Energy, age, body weight, ever smoked, history of diabetes, oral contraceptive use, hormone replacement therapy use, university education, live births, age at menarche	Population-based Response rate for cases 50% of potentially eligible, 70% of eligible with MD approval, for controls 41%
McCann et al., 2000, USA	232/639	Diet history (172, 18 fruits) self-administered, usual intake, portion size in relation to pictures	> 184 vs < 81 times/mo (4)	0.9 (0.5–1.7)	p = 0.97	Age, education, BMI, diabetes, hypertension, pack-years cigarette smoking, age at menarche, parity, oral contraceptive use, menopause status, hormone replacement therapy use, other food groups	Population-based Response rate for cases 51%, for controls 51%
Littman et al., 2001, USA	679/944	FFQ (98, 16 fruits), interviewed, frequency five years previously, portion size relative to three categories	> 2.3 vs < 0.8 servings/d (5)	0.67 (0.47–0.95)	p = 0.02	Age, county of residence, energy, unopposed estrogen use, smoking, BMI	Population-based Response rate for cases 72%, for controls 73% among those found eligible
Terry et al., 2002, Sweden	709/2887	FFQ, self-administered, nine frequency categories	> 21 vs < 2.5 servings/wk (median values (4)	0.9 (0.7–1.2)	p = 0.35	Age, BMI, smoking, physical activity, prevalence of diabetes, fatty fish consumption, quintiles of total food consumption, other dietary factors	Population-based Postmenopausal women with intact uterus, no history of endometrial or breast cancer Response rate for cases 75%

*p for trend when applicable

Table 74. Case–control studies of vegetable consumption and risk of endometrium cancer

Author, year, country	Cases/controls	Exposure assessment (no. of items)	Range contrasts (no. of categories)	Relative risk (95% CI)	Stat. sign.*	Adjustment for confounding	Comments
Zemla et al., 1986, Poland	173/346	No information	Raw veg.: Frequent vs never (3)	0.43	$p < 0.001$	None	Hospital-based cases, control selection not clear
La Vecchia et al., 1986, Italy	206/206	FFQ (10), frequency	Green veg.: ≥ 8 vs < 8 portions/wk (2)	0.24 (0.13–0.45)		Interviewer, age, marital status, years of education, BMI, parity, history of diabetes or hypertension, age at menarche, age at menopause, oral contraceptive use, other female hormone use	Hospital-based
Levi et al., 1993a, Switzerland, northern Italy	274/572	FFQ (50) interviewed, frequencies	Highest vs lowest (3)	0.38	$p < 0.01$	Age, study centre, energy	Hospital-based
Potischman et al., 1993, USA	399/296	FFQ (60, 13 veg.) open-ended frequency of intake, one of three portion sizes	> 21.0 vs < 11.1 times/wk (4)	1.0 (0.6–1.6)		Age-group, BMI, ever estrogen use, ever oral-contraceptive use, number of births, current smoking, education, energy	Population-based Response among eligible cases 87%, among eligible controls 66% Includes potatoes, pulses and legumes
Shu et al., 1993, China	268/268	FFQ (63, 23 veg.), interviewed, open-ended usual intake frequency, portion per unit time, 23 veg. (includes four legumes)	Highest vs lowest (4)	1.4	$p = 0.39$	Age, number of pregnancies, BMI, energy	Population-based Response rate for cases 91%, for controls 96%
Hirose et al., 1996, Japan	145/26 751	Questionnaire or frequency of intake	Raw veg.: Daily vs ≤ 3–4 servings/wk (2)	1.54 (1.11–2.13)	$p < 0.05$	Age and first-visit year	Hospital-based 98% of first-visit patients completed questionnaire
			Green veg.: > 5 vs ≤ 2 servings/wk (3)	1.12 (0.74–1.70)	NS		

Table 74 (contd)

Author, year, country	Cases/controls	Exposure assessment (no. of items)	Range contrasts (no. of categories)	Relative risk (95% CI)	Stat. sign.*	Adjustment for confounding	Comments
Tzonou et al., 1996b, Greece	145/298	Semi-quantitative FFQ, (115), 25 veg., interviewed	Highest vs lowest (4)	0.85 (0.66–1.11)	p = 0.24	Age, education, age at menopause, age at menarche, parity, miscarriages, abortions, oral contraceptive use, HRT, smoking, alcohol, coffee, height, BMI, energy	Hospital-based Response rate for cases 83%, for controls 88%
Goodman et al., 1997, USA	332/511	FFQ, (250), interviewed, open ended usual intake frequency, portion size from pictures of three different portions	> 272 vs < 132 g/d (4)	0.5	p = 0.02	Pregnancy history, oral contraceptive usage, history of diabetes, BMI, energy	Population-based Response rate for cases 66%, for controls 73%
Jain et al., 2000, Canada	552/563	Diet history, interviewed, usual frequency, usual amount in relation to food models	> 633 vs < 271 g/d (4)	0.65 (0.44–0.96)	p = 0.04	Energy, age, body weight, ever smoked, history of diabetes, oral contraceptive use, HRT, university education, live births, age at menarche	Population-based Response rate for cases 50% of potentially eligible, 70% of eligible with MD approval, for controls 41%
McCann et al., 2000, USA	232/639	Diet history (172, 34 veg.), self-administered, usual intake portion size in relation to pictures	> 221 vs < 127 times/mo (4)	0.5 (0.3–0.9)	p = 0.03	Age, education, BMI, diabetes, hypertension, pack-years cigarette smoking, age at menarche, parity, oral contraceptive use, menopause status, HRT, other food groups	Population-based Response rate for cases 51%, for controls 51%
Littman et al., 2001, USA	679/944	FFQ, (98, 19 veg.), frequency 5 y previous, portion size relative to three categories	> 3.1 vs < 1.5 servings/d (5)	0.69 (0.48–1.0)	p = 0.07	Age, county of residence, energy, unopposed estrogen usage, smoking, BMI	Population-based Response rate for cases 72%, for controls 73% among those found eligible Includes potatoes

*p for trend when applicable. HRT, hormone replacement therapy

Table 75. Cohort study of fruit and vegetable consumption and risk of endometrium cancer

Author, year, country	Cases/ cohort size (years follow-up)	Exposure assessment (no. of items)	Range contrasts (no. of categories)	Relative risk (95% CI)	Stat. sign.*	Adjustment for confounding	Comments
Terry et al., 1999, Sweden	133/11 659 25 y	Questionnaire (107, 1 fruit, 1 veg.), self-administered, four categories of contribution to total diet	Large vs very little or no part of the diet (4)	[0.32 (0.08–1.25)]	NS	Age, physical activity, weight at baseline, parity	Incidence Twin study

*p for trend when applicable

Table 76. Case–control studies of fruit and vegetable consumption and risk of endometrium cancer

Author, year, country	Cases/ controls	Exposure assessment (no. of items)	Range contrasts (no. of categories)	Relative risk (95% CI)	Stat. sign.*	Adjustment for confounding	Comments
Goodman et al., 1997, USA	332/511	FFQ (250), interviewed, open-ended usual intake frequency, portion size from pictures of three different portions (4)	> 553 vs < 259 g	0.6	p = 0.02	Pregnancy history, oral contraceptive use, history of diabetes, BMI, energy	Population-based Response rate for cases 66%, for controls 73%
Littman et al., 2001, USA	679/944	FFQ, (98, 16 fruit 19 veg.), interviewed, frequency 5 y previously, portion size relative to three categories	> 5.2 vs < 2.3 servings/d (5)	0.73 (0.50–1.1)	p = 0.13	Age, county of residence, energy, unopposed estrogen use, smoking, BMI	Population-based Response rate for cases 72%, for controls 73% among those found eligible
Terry et al., 2002, Sweden	709/2887	FFQ, self-administered, nine frequency categories	> 37 vs < 9.9 servings/wk (4) (median values)	0.9 (0.7–1.2)	p = 0.73	Age, BMI, smoking, physical activity, prevalence of diabetes, fatty fish consumption, quintiles of total food consumption, other dietary factors	Population-based Postmenopausal women with intact uterus, no previous history of endometrial or breast cancer. Response rate among cases 75%, among controls 80%

*p for trend when applicable

Cancer-preventive effects

Table 77. Cohort studies of fruit consumption and risk of ovary cancer

Author, year, country	Cases/ cohort size (years follow-up)	Exposure assessment (no. of items)	Range contrasts (no. of categories)	Relative risk (95% CI)	Stat. sign.*	Adjustment for confounding	Comments
Kushi et al., 1999, USA	139/29 083 10 y	Semi-quantitative FFQ (126), self-administered, nine frequency categories, validated	> 23 vs < 11 times/wk (4)	1.13 (0.66–1.93)	$p = 0.51$	Age, energy, number of live births, age at menopause, family history of ovarian cancer, hysterectomy/unilateral oophorectomy status, waist-to-hip ratio, physical activity, pack-years of smoking, education	Incidence Iowa Health Study
Fairfield et al., 2001, USA	301/80 326 16 y	Semi-quantitative FFQ (126), self-administered, nine frequency categories, validated	≥ 3.2 vs < 1.1 servings/d (5)	1.27 (0.80–2.02)	$p = 0.20$	Age, energy, duration of oral contraceptive use, parity, tubal ligation, BMI, smoking, dietary fibre	Incidence Nurses' Health Study Limited to epithelial cancers

*p for trend when applicable

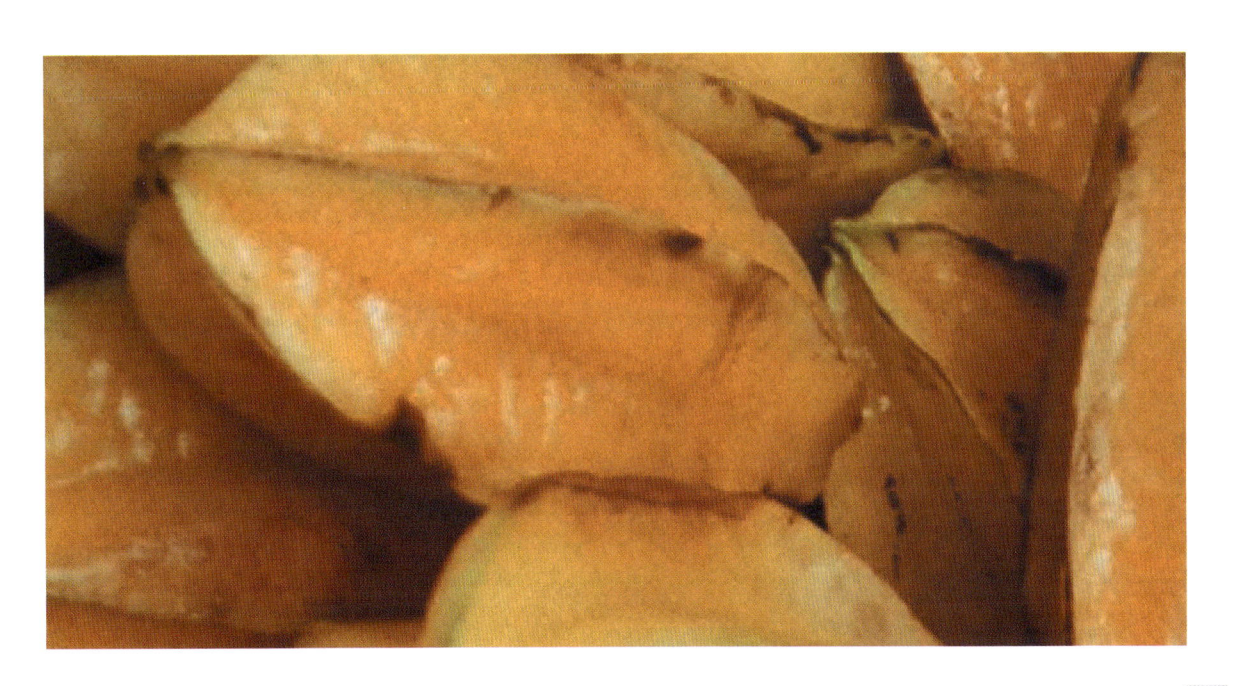

Table 78. Case–control studies of fruit consumption and risk of ovary cancer

Author, year, country	Cases/ controls	Exposure assessment (no. of items)	Range contrasts (no. of categories)	Relative risk (95% CI)	Stat. sign.*	Adjustment for confounding	Comments
Shu et al., 1989, China	172/172	FFQ (63, 4 fruits), interviewed, open-ended usual intake frequency, portion per unit time	Highest vs lowest (4)	0.9	$p = 0.68$	Education	Population-based Response rate for eligible cases 89%, for controls 100%
McCann et al., 2001, USA	496/1425	FFQ (44), self-administered, no portion size	Fruit and fruit juices: > 101 vs ≤ 48 times/mo (4)	0.85 (0.59–1.21)	$p = 0.40$	Age, education, region of residence, regularity of menstruation, family history of ovarian cancer, parity, age at menarche, oral contraceptive use, and remaining food groups	Hospital-based
Salazar-Martinez et al., 2002, Mexico	84/629	FFQ (116), interviewed, frequency of fixed portion for 10 intake frequencies, validated	Highest vs lowest (3)	2.43 (1.02–5.75)	$p = 0.004$	Age, energy, number of live births, recent change in weight, physical activity, diabetes	Hospital-based
Zhang et al., 2002b, China	254/652	FFQ (120), interviewed, portion size from eight categories, cooking method, vitamin and mineral supplements, validated	≥ 110.05 vs ≤ 32.60 kg/y (4)	0.36 (0.2–0.7)	$p < 0.001$	Age, education, area of residence, BMI five years previously, smoking, alcohol, tea, family income, marital status, menopausal status, parity, tubal ligation, oral contraceptive use, physical activity, family history of ovarian cancer, energy, other food groups	Hospital-based and population-based

* p for trend when applicable

Table 79. Cohort studies of vegetable consumption and risk of ovary cancer

Author, year, country	Cases/cohort size (years follow-up)	Exposure assessment (no. of items)	Range contrasts (no. of categories)	Relative risk (95% CI)	Stat. sign.*	Adjustment for confounding	Comments
Kushi et al., 1999, USA	139/29 083 10 y	Semi-quantitative FFQ (126), self-administered, nine frequency categories, validated	> 31 vs < 16 times/wk (4)	0.76 (0.42–1.37)	p = 0.21	Age, energy, number of live births, age at menopause, family history of ovarian cancer, hysterectomy/unilateral oophorectomy status, waist-to-hip ratio, physical activity, pack-years of smoking, education	Incidence Iowa Health Study
Fairfield et al., 2001, USA	301/80 326 16 y	Semi-quantitative FFQ (126), self-administered, nine frequency categories	> 4.4 vs < 1.8 servings/d (5)	0.77 (0.48–1.24)	p = 0.30	Age, energy, duration of oral contraceptive use, parity, tubal ligation, BMI, smoking, dietary fibre	Incidence Nurses' Health Study Limited to epithelial cancers

*p for trend when applicable

Table 80. Case–control studies of vegetable consumption and risk of ovary cancer

Author, year, country	Cases/controls	Exposure assessment (no. of items)	Range contrasts (no. of categories)	Relative risk (95% CI)	Stat. sign.*	Adjustment for confounding	Comments
Shu et al., 1989, China	172/172	FFQ (63, 18 veg.), interviewed, open-ended usual intake frequency, portion per unit time	Highest vs lowest (4)	0.8	p = 0.45	Education	Population-based Response rate for eligible cases 89%, for controls 100%
La Vecchia et al., 1987b, Italy	455/1385	FFQ (10), interviewed, three categories of frequency	Green veg.: ≥ 8 vs < 7 times/wk (3)	0.61 (0.46–0.82)	p < 0.001	Age, interviewer, marital status, social class, education, parity, age at first birth, age at menarche, menopausal status, age at menopause, BMI, oral contraceptive use, other female hormone use, retinol, carotene, added fat, alcohol, other foods	Hospital-based

Table 80 (contd)

Author, year, country	Cases/ controls	Exposure assessment (no. of items)	Range contrasts (no. of categories)	Relative risk (95% CI)	Stat. sign.*	Adjustment for confounding	Comments
Bosetti et al., 2001, Italy	1031/2411	FFQ, (78), interviewed, frequency only	Raw veg.: > 11.5 vs < 4.0 servings/wk (5)	0.47 (0.34–0.64)	p < 0.0001	Age, study centre, education, year of interview, parity, oral contraceptive use, energy	Hospital-based in four regions of Italy
			Cooked veg.: > 5.0 vs < 1.8 servings/wk (5)	0.65 (0.48–0.87)	p = 0.002		
McCann et al., 2001, USA	496/1425	FFQ (44), self-administered, no portion size	> 66 vs ≤ 24 times/mo (4)	0.76 (0.52–1.10)	p = 0.07	Age, education, region of residence, regularity of menstruation, family history of ovarian cancer, parity, age at menarche, oral contraceptive use, and remaining food groups	Hospital-based
Salazar-Martinez et al., 2002, Mexico	84/629	FFQ, (116), frequency of fixed portion for 10 intake frequencies, validated	Green leafy veg.: Highest vs lowest (3)	1.56 (0.67–3.64)	p = 0.14	Age, energy, number of live births, recent change in weight, physical activity, diabetes	Hospital-based
Zhang et al., 2002b, China	254/652	FFQ (120), interviewed, portion size from eight categories, cooking method, vitamin and mineral supplements, validated	≥ 180.55 vs ≤ 89.25 kg/y (4)	0.24 (0.1–0.5)	p < 0.001	Age, education, area of residence, BMI five years previously, smoking, alcohol, tea, family income, marital status, menopausal status, parity, tubal ligation, oral contraceptive use, physical activity, family history of ovarian cancer, energy, other food groups	Hospital-based and population-based

*p for trend when applicable

Cancer-preventive effects

Table 81. Cohort study of fruit and vegetable consumption and risk of ovary cancer

Author, year, country	Cases/cohort size (years follow-up)	Exposure assessment (no. of items)	Range contrasts (no. of categories)	Relative risk (95% CI)	Stat. sign.*	Adjustment for confounding	Comments
Fairfield et al., 2001, USA	301/80 325 16 y	FFQ (126), self-administered, nine frequency categories, validated	> 7.3 vs < 3.3 servings/d (5)	1.10 (0.64–1.90)	p = 0.84	Age, energy, duration or oral contraceptive use, parity, tubal ligation, BMI, smoking, dietary fibre	Incidence Nurses' Health Study Limited to epithelial cancers Inverse association with reported diet in adolescence

*p for trend when applicable

Table 82. Case–control study of fruit and vegetable consumption and risk of ovary cancer

Author, year, country	Cases/controls	Exposure assessment (no. of items)	Range contrasts (no. of categories)	Relative risk (95% CI)	Stat. sign.*	Adjustment for confounding	Comments
McCann et al., 2001, USA	496/1325	FFQ (44), self-administered, no portion size	> 164 vs ≤ 80 times/mo (4)	0.62 (0.42–0.92)	p = 0.09	Age, education, region of residence, regularity of menstruation, family history of ovarian cancer, parity, age at menarche, oral contraceptive use, remaining food groups	Hospital-based

*p for trend when applicable

Table 83. Cohort studies of fruit consumption and risk of prostate cancer

Author, year, country	Cases/cohort size (years follow-up)	Exposure assessment (no. of items)	Range contrasts (no. of categories)	Relative risk (95% CI)	Stat. sign.*	Adjustment for confounding	Comments
Mills et al., 1989, USA	180/14 000 6 y	FFQ (5 fruits)	≥ 60 vs < 12/mo (3)	1.07 (0.72–1.58)	NS	Age, education, other foods	Incidence Seventh-day Adventists
Severson et al., 1989, USA	174/8006 21 y	FFQ (20), interviewed	≥ 5 vs ≤ 1/wk (3)	1.57 (0.95–2.61)		Age	Incidence Men of Japanese ancestry in Hawaii
Hsing et al., 1990, USA	149/17 633 20 y	FFQ (35, 5 fruits), self-administered	> 67 vs < 29.3 times/mo (4)	0.9 (0.6–1.4)		Age, smoking	Mortality Policy holders
Shibata et al., 1992, USA	208/11 580 (women included), 9 y	FFQ (59, 23 fruits), self-administered	≥ 3.5 vs < 2.2 servings/d (3)	1.04 (0.74–1.46)	NS	Age, smoking	Incidence Retirement community
Le Marchand et al., 1994, USA	198/20 316 15 y	FFQ (13)	Fresh fruit: > 974 vs < 414 g/wk (4)	1.0 (0.7–1.6)	$p = 0.99$	Age, ethnicity, income	Incidence Men of various ethnicities in Hawaii
Giovannucci et al., 1995, USA	773/47 894 7 y	FFQ (131, 46 fruits and veg.), self-administered, validated	> 4 vs < 1 serving/d	0.84 (0.59–1.84)	$p = 0.21$	Age, energy	Incidence Health professionals
Schuurman et al., 1998, Netherlands	642/58 279 6.3 y	FFQ (150, 8 fruits), self-administered, validated	286.4 vs 34.0 g/d (median values) (5)	1.31 (0.96–1.79)	$p = 0.02$	Age, family history, socioeconomic status, veg.	Incidence Netherlands cohort study
Chan et al., 2000, Finland	184/27 062 8 y	FFQ (276), self-administered, validated	230 vs 25 g/d (median values) (5)	1.3 (0.8–2.2)	$p = 0.13$	Supplementation group, education, age, BMI, energy, smoking	Incidence Smokers, ATBC study
Appleby et al., 2002, UK	41/4325 25 y	FFQ	Fresh fruit: Daily vs < daily (2)	0.73 (0.35–1.50)	NS	Age, smoking, other foods	Mortality Cohort of health-food shoppers
Key et al., 2003, European countries	1104/130 544 (mean, 4.8 y)	FFQ, validated self-administered or interviewed	Highest vs lowest (5)	1.06 (0.84–1.34)	$p = 0.74$	Age, centre, height, weight, energy	Incidence

*p for trend when applicable

Table 84. Case–control studies of fruit consumption and risk of prostate cancer

Author, year, country	Cases/ controls	Exposure assessment (no. of items)	Range contrasts (no. of categories)	Relative risk (95% CI)	Stat. sign.*	Adjustment for confounding	Comments
Negri et al., 1991, Italy	107/2522	FFQ (13–37 depending on cancer site)	Highest vs lowest (3)	0.4 (0.3–0.8)	$p < 0.01$	Age, area, education, smoking, vegetables	Hospital-based Data from a network of case–control studies Response rate > 97%
Talamini et al., 1992, Italy	271/685	FFQ (14), interviewed	Fresh fruit: Highest vs lowest (3)	1.41 (0.96–2.07)	$p = 0.06$	Age, area, education, BMI	Hospital-based Response rate > 96%
De Stefani et al., 1995, Uruguay	156/302	FFQ, interviewed	≥ 261 vs ≤ 96 times/y (3)	1.7 (1.1–2.8)	$p = 0.04$	Age, residence, education, tobacco, beer	Hospital-based Response rate for cases 98%, controls not given
Deneo-Pellegrini et al., 1999, Uruguay	175/233	FFQ (64, 9 fruits), interviewed, not validated but reproducible	≥ 736 vs ≤ 270 times/y (4)	0.8 (0.4–1.4)	$p = 0.08$	Age, residence, urban/rural, education, family history, BMI, energy	Hospital-based Response rate for cases 92%, controls 97%
Hayes et al., 1999, USA	932/1201	FFQ (60, 10 fruits), interviewed	Highest vs lowest (4)	1.1	$p = 0.48$	Age, study site, race	Population-based Response rate for cases 76%, controls 70%
Jain et al., 1999, Canada	617/636	Diet history (1129), validated	> 514.4 vs < 183.3 g/d (4)	1.51 (1.14–2.01)	$p = 0.01$	Energy, vasectomy, age, smoking, marital status, area, BMI, education, multi-vitamins, other foods and nutrients	Population-based Response rate for cases 81%, controls 63%
Sung et al., 1999, Taiwan	90/180	FFQ, interviewed	≥ 2 vs < 2/wk (2)	1.16 (0.57–2.35)		None	Hospital-based Response rate for cases 93%, controls 92%
Tzonou et al., 1999, Greece	320/246	FFQ (120, 19 fruits), interviewed, validated	Quintile increment (median = 222.5 vs 64.5 times/mo)	0.98 (0.86–1.13)		Age, height, BMI, education, energy, other foods	Hospital-based Response rate for cases 86%, controls 80%

Table 84 (contd)

Author, year, country	Cases/ controls	Exposure assessment (no. of items)	Range contrasts (no. of categories)	Relative risk (95% CI)	Stat. sign.*	Adjustment for confounding	Comments
Villeneuve et al., 1999, Canada	1623/1623	FFQ (60), modified from validated FFQ, self-administered	Fruit and fruit juices ≥ 28 vs < 7/wk (4)	1.5 (1.1–1.9)	p = 0.03	Age, province, race, smoking, BMI, other foods, family history	Population-based Response rate for cases 69%, controls 69%
Cohen et al., 2000, USA	628/602	FFQ (99, 12 fruits), self-administered	≥ 21 vs < 7 servings/wk (4)	1.07 (0.72–1.60)	p = 0.96	Fat, energy, race, age, family history, BMI, PSA in previous five years, education	Population-based Response rate for cases 82%, controls 75%
Kolonel et al., 2000, USA and Canada	1619/1618	Diet history (147, 17 fruits), interviewed	> 360.9 vs ≤ 75.3 g/d (5)	1.01 (0.79–1.28)	p = 0.48	Age, education, ethnicity, geographical area, energy	Population-based, multicentre, multi-ethnic Response rate for cases 70%, controls 58%

*p for trend when applicable

Table 85. Cohort studies of vegetable consumption and risk of prostate cancer

Author, year, country	Cases/ cohort size, (years follow-up)	Exposure assessment (no. of items)	Range contrasts (no. of categories)	Relative risk (95% CI)	Stat. sign.*	Adjustment for confounding	Comments
Hirayama, 1990, Japan	183/265 118 17 y	FFQ (7)	Green yellow veg.: Daily vs non-daily (2)	0.95 (90% CI, 0.73–1.25)		Not reported	Mortality Census-based cohort in four prefectures
Hsing et al., 1990, USA	149/17 633 20 y	FFQ (35, 10 veg.), self-administered	> 99.1 vs < 56.8 times/mo (4)	0.7 (0.4–1.2)		Age and tobacco	Mortality Policy-holders Include potatoes
Shibata et al., 1992, USA	208/11 580 (women included) 9 y	FFQ (59, 21 veg.), self-administered	≥ 4.5 vs < 3.0 servings/d (3)	1.04 (0.74–1.46)	NS	Age and smoking	Incidence Retirement community
Le Marchand et al., 1994	198/20 316 15 y	FFQ (13)	Raw veg.: > 302 vs < 82 g/wk (4)	1.1 (0.7–1.7)	p = 0.69	Age, ethnicity, income	Incidence Men of various ethnicities in Hawaii

Table 85 (contd)

Author, year, country	Cases/ cohort size, (years follow-up)	Exposure assessment (no. of items)	Range contrasts (no. of categories)	Relative risk (95% CI)	Stat. sign.*	Adjustment for confounding	Comments
Giovannucci et al., 1995, USA	773/47 894 7 y	FFQ (131, 46 fruits and veg.), self-administered, validated	> 5 vs < 2 servings/d	1.04 (0.81–1.34)	$p = 0.68$	Age and energy	Incidence Health professionals
Schuurman et al., 1998, Netherlands	642/58 279 6.3 y	FFQ (150, 17 veg.), self-administered, validated	285 vs 100 g/d (median values) (5)	0.80 (0.57–1.12)	$p = 0.51$	Age, family history, socio-economic status, fruit	Incidence Netherlands cohort study
Chan et al., 2000, Finland	184/27 062 8 y	FFQ (276), self-administered, validated	204 vs 40 g/d (median values) (5)	0.8 (0.5–1.3)	$p = 0.84$	Supplementation group, education, age, BMI, energy, smoking	Incidence Smokers, ATBC study
Key et al., 2003, European countries	1104/130 544 (mean, 4.8 y)	FFQ, self-administered or interviewed, validated	Highest vs lowest (5)	1.00 (0.81–1.22)	$p = 0.74$	Age, centre, height, weight, energy	Incidence

* p for trend when applicable

Table 86. Case–control studies of vegetable consumption and risk of prostate cancer

Author, year, country	Cases/ controls	Exposure assessment (no. of items)	Range contrasts (no. of categories)	Relative risk (95% CI)	Stat. sign.*	Adjustment for confounding	Comments
Mishina et al., 1985, Japan	100/100	Questionnaire, interviewed	Green yellow veg. > occasionally vs ≤ occasionally (2)	0.5	NS	Matched by age	Mostly screening based
Oishi et al., 1988, Japan	100/100	FFQ (31)	Highest vs lowest (3)	0.87 (0.43–1.76)		Matched by age	Hospital-based
Negri et al., 1991, Italy	107/2522	FFQ (14–37 depending on cancer site)	Green veg.: Highest vs lowest (3)	0.3 (0.1–0.5)	$p < 0.01$	Age, area, education, smoking, fruit	Hospital-based Data from network of case–control studies Response rate > 97%
Talamini et al., 1992, Italy	271/685	FFQ (14), interviewed	Highest vs lowest (3)	1.39 (0.88–2.17)	$p = 0.17$	Age, area, education, BMI	Hospital-based Response rate > 96%

Table 86 (contd)

Author, year, country	Cases/ controls	Exposure assessment (no. of items)	Range contrasts (no. of categories)	Relative risk (95% CI)	Stat. sign.*	Adjustment for confounding	Comments
De Stefani et al., 1995, Uruguay	156/302	FFQ, interviewed	≥ 131 vs ≤ 51 times/y (3)	1.1 (0.6–1.9)	p = 0.71	Age, residence, education, tobacco, beer	Hospital-based Response rat for cases 98%, controls not given
Key et al., 1997, UK	328/328	FFQ (83), interviewed, validated	Cooked veg.: > 1/d vs ≤ 4/wk (4)	0.71 (0.34–1.48)	p = 0.415	Matched by age. Adjusted for social class	Population-based Potatoes excluded Response rate for cases 77%, for controls 81%
Deneo-Pellegrini et al., 1999, Uruguay	175/233	FFQ (64, 12 veg.), inteviewed, not validated but reproducible	≥ 697 vs ≤ 336 times/y (4)	0.6 (0.3–1.1)	p = 0.02	Age, residence, urban/rural, education, family history, BMI, energy	Hospital-based Response rate for cases 92%, for controls 97%
Hayes et al., 1999, USA	932/1201	FFQ (60, 21 veg.), interviewed	Highest vs lowest (4)	1.0	p = 0.89	Age, study site, race	Population-based Includes potatoes Response rate for cases 76%, for controls 70%
Jain et al., 1999, Canada	617/636	Diet history (1129), validated	> 594.6 vs < 286.5 g/d (4)	0.95 (0.68–1.33)	NS	Energy, vasectomy, age, smoking, marital status, area, BMI, education, multivitamins, other foods and nutrients	Population-based Response rate for cases 81%, for controls 63%
Tzonou et al., 1999, Greece	320/246	FFQ (120, 26 veg.), interviewed, validated	Quintile increment (median = 121.3 vs 48 times/mo)	0.94 (0.81–1.10)		Age, height, BMI, education, energy, other foods	Hospital-based Potatoes excluded Response rate for cases 86%, for controls 80%
Villeneuve et al., 1999, Canada	1623/1623	FFQ (60), modified from validated FFQ, self-administered	≥ 28 vs < 14/wk (4)	1.0 (0.8–1.3)	p = 0.79	Age, province, race, smoking, BMI, other foods, family history	Population-based Response rate for cases 69%, for controls 69%
Cohen et al., 2000, USA	628/602	FFQ (99, 21 veg.), self-administered	≥ 28 vs < 14 servings/wk (4)	0.65 (0.45–0.94)	p = 0.01	Fat, energy, race, age, family history, BMI, PSA in previous 5 y, education	Population-based Response rate for cases 82%, for controls 75%
Kolonel et al., 2000, USA, Canada	1619/1618	Diet history, 37 veg.	> 324.8 vs ≤ 101.3 g/d (5)	0.74 (0.58–0.96)	p = 0.04	Age, education, ethnicity, geographic area, energy	Population-bases, multicentre, multi-ethnic Response rate for cases 70%, for controls 58%

*p for trend when applicable

Cancer-preventive effects

Table 87. Cohort studies of fruit and vegetable consumption and risk of prostate cancer

Author, year, country	Cases/ cohort size, (years follow-up)	Exposure assessment (no. of items)	Range contrasts (no. of categories)	Relative risk (95% CI)	Stat. sign.*	Adjustment for confounding	Comments
Shibata et al., 1992, USA	208/11 580 (including women) 9 y	FFQ (59, 23 fruits, 21 veg.), self-administered	≥ 7.9 vs < 5.5 servings/d (3)	1.10 (0.78–1.55)	NS	Age and smoking	Incidence Retirement community
Schuurman et al., 1998, Netherlands	642/ 58 279 6.3 y	FFQ (150, 8 fruits, 17 veg.), self-administered	519 vs 177.7 g/d (median values) (5)	1.05 (0.76–1.45)	p = 0.58	Age, family history, socio-economic status	Incidence Netherlands cohort study

* p for trend when applicable

Table 88. Case–control study of fruit and vegetable consumption and risk of prostate cancer

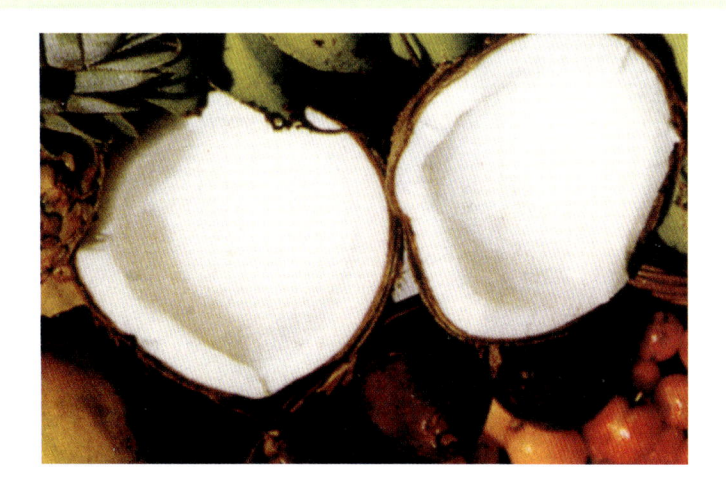

Author, year, country	Cases/ controls	Exposure assessment (no. of items)	Range contrasts (no. of categories)	Relative risk (95% CI)	Stat. sign.*	Adjustment for confounding	Comments
Deneo-Pellegrini et al., 1999, Uruguay	175/233	FFQ (64, 9 fruits, 12 veg.), interviewed, not validated, but reproducible	> 1390 vs < 685 times/y (4)	0.5 (0.3–0.9)	p = 0.04	Age, residence, urban/rural, education, family history, BMI, energy	Hospital-based

* p for trend when applicable

229

IARC Handbooks of Cancer Prevention Volume 8: Fruit and Vegetables

Table 89. Case-control studies of fruit and/or vegetable consumption and risk of testicular cancer

Author, year, country	Cases/ controls	Exposure assessment (no. of items)	Range contrasts (no. of categories)	Relative risk (95% CI)	Stat. sign.*	Adjustment for confounding	Comments
Sigurdson et al., 1999, USA	160 (82 non-seminomas, 46 seminomas, 32 mixed germ-cell)/136	FFQ (152), self-administered, validated	Fruit: > 147.2 vs < 29.7 g/1000 kcal (4) Non-seminoma Seminoma Mixed germ-cell Veg.: > 58.9 vs < 18.6 g/1000 kcal (4) Non-seminoma Seminoma Mixed germ-cell	 [0.9(0.3–2.5)] [0.4(0.1–1.4)] [0.3(0.1–1.3)] [0.8(0.3–2.5)] [1.7(0.5–5.0)] [1.4(0.4–5.0)]	 $p = 0.99$ $p = 0.29$ $p = 0.09$ $p = 0.81$ $p = 0.25$ $p = 0.48$	Age, education, income, ethnicity, cryptorchidism, energy	Hospital-based, friend-matched controls Response rates for cases 38%, for controls 73%
Swerdlow et al., 1999, UK	60 twin pairs	FFQ, self-administered	OR for having consumed more during childhood	Fruit: 1.0 (0.3–3.1) Veg.: 0.3 (0.1–1.0)			Study in twins

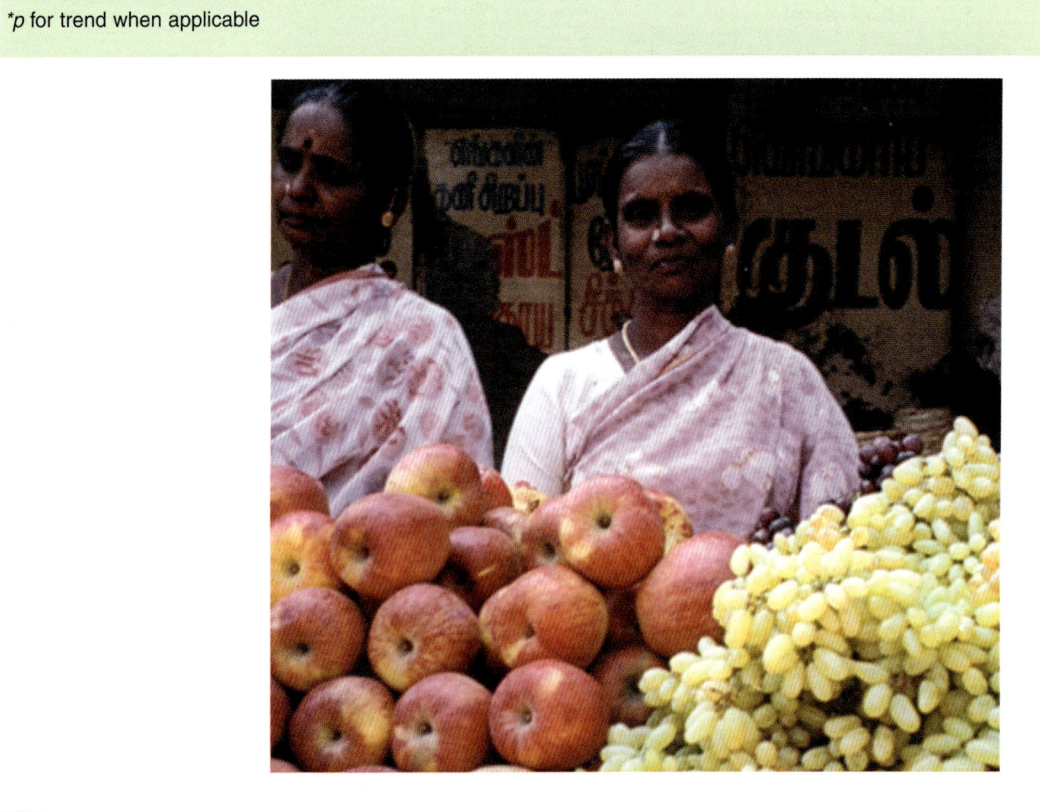

*p for trend when applicable

230

Table 90. Cohort studies of fruit consumption and risk of bladder cancer

Author, year, country	Cases/cohort size, gender (years follow-up)	Exposure assessment (no. of items)	Range contrasts (no. of categories)	Relative risk (95% CI)	Stat. sign.*	Adjustment for confounding	Comments
Chyou et al., 1993, USA	96/6790, M 22 y	FFQ (17) + 24-h dietary recall	≥ 5 vs ≤ 1/wk (3)	0.63 (0.37–1.08)	$p = 0.038$	Age, smoking	Incidence Japanese resident in Hawaii
Michaud et al., 1999, USA	252/47 909, M 10 y	FFQ (131), validated	> 3.5 vs ≤ 1 servings/d (5)	1.12 (0.70–1.78)	$p = 0.68$	Age, geographical region, smoking, fluid intake, energy	Incidence Health professionals study
Nagano et al., 2000, Japan	106/38 540, M, F 14 y	FFQ (22) self-administered	≥ 5 vs 0–1 times/wk (3)	0.75 (0.46–1.22)	$p = 0.29$	Age, gender, education, calendar time, radiation dose, smoking, BMI, green veg.	Incidence Atomic bombing survivors
Zeegers et al., 2001, Netherlands	569/120 852, M, F 6.3 y	FFQ (150, 9 fruits), self-administered	≥ 256 vs < 83 g/d (5)	0.74 (0.53–1.04)	$p = 0.02$	Sex, age, smoking, veg.	Incidence Netherlands cohort study
Michaud et al., 2002, Finland	344/27 111, M, smokers 13 y	FFQ (276, 45 fruits or veg.)	245.4 vs 25 g/d (median values) (5)	1.10 (0.77–1.57)	$p = 0.98$	Age, duration of smoking, smoking dose, energy, trial intervention	Incidence Follow-up of ATBC trial

Table 91. Case–control studies of fruit consumption and risk of bladder cancer

Author, year, country	Cases/controls, gender	Exposure assessment (no. of items)	Range contrasts (no. of categories)	Relative risk (95% CI)	Stat. sign.*	Adjustment for confounding	Comments
Riboli et al., 1991, Spain	432/789, M, F	Dietary history, interviewed	Highest vs lowest (4)	0.95 (0.67–1.35)	$p = 0.62$	Age, tobacco, gender, energy	Hospital-based and population-based Multicentre study
Bruemmer et al., 1996, USA	240/395, M, F	FFQ (71), self-administered	> 2.7 vs ≤ 0.9 times/d (4)	0.53 (0.30–0.93)	$p = 0.01$	Age, gender, county, smoking, energy	Population-based
Wakai et al., 2000, Japan	297/295, M, F	FFQ (97), interviewed	Highest vs lowest (4)	All: 0.65 (0.40–1.06) M: 0.52 (0.30–0.90)	$p = 0.09$ $p = 0.03$	Age, gender, hospital, smoking, occupation	Hospital-based
Balbi et al., 2001, Uruguay	144/576, M, F	FFQ (64, 8 fruits)	Highest vs lowest (3)	0.65 (0.40–1.04)	$p = 0.06$	Age, gender, urban/rural status, residence, education, BMI, smoking, energy, mate drinking	Hospital-based

*p for trend when applicable

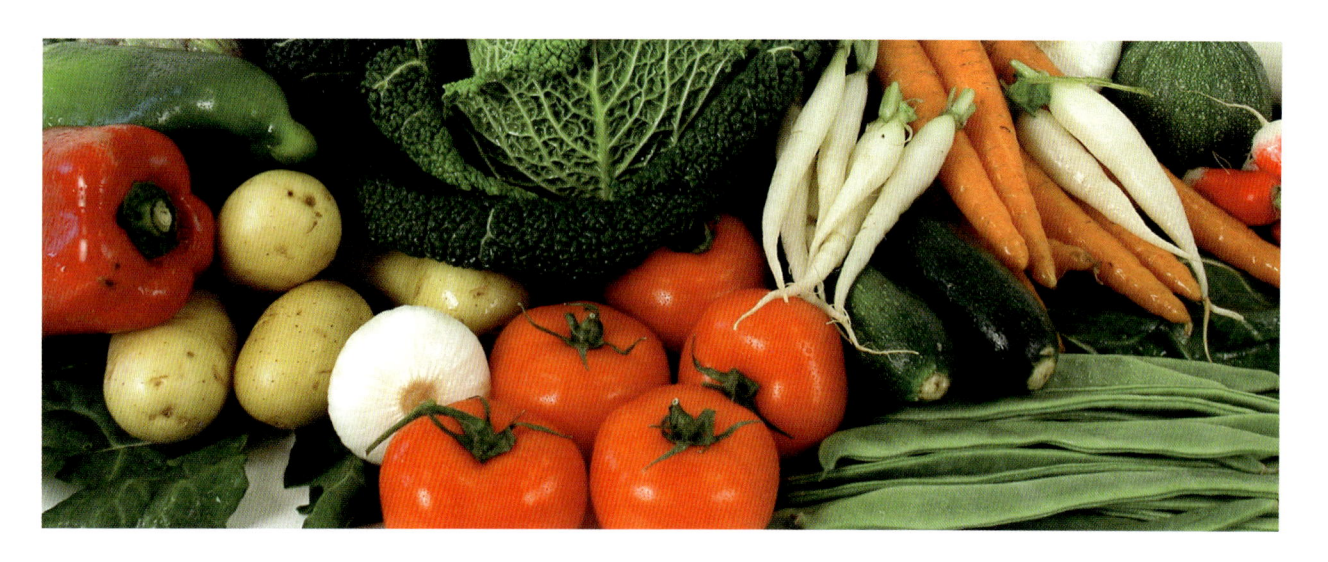

Table 92. Cohort studies of vegetable consumption and risk of bladder cancer

Author, year, country	Cases/cohort size, gender (years follow-up)	Exposure assessment (no. of items)	Range contrasts (no. of categories)	Relative risk (95% CI)	Stat. sign.*	Adjustment for confounding	Comments
Michaud et al., 1999, USA	252/47 909, M, 10 y	FFQ (131), validated	≥ 5 vs < 2 servings/d (5)	0.72 (0.47–1.09)	p = 0.09	Age, geographical region, smoking, fluid intake, energy	Incidence Health professionals study Statistically significant association for cruciferous veg.
Nagano et al., 2000, Japan	95/38 540, M, F, 14 y	FFQ (22), self-administered	Green-yellow veg.: ≥ 5 vs 0–1 times/wk (3)	0.60 (0.33–1.07)	p = 0.07	Age, gender, education, calendar time, radiation dose, smoking, BMI, fruit	Incidence Atomic bombing survivors
Zeegers et al., 2001, Netherlands	538/120 852, M, F, 6.3 y	FFQ (150, 21 veg.), self-administered	≥ 242 vs < 126 g/d (5)	0.91 (0.65–1.27)	p = 0.38	Sex, age, smoking, fruit	Incidence Netherlands cohort study
Michaud et al., 2002, Finland	344/27 111, M, smokers, 13 y	FFQ (276, 45 fruits or veg.)	205.3 vs 39.5 g/day (median values) (5)	1.16 (0.82–1.63)	p = 0.14	Age, duration of smoking, smoking dose, energy, trial intervention	Incidence Follow-up of ATBC trial

*p for trend when applicable

Table 93. Case–control studies of vegetable consumption and risk of bladder cancer

Author, year, country	Cases/ controls, gender	Exposure assessment (no. of items)	Range contrasts (no. of categories)	Relative risk (95% CI)	Stat. sign.*	Adjustment for confounding	Comments
Riboli et al., 1991, Spain	432/789, M, F	Dietary history, interviewed	Highest vs lowest (4)	1.04 (0.73–1.48)	$p = 0.45$	Age, gender, tobacco, energy	Hospital-based and population-based Multicentre study
Bruemmer et al., 1996, USA	240/395, M, F	FFQ (71), self-administered	> 3.6 times/d vs ≤ 1.3 times/d (4)	0.87 (0.52–1.45)	$p = 0.65$	Age, gender, county, smoking, energy	Population-based
Wakai et al., 2000, Japan	297/295, M, F	FFQ (97), interviewed	Green-yellow veg.: Highest vs lowest (4) Other veg.: Highest vs lowest (4)	0.73 (0.45–1.20) 1.04 (0.62–1.73)	$p = 0.20$ $p = 0.73$	Age, gender, hospital, smoking, occupation	Hospital-based
Balbi et al., 2001, Uruguay	144/576, M, F	FFQ (64, 11 veg.)	Highest vs lowest (3)	0.66 (0.40–1.09)	$p = 0.12$	Age, gender, residence, urban/rural status, education, BMI, smoking, energy, mate drinking	Hospital-based

*p for trend when applicable

Table 94. Cohort studies of total fruit and vegetable consumption and risk of bladder cancer

Author, year, country	Cases/cohort size, gender (years follow-up)	Exposure assessment (no. of items)	Range contrasts (no. of categories)	Relative risk (95% CI)	Stat. sign.*	Adjustment for confounding	Comments
Steineck et al., 1988, Sweden	70/16 477 14 y	FFQ (8), self-administered	"Exposed to fruit and veg."	1.0 (0.6–1.6)		Age, sex, smoking	Incidence Twin study
Zeegers et al., 2001, Netherlands	538/120 852, M, F 6.3 y	FFQ (150, 9 fruits, 21 veg.), self-administered	≥ 471 vs <241 g/d (5)	0.98 (0.60–1.61)	$p = 0.39$	Age, sex, smoking	Incidence Netherlands cohort study

* p for trend when applicable

Table 95. Case–control studies of total fruit and vegetable consumption and risk of bladder cancer

Author, year, country	Cases/ controls, gender	Exposure assessment (no. of items)	Range contrasts (no. of categories)	Relative risk (95% CI)	Stat. sign.*	Adjustment for confounding	Comments
Claude et al., 1986, Germany	531/531, M, F	FFQ, interviewed	Eaten regularly	M: 0.59 (0.37–0.95) F: 0.90 (0.37–2.21)		Age, smoking	Hospital-based
De Stefani et al., 1991, Uruguay	111/222, M, F	FFQ, interviewed		"Moderately elevated OR for infrequent consumers of green and yellow veg. and raw fruits"		Age, gender, residence, social class	Hospital-based
Balbi et al., 2001, Uruguay	144/576 M, F	FFQ (64, 8 fruits, 11 veg.)	Highest vs lowest (3)	0.67 (0.41–1.09)	$p = 0.11$	Age, gender, urban/rural status, residence, education, BMI, smoking, energy, mate drinking	Hospital-based

*p for trend when applicable

Table 96. Cohort studies of total fruit consumption and risk of renal-cell cancer

Author, year, country	Cases/cohort size, gender (years follow-up)	Exposure assessment (no. of items)	Range contrasts (no. of categories)	Relative risk (95% CI)	Stat. sign.*	Adjustment for confounding	Comments
Fraser et al., 1990, USA	14/34 198, M, F 6 y	FFQ (51)	> 3 vs < 3/wk (2)	0.21 (0.05–1.45)	$p = 0.097$	Age, sex	Incidence Seventh-Day Adventists (58% lactoovo vegetarians), 3.7% current smokers
Prineas et al., 1997, USA	62/35 192, F 8 y	FFQ (127)	> 15 vs < 9 servings/wk (3)	1.00 (0.55–1.80)		Age	Incidence Postmenopausal women

*p for trend when applicable

Table 97. Case–control studies of fruit consumption and risk of renal-cell cancer

Author, year, country	Cases/ controls, gender	Exposure assessment (no. of items)	Range contrasts (no. of categories)	Relative risk (95% CI)	Stat. sign.*	Adjustment for confounding	Comments
Talamini et al., 1990, Italy	240/665, M, F	FFQ (14), interviewed	≥ 14 servings/wk vs lowest (3)	0.92 (0.63–1.35)		Age, sex, education, area of residence, BMI	Hospital-based Response rate for cases 97%, for controls 96%
Negri et al., 1991, Italy	147/6147, M, F	FFQ (24–37, depending on cancer site)	Highest vs lowest (3)	0.6 (0.4–1.0)	$p < 0.05$	Age, area of residence, education, smoking, veg. consumption	Hospital-based, data from a network of case–control studies Response rate 97%
McLaughlin et al., 1992, China	154 (90 M, 64 F)/157	Structured questionnaire, interviewed	Highest vs lowest (4)	M: 0.2 (0.0–0.5) F: 0.7 (0.2–2.0)	$p < 0.001$ $p = 0.07$	Age, education, smoking, BMI	Population-based Response rate for cases 87%, for controls 100%
Chow et al., 1994, USA**	415/650, M, F	FFQ (65, 8 fruits), self-administered	Highest vs lowest (4)	1.2 (0.8–1.7)		Age, sex, smoking, BMI	Population-based Next-of-kin interviews for 117 cases Response rate 79%
Mellemgaard et al., 1996, Denmark**	351 (216 M, 135 F)/340	FFQ (92), interviewed, validated	> 3 vs ≤ 1 times/wk (4)	M: 0.6 (0.3–1.4) F: 0.9 (0.4–2.3)	$p = 0.34$ $p = 0.73$	Age, smoking, BMI, socio-economic status	Population-based Response rate for cases 73%, for controls 68%
Boeing et al., 1997, Germany	155/212, M, F	FFQ (122), self-administered	Highest vs lowest (3)	0.40 (0.23–0.69)	$p = 0.001$	Age, sex, education, smoking, alcohol	Population-based Response rate for cases 47%, for controls 56%
Lindblad et al., 1997, Sweden**	378/350, M, F	FFQ (63, 8 fruits), interviewed	≥ 1907 vs ≤ 576 g/wk (4)	0.65 (0.42–1.02) Non-smokers: 0.37 (0.19–0.72) Smokers: 1.08 (0.58–2.02)	$p = 0.05$ $p = 0.003$ $p = 0.94$	Age, sex, BMI, smoking, education	Population-based Response rate for cases 70%, for controls 72%
Wolk et al., 1996, Australia, Denmark, USA, Sweden	1185/1526, M, F	FFQ (63–205, depending on study centre), interviewed or self-administered	Highest vs lowest (4)	0.85 (0.66–1.10) Non-smokers: 0.6 (0.4–0.9)		Age, sex, study centre, BMI, smoking, energy	Population-based. Multicentre analysis Response rate for cases 54–72%, for controls 53–78%

*p for trend when applicable
**Substudy in the multicentre analyses (Wolk et al., 1996)

Table 98. Cohort study of vegetable consumption and risk of renal-cell cancer

Author, year, country	Cases/cohort size, gender (years follow-up)	Exposure assessment (no. of items)	Range contrasts (no. of categories)	Relative risk (95% CI)	Stat. sign.	Adjustment for confounding	Comments
Prineas et al., 1997, USA	62/35 192, F 8 y	FFQ (127)	> 27 vs < 17 servings/wk (3)	1.44 (0.80–2.59)		Age	Incidence Postmenopausal women

Table 99. Case–control studies of vegetable consumption and risk of renal-cell cancer

Author, year, country	Cases/ controls, gender	Exposure assessment (no. of items)	Range contrasts (no. of categories)	Relative risk (95% CI)	Stat. sign.*	Adjustment for confounding	Comments
McLaughlin et al., 1992, China	154/157, M, F	Structured questionnaire, interviewed	Highest vs. lowest (4)	M 0.3 (0.1–0.7) F 1.6 (0.6–4.6)	$p = 0.01$ $p = 0.33$	Age, education, smoking, BMI	Population-based Response rate for cases 87%, for controls 100%
Chow et al., 1994, USA**	415/650, M, F	FFQ (65, 9 veg.), self-administered	M: ≥ 12.4 vs ≤ 5.1 servings/wk (4) F: ≥ 14.1 vs. ≤7.3 servings/wk (4)	1.0 (0.7–1.5)		Age, sex, smoking, BMI	Population-based Response rate 79%
Boeing et al., 1997, Germany	155/212	FFQ (122), self-administered	Highest vs. lowest (3)	0.75 (0.44–1.27) $p = 0.285$		Age, sex, education, smoking, alcohol	Population-based Response rate for cases 47%, for controls 56%
Lindblad et al.,1997, Sweden**	378/350	FFQ (63, 13 veg.), interviewed	≥ 816 vs < 290 g/wk (4)	0.84 (0.53–1.31) $p = 0.74$ Non-smokers: 0.60 (0.30–1.16) $p = 0.35$ Smokers: 1.04 (0.56–1.94) $p = 0.72$		Age, sex, BMI, smoking, education	Population-based Response rate for cases 70%, for controls 72%
Yuan et al., 1998, USA	1204/1204 M, F	FFQ (40), interviewed	Dark-green veg.: ≥ 13.1 vs ≤ 2.0 times/mo (5) Yellow-orange veg.: ≥ 17.1 vs ≤ 4.3 times/mo (5)	0.51 (0.38–0.69) $p < 0.001$ 0.64 (0.48–0.86) $p < 0.001$		Age, sex, education, BMI, hypertension, smoking, analgesics, amphetamines	Population-based, neighbourhood controls
Wolk et al., 1996, Australia, Denmark, USA, Sweden	1185/1526, M, F	FFQ (63–205, depending on study centre), interviewed or self-administered	Highest vs lowest (4)	0.81 (0.61–1.08)		Age, sex, study centre, BMI, smoking, energy	Population-based Multicentre analysis Response rate for cases 54–72%, for controls 53–78%

* p for trend when applicable. **Substudy in the multicentre analyses (Wolk et al., 1996)

Cancer-preventive effects

Table 100. Cohort study of fruit and vegetable consumption and risk of renal-cell cancer

Author, year, country	Cases/ cohort size, gender (years follow-up)	Exposure assessment (no. of items)	Range contrasts (no. of categories)	Relative risk (95% CI)	Stat. sign.	Adjustment for confounding	Comments
Prineas et al., 1997, USA	62/35 102. F 8 y	FFQ (127)	> 42 vs < 28 servings/wk (3)	1.56 (0.83–2.92)		Age	Incidence Postmenopausal women

Table 101. Case-control studies of fruit and vegetable consumption and risk of renal cell cancer

Author, year, country	Cases/ controls, gender	Exposure assessment (no. of items)	Range contrasts (no. of categories)	Relative risk (95% CI)	Stat. sign.*	Adjustment for confounding	Comments
McLaughlin et al., 1984, USA	M 313/428 F 182/269	FFQ (28), interviewed	Highest vs lowest (4)	M: 1.5 F: 0.7	NS NS	Age, cigarette smoking, relative weight	Population-based Response rate 98%
Yu et al., 1986, USA	160/160 M, F	FFQ, interviewed		No difference in consumption of fresh fruit and veg. between cases and controls		Matched by age	Population-based, neighbourhood controls Response rate for cases 73%

* p for trend when applicable

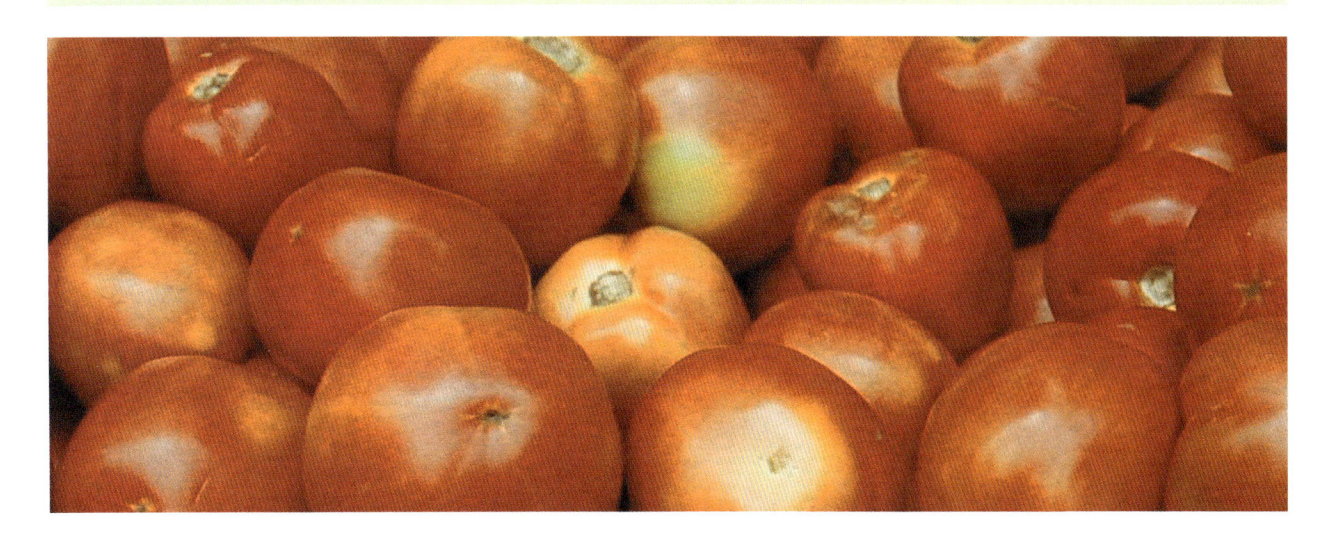

Table 102. Case–control studies of fruit consumption and risk of adult brain cancer

Author, year, country	Cases/ controls, gender	Exposure assessment (no. of items)	Range contrasts (no. of categories)	Relative risk (95% CI)	Stat. sign.*	Adjustment for confounding	Comments
Hu et al., 1998, China	218 (glioma)/ 436, M, F	FFQ (15 fruit and veg.), interviewed	≥ 46 vs ≤ 19 kg/y (4)	0.28 (0.16–0.51)	p = 0.0005	Income, education, alcohol, selected occupational exposures, veg.	Hospital-based
Hu et al., 1999, China	129 (73 glioma, 56 meningioma)/258, M, F	FFQ (57, 5 fruits), interviewed	Highest vs lowest (4)	0.15 (0.1–0.4)	p < 0.01	Income, education, cigarette smoking, alcohol, selected occupational exposures, energy	Hospital-based Continuation of study of Hu et al., 1998 with more comprehensive questionnaire

* p for trend when applicable

Table 103. Case–control studies of vegetable consumption and risk of adult brain cancer

Author, year, country	Cases/ controls, gender	Exposure assessment (no. of items)	Range contrasts (no. of categories)	Relative risk (95% CI)	Stat. sign.*	Adjustment for confounding	Comments
Hu et al., 1998, China	218 (glioma)/ 436, M, F	FFQ (15 fruit and veg.), interviewed	≥ 125 vs ≤ 84 kg/y (4)	0.51 (0.29–0.89)	p = 0.009	Income, education, alcohol, selected occupational exposures, fruit	Hospital-based
Hu et al., 1999, China	129 (73 glioma, 56 meningioma)/ 258, M, F	FFQ (57, 17 veg.), interviewed	Fresh veg.: Highest vs lowest (4)	0.29 (0.1–0.7)	p < 0.01	Income, education, cigarette smoking, alcohol, selected occupational exposures, energy	Hospital-based Continuation of study of Hu et al. (1998) with more comprehensive questionnaire
Chen et al., 2002b, USA	236 (glioma)/ 449, M, F	FFQ (48), interviewed by telephone	Highest vs lowest (4)	0.5 (0.3–1.0)	p = 0.06	Age, gender, energy, respondent type, education level, family history, farming experience	Population-based Response rate for cases 90%, for controls 71%, reinterviewed following a previous study

*p for trend when applicable

Table 104. Case–control studies of fruit consumption and risk of childhood brain cancer

Author, year, country	Cases/ controls, gender	Exposure assessment (no. of items)	Range contrasts (no. of categories)	Relative risk (95% CI)	Stat. sign.*	Adjustment for confounding	Comments
Bunin et al., 1993, USA	166/166	FFQ, interviews of mothers regarding their diet during pregnancy	Fruit and fruit juices: Highest vs lowest (4)	0.28 (0.14–0.59)	$p = 0.003$	Sex, birth order, birth weight, duration of breast feeding for child, age, history of miscarriage, month of first prenatal visit, educational level, income level for mother, use during pregnancy of cigarettes, bottled water, electric blanket, duration of nausea, child's diet in first year of life	Population-based Study of primitive neuroectodermal tumours (mostly medulloblastomas) 74% first eligible control contacted
Cordier et al., 1994, France	75/113, M, F	Interview on maternal diet during pregnancy	Fresh fruit: Highest vs lowest (4)	0.6 (0.1–3.0)		Child's age and sex, maternal age, number of years of schooling of the mother	Population-based Response rate for identified cases 69%, for eligible controls contacted 71.5%
McCredie et al., 1994a, Australia	82/164, M, F	FFQ based on maternal diet during pregnancy, interviewed	> 952.3 vs < 299.7 items/y (4)	1.5 (0.6–3.7)	$p = 0.39$	Age, sex, mother's education, mother's BMI before pregnancy, vegetables, cured meats	Population-based Response rate for eligible cases 85%, for controls 60%
McCredie et al., 1994b, Australia	82/164, M, F	FFQ based on child's diet in the perinatal and early postnatal period, interviewed	Blended or solid fruit: > 240 vs < 154.8 times/first year (4)	0.4 (0.1–1.1)		Age, sex, mother's education, ever/never use of a dummy, other food groups	Population-based Response rate for eligible cases 85%, for controls 60%
Lubin et al., 2000, Israel	300/574, under age 10 y, M, F	FFQ (100), interviewed	Highest vs lowest (3)	During gestation: 1.24 (0.7–1.8) As a child: 1.24 (0.8–2.1)	$p = 0.50$ $p = 0.39$	Energy	Population-based

*p for trend when applicable

Table 105. Case–control studies of vegetable consumption and risk of childhood brain cancer

Author, year, country	Cases/ controls gender	Exposure assessment (no. of items)	Range contrasts (no. of categories)	Relative risk (95% CI)	Stat. sign.*	Adjustment for confounding	Comments
Bunin et al., 1993, USA	166/166	FFQ, interviews of mothers regarding their diet during pregnancy	Highest vs lowest (4)	0.37 (0.19–0.72)	p = 0.005	Sex, birth order, birth weight, duration of breast feeding for child, age, history of miscarriage, month of first prenatal visit, educational level, income level for mother, use during pregnancy of cigarettes, bottled water, electric blanket, duration of nausea, child's diet in first year of life	Population-based Study of primitive neuroectodermal tumours (mostly medulloblastomas) 74% first eligible control contacted
McCredie et al., 1994a, Australia	82/164, M, F	FFQ based on maternal diet during pregnancy, interviewed	> 1109.9 vs < 597.6 items/y (4)	0.4 (0.1–1.0)	p = 0.06	Age, sex, mother's education, mother's BMI before pregnancy, fruit, cured meats	Population-based Response rate for eligible cases 85%, for controls 60%
Lubin et al., 2000, Israel	300/574, under age 10, M, F	FFQ (100), interviewed	Highest vs lowest (3)	During gestation: 1.25 (0.8–1.9) As a child: 1.30 (0.8–2.3)	p = 0.35 p = 0.24	Energy	Population-based

* p for trend when applicable

Table 106. Case–control studies of fruit consumption and risk of thyroid cancer

Author, year, country	Cases/ controls, gender	Exposure assessment (no. of items)	Range contrasts (no. of categories)	Relative risk (95% CI)	Stat. sign.*	Adjustment for confounding	Comments
Franceschi et al., 1991b, Italy and Switzerland	385/798, M, F	FFQ (30–38)	Fresh fruit: Highest vs lowest (3)	0.9	NS	Centre, age, sex, education	Hospital-based Pool of three studies from northern Italy, and one from Swiss Canton Vaud Response rates in cases and controls > 95%
Galanti et al., 1997, Sweden and Norway	246/440, M, F	FFQ (56), self-administered	> 42 vs < 19 pieces/mo (3)	1.0 (0.6–1.5)	NS	Univariate analysis	Population-based Response rates for cases/controls: Norway, 75%/56%; Sweden, 86%/69%

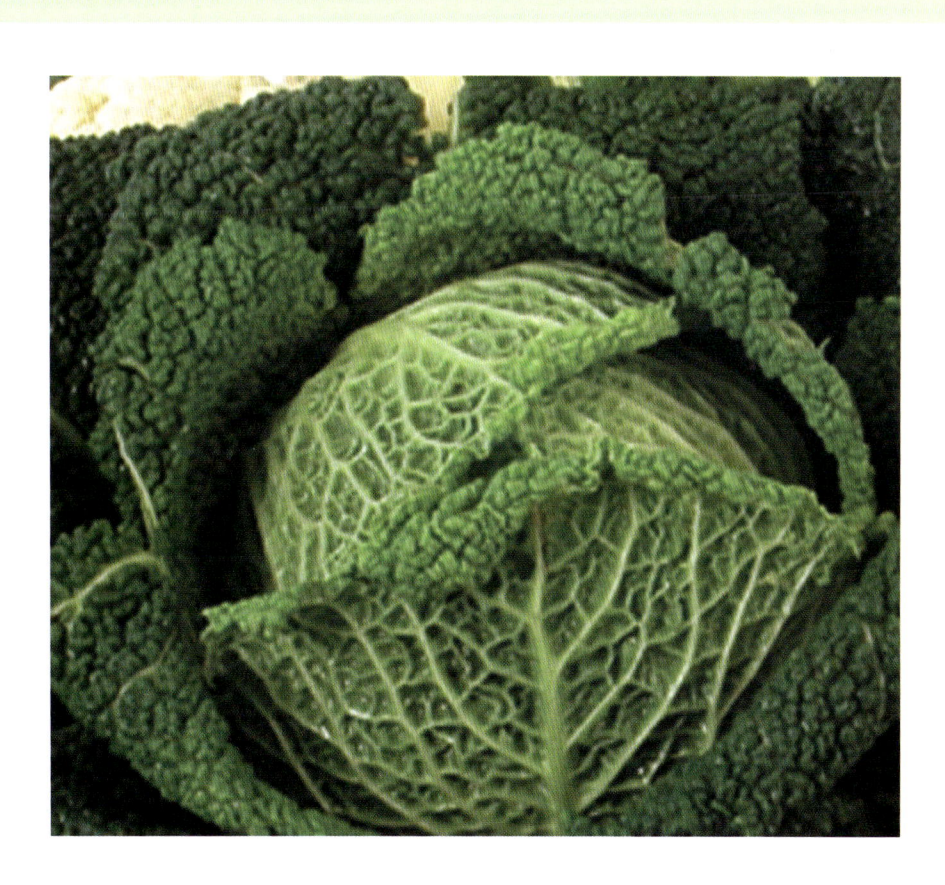

*p for trend when applicable

Table 107. Case–control studies of vegetable consumption and risk of thyroid cancer

Author, year, country	Cases/ controls, gender	Exposure assessment (no. of items)	Range contrasts (no. of categories)	Relative risk (95% CI)	Stat. sign.*	Adjustment for confounding	Comments
Franceschi et al., 1991b, Italy and Switzerland	385/798, M, F	FFQ (30–38)	Green veg.: Highest vs lowest (3)	0.9	NS	Centre, age, sex, education	Hospital-based Pool of three studies from northern Italy and one from Swiss Canton Vaud Response rates in cases and controls > 95%
Hallquist et al., 1994, Sweden	171/325, M, F	FFQ, self-administered	Green veg.: Several vs some times/week (3)	Age ≤ 20 y: 0.8 (0.5–1.4) Age > 20 y: 0.7 (0.3–1.6)		Age, gender	Population-based Response for cases 95%, for controls 90%
Galanti et al., 1997, Norway and Sweden	246/440, M, F	FFQ (56), self-administered	> 60 vs ≤ 40 portions/mo (3)	0.9 (0.6–1.4)	NS	Univariate analysis	Population-based Response rates in cases/controls: Norway, 75%/56%; Sweden, 86%/69%
Bosetti et al., 2002b	2241/3716, M, F	Different information in each study	Other than cruciferous veg.: Highest vs lowest (3)	0.82 (0.69–0.98)		Age, sex, prior radiotherapy, thyroid nodules, goitre	Collaborative re-analysis of 11 case–control studies from USA (3), Asia (1), and Europe (7) Weighted mean of OR from each study Test for heterogeneity between studies: $p < 0.02$ for both

* p for trend when applicable

Table 108. Cohort studies of fruit consumption and risk of non-Hodgkin lymphoma

Author, year, country	Cases/ cohort size, gender (years follow-up)	Exposure assessment (no. of items)	Range contrasts (no. of categories)	Relative risk (95% CI)	Stat. sign.*	Adjustment for confounding	Comments
Chiu et al., 1996, USA	104/35 156, F 7 y	Semi-quantitative FFQ (126)	> 84 vs < 54 servings/mo (3)	0.67 (0.41–1.08)	p = 0.09	Age, energy	Incidence Iowa Women's Health Study
Zhang et al., 2000, USA	199/88 410, F 14 y	Semi-quantitative FFQ (61)	≥ 3 vs < 1 servings/d (4)	0.79 (0.49–1.27)	p = 0.39	Age, energy, length of follow-up, geographical region, cigarette smoking, height, beef, pork or lamb as a main dish	Incidence Nurses' Health Study

* p for trend when applicable

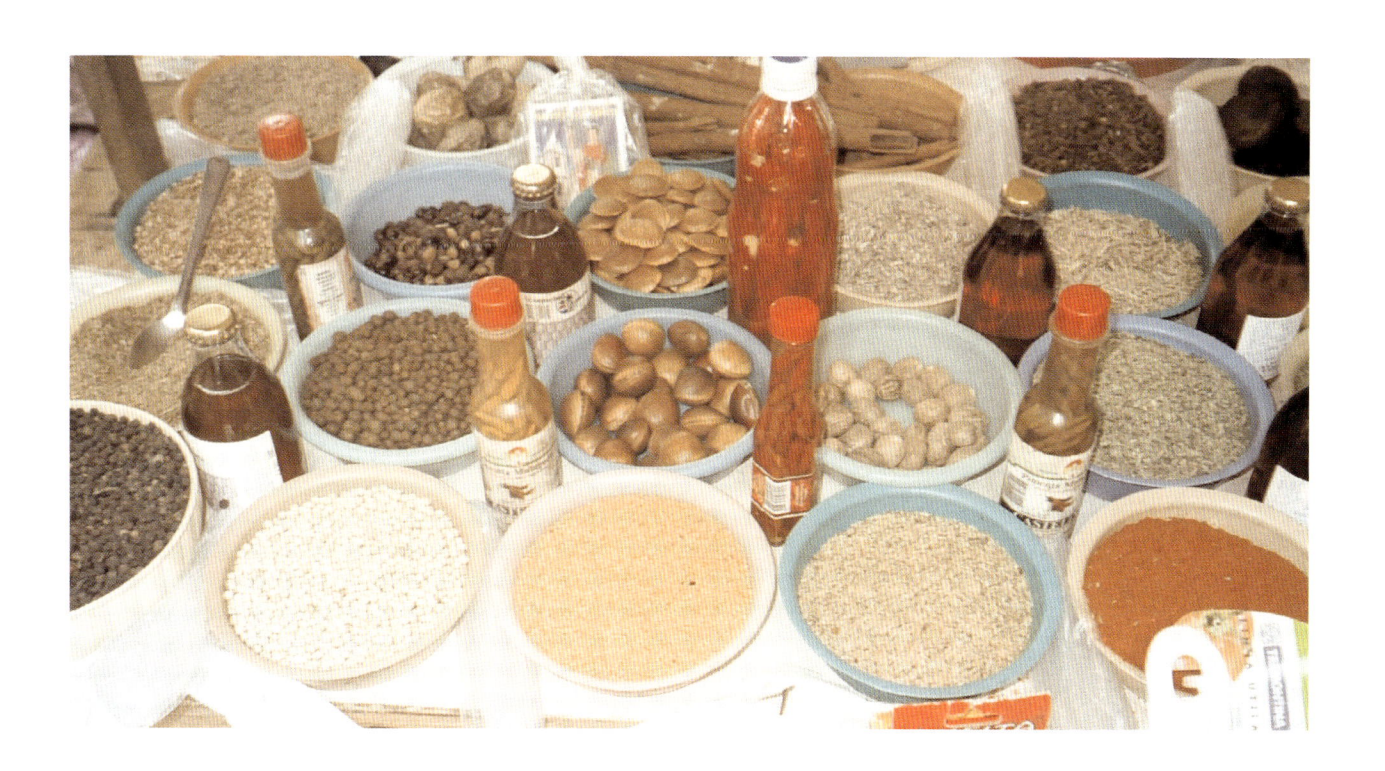

Table 109. Case–control studies of fruit consumption and risk of non-Hodgkin lymphoma

Author, year, country	Cases/controls, gender	Exposure assessment (no. of items)	Range contrasts (no. of categories)	Relative risk (95% CI)	Stat. sign.	Adjustment for confounding	Comments
Tavani et al., 1997, Italy	429/1157 M, F	FFQ (14)	Highest vs lowest (3)	0.9	NS	Centre, age, sex	Hospital-based Response rates ~97%

Table 110. Cohort studies of vegetable consumption and risk of non-Hodgkin lymphoma

Author, year, country	Cases/cohort size, gender (years follow-up)	Exposure assessment (no. of items)	Range contrasts (no. of categories)	Relative risk (95% CI)	Stat. sign.*	Adjustment for confounding	Comments
Hirayama, 1990, Japan	219 lymphosarcoma, 29 other lymphoma/265 118, M, F 17 y	FFQ (7)	Green-yellow veg.: Daily vs non-daily (2)	1.15 (90% CI, 0.95–1.40)		Not reported	Mortality Census-based cohort in seven prefectures
Chiu et al., 1996, USA	104/35 156, F 7 y	Semi-quantitative FFQ (126)	> 98 vs < 62 servings/mo (3)	0.96 (0.58–1.60)	$p = 0.88$	Age, energy	Incidence Iowa Women's Health Study
Zhang et al., 2000, USA	199/88 410, F 14 y	Semi-quantitative FFQ (61)	≥ 3 vs < 1 servings/d (4)	0.65 (0.37–1.13)	$p = 0.04$	Age, energy, length of follow-up, geographical region, cigarette smoking, height, beef, pork or lamb as a main dish	Incidence Nurses' Health Study

* p for trend when applicable

Table 111. Case–control study of vegetable consumption and risk of non-Hodgkin lymphoma

Author, year, country	Cases/controls, gender	Exposure assessment (no. of items)	Range contrasts (no. of categories)	Relative risk (95% CI)	Stat. sign.*	Adjustment for confounding	Comments
Ward et al., 1994, USA	315 (171 M, 144 F)/1075	FFQ (30), interviewed by telephone	> 27 vs < 16 times/wk (4)	M: 1.0 (0.6–1.6) F: 0.9 (0.5–1.7)	NS NS	Age	Population-based Response rate for cases 90%, for controls 84%

* p for trend when applicable

Table 112. Cohort study of vegetable consumption and risk of leukaemia

Author, year, country	Cases/ cohort size, gender (years follow-up)	Exposure assessment (no. of items)	Range contrasts (no. of categories)	Relative risk (95% CI)	Stat. sign.	Adjustment for confounding	Comments
Hirayama, 1990, Japan	206/265 118, M, F 17 y	FFQ (7)	Green-yellow veg.: Daily vs non-daily (2)	0.92 (90% CI, 0.71–1.18)		Not reported	Mortality Census-based cohort in seven prefectures

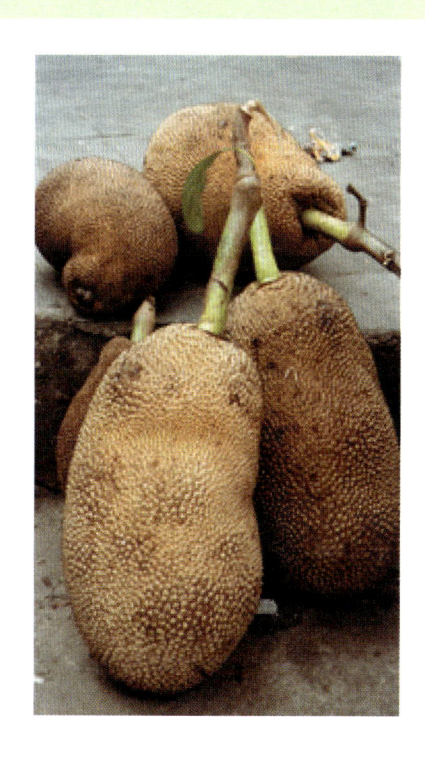

Preventable fraction

The proportion of any disease potentially preventable by modification of a risk factor in a population is determined by both the strength of the risk factor, as represented by the relative risk, and the prevalence of the risk factor. This proportion is commonly known as the "preventable fraction" (also sometimes called the "population attributable risk") (WHO, 2002). The certainty in any estimate of preventable fraction, including that for the fraction of cancers that is due to low intake of fruit and vegetables, is dependent on the precision of both the relative risk associated with low intake and the proportion of the population consuming low levels. The review presented earlier in this chapter makes it clear that many of the relative risk estimates are uncertain and that the prevalence of exposure to low intake varies widely across studies and cancer sites. Therefore, confidence in an estimate of any particular cancer's preventable fraction for low fruit and vegetable intake must be low.

Nevertheless, the Working Group calculated the preventable fractions for cancer sites for which it judged there was at least limited support for a causal association, in order to estimate the approximate extent of the potential prevention that could be linked to increasing fruit and vegetable intake. Although the relative risks and prevalences of low intake vary widely between studies, in many of the studies reviewed, the levels of fruit and vegetable intake being compared were the highest versus lowest quartiles or tertiles (i.e., range of prevalence of low intake 25% to 33%), and the relative risk estimates were generally in the range of 20% to 30% lower risk for subjects in the highest category of intake. Applying this range of risk difference to the range of prevalence of low intake, the preventable fraction for low fruit and vegetable intake would fall into the range of 5–12%. It is important to recognize that this is only a crude range of estimates and that the proportion of cancers that might be preventable by increasing fruit and vegetable intake may vary beyond this range for specific cancer sites and across different regions of the world.

There have been many estimates of the fraction of cancer preventable by increasing fruit and vegetable intake based on individual case–control studies, but only two based on meta-analyses. Van't Veer *et al.* (2000) reviewed published studies and estimated the population attributable risks for all cancer sites due to consumption of 250 grams of fruit and vegetables per day as compared to the recommended 400 grams per day. They made three estimates based on different assumptions of the size of the relative risks: a "best guess" estimate (19%), an "optimistic" estimate (28%), and a "conservative" estimate (6%). Norat and Riboli (2002) estimated the preventable fractions for oesophageal, stomach and colorectal cancers in various populations around the world using relative risks derived from a meta-analysis of published studies (largely from developed countries), coupled with regional prevalence estimates derived from sources including FAO data. This approach led to estimates of the proportion of cancers preventable by increasing fruit and vegetable intake from current levels to 350 grams per day in the range of 8–16% for colorectal cancer and 20–30% for oesophageal and gastric cancers; these estimates varied substantially in different regions of the world.

The preventable fraction estimates of 5–12% for the groups of cancers evaluated here as having limited evidence for an inverse association with fruit and vegetable consumption are similar to the estimates for all cancer sites made by van't Veer *et al.*, and to the estimates for colorectal cancer by Norat and Riboli, but they are lower than the Norat and Riboli estimates for oesophageal and stomach cancers. The range of estimates of the fraction of selected cancers preventable by increasing intake of fruit and vegetables is only an approximation. The true relative risk for low intake is quite uncertain given limitations in dietary assessment and in study designs. In addition, the mix of various cancers as well as the prevalence of low intake can vary substantially across different populations.

The present estimates for the fraction of selected cancers preventable by increasing fruit and vegetable intake could be either high or low. They would be too high if the relative risk estimates on which the measure is based are inflated by biases in study design and/or uncontrolled confounding by other factors. On the other hand, they would be too low if the relative risks were underestimated because of misclassification arising from random errors in estimating dietary intake. In addition, benefits of increasing fruit and vegetable intake may well extend beyond those at the lowest levels of intake. Shifting the diets of entire populations over long periods to lower levels of risk can have a greater impact on population health than reducing risk only for a subgroup at highest risk (Rose, 1985). Increasing fruit and vegetable intake in populations is likely also to be accompanied by other beneficial changes in diet composition and in other chronic diseases.

Ecological studies

Ecological studies are analyses of associations between characteristics of populations and disease rates in populations. The essential feature of an ecological study is that *populations*, rather than *individuals*, are the unit of analysis. Populations compared with the ecological design can be populations in different countries, populations in different regions within a single country, or the same population across different times. Ecological studies can also compare populations defined by characteristics such as religion, racial/ethnic characteristics or special historical circumstances, such as the experience of famine. Thus, ecological studies, also referred to sometimes as *correlational* studies, can be cross-sectional or longitudinal.

The study of changing disease risk among people who migrate from one country to another combines the elements of geography and time in ecological analysis. Migrant studies build on geographical studies, as they are uncontrolled experiments in which presumed changes in lifestyle related to migration (notably diet) can be assessed as affecting cancer risk. The appeal of migrant studies is the internal control for the many characteristics of people that are unchanged after migration, notably the inherited genotype of individuals. Changes in cancer risk with migration have therefore been critical observations for estimating the proportion of differences in cancer risk between countries that may be due to genetic rather than non-genetic etiology (Doll & Peto, 1981).

The main weakness of ecological studies is suggested by their inherent design – that the characteristics being examined are population-level characteristics and cannot be directly linked to individual disease risk. Confounding at the population level between a suspected risk factor and disease cannot be accounted for properly in ecological studies (Morgenstern, 1995; Greenland, 2001). Thus, ecological studies may result in biased estimates of the true individual-level relationship between exposure and disease risk – a problem that is known as the "ecological fallacy" – and group-level associations may be reflective only of the spurious association between the factor of interest and other truly causal factors.

Ecological studies of differences diet and disease between regions within a single country and ecological studies comparing changes in diet with changes in disease across time within a single population are somewhat less susceptible to the ecological fallacy than are international ecological studies. This is because cultural differences apart from diet may be fewer across regions within a single country or across time in a single population. However, the very presence of variation between regions or over time in diet and disease suggests that there may also be other differences that could confound the association. Because of this important limitation, ecological studies have usually been regarded solely as hypothesis-generating.

Despite these weaknesses, ecological studies do offer substantial strengths for elucidating relationships between diet and cancer. If factors in the diet affect cancer risk only over long periods of time, perhaps even across generations, it becomes very difficult or impossible to estimate the relevant exposures to diet at the individual level. The ecological study design, in which long-term diet differences between populations can be examined, may offer a better means to observe hypothesized associations between long-term dietary exposures and cancer risk. When a hypothesized dietary exposure is very specific and discrete (e.g., soy), ecological studies can be more useful. When the exposure is less specific, such as total fruit and vegetable intake, ecological studies are less useful. The presence of a biologically plausible link between aspects of diet and particular cancers can help to strengthen the internal consistency of ecological studies. With fruit and vegetables and cancer, however, there is little specificity for cancer types that can be useful in this regard.

Ecological studies can be refined by correlating disease rates and dietary exposures within specific subgroups of the population for which both disease rates and diet can be stratified, such as age and gender. This type of detail is usually available for disease rates, but is often lacking in the dietary data used in ecological analyses. If ecological associations are to be interpreted as causal, the argument for the proper temporality of the relationship between diet and disease can be strengthened by lagging the analysis so that the dietary measures precede the disease rates. Information on diet lagged by 10 years or more may be more relevant than contemporaneous information to cancer rates in a population. This type of lagging of analyses is often not possible, however, due to insufficient historical information.

Cancer rates used in ecological analyses can be either mortality rates or incidence rates. In either case, attention to the quality of the cancer data is important, especially for comparisons between countries or across long time periods. Equally important is attention to the quality of the dietary data. Indicators as crude as the population-level estimates of food intake derived from crude agricultural data sources, or as refined as population-representative diet surveys, have been used. Even with the best possible measures of cancer risk and food intake, however, the fundamental problem of the ecological fallacy will render any association observed in an ecological study no more than suggestive of a causal relationship.

Table 113 summarizes findings from two types of study – cross-sectional ecological studies comparing countries and those comparing regions within countries. Table 114 summarizes studies that analysed the relationship between fruit and vegetable intake and changes in cancer risk within single populations over time.

Cross-sectional studies between countries

International cross-sectional studies look for relationships between levels of fruit and vegetable intake and cancer rates among populations defined by national boundaries. In such studies, the cancer rates are either mortality or incidence rates as collected by each country, and the dietary data are typically crude food disappearance estimates from agricultural sources such as the food balance sheets, which are country-level estimates of food consumption at the population level as estimated by the Food and Agricultural Organization (FAO) (see Chapter 3).

A classic analysis of the association between food consumption patterns and cancer rates between countries (Armstrong & Doll, 1975) showed rather strong associations of several factors, such as fat, in the diet with several common cancers. Associations with fruit and/or vegetable intake were reported for cancers of the liver, breast, ovary and kidney. Positive associations were seen between fruit intake and cancers of the breast and ovary, while inverse associations were seen between fruit intake and liver cancer, and between vegetable intake and kidney cancer. In a similar analysis by Rose et al. (1986), inverse associations were observed between fruit intake and ovarian cancer, and between vegetable intake and cancers of the colon (for women only), breast, ovary and prostate. Thouez et al. (1990) reported an inverse association between energy intake from vegetables and oesophageal and pancreatic cancer across 29 countries, and a study by Hebert et al. (1993) including 59 countries showed inverse associations of both fruit and vegetables with oesophageal and oral cancers. A positive association between calorie intake from vegetables and cancer of the stomach was reported by Thouez et al. (1990), but that association was diminished after adjustment for age differences between countries. The rates of lung cancer across 10 nations in the South Pacific were found to be inversely associated with the intake of yellow-orange vegetables in models that adjusted for demographic differences as well as tobacco use and other dietary factors (Le Marchand et al., 1995). Hebert and collaborators reported little relationship between fruit and vegetable intake and cancer of the bladder across 50 countries (Hebert & Miller, 1994) and little relationship between breast cancer and fruit intake across 66 countries (Hebert & Rosen, 1996), but there was a modest inverse association between cabbage intake and breast cancer (Hebert & Rosen, 1996). Another ecological study across 28 countries showed an inverse association between tomato consumption and prostate cancer risk (Grant, 1999), though this was found only with multivariate models also containing non-fat milk intake (data not shown). This analysis was inspired by observations from case–control and cohort studies of a protective association between tomato intake and prostate cancer risk, and provides a good example of the use of ecological studies to support or refute hypotheses emerging from studies with other designs.

In sum, the international studies tend to report more inverse associations than positive associations between cancer rates and intake of fruit and vegetables. These associations are generally stronger for vegetables than for fruit. There are many reported associations that are null, however, and the various reports cannot be easily compared due to different methods of analysis, different time periods of collection of cancer and diet data, the high likelihood of selective reporting of findings by cancer site, by food type, and according to the strength and statistical significance of the observations. It is quite possible, therefore, that the number of null associations is greater than the selective literature suggests.

Cross-sectional studies between regions within countries

Regional cross-sectional studies look for relationships between levels of fruit and vegetable intake and cancer rates across populations defined by regional boundaries within countries. In such studies, the cancer mortality or incidence data are usually collected in a uniform way across regions, and the dietary data are usually much more detailed and reliable than the FAO data, often being derived from national surveys of food intake as reported by individuals.

Bingham et al. (1979) reported strong inverse associations between intake of vegetables (other than potatoes) and colon cancer, using data from diet surveys in nine different regions of the United Kingdom. Shimada (1986) used similar methods to show an inverse association between vegetable intake and stomach cancer in five regions of Japan. The most extensive within-country ecological study ever conducted is the analysis of cancer rates in relation to diet across 65 counties in China (Zhuo & Watanabe, 1999). In this ambitious project, two communes in each of 65 Chinese counties were selected for dietary assessments, which included not only dietary measurements from households but also collection of samples from individuals for nutritional biomarker measurements. The study was substantially weakened by the use of cancer rates for a time period preceding the dietary assessments. Modest correlations, either positive or inverse, with fruit and

Table 113. Cross-sectional ecological studies of fruit and vegetables as related to cancer risk both between several countries and within single countries

Cancer site	Reference	Populations compared	Findings: correlation coeffecient Fruit	Vegetables	Comments
Oesophagus	Thouez et al., 1990	29 countries		Energy from veg.: −0.21 (men) −0.46 (women)	Mortality Adjusted for age
	Hebert et al., 1993	59 countries	−0.34 (men) −0.27 (women)	−0.33 (men) −0.09 (women)	Mortality
	Zhuo & Watanabe, 1999	65 counties in China	−0.13	0.04	Mortality
Stomach	Shimada, 1986	5 areas in Japan		Inversely associated with risk	Mortality
	Chen et al., 1990	65 counties in China	0.17	Green veg.: 0.05	Mortality
	Thouez et al., 1990	29 countries		Energy from veg.: 0.34 (men) 0.42 (women)	Mortality Adjusted for age
	Corella et al., 1996	50 provinces in Spain	−0.57 (men) −0.58 (women)	−0.61 (men) −0.67 (women)	Mortality Analysis lagged 20 years
	Sichieri et al., 1996	10 state capitals of Brazil	−0.62	−0.28	Mortality Adjusted for sex and tobacco
	Tsubono et al., 1997	5 areas in Japan	0.35	Green veg.: −0.88 Yellow veg.: −0.57	Mortality Adjusted for sex and tobacco
	Azevedo et al., 1999	18 districts in Portugal	−0.69 (men) −0.65 (women)	−0.81 −0.74	Mortality Intake of 100 g veg./person/day predicted 10 fewer deaths per 100 000 persons/year among men (95% CI 6–14) and 5 fewer death among women (95% CI 3–7)
	Takezaki et al., 1999	China (low vs high risk area)	Consumption higher in lower-risk area	Consumption higher in lower-risk area	
	Zhuo & Watanabe, 1999	65 counties in China	0.18	−0.11	Mortality

Table 113 (contd)

Cancer site	Reference	Populations compared	Findings: correlation coeffecient Fruit	Vegetables	Comments
Colon	Bingham et al., 1979	9 regions in Great Britain		−0.94	Mortality
	Rose et al., 1986	30 countries	0.03 (men) −0.03 (women)	0.06 (men) −0.17 (women)	Mortality Adjusted for age
	Chen et al., 1990	65 counties in China	−0.08	Green veg.: −0.03	Mortality
	Sichieri et al., 1996	10 state capitals of Brazil	−0.05	0.09	Mortality Adjusted for sex and tobacco
	Zhuo & Watanabe, 1999	65 counties in China	−0.08	−0.13	Mortality
Liver	Armstrong & Doll, 1975	23 countries	−0.38 (men) −0.46 (women)		Incidence
	Chen et al., 1990	65 counties in China	−0.06	Green veg.: 0.11	Mortality
Pancreas	Thouez et al., 1990	29 countries		Calories from veg.: −0.58 (men) −0.56 (women)	Adjusted for age
	Vioque et al., 1990	Regions of Spain	Fruits, other than citrus: −2.01 (men)		
Lung	Le Marchand et al., 1995	10 island nations of the South Pacific		Yellow-orange veg.: associated with decreased risk (p=0.06)	Incidence Multivariate models adjusting for age, sex, tobacco, and selected other dietary factors
	Chen et al., 1990	65 counties in China	−0.22 (men) −0.20 (women)	Green veg.: 0.15 (men) 0.22 (women)	Mortality
Breast	Armstrong & Doll, 1975	32 countries	0.44		Mortality
	Rose et al., 1986	30 countries	0.09	−0.11	Mortality Adjusted for age
	Chen et al., 1990	65 counties in China	−0.09	Green veg.: −0.16–0.02	Mortality

Cancer-preventive effects

Table 113 (contd)

Cancer site	Reference	Populations compared	Findings: correlation coeffecient Fruits	Vegetables	Comments
Breast (contd)	Ishimoto et al., 1994	12 districts in Japan	0.62	Green-yellow veg.: −0.02	Mortality Adjusted for age
	Hebert & Rosen, 1996	66 countries	−0.05	−0.23 (cabbage)	Mortality
Ovary	Armstrong & Doll, 1975	21 countries	0.31		Mortality
	Rose et al., 1986	26 countries	−0.26	−0.54	Mortality Adjusted for age
Prostate	Rose et al., 1986	29 countries	−0.09	−0.38	Mortality Adjusted for age
Bladder	Hebert & Miller, 1994	50 countries	−0.09 (men) −0.05 (women)	0.20 (men) −0.04 (women)	Mortality
Kidney	Armstrong & Doll, 1975	21 countries		−0.43 (men) −0.51 (women)	Mortality
All sites	Farchi et al., 1996	Regions of Italy		1 g increase veg. proteins associated with reduction of 2.5 cases per 100	Mortality

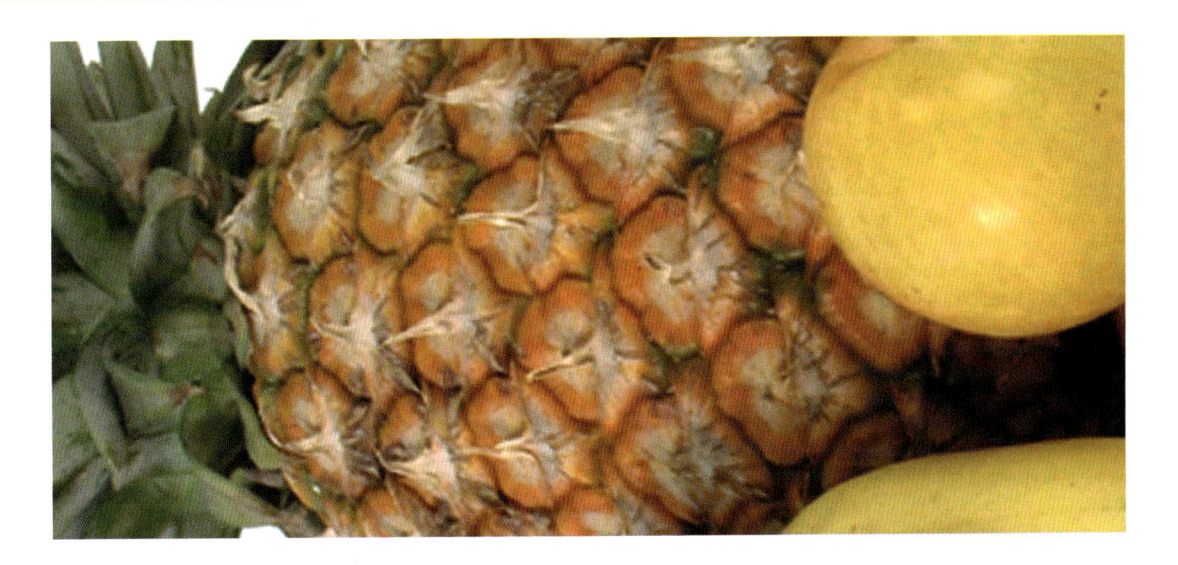

251

vegetable intake were found for several cancer sites. Fruit intake was inversely associated with risk of stomach cancer across 50 provinces in Spain (Corella et al., 1996), 10 states in Brazil (Sichieri et al., 1996) and 18 districts in Portugal (Azevedo et al., 1999), and between high- versus low-risk areas in China (Takezaki et al., 1999); but the corresponding association was positive with stomach cancer across the 65 counties in China (Chen et al., 1990) and across five areas in Japan (Tsubono et al., 1997). Vegetable intake has been consistently observed to be inversely associated with risk for stomach and colon cancers in many countries (Bingham et al., 1979; Shimada, 1986; Corella et al., 1996; Sichieri et al., 1996; Tsubono et al., 1997; Azevedo et al., 1999; Zhuo & Watanabe, 1999).

In sum, studies of correlations between cancer rates and diet within countries also tend to show inverse associations between fruit and vegetable intake and many cancers, especially cancers of the stomach and colon.

Time trend studies
Analyses of time trends are ecological studies correlating fruit and vegetable intake with cancer rates over time either within a single population or across several populations. These studies suffer from the same ecological fallacy as the cross-sectional studies among and within countries, but they have the advantage of following the same population over time. Since many characteristics of the population do not change over time, the number of potential confounding factors is reduced. Table 114 summarizes findings from the few such studies that have examined fruit and vegetables specifically. The analyses of temporal relationships between fruit and vegetables and cancer have had a variety of methods and mixed findings. The most consistently reported inverse associations have been for stomach cancer (Jedrychowski & Popiela, 1986; Swistak et al., 1996; Tominaga & Kuroishi, 1997). The interpretation of these observations is particularly difficult, however, due to potential confounding by improving socioeconomic conditions that have led to both a more varied diet and a lower risk of infection with *Helicobacter pylori*.

Migrant studies
Migrant studies are ecological studies examining cancer rates in relation to migration of people from countries of differing cancer rates. Studies of migrants from Asia to America (Ubukata et al., 1986; Story & Harris, 1989) showed that migrants themselves tended to retain Asian dietary patterns, whereas their children acquired the food preferences of America. Such changes, either within the generation of migrants or in subsequent generations of their offspring, feature increased intake of meats and fats and decreased intake of vegetables (Lee et al., 1999). This shift to a more "western" diet is associated with substantial increases in the risk of cancers of the breast (Wu & Bernstein, 1998) and colon (Bernstein & Wu, 1998). Ziegler et al. (1993) conducted a large, population-based case–control study that in many ways serves as an example of how migration can be better studied. They assessed migration effects on breast cancer for childhood, adolescent and adult exposures among Asian-American women in California by interviewing both study participants and their mothers. They found a gradient in breast cancer risk related to migration history that was quite comparable with the international differences in breast cancer incidence rates.

Summary
Ecological analyses have been generally consistent with the hypothesis that increased fruit and vegetable intake is associated with lower risk of cancer at many sites. International correlational studies, studies across regions in single countries and studies of time trends and migrating populations are all congruent in this conclusion.

Ecological studies offer both limitations and advantages for assessing the relationship between fruit and vegetable intake and cancer risk. The large contrasts between countries in diet that reflect long-term dietary differences over decades or entire lifetimes are difficult to measure in studies based on assessments of dietary exposures in individuals. The strength of ecological studies is their ability to examine such long-term differences. Their weakness is that there are many confounding factors that limit the ability to conclude causality attributable to any particular dietary factor. As fruit and vegetable intake varies substantially along with many other factors, including both dietary and non-dietary factors, any association between fruit and vegetable intake and cancer risk emerging from ecological analyses cannot be interpreted as causal. Another limitation is the apparently selective reporting of findings by cancer site, food type, or non-null results.

Intermediate markers of cancer
Experimental dietary studies in humans serve as an important link between the nutritional epidemiological studies and experiments conducted in animal models. They rely on intermediate end-points related to disease risk, using biological markers that may also provide insight into the modes of action of fruit and vegetable constituents in humans. At the same time, they are limited by the sensitivity

Table 114. Studies of trends in fruit and vegetable consumption as related to cancer trends

Cancer site	Reference	Country or areas studied	Years of trend	Findings: correlation coefficient — Fruit	Vegetables	Comments
Stomach	Jedrychowski & Popiela, 1986	Poland	1951–83	Fruit increased 87%, while mortality decreased about 50%	Veg. increased 14%, while mortality decreased about 50%	
	Swistak et al., 1996	4 European countries	1970–92	Mortality decreased as fruit increased	Mortality decreased as veg. increased	
	Tominaga & Kuroishi, 1997	Japan	1955–93	−0.83 (men) −0.82 (women)	Green yellow veg.: −0.38 (men) −0.40 (women) Other veg.: −0.61 (men) −0.62 (women)	10-year time lag between diet and cancer. Adjusted for age
Colon/rectum	McMichael et al., 1979	4 countries	1921–74	Fruit tended to be relatively stable, while mortality varied depending on country, age, sex	Veg. tended to be relatively stable, while mortality varied depending on country, age, sex	
	Holmqvist, 1997	15 European countries	1961–90	No consistent pattern of association	No consistent pattern of association	
	Tominaga & Kuroishi, 1997	Japan	1955–93	0.81 (men) 0.83 (women)	Green-yellow veg.: 0.44 (men) 0.40 (women) Other veg.: 0.59 (men) 0.62 (women)	10-year time lag between diet and cancer. Adjusted for age
Breast	Prieto-Ramos et al., 1996	50 provinces in Spain	30 years	Correlation between breast cancer mortality rates in 1981–85 and fruit intake in 1964–65 Citrus fruit: −0.10 Other fresh fruit: −0.16	Provinces with highest increase in veg. consumption from 1964 to 1981 had lowest breast cancer mortality level in 1981–85	

and specificity of the biological markers, access to relevant biological specimens and the logistics of conducting experimental studies in humans. Most of the markers reflect very early processes in the pathways of carcinogenesis (e.g., carcinogen metabolism, adduct formation), since downstream signal-transduction markers relevant to cancer progression are lacking. These early markers may not associate directly with cancer risk.

Dietary intervention studies in humans using disease end-points would provide the strongest evidence for an effect of fruit and vegetables on disease risk. However, such dietary intervention studies need to have thousands of participants in order to have sufficient statistical power and are very expensive. Issues such as timing and dose of the intervention, choice of study populations and compliance also influence interpretation of the results. As a result, no fruit and vegetable interventions have yet been conducted with cancer as the outcome.

Intervention studies

This section reviews the human experimental studies that have examined the capacity of fruit and vegetables to modulate biological processes relevant to cancer (Table 115–119). Several of these studies were designed to test the effect of fruit and vegetables on biomarkers of cardiovascular or other diseases. Results of these studies are applicable to cancer in so far as the markers are shared. The interventions differ greatly in duration, sample size and study design. Study duration ranges from single doses to months or years of intervention and is typically determined by the biology of the marker and its responsiveness to change. Ideally, sample size is dictated by the variance associated with the biomarker and the statistical power needed to detect an effect of intervention, but in practice, logistic and cost considerations often limit the sample size, so that the studies may be statistically underpowered to test effectively the fruit and vegetable treatments. The majority of intervention studies in humans have been of short duration and sample sizes have been small. No long-term, randomized clinical trials have tested solely the effects of increasing fruit and vegetable intake on intermediate cancer markers. Those that have included other diet alterations as part of the treatment, e.g., reduced energy intake from fat and/or increased whole grain intake (Schatzkin et al., 2000), have limited capacity to examine the effects of fruits and vegetables alone.

A variety of study designs have been used. Study designs described in the table as "crossover" or "x-arm trial" refer to randomized intervention studies in which participants are recruited, screened for eligibility and interest in participating, randomly assigned to one or more interventions and/or control groups and followed over time until the end of the study. Crossover studies may or may not include washout periods between different treatments. Crossover designs lacking washout periods of sufficient duration are prone to carryover effects that can jeopardize interpretation of the results. Numerous studies examining effects of fruit and vegetables have employed less stringent designs that do not use randomization or a control group. These designs include taking measurements before and after the intervention (e.g., "pre–post") or the sequential addition of treatments (tx) after an initial, dietary-restricted control period (e.g., "control–tx1–tx2"). Interventions such as these have the potential to produce biased results.

The degree of dietary control also varies. In the following tables, "controlled intervention" refers to a study in which the diet is provided to study participants. In this type of study, volunteers may be free-living, eating the food at a feeding centre or taking it home, or they may be housed in a metabolic ward. There are also different degrees of control within these types of study; the loosening of control (e.g., including free days on which participants can deviate from the study diet, drink alcohol, etc.) is more characteristic of studies of longer duration, where long-term participant retention is often most challenging. The term "supplementation of habitual diet" refers to addition of fruit or vegetables to a participant's usual diet. This common approach allows participants more control over their diets and minimizes metabolic effects of drastic changes in diet that are a potential problem with controlled interventions. In some cases, habitual diets may be modified to restrict particular foods (e.g., certain fruits and vegetables) that may influence the outcome of the study.

The following review is limited to plant foods, excluding grains, nuts, seeds, dried legumes, starchy tubers, spices and products used for infusions (e.g., teas).

Antioxidant effects (Table 115)

Oxidative damage, resulting from an imbalance between free-radical generation and antioxidant defence, has been hypothesized to play a role in cancer (Rock et al., 1996). The antioxidant defence system has both enzymatic and non-enzymatic components that prevent radical formation and remove radicals before damage can occur.

Antioxidant enzymes

Several studies have reported altered activities of antioxidant enzymes in red blood cells (RBC) after fruit and vegetable interventions; however, the responses have varied widely according to the type and dose of fruit or vegetable and only a few very different foods have been tested. In three studies, RBC glutathione reductase activities increased with spinach, parsley and grape-skin extract supplementation (Castenmiller et al., 1999; Nielsen et al., 1999; Young et al., 2000). RBC glutathione peroxidase activity increased in interventions using grape-skin extract (Young et al., 2000) and blackcurrant and apple juice (Young et al., 1999) and was unchanged with onion and parsley (Lean et al., 1999; Nielsen et al., 1999). RBC superoxide dismutase activity increased with parsley (Nielsen et al., 1999) and was unchanged with onion (Lean et al., 1999) and with blackcurrant and apple juice (Young et al., 1999). Catalase activity decreased with spinach (Castenmiller et al., 1999) and was unchanged with parsley (Nielsen et al., 1999), blackcurrant and apple juice (Young et al., 1999) and grape-skin extract (Young et al., 2000).

Total antioxidant capacity
The antioxidant capacity of fruits and vegetables has been measured in human intervention studies. Most interventions relied on effects detectable in blood samples. Several assays measure serum total antioxidant capacity *ex vivo*. These include oxygen radical absorbance capacity (ORAC), ferric-reducing ability (FRAP) and Trolox equivalent antioxidant capacity (TEAC). Typically, these markers are indicative of recent exposure to antioxidants (Mayne, 2003). Interventions with fruits and fruit juices led to an increase in total antioxidant capacity (Day et al., 1997; Cao et al., 1998a,b; Serafini et al., 1998; Aviram et al., 2000; Marniemi et al., 2000; Pedersen et al., 2000; van den Berg et al., 2001; Kay & Holub, 2002), whereas those with cruciferous and allium vegetables, spinach and tomatoes had no effect (Zhang et al., 1997; Cao et al., 1998b; Castenmiller et al., 1999; Lean et al., 1999; Bub et al., 2000; Pellegrini et al., 2000).

Oxidative damage
If not quenched by antioxidants, free radicals react with, and may alter, the structure and function of a number of cellular components, such as lipid-containing cell membranes, lipoproteins, proteins, carbohydrates, RNA and DNA.

Lipids
Effects of fruits and vegetables on the susceptibility to oxidation of serum lipoprotein *ex vivo* have been explored extensively in relation to cardiovascular disease; however, since lipid peroxidation products form adducts with DNA, they may also increase cancer risk (see section on mechanisms in this chapter). The majority of intervention studies found that low-density lipoprotein (LDL) oxidation was decreased and lag time to oxidation increased following supplementation of a wide range of fruits and vegetables, including tomato products and juice at various doses (Agarwal & Rao, 1998; Bub et al., 2000), orange (Harats et al., 1998), grape (Day et al., 1997) and pomegranate juices (Aviram et al., 2000), a mixture of vegetables (Hininger et al., 1997) and garlic powder (Phelps & Harris, 1993). Tomato or orange juice was not consistently effective; two studies reported no change in LDL oxidation with these juices (Abbey et al., 1995; Maruyama et al., 2001). Other treatments that did not significantly alter these markers included sea buckthorn juice (Eccleston et al., 2002) and aged garlic extract (Steiner & Lin, 1998). O'Reilly et al. (2001), testing the effects of onion and black tea supplementation, found no change in plasma F2-isoprostane or malondialdehyde–LDL autoantibody titre, suggesting no alteration in LDL oxidation *in vivo*. In addition, two studies have reported no change in urinary malondialdehyde with onion supplementation (Boyle et al., 2000) and with increasing fruit and vegetable intake to twelve servings per day (Thompson et al., 1999a).

Proteins
Five studies have tested the effects of fruit and vegetable interventions on plasma protein oxidation, specifically protein carbonyl formation. Three found no effect of intervention (Castenmiller et al., 1999; Nielsen et al., 1999; van den Berg et al., 2001). One reported an increase in formation of plasma 2-aminoadipic semialdehyde (a specific carbonyl at lysine residues) with a blackcurrant–apple juice mixture (Young et al., 1999)—a prooxidant effect significantly positively correlated with plasma vitamin C concentrations (Castenmiller et al., 1999; Dragsted et al., 2001). Another study reported a non-significant increase in oxidation with grape-skin extract (Young et al., 2000).

DNA oxidation and adduct formation
Interaction of reactive oxygen or nitrogen species with DNA bases can result in the formation of adducts, which, during the course of attempted repair or replication, can lead to mutations that may contribute to the development of neoplastic cells (see section on mechanisms in this chapter). To test whether antioxidant scavenging of free radicals diminishes the production of DNA adducts, studies have measured oxidative DNA damage in humans in relation to various fruit and vegetable treatments. Urinary and/or peripheral blood leukocyte concentrations of 8-hydroxydeoxyguanosine (8-OHdG) were decreased after interventions with Brussels sprouts (Verhagen et al., 1995, 1997), various tomato products (Rehman et al., 1999; Chen et al., 2001b), vegetable juice (Fan et al., 2000) and a diet high in fruit and vegetables (Thompson et al., 1999a). Results have been inconsistent for allium interventions (Hageman et al., 1997; Beatty et al., 2000; Boyle et al.,

Table 115. Studies of effects of fruit and vegetable interventions on antioxidant activity in humans

Author, year, country	Subjects, age (mean or range)	Study design	Daily dose of food/agent	Duration of intervention	Treatment outcomes
Antioxidant enzymes					
Castenmiller et al., 1999, Netherlands	Healthy NS normolipidaemic, 30 M, 42 F; 18–58 y	Parallel arm; controlled intervention	Tx1: carotenoid supplement; tx2: whole-leaf spinach 20 g/MJ, tx3: minced spinach 20 g/MJ, tx4: liquefied spinach 20 g/MJ, tx5: liquefied spinach 20 g/MJ + beetroot fibre 10 g/kg	3 wk	Increased RBC glutathione reductase and decreased catalase activities with spinach. No effect on SOD.
Lean et al., 1999, UK	Type II diabetics, 5 M, 5 F; 50–74 y	Crossover, two-arm trial; supplementation of restricted habitual diet	Onion 400 g + tea 250 mL or onion 400 g + ketchup 20 g + Italian seasoning herbs 1 g + tea 250 mL	14 d	No effect on plasma SOD or glutathione peroxidase activity
Nielsen et al., 1999, Denmark	NS, 7 M, 7 F; 20–31 y	Crossover; controlled intervention	Parsley 20 g/10 MJ	1 wk each tx	Increased RBC glutathione reductase and SOD activities; no effect on RBC catalase and glutathione peroxidase
Young et al., 1999, Denmark	Healthy NS 4 F, 1 M; 22–28 y	Crossover; supplementation of restricted habitual diet	Fruit juice (blackcurrant and apple juice, 1:1): 750, 1000 and 1500 mL	1 wk each tx	Increased RBC glutathione peroxidase activity with juice. No effect on glutathione reductase, catalase and SOD
Young et al., 2000, Denmark	Healthy NS 9 F, 6 M; 21–33 y	Crossover; supplementation of restricted habitual diet	Grape-skin extract 600 mg	1 wk each tx	Increased RBC glutathione reductase and glutathione peroxidase activities. No effect on catalase and SOD
Aviram et al., 2000, Israel	NS; Study 1: 13 Study 2: 3 20–35 y	Study 1: pre–post; supplementation of habitual diet Study 2: pre–post; supplementation of habitual diet	Study 1: 50 mL pomegranate juice Study 2: increasing doses of pomegranate juice 20–80 mL	Study 1: 2 wk Study 2: 10 wk	Increased serum paraoxonase
Total antioxidant capacity					
Day et al., 1997, UK	Healthy adults, 6 M, 1 F	Pre–post; supplementation of habitual diet	Red grape juice concentrate 125 mL	1 wk	Increased serum TAC
Zhang et al., 1997, UK	Healthy, 52 M, F	3-arm trial; supplementation of habitual diet	8 mg garlic oil or 1.0 g garlic powder	11 wk	Increased plasma TAC at 4 and 6 wk, but no difference at 11 wk
Cao et al., 1998a, USA	Healthy NS, 8 F; mean age 66.9 y	5 treatments assigned to each subject in a random sequence	Coconut drink or coconut drink + strawberries 240 g; ascorbic acid 1250 mg; raw spinach 294 g; red wine 300 mL	Single dose, each 2 wk apart	Increased serum TAC (ORAC, TEAC and FRAP) with all tx and increased urinary TAC (ORAC) with strawberries, spinach and ascorbic acid

Table 115 (contd)

Author, year, country	Subjects, age (mean or range)	Study design	Daily dose of food/agent	Duration of intervention	Treatment outcomes
Cao et al., 1998b, USA	Healthy, 17 M, 17 F; 20–40 y and 60–80 y	Crossover; controlled intervention	Tx1: fruit and vegetables 10 servings tx2: fruit and vegetables 10 servings + broccoli 2 servings (205 g) days 6–10	15 d per tx	Increased plasma TAC (ORAC) on both tx; no further effect of broccoli
Serafini et al., 1998, Italy	Healthy non-smokers, 6 F, 4 M; 25–50 y	Tx1–tx2–tx3	Tx1: dealcoholized red wine 113 mL; tx2: dealcoholized white wine; tx3: tap water	Single doses per tx	Increased plasma TRAP with dealcoholized red wine
Castenmiller et al., 1999, Netherlands	Healthy non-smokers, normo-lipidaemic, 42 F, 30 M; 18–58 y	Parallel arm; controlled intervention	Tx1: carotenoid supplement; tx2: whole-leaf spinach 20 g/MJ, tx3: minced spinach 20 g/MJ, tx4: liquefied spinach 20 g/MJ, tx5: liquefied spinach 20 g/MJ + beetroot fibre 10 g/kg	3 wk	No effect on plasma FRAP
Lean et al., 1999, UK	Type II diabetics, 5 M, 5 F; 50–74 y	Crossover, two-arm trial; supplementation of restricted habitual diet	Onion 400 g + tea 250 mL or onion 400 g + ketchup 20 g + Italian seasoning herbs 1 g + 250 mL	14 d	No effect on plasma TEAC
Leighton et al., 1999, Chile	Healthy omnivorous 42 M; 20–27 y	2-arm trial; controlled intervention	Mediterranean diet or high fat diet; red wine 240 mL/d added	3 months; during the second month wine added	Increased plasma TAC with Mediterranean diet and with wine in both diets
Young et al., 1999, Denmark	Healthy non-smokers, 4 F, 1 M; 22–28 y	Crossover; supplementation of restricted habitual diet	Fruit juice (blackcurrant and apple juice 1:1): 750, 1000 and 1500 mL	1 wk each tx	No effect on plasma TEAC and FRAP
Aviram et al., 2000, Israel	Non-smokers M; Study 1: 13 Study 2: 3 20–35 y	Study 1: pre–post; supplementation of habitual diet Study 2: pre–post; supplementation of habitual diet	Study 1: 50 mL pomegranate juice Study 2: increasing doses of pomegranate juice 20–80 mL	Study 1: 2 wk Study 2: 10 wk	Increased serum TAC
Bub et al., 2000, Germany	Healthy non-smoking 23 M; 27–40 y		Tx1: tomato juice 330 mL; tx2: carrot juice 330 mL; tx3: dried spinach powder 10 g	2 wk each tx	No effect on plasma FRAP
Lee et al., 2000, UK	Healthy, 5 F, 1 M; 20–24 y		Tx1: tomato soup 200 g + canned tomatoes 230 g + olive oil 20 mL Tx2: tomato soup 200 g + canned tomatoes 230 g + sunflower oil 20 mL	7 d each tx	Increased plasma FRAP with tomatoes + olive oil

Table 115 (contd)

Author, year, country	Subjects, age (mean or range)	Study design	Daily dose of food/agent	Duration of intervention	Treatment outcomes
Marniemi et al., 2000, Finland	Study 1: healthy, 60 M; 60 y Study 2: healthy, 6 M; mean age 48.7 y	Study 1: 3-arm trial; supplementation of habitual diet Study 2: pre–post; fasting	Study1: berries (bilberries or lingonberries or blackcurrants) 100 g ; tocopherol 100 mg + ascorbic acid 500 mg ; calcium gluconate 500 mg Study 2: berries 240 g	Study 1: 8 wk Study 2: single dose	Study 1: Increased serum TRAP with berries and LDL TRAP with supplement. Study 2: Increased LDL TRAP
Pedersen et al., 2000, UK	Healthy, 9 F; 23–41 y	Crossover; fasting	Blueberry juice 500 mL; vitamin-C fortified cranberry juice 500 mL	Single dose	Increased plasma TAC (ESR spectroscopy and FRAP) with cranberry
Pellegrini et al., 2000, Italy	Healthy, non-smokers, 11 F; mean age 25.4 y	Pre–post; supplementation of restricted habitual diet	Tomato puree 25 g	14 d	No change in plasma TAC (TRAP)
Record et al., 2001, Australia	Healthy, non-smokers, 25 M; 25–60 y	Crossover; modification/supplementation of habitual diet	Fruit and vegetables 5–7 servings ; spray-dried fruit and vegetable supplement 30 g	2 wk each tx	No effect on plasma TAC
van den Berg et al., 2001, Netherlands	Healthy, smokers, 22 M; 18–50 y	Crossover; supplementation of habitual diet	Veg. burger (lyophilized tomatoes, carrots, onions, broccoli, sweet red pepper; equivalent of 500 g mixed fresh veg.) and mixed fruit drink (orange, apple, blueberry, lemon, lime) 330 mL	3 wk each tx	Increase of plasma TAC (TEAC)
Kay & Holub 2002, Canada	Healthy, non-smokers, 8 M; 38–54 y	Crossover; fasting	Freeze-dried wild blueberry powder 100 g	Single dose with high-fat meal	Increased serum TAC (ORAC)

Oxidative damage - lipids

Author, year, country	Subjects, age (mean or range)	Study design	Daily dose of food/agent	Duration of intervention	Treatment outcomes
Phelps & Harris 1993, USA	Healthy, 5 M, 5 F; mean age 32 y	Crossover; supplementation of habitual diet	Garlic powder 600 mg	2 wk	Decreased susceptibility of apolipoprotein B-containing lipoproteins to oxidation
Abbey et al., 1995, Australia	Normocholesterolaemic smokers, 15 M; mean age 41.3 y	Pre–post; supplementation of habitual diet	Orange juice 250 mL + carrot juice 300 mL	3 wk of control; 3 wk of tx	Decreased MDA in copper-oxidized LDL; no effect on rate of LDL oxidation or lag time
Day et al., 1997, UK	Healthy adults, 6 M, 1 F	Pre-post: supplementation of habitual diet	Red grape juice concentrate 125 mL	1 wk	Decreased LDL oxidation
Hininger et al., 1997, France	Health smokers and non-smokers, 11 M, 11 F, 25–45 y	Pre-post; modification of habitual diet	Carrots 150 g + tomatoes 200 g + French beans, cabbage and/or spinach 300 g	2 wk	Lengthened lag time before the onset of LDL oxidation

Table 115 (contd)

Author, year, country	Subjects; age (mean or range)	Study design	Daily dose of food/agent	Duration of intervention	Treatment outcomes
Agarwal & Rao, 1998, Canada	Healthy non-smokers, 10 M, 9 F; 25–40 y	Crossover; standardized breakfast with habitual diet	Tomato sauce 126 g; tomato juice 540 mL; lycopene 1.243 g	1 wk each tx	Decreased LDL oxidation (TBARS and conjugated dienes) with all tx
Harats et al., 1998, Israel	Healthy 36 M; 18–23 y	2-arm trial; controlled intervention	Orange juice providing ~500 mg vitamin C	2 mo	Increased lag time of LDL oxidation
Rao & Agarwal, 1998, Canada	Healthy non-smokers, 10 M, 10 F; 25–40 y	Crossover; standardized breakfast with habitual diet	5 tx: tomato sauce 126 g; high-lycopene tomato sauce 126 g; tomato juice 540 mL; lycopene 1.232 g; lycopene 2.486 g	1 wk per tx	Decreased serum TBARS
Steiner & Lin, 1998, USA	Hypercholesterolaemic, 15 M; 30–65 y	Crossover; supplementation of habitual diet	Aged garlic extract 800 mg	6 mo one tx, 4 mo other	Decreased (not significant) susceptibility of LDL to oxidation
Young et al., 1999, Denmark	Healthy non-smokers, 1 M, 4 F; 22–28 y	Crossover; supplementation of restricted habitual diet	Fruit juice (blackcurrant and apple juice 1:1): 750, 1000 and 1500 mL	1 wk each tx	Decreased plasma MDA with 1500 mL
Thompson et al., 1999a, USA	Healthy, 28 F; 27–80 y	Pre–post; recipe-defined modification of habitual diet	12 servings of fruit and veg.	14 days	No change in urinary MDA; increase of urinary EPG
Aviram et al., 2000, Israel	Non-smokers; M Study 1: 13 Study 2: 3 20–35 y	Study 1: pre–post; supplementation of habitual diet Study 2: pre–post; supplementation of habitual diet	Study 1: 50 mL pomegranate juice Study 2: increasing doses of pomegranate juice 20–80 mL	Study 1: 2 wk Study 2: 10 wk	Decreased lipid peroxidation; prolonged lag time of LDL oxidation
Boyle et al., 2000, UK	Healthy non-smokers, 6 F; 20–44 y	Crossover; supplementation of restricted habitual diet	Onion 200 g ; onions 200 g + uncooked tomatoes 100 g	Single dose	No effect on urinary MDA
Bub et al., 2000, Germany	Healthy non-smokers, 23 M; 27–40 y	Control–tx1–tx2–tx3; supplementation of restricted habitual diet	Tx1: tomato juice 330 mL; tx2: carrot juice 330 mL; tx3: dried spinach powder 10 g	2 wk each tx	Tomato juice reduced plasma TBARS and LDL oxidation; no effect of other tx
Caccetta et al., 2000, Australia	Healthy non-smokers, 12 M; 40–63 y	Crossover; supplementation of restricted habitual diet	Tx1: red wine; tx2: dealcoholized red wine; tx3: phenol-stripped red wine; tx4: water. Dose: 5 mL red wine equivalents/kg bw	Single dose after 12-h fast	No effect of any tx on serum or LDL oxidation

Table 115 (contd)

Author, year, country	Subjects; age (mean or range)	Study design	Daily dose of food/agent	Duration of intervention	Treatment outcomes
Chopra et al., 2000, UK	18 non-smokers and 14 smokers, F; 24–52 y	Crossover; supplementation of habitual diet	Creamed spinach 200 g and mango puree 100 g; tomato puree 200 g and watermelon 100 g/d	1 wk each tx	Increased lag-phase of LDL oxidation only in non-smokers on tomato and watermelon tx
Fuhrman et al., 2000, Israel	Healthy non-smokers, 4; 30–45 y	Pre–post	Tomato oleoresin (lycopene 30 mg)	Single dose with high-fat meal	Reduced susceptibility of LDL to oxidation
Young et al., 2000, Denmark	Healthy non-smokers, 6 M, 9 F; 21–33 y	Crossover; supplementation of restricted habitual diet	Grape-skin extract 600 mg	1 wk each tx	No effect on plasma- or LDL-MDA
Böhm et al., 2001, Germany	Not reported	Pre–post	Tomato juice 500 mL	2 wk	Decreased ex vivo lymphocyte membrane damage by reactive oxygen species
Lau, 2001, USA	4 M, 4 F; mean age 68 y	Placebo-controlled crossover; supplementation of habitual diet	Aged garlic extract 3.6 g	2 wk	Increased resistance to LDL oxidation
Maruyama et al., 2001, Japan	Healthy, 31 F; mean age 21.3 y	3-arm trial; supplementation of habitual diet	Tomato juice 160 g; tomato juice 480 g	1 menstrual cycle	No change in lag time of LDL oxidation
O'Reilly et al., 2001, UK	Healthy non-smokers, 20 M, 22 F; 20–60 y	Crossover; supplementation of restricted habitual diet	Onion 150 g + black tea 300 mL	2 wk	No effect on plasma F2-isoprostane or MDA-LDL autoantibody titre
van den Berg et al., 2001, Netherlands	Healthy smokers, 22 M; 18–50 y	Crossover; supplementation of habitual diet	Veg. burger (lyophilized tomatoes, carrots, onions, broccoli, sweet red pepper; equivalent of 500 g mixed fresh veg.) and mixed fruit drink (orange, apple, blueberry, lemon, lime) 330 mL	3 wk each tx	No effect on MDA or F2-isoprostane
Eccleston et al., 2002, UK	Healthy non-smokers, 20 M; 18–55 y	2-arm trial; supplementation of habitual diet	Sea buckthorn juice 300 mL	8 wk	Increased (not significant) lag time of LDL oxidation

Oxidative damage – proteins

Castenmiller et al., 1999, Netherlands	Healthy non-smokers, normolipidaemic, 30 M, 42 F; 18–58 y	Parallel arm; controlled intervention	Tx1: carotenoid supplement; tx2: whole leaf spinach 20 g/MJ, tx3: minced spinach 20 g/MJ, tx4: liquefied spinach 20 g/MJ, tx5: liquefied spinach 20 g/MJ + beetroot fibre 10 g/kg	3 wk	No effect on plasma 2-aminoadipic semialdehyde formation

Table 115 (contd)

Author, year, country	Subjects; age (mean or range)	Study design	Daily dose of food/agent	Duration of intervention	Treatment outcomes
Nielsen et al., 1999, Denmark	Non-smokers, 7 M, 7 F; 20–31 y	Crossover; controlled intervention	Parsley 20 g/10 MJ	1 wk each tx	No effect plasma 2-aminoadipic semialdehyde formation
Young et al., 1999, Denmark	Healthy non-smokers, 1 M, 4 F; 22–28 y	Crossover; supplementation of restricted habitual diet	Fruit juice (blackcurrant and apple juice 1:1): 750, 1000 and 1500 mL	1 wk each tx	Increased plasma 2-aminoadipic semialdehyde formation with juice dose; no effect on RBC 2-aminoadipic semialdehyde and γ-glutamyl semialdehyde formation.
Young et al., 2000, Denmark	Healthy non-smokers, 6 M, 9 F; 21–33 y	Crossover; supplementation of restricted habitual diet	Grape-skin extract 600 mg	1 wk each tx	Non-significant increase in plasma 2-aminoadipic semialdehyde formation
van den Berg et al., 2001, Netherlands	Healthy smokers, 22 M; 18–50 y	Crossover; supplementation of habitual diet	Veg. burger (lyophilized tomatoes, carrots, onions, broccoli, sweet red pepper; equivalent of 500 g mixed fresh veg.) and mixed fruit drink (orange, apple, blueberry, lemon, lime) 330 mL	3 wk each tx	No effect on protein carbonyl formation

Oxidative damage and adduct formation – DNA

Author, year, country	Subjects; age (mean or range)	Study design	Daily dose of food/agent	Duration of intervention	Treatment outcomes
Verhagen et al., 1995, Netherlands	Healthy non-smokers, 10 M; 20–28 y	2-arm trial; controlled intervention	Brussels sprouts 300 g	3 wk	Decreased urinary 8-OHdG
Hageman et al., 1997, Netherlands	Healthy non-smokers, 9 M	Crossover; supplementation of habitual diet	Cucumber salad 100 g; cucumber salad 100 g + raw garlic 3 g	8 d each tx	Decreased ex vivo PBL benzo[a]pyrene–DNA adduct formation and PBL 8-OHdG with both tx. Additional decrease of benzo[a]pyrene–DNA adduct with garlic
Pool-Zobel et al., 1997, Germany	Healthy non-smokers, 23 M; 27–40 y	Control–tx1–tx2–tx3; supplementation of restricted habitual diet	Tx1: tomato juice 330 mL; tx2: carrot juice 330 mL; tx3: dried spinach powder 10 g	2 wk each tx	Decreased lymphocyte DNA strand breaks (comet assay) with all tx and decreased oxidative DNA base damage (endonuclease III assay) with carrot juice only
Verhagen et al., 1997, Netherlands	Healthy non-smokers, 5 M, 5 F	Crossover; supplementation of restricted habitual diet	Brussels sprouts 300 g	1 wk per tx	Decreased urinary 8-OHdG in 4/5 men; no effect in women
Rao & Agarwal 1998, Canada	Healthy non-smokers, 10 M, 10 F; 25–40 y	Crossover; standardized breakfast with habitual diet	Tomato sauce 126 g; high-lycopene tomato sauce 126 g; tomato juice 540 mL; lycopene 1.232 g; lycopene 2.486 g	1 wk per tx	No significant change in lymphocyte 8-OHdG

Table 115 (contd)

Author, year country	Subjects; age (mean or range)	Study design	Daily dose of food/agent	Duration of intervention	Treatment outcomes
Lein et al., 1999, UK	Type II diabetics, 5 M, 5 F; 50–74 y	Crossover, 2-arm trial; supplementation of restricted habitual diet	Onion 400 g + tea 250 mL; onion 400 g + ketchup 20 g + Italian seasoning herbs 1 g + tea 250 ml	14 d	Increased *ex vivo* antioxidant resistance (comet assay with H_2O_2 with tx; no effect on oxidative DNA base damage (endonuclease III assay)
Leighton et al., 1999, Chile	Healthy omnivorous, 42 M; 20–27y	2-arm trial; controlled intervention	Mediterranean diet; high fat diet; red wine 240 mL/d added	3 mo; wine added during month 2	No change in PBL 8-OHdG with Mediterranean diet; increased with high-fat diet; decreased with wine with both diets
Rehman et al., 1999, UK	Healthy volunteers, 1 M, 4 F; mean age 27.2 y	Pre–post; restricted habitual diet	Tomatoes 360–728 g (8 g/kg bw)	Single dose	Decreased 8-hydroxyguanine in individuals with high baseline values; increase of 8-hydroxyadenine; no effect on damage of other bases or on total damage
Riso et al., 1999, Italy	Healthy, 10 F; mean age 23.1 y	Crossover; supplementation of restricted habitual diet	Tomato puree 60 g	21 d each tx	Increased *ex vivo* antioxidant resistance (comet assay with H_2O_2)
Thompson et al., 1999a, USA	Healthy 28 F; 27–80 y	Pre–post; recipe-defined modification of habitual diet	12 servings of fruit and veg.	14 d	Decreased lymphocyte and urinary 8-OHdG
Beatty et al., 2000, UK	Healthy non-smokers, 16 M, 20 F; 21–57 y	Crossover; supplementation of restricted habitual diet	Onion 150 g + black tea 300 mL	14 d	No effect on leukocyte DNA damage (individual bases and total damage)
Boyle et al., 2000, UK	Healthy non-smokers, 6 F; 20–44 y	Crossover; supplementation of restricted habitual diet	Onion 200 g ; onions 200 g + uncooked tomatoes 100 g	Single dose	No effect on lymphocyte DNA damage (comet assay); increased *ex vivo* antioxidant resistance (comet assay with H_2O_2) on onion tx; decreased oxidative DNA base damage (endonuclease III assay) with both tx; decreased urinary 8-OHdG after onion, but not onion + tomato, meal
Fan et al., 2000, Japan	Healthy athletes, 11 M; mean age 21.0 y	2-arm trial; controlled intervention	Veg. juice 480 mL	4 d	Decreased urinary 8-OHdG
Porrini & Riso, 2000, Italy	Healthy, 9 F; mean age 25.4 y	Pre–post; supplementation of restricted habitual diet	Tomato puree 25 g	14 d	Increased *ex vivo* antioxidant resistance (comet assay with H_2O_2)

Table 115 (contd)

Author, year, country	Subject; age (mean or range)	Study design	Daily dose of food/agent	Duration of intervention	Treatment outcomes
Chen et al., 2001b, USA	32 M, localized prostate adeno-carcinoma; mean age, 65.7	Pre-post; substitution in habitual diet	Tomato sauce 200 g incorporated into pasta dishes	3 wk	Decreased leukocyte and prostate tissue 8-OHdG
Collins et al., 2001, UK	Healthy, non-smokers, 6 M, F; 24–55 y	Crossover; supplementation of habitual diet	Homogenized kiwi fruit 500 mL	Single dose	No effect on endogenous lymphocyte DNA damage (comet assay) or oxidative DNA base damage (endonuclease III assay), but increased *ex vivo* antioxidant resistance (to H_2O_2)
Dragsted et al., 2001, Denmark	Healthy non-smokers, 4 F, 1 M; 22–28 y	Crossover; supplementation of restricted habitual diet	Fruit juice (blackcurrant and apple juice 1:1): 750, 1000 and 1500 mL	1 wk each tx	No effect on urinary 8-OHdG
van den Berg et al., 2001, Netherlands	Healthy smokers, 22 M; 18–50 y	Crossover; supplementation of habitual diet	Veg. burger (lyophilized tomatoes, carrots, onions, broccoli, sweet red pepper; equivalent of 500 g mixed fresh veg.) and mixed fruit drink (orange, apple, blueberry, lemon, lime) 330 mL	3 wk each tx	No effect on PBMC DNA damage (comet with and without H_2O_2; endonuclease III)
Porrini et al., 2002, Italy	Healthy non-smokers, 9 F; mean age 25.2 y	Control–tx1–washout–tx2; supplementation of restricted habitual diet	tx1: spinach 150 g per day tx2: spinach 150 g + tomato puree 25 g	3 wk each tx	Increased *ex vivo* antioxidant resistance (comet assay with H_2O_2) with both tx; no additional effect of tomato
Vogel et al., 2002, Denmark	Healthy non-smokers, 22 M, 21 F; 21–56 y	Controlled intervention; parallel arm	Flavonoid-food free basal diet + tx1: fruits and vegetables 600 g; tx2: vitamin-mineral tablets; tx3: placebo tablets	25 d	No effect of fruit and vegetables on PBL DNA-repair enzyme expression (OGG1 and ERCC1)

bw, body weight; EPG, 8-isoprostane; ESR, electron spin resonance spectroscopy; FRAP, ferric-reducing ability of plasma; LDL, low-density lipoprotein; MDA, malondialdehyde; ORAC, oxygen radical absorbance capacity; 8-OHdG, 8-hydroxydeoxyguanosine; PBL, peripheral blood lymphocyte; RBC, red blood cell; SOD, superoxide dismutase; TAC, total antioxidant capacity; TBARS, thiobarbituric acid reactive substances; TEAC, trolox equivalent antioxidant capacity; TRAP, antioxidant potential; tx or Tx, treatment

2000), which ranged in length from a single dose to 14 days. In addition, Chen et al. (2001b) reported concomitantly decreased levels of 8-OHdG in both peripheral leukocytes and in prostate tissue of prostate adenocarcinoma patients whose diets were supplemented with tomato sauce (200 g/d) for three weeks.

The other main approach to study DNA damage in response to interventions has been to measure lymphocyte damage *ex vivo*, using a single-cell gel electrophoresis or "comet" assay. Two modifications of this assay, hydrogen-peroxide-induced DNA damage and endonuclease III cleavage to determine the presence of oxidized pyrimidines, indicate the susceptibility of lymphocyte DNA to oxidative damage. Using the comet assay, several studies (Pool-Zobel et al., 1997; Lean et al., 1999; Riso et al., 1999; Boyle et al., 2000; Collins et al., 2001; Porrini et al., 2002), but not all (van den Berg et al., 2001), have shown that various fruits and vegetables (e.g., tomato products, onions, carrot juice and kiwi fruit) reduce endogenous and/or hydrogen-peroxide-induced DNA strand breaks; however, these treatments do not always concurrently inhibit base oxidation. Another study showed that addition of raw garlic to a cucumber salad intervention for eight days further inhibited *ex vivo* lymphocyte benzo[a]-pyrene–DNA adduct formation (Hageman et al., 1997).

Nitrosation (Table 116)
Some of the same factors that contribute to oxidative damage and the production of reactive oxygen species can also lead to production of reactive nitrogen species. A wide range of nitrogen-containing compounds and nitrosating agents to which humans are exposed react *in vivo* to form potentially carcinogenic *N*-nitroso, *C*-nitroso and reactive diazo compounds (Bartsch & Frank, 1996). Nitrosating agents can also be synthesized endogenously by bacteria in the gut and activated macrophages.

Nitrosation in humans can be estimated quantitatively by monitoring urinary excretion of *N*-nitrosoproline (NPRO) after an oral dose of L-proline (Ohshima & Bartsch, 1981). Various studies have shown reduced urinary excretion of nitrosation products after single doses or one-week interventions of vitamin-C-rich fruits, vegetables and juices (Knight & Forman, 1987; Helser et al., 1992; Xu et al., 1993; Chung et al., 2002). In contrast, a longer-term (15-day) intervention of broccoli, green peas (*Pisum sativum*) and Brussels sprouts had no effect on *N*-nitrosation, particularly in the large intestine (Hughes et al., 2002). Some vegetables that are significant sources of nitrate and certain vegetable-canning methods increase body nitrite load (Lowenfels et al., 1978; Xu et al., 1993).

Modulation of biotransformation enzymes (Table 117)
Drug-metabolizing enzymes metabolize many endogenous compounds and detoxify numerous xenobiotics (Yang et al., 1994). Phase I enzymes such as cytochrome P450-dependent monooxygenases (CYP) catalyse oxidation, hydroxylation and reduction reactions, converting hydrophobic compounds to reactive electrophiles in preparation for reaction with water-soluble moieties (conjugation) to enhance their excretion. Phase II enzymes, such as UDP-glucuronosyltransferases (UGT), sulfotransferases and glutathione *S*-transferases (GST), catalyse these conjugation reactions.

Research efforts on effects of constituents of fruit and vegetables on biotransformation enzymes have focused particularly on the phase II conjugating enzymes. These enzyme systems are rapidly induced; enzymatic activities rose and reached a plateau within five days of continued daily ingestion of a food with inducing capacity (coffee or broccoli) and dropped rapidly when the food was removed from the diet (Sreerama et al., 1995). This suggests that most of the interventions to date, which have been short (one to two weeks), are of sufficient duration to evaluate the initial effect of diet on these enzyme systems. Several controlled dietary interventions have shown that cruciferous vegetables at doses of at least 300 g per day increase plasma (Bogaards et al., 1994; Nijhoff et al., 1995a; Lampe et al., 2000a) and rectal (Nijhoff et al., 1995b) GST-α concentrations. A lower dose of broccoli (~85 g) as part of a lyophilized mixed-vegetable treatment had no effect on plasma GST-α (van den Berg et al., 2001). GST-π in plasma and peripheral white blood cells did not respond to a cruciferous vegetable intervention, although rectal GST-π increased after feeding with Brussels sprouts (Nijhoff et al., 1995a, b). In two other studies, GST-π mRNA and/or protein in white blood cells decreased when participants were fed mixtures of vegetables of which Cruciferae were a minor component (Persson et al., 2000; van den Berg et al., 2001). However, another study reported a trend towards higher lymphocyte GSTP1 with high-carotenoid vegetable juices (Pool-Zobel et al., 1998), suggesting that responses vary extensively depending on the treatment.

Biotransformation of xenobiotics and that of therapeutic drugs share many of the same enzyme systems; therefore, drug metabolites can be monitored in intervention studies designed to test the effects of exposures on these systems. This is useful because in human studies it is often difficult to obtain particular tissue samples to measure enzyme activities directly. Five studies have used caffeine metabolite ratios to test broccoli, Brussels sprouts or mixed cruciferous vegetables and found increased CYP1A2 activity (McDanell et al., 1992; Vistisen et al., 1992; Kall et al., 1996; Lampe et al., 2000b; Murray et al., 2001), slightly increased CYP2E1 activity (Kall et al., 1996) and no change in N-acetyltransferase (NAT) 2 or xanthine oxidase (XO). In contrast, single doses of watercress modestly reduced activities of CYP2E1 (Leclercq et al., 1998) and CYP2A6 (Murphy et al., 2001) and oxidation of acetaminophen (paracetamol) (Chen et al., 1996), but had no effect on CYP2D6 (Caporaso et al., 1994). Few studies have examined effects of non-cruciferous vegetables on phase I metabolism; however, one reported inhibition of CYP1A2 with a six-day apiaceous vegetable intervention (Lampe et al., 2000b) and another reported that garlic increased NAT activity without changes in CYP1A2, CYP2A6 or XO (Hageman et al., 1997). Numerous studies have reported inconsistent effects of acute grapefruit juice dosing on phase I metabolism of a wide variety of drugs (Bailey et al., 1994). Phase II conjugation also is affected by cruciferous vegetables (including watercress); increased glucuronidation of several drugs has been reported (Pantuck et al., 1979, 1984), although there are no studies on induction of specific UGT families. Garlic did not appear to alter glucuronidation of acetaminophen, but slightly increased its sulfation (Gwilt et al., 1994).

Human intervention studies have also examined direct effects of supplementation with cruciferous vegetables on metabolism of carcinogens. Addition of watercress to diets of smokers significantly increased glucuronidation of nicotine and tobacco-carcinogen metabolites, while having modest effects on oxidative metabolism of these compounds (Hecht et al., 1999). Similarly, broccoli and Brussels sprouts increased the metabolism of cooked meat-derived heterocyclic aromatic amines (i.e., reduced urinary excretion of MeIQx and PhIP), implicating the induction of both CYP1A2 and phase II enzymes that are involved in heterocyclic amine metabolism (Murray et al., 2001; Knize et al., 2002).

Urinary mutagenicity (Table 118)
Bacterial assays (Ames et al., 1975) can be used to detect mutagenicity of human urine as a biomarker of exposure to carcinogens in cooked meats, cigarette smoke and certain occupational agents (see Ohyama et al., 1987a). This biomarker has been used to evaluate the effects of vegetables and grape juice on clearance of mutagens after interventions varying in length from a single dose to six weeks. Cabbage consumed as a single dose concurrently with fried salmon had no effect on urinary mutagenicity (Ohyama et al., 1987a). However, longer-term cruciferous vegetable supplementation increased mutagenicity in two separate studies (DeMarini et al., 1997; Murray et al., 2001), supporting the hypothesis that induction of biotransformation enzymes by cruciferous vegetables leads to increased excretion of mutagens. The decreased mutagenic activity of urine after a single dose of parsley (Ohyama et al., 1987b) suggests that constituents of parsley directly inhibit activity of enzymes involved in mutagen metabolism.

Other biomarkers (Table 119)
Steroid hormone metabolism
Cytochrome P450 enzymes that metabolize, and/or are modulated by, constituents of vegetables and fruit have the capacity to alter the potency of testosterone, estrogens and their derivatives via oxidation and hydroxylation reactions (Aoyama et al., 1990). This has been evaluated in relation to formation of specific 2-hydroxy- and 16α-hydroxy-estrogen metabolites, which have been hypothesized to affect breast cancer risk (Bradlow, 1986). Cruciferous vegetables fed at levels of at least 200 g/d increased the urinary ratio of 2-hydroxy- to 16α-hydroxyestrone in men and women (Kall et al., 1996; Fowke et al., 2000).

Tissue markers and clinical markers of cancer risk
Very few studies have examined the effects of fruit and vegetables on tissue markers or established clinical markers of cancer risk. In one pre–post study in the USA, serum concentrations of prostate-specific antigen (PSA) decreased with tomato-sauce supplementation in patients with prostate adenocarcinoma (Chen et al., 2001b). To date, the largest and longest intervention involving fruit and vegetables and using a clinical marker of cancer risk is the Polyp Prevention Trial (Schatzkin et al., 2000), described under Colon and rectum in the section of this chapter on cancer-preventive effects in humans. Four years of this dietary intervention had no protective effect; polyp recurrence did not differ between the treatment and control groups.

Immune function
Immune status has not been clearly linked to cancer etiology; however, it is biologically plausible that immune function is important in cancer development and growth (see section on mechanisms in this chapter). Three interventions, ranging in duration from two to eight weeks, have demonstrated modest changes in markers of cell-mediated immunity. Tomato-juice supplementation in young men consuming a low-carotenoid diet significantly increased interleukin (IL)-2 and IL-4 secretion but had no effect on lymphocyte proliferation (Watzl et al., 1999). In contrast, in older individuals consuming their habitual diet, addition of tomato juice for eight weeks had no effect on a panel of immune function

Table 116. Studies of effects of fruit and vegetable interventions on nitrosation in humans

Author, year, country	Subjects; age (mean or range)	Study design	Daily dose of food/agent	Duration of intervention	Treatment outcomes
Lowenfels et al., 1978, France	Oesophageal cancer patients, 20 M (cases) 39–78 y and hospital employees, 15 M (control) 20–50 y	Pre–post; controlled meal	Beet juice 100 mL	Single dose	Increased salivary nitrite
Knight & Forman 1987, UK	19 F; 20–28 y	Control–tx1 3-arm trial (tx2, tx3 or tx4); supplementation of restricted habitual diet	Control : test meal (high nitrate salad) Tx1: test meal + foods rich in vitamin C (green pepper, strawberries and blackcurrant drink) Tx2: tx1 + high-fat cheese and salad dressing Tx3: tx1 + white wine 225 mL Tx4: tx1 + coffee 2 cups	1 wk per tx	Decreased urinary NPRO with tx1; no effect of tx2, tx3 and tx4
Helser et al., 1992, USA	Healthy non-smokers, 16 M; 22–38 y	Crossover; controlled intervention	Juices (carrot, strawberry, pineapple, tomato, green pepper, or celery) 100 mL	Single dose each day	Decreased urinary NPRO with green pepper, tomato, pineapple, strawberry and carrot juices
Xu et al., 1993, China	Subjects from a high-risk area for gastric cancer, 44 M, 42 F; mean age 53 y	Pre–post; parallel arm; controlled intervention	Tx1: *Phylanthus emblica* juice 16.5 mL Tx2: kiwi juice 30 mL on day 6, processed vegetable juice 300 mL on day 8, and Cili juice 30 mL on day 10 Tx3: green tea extract 4.65 g on day 6, orange peel powder 6 g on day 8 and *Rosa laevigata* juice 57 mL on day 10	1 d tx separated by 1 d	Decreased urinary NPRO with fruit juices and orange-peel powder; increased NPRO with heat-processed juice
Chung et al., 2002, Republic of Korea	Healthy non-smokers; 27 M, 13 F, 17–30 y	Pre–post; restricted habitual diet and controlled intervention	Whole strawberries 300 g or garlic juice 75 g or kale juice 200 g	Single doses	Decreased urinary NDMA; no change in salivary nitrite
Hughes et al., 2002, UK	Healthy, 11 M; 30–59 y	Crossover; 7 subjects completed Tx4; controlled intervention	Tx1: vegetable (broccoli, green peas and Brussels sprouts) 400 g Tx 2: tea (500 mg tea extract per cup) 6 cups Tx3: vegetables + tea Tx4: soy beans 100 g	15 d each tx	No effect of vegetables alone on faecal or urinary markers

NDMA, *N*-nitrosodimethylamine; NPRO, *N*-nitrosoproline

Table 117. Studies of effects of fruit and vegetable interventions on biotransformation enzymes

Author, year, country	Subjects: age (mean or range)	Study design	Daily dose of food/agent	Duration of intervention	Treatment outcomes
Pantuck et al., 1979, USA	Healthy non-smokers, 7 M, 3 F; 21–32 y	Control–tx–control; controlled intervention	Brussels sprouts 300 g + cabbage 200 g	7 d	Increased metabolism of antipyrine and conjugation of phenacetin metabolite
Pantuck et al., 1984, USA	Healthy non-smokers, 10 M; 23–35 y	Control–tx–control; controlled intervention	Brussels sprouts 300 g + cabbage 200 g	7 d	Increased acetaminophen glucuronidation, but not sulfation. No effect on oxazepam conjugation
McDanell et al., 1992, UK	Healthy non-smokers, Study 1: 4 M Study 2: 3 M, 3 F; 20–57 y	Study 1: pre–post; Study 2: pre–post; controlled intervention	Study 1: cabbage 200 g each meal Study 2: Brussels sprouts 200 g each meal	Study 1: 2 days (3 meals on day 1 and breakfast on d 2); Study 2: 1 day (2 meals)	Reduced mean plasma half-life of caffeine
Vistisen et al., 1992, Denmark	Healthy, 4 M, 5 F; mean age 33 y	Pre–post; supplementation of habitual diet	Broccoli 500 g or non-cruciferous veg. 500 g	10 d	Increased CYP1A2 with broccoli compared to non-cruciferous veg.; no effect on XO or NAT2 (caffeine)
Bogaards et al., 1994, Netherlands	Healthy non-smokers, 10 M; 20–28 y	2-arm trial; controlled intervention	Brussels sprouts 300 g	3 wk	Increased plasma GST-α
Caporaso et al., 1994, USA and UK	15 M, 16 F; 21–42 y	Pre–post; controlled meal	Watercress 50 g	Single dose	No effect on CYP2D6 (debrisoquine)
Gwilt et al., 1994, USA	Non-smokers, 16 M; mean age 25.7 y	Pre–post; supplementation of restricted habitual diet	10 mL aged garlic extract with 120 mL orange juice	12 wk	No effect on oxidative metabolism of acetaminophen and glutathione conjugation of reactive metabolites; slight increase in sulfate conjugation
Hecht et al., 1995, USA	Healthy smokers, 5 M, 6 F; 24–48 y	Control–tx–control; supplementation of *Brassica*-restricted habitual diet	Watercress 170.4 g	3 d	Increased urinary NNAL and NNAL-glucuronide
Nijhoff et al., 1995a, Netherlands	Healthy non-smokers, 5 M, 5 F; 21–29 y	Crossover; supplementation of *Brassica*-restricted habitual diet	Brussels sprouts 300 g	1 wk each tx	Increased plasma GST-α in men; no change in plasma GST-π

Table 117 (contd)

Author, year country	Subjects: age (mean or range)	Study design	Daily dose of food/agent	Duration of intervention	Treatment outcomes
Nijhoff et al., 1995b, Netherlands	Healthy non-smokers, 5 M, 5 F; mean age 24 y	Crossover; supplementation of Brassica-restricted habitual diet	Brussels sprouts 300 g	1 week each tx	Increased rectal GST-α and GST-π; no effect on duodenal or lymphocyte GST
Sreerama et al., 1995, USA	Healthy, 1 F; 28 y	Control–tx–control; supplementation of restricted habitual diet	Broccoli 300 g	12 d	Increased activities of GST, class 3 aldehyde dehydrogenase and DT-diaphorase (NAD(P)H:quinone oxido-reductase) in saliva
Chen et al., 1996, USA	Healthy non-smokers, 7 M, 3 F, 23–48 y	Crossover; fasting	Watercress 50 g	Single dose	Decreased oxidative metabolites of acetaminophen
Kall et al., 1996, Denmark	Healthy non-smokers, 2 M, 14 F; 21–35 y	Control–tx1–tx2; supplementation of modified habitual diet	Tx1: standard diet avoiding GST inducers Tx2: standard diet + broccoli 500 g	Tx 1: 6 d; Tx 2: 12 d	Increased CYP1A2 (caffeine); non-significant increase in CYP2E1 (chlorzoxazone)
Hageman et al., 1997, Netherlands	Healthy non-smokers, 9 M	Pre–post; supplementation of habitual diet	Raw garlic 3 g	8 d	Increased NAT activity; no change in CYP1A2, XO, or CYP2A6 (caffeine)
Pool-Zobel et al., 1998, Germany	Healthy non-smokers, 23 M; 27–40 y	Control–tx1–tx2–tx3; supplementation of restricted habitual diet	Tx1: tomato juice 330 mL; tx2: carrot juice 330 mL; tx3: dried spinach powder 10 g	2 wk each tx	Increased lymphocyte cytosolic protein and GSTP1 with tomato and carrot juice, but not spinach
Leclercq et al., 1998, Belgium	Healthy, 6 M, 4 F; 26–55 y	Pre–post; fasting	Watercress 50 g	Single dose	Decreased CYP2E1 (chlorzoxazone)
Hecht et al., 1999, USA	Healthy smokers, 5 M, 6 F; 24–48 y	Control–tx–control; supplementation of Brassica-restricted habitual diet	Watercress 170.4 g	3 d	Increased urinary glucuronides of cotinine and trans-3'-hydroxycotinine; no effect on oxidative metabolism of nicotine and cotinine
Lampe et al., 2000b, USA	Healthy non-smokers, 19 M, 17 F; 20–40 y	Randomized crossover; controlled intervention	Brassica vegetables 436 g; allium veg. 190 g; apiaceous veg. 265 g	6 d each tx	Brassica increased and apiaceous decreased CYP1A2 compared with basal and allium diets; no effect on NAT2 and XO activities (caffeine)
Lampe et al., 2000a, USA	Healthy non-smokers, 21 M, 22 F; 20–40 y	Crossover; controlled intervention	Brassica vegetables 436 g; allium veg. 190 g; apiaceous veg. 265 g	6 d each tx	Increased GST-α and GST activity with Brassica in GSTM1-null individuals; decreased GST-α with apiaceous in GSTM1+ men; increased GST-μ activity with Brassica and Allium in GSTM1+ women

Table 117 (contd)

Author, year, country	Subjects; age (mean or range)	Study design	Daily dose of food/agent	Duration of intervention	Treatment outcomes
Persson et al., 2000, China	Healthy non-smokers, 6 M; 20–30 y	Pre–post; supplementation of habitual diet	Mixed veg. (peppers, onions, white cabbage, carrots, peas, corn, and tomatoes) 250 g	3 wk	Decreased lymphocyte GSTP1 mRNA and protein
Murphy et al., 2001, USA	Healthy non-smokers, 8 M, 7 F; 19–30 y	Pre–post; supplementation of restricted habitual diet	Watercress 170.4 g	2 d and breakfast on the third day	Marginal inhibition of CYP2A6 (coumarin)
Murray et al., 2001, UK	Healthy non-smokers, 20 M; 22–46 y	Control–tx–control; supplementation of restricted habitual diet	Brussels sprouts 250 g and broccoli 250 g	12 d	Increased CYP1A2 (caffeine) and reduced urinary excretion of MeIQx and PhIP
van den Berg et al., 2001, Netherlands	Healthy smokers, 22 M; 18–50 y	Crossover; supplementation of habitual diet	Vegetable burger (lyophilized tomatoes, carrots, onions, broccoli, sweet red pepper; equivalent of 500 g mixed fresh veg.) and mixed fruit drink (orange, apple, blueberry, lemon, lime) 330 mL	3 wk each tx	Decreased PBMC GSTπ; no effect on plasma GSTα or erythrocyte GSH or GSSG
Knize et al., 2002, USA	Healthy non-smokers; 6; age NA	Control–tx–control; supplementation of restricted habitual diet	Broccoli 1 cup	3 d	Increased urinary excretion of PhIP metabolites in 5 of 6 subjects

CYP, cytochrome P450; GSH, reduced glutathione; GST, glutathione S-transferase; GSSG, oxidized glutathione; MeIQx, 2-amino-3,8-dimethylimidazo(4,5-f)quinoxaline; NAT, N-acetyltransferase; NNAL, 4-(methylnitrosamino)-1-(3-pyridyl)-1-butanol; PhIP, 2-amino-1-methyl-6-phenyl-imidazo(4,5-b)pyridine; XO, xanthine oxidase

Table 118. Studies of effects of fruit and vegetable interventions on urinary mutagenicity in humans

Author, year, country	Subjects; age (mean or range)	Study design	Daily dose of food/agent	Duration of intervention	Treatment outcomes
Sousa et al., 1985, USA	Non-smokers, 3 M, 2 F; age N/A	Pre–post; restricted diet and fasting	Grape juice 1180 mL	Single dose	No effect on mutagenic activity of urine concentrates (in S. typhimurium TA98 and TA100)
Ohyama et al., 1987a, Japan	Non-smokers, 3 M, 1 F; 25–42 y	Control–tx1–control–tx2; controlled intervention	Tx1: fried salted salmon 120 g Tx2: fried salted salmon 120 g + cabbage 240 g	2 d per tx	No change in mutagenic activity of urine concentrate with cabbage (in S. typhimurium TA98, 100, 1535, 1538)
Ohyama et al., 1987b, Japan	Healthy non-smokers, 3 M; 27–42 y	Tx1–tx2–controlled intervention	Tx 1: fried salmon 150 g. Tx 2: fried salmon 150 g + parsley 70 g	Single dose: tx 1 on d 1 and tx 2 on d 2	Decreased mutagenic activity of urine concentrate with parsley (S. typhimurium TA98)
DeMarini et al., 1997, USA	Healthy non-smokers, 3 M, 5 F; 40–65 y	2-arm trial; controlled intervention	Tx1: fried meat + cruciferous veg. or Tx2: fried meat + non-cruciferous veg.	6 wk	Increased (non-signficant) conjugated urinary mutagenicity with cruciferous veg. (in S. typhimurium YG1024)
Murray et al., 2001, UK	Healthy non-smokers, 20 M; 22–46 y	Control–tx–control; sup. of restricted habitual diet	Brussels sprouts 250 g and broccoli 250 g	12 d	Increased urinary mutagenicity with cruciferous veg. (in S. typhimurium YG1024)

Table 119. Studies of effects of fruit and vegetable interventions on other intermediate end-points in humans

Author, year, country	Subjects; age (mean or range)	Study design	Daily dose of food/agent	Duration of intervention	Treatment outcomes
Steroid hormone metabolism					
Kall et al., 1996, Denmark	Healthy, non-smokers, 2 M, 14F; 21–35 y	Control–tx1–tx2; supplementation of restricted habitual diet	Tx1: standard diet avoiding GST inducers Tx2: standard diet + broccoli 550 g	Tx 1: 6 d; Tx 2: 12 d	Increased urinary 2-OH-E1: 16α-OH-E1 ratio with broccoli
Fowke et al., 2000, USA	Healthy postmenopausal, 34 F; 49–77 y	Pre–post; supplementation of habitual diet through counselling	*Brassica* vegetable up to 193 g	4 wk	Increased urinary 2-OH-E1: 16α-OH-E1 ratio
Tissue markers and clinical markers of cancer risk					
Schatzkin et al., 2000, USA	1228 M, 677 F; one or more histologically-confirmed colorectal adenoma; >35 y	2-arm trial; modification of diet through counselling	20% energy from fat + dietary fibre 18 g/1000 kcal, + fruit and veg. 3.5 servings/1000 kcal	4 y	No difference in rate of recurrence of colorectal adenomas
Chen et al., 2001b, USA	32 M; localized prostate adenocarcinoma; mean age 65.7 y	Pre–post; substitution in habitual diet	Tomato sauce 200 g incorporated into pasta dishes	3 wk	Decreased serum PSA levels
Immune function					
Kandil et al., 1988	HIV+ men	2-arm trial; supplementation of habitual diet	0.5 g raw garlic/kg bw; 1800 mg garlic powder	3 wk	Enhanced NK cell activity
Watzl et al., 1999, Germany	Healthy non-smokers, 23 M; 27–40 y	Non-randomized trial; supplementation to diet restricted in high carotenoid veg. and fruit	Tomato juice 330 mL; carrot juice 330 mL; spinach powder 10 g	8 wk: 2 wk per tx	Tomato juice consumption significantly enhanced IL-2 and IL-4 secretion compared to restricted diet. No change in lymphocyte proliferation
Watzl et al., 2000, Germany	Healthy, 18 M, 32 F; 63–86 y	2-arm trial; supplementation to	Tomato juice 330 mL	8 wk	No change in: number or lytic activity of NK cells; IL-2 or –4 or TNF-α secretion by activated PBMC; lymphocyte proliferation; or delayed hypersensitivity skin response

Table 119 (contd)

Author, year country	Subjects; age (mean or range)	Study design	Daily dose of food/agent	Duration of intervention	Treatment outcomes
Antibacterial activity					
Aydin et al., 1997, Turkey	H. pylori-positive dyspeptic patients, 5 M, 15 F; 21–61 y	2-arm trial; supplementation of habitual diet	Garlic oil 275 mg capsules (800 µg allicin) 3 times or garlic-oil capsules 3 times + omeprazole 20 mg 2 times	2 wk	No change in grade of gastritis or H. pylori-positivity (gastric mucosal urease test)
Graham et al., 1999, USA	Healthy, 7 M, 5 F, proven H. pylori infection; 18–75 y	Crossover; controlled test meals	Tx1: fresh garlic (10 sliced cloves);Tx2: capsaicin (6 sliced fresh jalapenos peppers); Tx3 (+ control): bismuth subsalicylate 2 tablets	1 meal per tx	No effect of garlic or capsaicin on H. pylori (urea breath test)
McNulty et al., 2001, UK	Dyspeptic patients with positive serology for H. pylori, 5; 18–75 y	Pre–post; supplementation of habitual diet	Garlic oil (4 mg) capsule 4 times	14 d	No eradication or suppression of H. pylori (urea breath test) or symptom improvement
Other biomarkers					
Ross et al., 1995, USA	Healthy, 19 M, F, ages N/A	Crossover; controlled intervention	Carrot coins 165 g + carrot puree 125 g + chopped spinach 250 g; broccoli 390 g + cauliflower 300 g; tofu and textured vegetable protein product 45 g	9 d each tx	No effect of vegetable tx on PDGF and mitogenic activity
Jenkins et al., 2001, Canada	Healthy, 8 M, 2 F; 24–60 y	Crossover; controlled intervention	Tx1: high-fruit and veg. diet (63 servings/2500 kcal diet); Tx2: starch-based diet (11 servings of fruit and veg.) Tx3: low-saturated fat diet (5 servings of fruit and veg.)	2 wk each tx	High-fruit and veg. diet resulted in: greatest faecal bile acid output, faecal bulk, and faecal short-chain fatty acid outputs; lowest concentrations of faecal bile acids; and increased urinary mevalonic acid excretion

bw, body weight; E1, estrone; IL, interleukin; NK, natural killer; PBMC, peripheral blood mononuclear cells; PDGF, platelet-derived growth factor; PSA, prostate-specific antigen; TNF, tumour necrosis factor

markers: number or lytic activity of natural killer (NK) cells, IL-2, IL-4 and tumour necrosis factor (TNF)-α secretion by activated mononuclear cells, lymphocyte proliferation or delayed hypersensitivity skin response (Watzl et al., 2000). One small study using garlic suggested that natural killer (NK) cell activity can be increased in immunocompromised individuals (e.g., human immunodeficiency virus (HIV)-positive patients) (Kandil et al., 1988).

Antibacterial activity
Garlic has received attention as a potential antibacterial agent, particularly in the treatment of *Helicobacter pylori* infection. This Allium vegetable has long been used as an antibiotic, antiviral and antifungal agent and in countries where modern medicines are scarce, it remains a treatment for various infections (Reuter et al., 1996); however, few clinical interventions have been conducted to test its efficacy. Three studies using garlic or garlic oil have been unsuccessful in eradicating existing *H. pylori* infection or associated gastrointestinal symptoms (Aydin et al., 1997; Graham et al., 1999; McNulty et al., 2001). These studies were small and of short duration – from a single meal up to two weeks – possibly not long enough to assess therapeutic efficacy (Mahady & Pendland, 2000).

Observational studies
Some biomarkers have been determined as part of case–control studies in order to evaluate possible carcinogenic mechanisms in relation to the observed cases.

Hemminki et al. (2002) investigated whether high consumption of fruit and vegetables can reduce mutations in the *von Hippel-Lindau* (*VHL*) gene, a gatekeeper gene for renal-cell cancer. Somatic *VHL* mutations appear to be associated with some 50% of sporadic renal-cell cancer (Gnarra et al., 1994; Prowse et al., 1997; Yang et al., 1999; Brauch et al., 2000). In a molecular epidemiological sub-study of 102 Swedish patients with renal-cell cancer, within a previously reported case–control study (Lindblad et al., 1997), consumption of total fruits was not associated with mutation, but consumption of citrus fruit (≥ 421 versus < 421 g/mo) was protective against mutation in both smokers and all subjects. Among smokers, vegetable intake (> 1039 versus < 1039 g/mo) also was significantly protective (Hemminki et al., 2002).

In a study on total aromatic DNA adducts in human white blood cells (Peluso et al., 2000), among 162 bladder cancer cases and 104 hospital controls, high consumption of fruit and vegetables during the previous 24 h decreased the strength of the association between adducts and the risk for bladder cancer: for vegetables, OR for 0–1 servings: 7.80, 95% CI 3.00–20.30; OR for two servings: 4.98; 95% CI 1.56–15.92; OR for 3 servings: 1.97 95% CI 0.48–8.02. In a study on 4-aminobiphenyl–DNA adducts in bladder biopsies, high consumption of fruit and vegetables was non-significantly associated with lower levels of adducts (Airoldi et al., 2002).

In approximately 100 volunteers in Italy, a strong inverse association between lymphocyte bulky DNA adducts and frequency of consumption of fresh fruit (*p* for trend = 0.04) and vegetables (*p* for trend = 0.01) was reported (Palli et al., 2000). Also in Italy, oxidative DNA damage, measured by comet assay with formamidopyrimidine DNA glycosylase in lymphocytes from 71 healthy adults, was inversely associated with tomato consumption (*p* for trend = 0.05) (Giovannelli et al., 2002). Regarding DNA adducts derived from lipid peroxidation products, levels of 1,N^6-ethenodeoxyadenosine in white blood cells were inversely correlated with vegetable consumption (*p* = 0.02) among 42 healthy female volunteers (Hagenlocher et al., 2001) and levels of malondialdehyde-deoxyguanosine were inversely, although non-significantly, associated with fruit and salad consumption in colorectal biopsies from normal mucosa in men (Leuratti et al., 2002).

Experimental studies

Animal studies
The review in this section covers studies on the effects of fruit and vegetables administered individually or in combination during the initiation stage of carcinogenesis (just before and during the carcinogen treatment), during the post-initiation and progression stages (after carcinogen treatment until the end of the study) and during the initiation, post-initiation and progression stages (Table 120). Also, the effects of mixtures of fruit and vegetables on intestinal tumours in transgenic mouse models are reviewed. As elsewhere in this volume, fruit and vegetables are taken to include edible plant foods, excluding cereal grains, nuts, seeds, dried beans, starchy roots, spices and products used mainly as infusions.

Both cereal-based and semi-purified diets have been used in studies of the effects of diet on carcinogenesis. Cereal-based diets include the dietary ingredients from whole-grain cereals and protein-rich foods. Semi-purified diets include defined ingredients such as casein, soybean protein, starch, sucrose and vitamins. Semi-purified diets have the advantage that each component can be modulated independently of the others in a controlled manner.

Effects on spontaneous tumours
The influence of dietary factors such as total composition, thermal pro-

Cancer-preventive effects

Table 120. Effect of vegetables, fruits, berries or their extracts on carcinogenesis in experimental animals

Organ, species, strain (sex)	Age at beginning of study	No. of animals per group	Carcinogen (dose, route, duration)	Vegetables, fruit, berries, or their extract (dose)	Treatment (route, and duration duration of study*)	Preventive effect	Reference
Numerous[a] *Rat* Wistar (M + F)	4	50	None (spontaneous tumours)	19.5% fruit and veg. mixture added to animal diet or to a human diet composed of meat, bread and eggs (raw or cooked)	Fed *ad libitum* for 142 wks	No effect on tumour incidence	Alink et al. (1989)
Oral cavity *Hamster* Syrian golden (sex not specified)	Not reported	5–8	0.5% DMBA painted on buccal pouches, 3/wk, 10 wk	Ground garlic, 10% in diet	Fed for 8 wk beginning 1 wk before DMBA treatment; control diet for 18 wk (initiation)	Reduced multiplicity and volume of tumours per pouch (S)	Shyu & Meng (1987)
Syrian golden (sex not specified)	Not reported	5–8	0.5% DMBA painted on buccal pouches, 3/wk, 10 wk	Garlic extract, 0.5, 25 or 50% in mineral oil	Applied topically to buccal pouches 3/wk for 3 wk starting 14 wk before DMBA treatment; experiment terminated at wk 30	Increased latency of tumour appearance in all treated groups; reduced tumour multiplicity and volume in animals treated with 25 and 50% garlic extract (all S)	Meng & Shyu (1990)
Syrian golden (M)	4–5	15	0.2% DMBA painted on buccal pouches 3/wk, 8 wk	Lyophilized black raspberries, 5 or 10% in diet	Fed for 12–13 wk starting 2 wk before DMBA treatment	No effect on size or incidence; reduced tumour multiplicity (S) in animals fed 5% berries	Casto et al., (2002)
Oesophagus *Rat* Fischer 344 (M)	5–6	15	NMBA, 0.25 mg/kg s.c., 1/wk, 15 wk	Freeze-dried strawberries, 5 or 10% in diet	Fed for 32 wk starting 2 wk before NMBA treatment	No effect on tumour incidence; reduced tumour multiplicity (papillomas) (S)	Stoner et al., (1999)
			NMBA, 0.5 mg/kg s.c., 3/wk, 5 wk	Freeze-dried strawberries, 5 or 10% in diet	Fed for 25 wk starting 24 h after last NMBA dose	Reduced tumour multiplicity (S)	Carlton et al. (2001)

Table 120 (contd)

Organ, species, strain (sex)	Age at beginning of study	No. of animals per group	Carcinogen (dose, route, duration)	Vegetables, fruit, berries, or their extract (dose)	Treatment (route, and duration; duration of study*)	Preventive effect	Reference
Fischer 344 (M)	7–8	15	NMBA, 0.25 mg/kg s.c., 1/wk, 15 wk	Lyophilized black raspberries, 5 or 10% in diet	Fed for 30 wk starting 2 wk before NMBA treatment	Reduced tumour multiplicity (S)	Kresty et al., (2001)
	5–8	8–15	NMBA, 0.25 mg/kg s.c., 3/wk, 5 wk	Lyophilized black raspberries, 5 or 10% in diet	Fed for 15, 25, 35 wk starting 3 d after last NMBA dose	Decreased tumour incidence and multiplicity and high-grade dysplasia after 25 wk with both treatments (all S)	
Fischer 344 (M)	6–7	10–25	NMBA, 0.25 mg/kg s.c., 1/wk, 15 wk	Freeze-dried blueberries, 5 or 10% in diet	Fed for 25 wk starting 2 wk before NMBA treatment	No effect on incidence, size or multiplicity	Aziz et al., (2002)

Colon
Mouse

Swiss ICR (M+F)	5–7	14–17	DMH, 23–56 mg/kg s.c., 1/wk, 7 wk, (total dose 320 mg/kg)	Fresh cabbage, 13% in diet	Fed for 21.5 wk starting 31 d before DMH treatment	Slight increase in tumour incidence in females (NS)	Temple & El-Khatib (1987)
Swiss ICR (F)	5–7	20–40	DMH 17–65 mg/kg s.c., 1/wk 8 wk (total dose, 291 mg/kg)	Fresh cabbage, 13% in diet	(a) Fed beginning 5 wk before DMH treatment until 3 d after last DMH dose (initiation); control diet for 19.5 wk (b) Fed for 19.5 wk beginning 3 d after last DMH dose (promotion)	(a) Slight increase in tumour incidence (NS) (b) Reduction in tumour multiplicity (S)	Temple & Basu (1987)
Apc^Min mice (M + F)	Weanlings	14–17	None (spontaneous tumours)	Low- or high-fat diet with 19.5 or 22.3% freeze-dried fruit-veg. mixture, respectively	Exposure in utero until around day 90 of life	Inhibited multiplicity of intestinal polyps in M fed low-fat (S). Increased multiplicity of intestinal polyps in M and F fed high-fat diet (S)	Van Kranen et al., (1998)

Table 120 (contd)

Organ, species, strain (sex)	Age at beginning of study	No. of animals per group	Carcinogen (dose, route, duration)	Vegetables, fruit, berries, or their extract (dose)	Treatment (route, and duration; duration of study*)	Preventive effect	Reference
Rat Wistar (M)	4	36–43	DMH, 50 mg/kg s.c., 1 wk, 10 wk	19.5% fruit and veg. mixture added to animal diet or to a human diet composed of meat, bread and eggs (raw or cooked)	Fed for 8 months starting 4 wk before DMH treatment	Reduction in polypoid adenomas in animals fed animal diet (S); increase in adenocarcinomas in animals fed human diet(s)	Alink et al. (1993)
Wistar (M)	5	30	DMH, 50 mg/kg, s.c., 1/wk, 10 wk	Low- or high-fat diet containing 19.5% fruit-veg. mixture	Fed for up to 35 wk beginning 4 wk before DMH treatment	Slight decrease in incidence of colorectal adenomas with low- or high-fat diet (NS)	Rijnkels et al., (1997a,b)
Wistar (M)	5	30	MNNG, 6 mg/kg, intrarectally, 1wk, 5 wks	Low- or high-fat diet containing 19.5% fruit-veg. mixture	Fed for 35 wk starting 4 wk before MNNG treatment	Reduced incidence of colon adenocarcinomas in animals fed high-fat diet	Rijnkels et al. (1997c)
Fischer 344 (M)	5	30	AOM, 15 mg/kg bw, s.c., 1/wk, 3 wk	Low- or high-fat diet containing 19.5% fruit-veg. mixture	(a) Fed for 8 wk beginning 4 wk before AOM treatment, control diet for 28 wk (initiation) (b) Fed for 2 wk starting 2 wk after last AOM dose (promotion)	No effect on colon carcinogenesis	Rijnkels et al., (1998)
Fischer 344/ NSlc (F)	7	24–25	MNU, 0.5 mL of 0.4% or 0.8%, intrarectally, 3/wk, 3 wk	Tomato juice diluted 1:2 or 1:14 (17 or 3.4 ppm lycopene) in drinking water	Given for 35 wk starting together with MNU treatment	Reduced colon incidence and multiplicity in animals given tomato juice diluted 1:2 (S)	Narisawa (1998)
Fischer 344 (M)	3	30	AOM, 15mg/kg, s.c., 1/wk, 2 wk	Orange juice in place of drinking water	Given for 28 wk beginning 1 wk after last AOM (post-initiation)	Reduced colon tumour incidence (S)	Miyagi et al. (2000)

Table 120 (contd)

Organ, species, strain (sex)	Age at beginning of study	No. of animals per group	Carcinogen (dose, route, duration)	Vegetables, fruit, berries, or their extract (dose)	Treatment (route, and duration; duration of study*)	Preventive effect	Reference
Fischer 344 (M)	7	20–29	AOM, 20 mg/kg, s.c., 1/wk, 2 wk	Mandarin juice in drinking-water at night	Given for 36 wk beginning 1 wk after last AOM dose (post-initiation)	Reduced incidence and multiplicity of colon adenocarcinoma (S)	Tanaka et al., (2000)
Sprague-Dawley (sex not specified)	5	30–42	DMH, 20 mg/kg 1/wk, 6 wk (route not specified)	Orange pulp, 15% in diet	Fed for 8 months starting together with DMH treatment	Colon adenocarcinoma incidence not affected; decreased incidence of endophytic adenocarcinomas (S); increased incidence of exophytic adenocarcinomas (S)	Kossoy et al., (2001)
Fischer 344 (M)	8–9	18	AOM 15 mg/kg i.p. 1/wk, 2 wk	Lyophilized black raspberries, 2.5, 5 or 10% in diet	Starting 24 h after last AOM dose; 9 wk for aberrant crypt foci and for 33 wk for tumours	Decreased total tumour multiplicity (all S); decreased multiplicity of adenocarcinoma (S for 10% raspberry group) and of aberrant cryptfoci (all S)	Harris et al., (2001)

Liver
Rat

Fischer 344 (M)	Weanling	8–11	1 ppm AFB_1 in the diet for 26 wk	Freeze-dried ground beets or cabbage, 25% in diet	Fed together with carcinogen for 26 wk; control diet for 16 wk	Decreased tumour incidence with cabbage (S); increased incidence and size with beet (S)	Boyd et al., (1982)
Sprague-Dawley (M)	8	25	NDEA in drinking water for 10 wk (total dose, 500 mg/kg bw)	120 or 160 g carrots 4 or 5 d/wk, respectively, without any other diet	Fed together with carcinogen for at least 14 wk	Delayed tumour occurrence and prolonged survival (S)	Rieder et al. (1983)
	16	30	NDEA, i.p., 1/wk, 8 wk (total dose, 400 mg/kg bw)	160 g carrots/wk, 5 d/wk without any other diet	Fed for 14 wk Starting 2 wk before NDEA treatment	Delayed appearance of tumours and prolonged survival (S)	

Cancer-preventive effects

Table 120 (contd)

Organ, species, strain (sex)	Age at beginning of study	No. of animals per group	Carcinogen (dose, route, duration)	Vegetables, fruit, berries, or their extract (dose)	Treatment (route, and duration; duration of study*)	Preventive effect	Reference
Toad *Bufo viridis* (M + F)	Sexually mature	50 M, 50 F	DMBA, 0.5 mg/toad, into dorsal lymph sac, 3/wk, 12 wk	Ground cabbage solution, 1 or 2 mL/day	Fed for 12 wk starting 3 h before or 3 h after DMBA treatment for 3 months	Reduced tumour incidence in animals treated before DMBA administration (S); no effect after DMBA administration	Sadek et al. (1995)
Lung Mouse A/J sex not specified)	5–6	20	NNK, 0.414 mg × 5 i.p or B[a]P 0.2 mg × 5 by gavage, over 2 wk	Freeze-dried strawberries, 10% in diet	Fed for 20 wk or 24 wk starting 1 wk before NNK or B[a]P treatment, respectively	No effect on incidence or multiplicity of lung tumours	Carlton et al. (2000)
A/J (M)	7	20–23	NNK, 10 µmol per mouse, i.p. single dose	Mandarin juice in place of drinking water at night	Given for 21 wk starting 1 wk after NNK injection (post-initiation)	No effect on lung tumour incidence or multiplicity or on alveolar cell hyperplasia	Kohno et al. (2001)
Skin Mouse Swiss albino (F)	4–5	25	1% DMBA (topical) (3x), followed by croton oil 2/wk, 2 months	Bitter gourd extract, 5% in water	50 µL/mouse/day, 12 wk, orally, starting together with DMBA-croton oil treatment	Skin papilloma incidence decreased (S); no effect on multiplicity	Ganguly et al. (2000)
Mammary gland Rat Sprague-Dawley (F)	5	15	DMBA, 60 mg/kg, orally, single dose	Freeze-dried Brussels sprouts, 20% in diet	For 4 wk beginning 2 wk before DMBA treatment; control diet for 48 wk (initiation)	Reduced incidence of mammary tumours 15 wk after dosing and of adenocarcinomas 50 wk after dosing (S)	Stoewsand et al., (1988)

277

Table 120 (contd)

Organ, species, strain (sex)	Age at beginning of study	No. of animals per group	Carcinogen (dose, route, duration)	Vegetables, fruit, berries, or their extract (dose)	Treatment (route, and duration; duration of study*)	Preventive effect	Reference
Sprague-Dawley (F)	4	16–20	DMBA, 50 mg/kg, orally, single dose	Freeze-dried Brussels sprouts, 20% in diet	For 4 wk beginning 2 wk before DMBA treatment; control diet for 25 wk (initiation)	Slightly reduced incidence and multiplicity of papillary carcinomas and adeno-carcinomas (NS)	Stoewsand et al. (1989)
Sprague-Dawley (F)	7	25–35	MNU, 50 mg/kg, i.v., single dose	5% or 10% dried cabbage, or 3.2% extracted residue, or 5% dried collards in low-fat diet; 5% cabbage or 5% collards in high-fat diet	Fed for up to 24 wk directly following MNU treatment	Low-fat diet containing 5% cabbage or cabbage residue inhibited mammary carcinogenesis (S); no effect with high-fat diet	Bresnick et al. (1990)
Sprague-Dawley (F)	6	20	DMBA, 25 mg/kg, orally, single dose	Garlic powder, 1, 2 or 4% in diet	(a) For 4 wk starting 2 wk before DMBA treatment; control diet for 20 wk (initiation) (b) Fed 2% garlic diet continuously for 24 wk* (initiation and post-initiation)	(a) inhibited tumour incidence and multiplicity in animals treated with 4% garlic (S) (b) Suppressed tumour incidence and multiplicity (S)	Liu et al., (1992)
Sprague-Dawley (F)	6	25	DMBA, 10 mg, intragastric, single dose	Garlic powder, 2% in diet	(a) Fed for 3 wk starting 2 wk before DMBA treatment (initiation) (b) Fed continuously for 26 wk (initiation and post-intiation)	(a) Slight reduction in tumour incidence and multiplicity (NS) (b) Inhibited tumour incidence and multiplicity (S)	Ip et al. (1992)
Sprague-Dawley (F)	6	21	MNU, 15 mg/kg i.p., single dose	Garlic powder, 2% in diet	For 27 wk beginning 14 d before MNU treatment	Reduced incidence and multiplicity of mammary tumours (S)	Schaffer et al. (1996)

Table 120 (contd)

Organ, species, strain (sex)	Age at beginning of study	No. of animals per group	Carcinogen (dose, route, duration)	Vegetables, fruit, berries, or their extract (dose)	Treatment (route, and duration; duration of study*)	Preventive effect	Reference
Sprague-Dawley (F)	6	26	DMBA, 50 mg/kg, orally, single dose	Freeze-dried bitter gourds, 6.25 or 12.5% in diet	Fed for 3 wk beginning 2 wk before DMBA treatment; control diet for 24 wk initiation	Both diets reduced multiplicity of mammary tumours (S); no effect on incidence	Kusamran et al. (1999a)
Uterine cervix *Mouse* Swiss albino (F)	8–10	25–30	3-MC, 600 µg into uterine cervix canal by laparotomy	Ground garlic in water, 400 mg/kg/d, orally	For 6 wk beginning 2 wk before 3-MC thread insertion; experiment ended after 14 wk	Reduced incidence of squamous cell carcinoma (S); no effect on hyperplasia or dysplasia	Hussain et al. (1990)
Bladder *Mouse* C3H/HeN (F)	Age not reported	20	10^3 MBT2 bladder cancer cells in 0.1 mL culture medium s.c., into right thigh	Garlic extract, 5, 50 and 500 mg garlic/100mL in drinking water	Given for 53 or 65 d beginning 1 month before MDT2 tumour transplantation	Dose-dependent decrease in tumour volume with 50 and 500 mg mg garlic extract (S)	Riggs et al. (1997)
Rat Fischer 344 (M)	6	24	BBN, 0.05% in drinking water for 8 wk	Tomato juice diluted 1:4 in drinking water (25 ppm lycopene)	For 12 wk starting directly after BBN treatment	Decreased multiplicity of transitional-cell carcinomas (S); no effect on incidence	Okajima et al. (1998)

AFB$_1$, aflatoxin B$_1$; AOM, azoxymethane; B[a]P, benzo[a]pyrene; BBN, N-butyl-N-(4-hydroxybutyl)nitrosamine; DMBA, 7,12-dimethylbenz[a]anthracene; DMH, 1,2-dimethylhydrazine; i.p., intraperitoneal; 3-MC, 3-methylcholanthrene; MNNG, N-methyl-N'-nitro-N-nitrosoguanidine; MNU, N-methyl-N-nitrosourea; NDEA: N-nitrosodiethylamine; NMBA: N-nitrosomethylbenzylamine; NNK, 4-(methylnitrosamino)-1-(3-pyridyl)-1-butanone; NS, not significant; p.c., percutaneous; S, significant, s.c., subcutaneous

[a] Abdominal cavity, adrenal glands, bone, brain, haemotopoietic system, liver, mammary glands, ovaries, pancreas, pituitary gland, skin, soft tissues, thymus, thyroid, uterus, other sites

*When study continued beyond last carcinogen or fruit/vegetable treatment. The number of weeks is counted from the beginning of the study (and not from beginning of carcinogen treatment).

cessing and the presence of fruit and vegetables on tumour incidence was studied in a long-term experiment in rats (Alink et al., 1989). Groups of 50 male and 50 female Wistar rats were fed one of the following diets: a semi-purified animal diet (A, control); diet A in which fruit and vegetables replaced macro- and micronutrients (B); an uncooked human diet (meat, bread and eggs) supplemented with semi-purified micronutrients (C); diet C with fried or baked products (D); or a complete human diet consisting of cooked products, fruit and vegetables (E). Diets B, C, D and E were prepared according to mean dietary composition figures for the Netherlands. The animal diets contained 21.6% energy fat and the human diets contained 40.6% energy fat. Rats were fed *ad libitum* for 142 weeks. Male but not female rats fed the human diets (C, D or E) had a significantly higher incidence of epithelial tumours ($p < 0.02$) than those fed the animal diets (A or B), mainly accounted for by tumours of the pituitary and thyroid glands. Compared with the uncooked human diet (diet C), frying and baking of food products (diet D) and the addition of fruit and vegetables (diet E) induced minor, non-significant differences in the tumour incidence in over 20 tissues examined.

Effects on carcinogen-induced tumours
Oral cavity
Hamster
Shyu & Meng (1987) studied the inhibitory effect of garlic (*Allium sativum*) administered during the initiation stage of carcinogenesis induced by 7,12-dimethylbenz[a]anthracene (referred to as 9,10-dimethyl-1,2-benzanthracene; DMBA) in the buccal pouch of hamsters. Groups of 5–8 Syrian golden hamsters [age and sex not reported] received a diet containing 10% (w/w) peeled and ground garlic for eight weeks. Painting of 0.5% DMBA on the buccal pouches began in the second week, three times per week for 10 weeks. Animals were killed after 26 weeks. Garlic administration significantly reduced the number and total volume of DMBA-induced tumours per buccal pouch three- and four-fold, respectively [values read from diagrams].

In another study (Meng & Shyu, 1990), groups of 5–8 golden Syrian hamsters [age and sex not specified] were painted with 0.5, 25 or 50% garlic extract in mineral oil three times per week for three weeks and, after a lag period of 11 weeks, with 0.5% DMBA on the right pouch three times per week for 10 weeks. The animals were killed at week 30. Garlic extract treatment increased the latency period of tumour appearance in DMBA-treated animals (8–10 weeks after DMBA painting versus six weeks in controls). The numbers of tumours per pouch in animals treated with DMBA alone and with 25% and 50% garlic extract were 4.6, 1.1 and 1.4, respectively ($p = 0.01$ and 0.003, respectively). The average tumour volume per pouch was also significantly reduced in animals treated with 25% and 50% garlic extract (26.5 and 7.8 mm^3, respectively, versus 72.6 mm^3; $p < 0.01$). [The Working Group noted that the effect could be either local or systemic.]

The ability of black raspberries (*Rubus occidentalis*) of the Jewel variety to inhibit DMBA-induced tumorigenesis in the hamster cheek pouch was evaluated (Casto et al., 2002). Male Syrian golden hamsters, 4–5 weeks of age, were fed 0, 5 or 10% freeze-dried black raspberries in AIN-76A diet for 12 weeks. The concentration of corn starch was adjusted to maintain an isocaloric diet among all groups. Beginning after two weeks, hamster cheek pouches were painted with 0.2% DMBA in dimethylsulfoxide (DMSO) three times per week for eight weeks. The animals were killed after 12–13 weeks and the number and volume of tumours determined. There was no difference in tumour size or incidence between groups. Treatment with 5% but not 10% raspberries resulted in a significant reduction in the multiplicity of tumours relative to DMBA controls (1.9 versus 3.2 tumours per animal; $p = 0.02$). [The Working Group noted inconsistencies between the text and table for the duration of treatment].

Oesophagus
Rat
The effect of strawberries (*Fragaria ananassa*) of the Commander variety on *N*-nitrosomethylbenzylamine (NMBA)-induced tumorigenesis in the oesophagus of male Fischer 344 rats was examined. In a first experiment (Stoner et al., 1999), 5–6-week-old rats (15 animals per group) were placed on AIN-76A diet or a diet containing 5 or 10% freeze-dried strawberries and were maintained on these diets for the duration of the study. The energy content of the berry diets was maintained by appropriately reducing the corn starch content. From two weeks after diet initiation, rats were given a subcutaneous injection of NMBA (0.25 mg/kg bw) once per week for 15 weeks. Controls received either the vehicle (20% DMSO in water) or a diet containing 10% freeze-dried strawberries. Thirty weeks after initiation of NMBA treatment, the rats were killed and oesophageal tumours (papillomas) counted. The 5 and 10% strawberry diets had no effect on tumour incidence but reduced oesophageal tumour multiplicity by 24% ($p < 0.05$) and 56% ($p < 0.01$), respectively, relative to NMBA controls. In addition, both strawberry diets significantly reduced the incidence of lesions classified as dysplastic leukoplakia ($p < 0.05$), while significantly increasing that of lesions classified as simple leukoplakia ($p < 0.05$). In a post-initiation experiment (Carlton et

al., 2001), rats were fed AIN-76A diet and given subcutaneous injections of NMBA (0.5 mg/kg bw) three times per week for five weeks. Immediately after NMBA treatment, animals were placed on control diet or a diet containing 5 or 10% strawberries. The 5 and 10% strawberry diets reduced oesophageal tumour multiplicity at 25 weeks by 38 and 31%, respectively. Both reductions were statistically significant ($p < 0.05$), although there was not a significant dose–response relationship. [The Working Group noted discrepancies between the text and figure for the treatment regimen.]

Their ability of black raspberries of the Driscol and Bristol varieties to inhibit NMBA-induced tumorigenesis in the rat oesophagus was evaluated in both initiation and post-initiation bioassays (Kresty et al., 2001). Groups of 15 male Fischer 344 rats, 7–8 weeks old, were given AIN-76A diet or AIN-76A diet containing 5 or 10% freeze-dried black raspberries. The energy content of the berry diets was maintained by appropriately reducing the corn starch content. Animals were maintained on their respective diets throughout the 30-week study. Starting two weeks after initiation of the experimental diets, rats were given subcutaneous injections of NMBA (0.25 mg/kg bw) once per week for 15 weeks. Controls received either the vehicle (20% DMSO in water) or a diet containing 10% black raspberries. At 30 weeks, the animals were killed and oesophageal papillomas counted. Control animals had no tumours. Feeding 5 and 10% black raspberries significantly reduced the multiplicity of NMBA-induced oesophageal tumours by 39 and 49%, respectively ($p < 0.05$). In a post-initiation bioassay, black raspberries were administered in the diet at 5 and 10% after completion of NMBA treatment. Animals were given subcutaneous injections of NMBA (0.25 mg/kg bw) three times per week for five weeks and maintained on their respective diets until killed at 15, 25 or 35 weeks of the study. Both 5 and 10% black raspberry diets reduced tumour incidence at 25 weeks by 54 and 46%, respectively, tumour multiplicity by 62 and 43%, respectively, and high-grade dysplastic lesions by 43 and 32%, respectively. After 35 weeks, similar significant reductions were seen only with the diet containing 5% black raspberries.

The effect of blueberries (*Vaccinium corymbosum*) of the Rubel variety on NMBA-induced tumorigenesis in the rat oesophagus was investigated (Aziz et al., 2002). Male Fischer 344 rats, 6–7 weeks old, were placed on AIN-76A diet or AIN-76A diets containing 5 or 10% freeze-dried blueberries. The energy content of the berry diets was maintained by appropriately reducing the corn starch content. Animals were maintained on the respective diets throughout the study. Two weeks after initiation of the experimental diets, three groups of rats (25 animals per group) were given subcutaneous injections of NMBA (0.25 mg/kg bw) once per week for 15 weeks. Control groups received either the vehicle (20% DMSO in water) or a diet containing 10% blueberries only. At 25 weeks, the rats were killed and oesophageal tumours were counted and sized. There were no significant differences in tumour incidence, multiplicity or size in berry-fed animals versus animals treated with NMBA only. The authors concluded that the lack of tumour-inhibitory effect of blueberries, in contrast to that of strawberries and black raspberries under similar conditions, might be explained, at least in part, by their relatively low content of ellagic acid.

Colon
Mouse
Mice were treated with 1,2-dimethylhydrazine (DMH) to induce colon tumours and fed cabbage during the initiation and/or post-initiation periods (Temple & El-Khatib, 1987; Temple & Basu, 1987). In the first study, groups of 14–17 male and female Swiss ICR mice, aged 5–7 weeks, were fed control diet or a diet containing 13% cabbage throughout the study. After 31 days, the mice received weekly subcutaneous injections of DMH at gradually increased doses of 23–56 mg/kg bw for seven weeks. All animals were killed 17 weeks after the first dose of DMH. Feeding of the cabbage diet had no significant effect on colon tumour incidence or multiplicity (Temple & El-Khatib, 1987). In the second experiment, cabbage was fed (*a*) starting five weeks before the first injection of DMH until three days after the last (initiation period) or (*b*) starting three days after the first DMH injection for 19.5 weeks (promotion period). DMH was injected once weekly for eight weeks at doses increasing from 17 to 65 mg/kg bw. Feeding of cabbage during the initiation period led to a modest increase in incidence of adenocarcinomas. In contrast, the incidence of adenomas was reduced by 30% and multiplicity by 50% ($p < 0.05$) when cabbage was given during the promotion period (Temple & Basu, 1987).

Van Kranen et al. (1998) evaluated the effect on intestinal neoplasia of the amount of dietary fat and a fruit–vegetable mixture. Groups of 14–17 male and female weanling *Apc*^{Min} mice, a model for multiple intestinal neoplasia, were fed a low-fat (20% fat energy) or a high-fat (40% fat energy) diet with or without a freeze-dried fruit–vegetable mixture (19.5 and 22.3% w/w, respectively). The choice of fruits and vegetables was based on the mean fruit and vegetable consumption in The Netherlands. The composition of the high-fat diets was adjusted to allow for decreased food consumption in these groups. Because of the early onset of tumours in these mice, exposure to the diets was started *in utero* and continued until around day 90 after birth. The fruit–vegetable mixture added to the low-fat diet significantly lowered the multiplicity of polyps in the small intestine (from 16.2 to 10.2 per mouse) but not in the colon, in male mice only. Surprisingly, the multiplicity of intestinal polyps was significantly increased in both male and female mice on the high-fat diet containing fruit–vegetable mixture (from 16.5 to 26.8 polyps per mouse on average).

Rat
Alink *et al.* (1993) studied the modulating effect of heat processing of and addition of fruit and vegetables to human diets on DMH-induced colon tumours in male Wistar rats. The same diets as in the chronic study were used, which included 19.5% of fruit and vegetable mixture (Alink *et al.*, 1989; see Effects on spontaneous tumours above). These diets were fed throughout the study. After four weeks, each rat was given one weekly subcutaneous injection of DMH (50 mg/kg bw) for 10 weeks. Animals were killed after eight months. A lower multiplicity of polypoid adenomas was found in rats consuming the animal diet with fruit and vegetables compared with the control animal diet (1.4 versus 2.6; $p < 0.01$). In contrast, adding fruit and vegetables to the fried or baked human diet increased the multiplicity of adenocarcinomas (2.9 versus 2.1; $p < 0.05$). The authors hypothesized that this might be due to an interaction between fat and non-nutrient components of the fruit and vegetables.

In a further experiment, the effect of low- and high-fat diets in combination with a fruit–vegetable mixture on DMH-induced colon carcinogenesis was studied (Rijnkels *et al.*, 1997a, b). Groups of 30 five-week-old male Wistar rats were maintained on low-fat (20% fat energy) or high-fat (40% fat energy) diets with or without 19.5% of fruit–vegetable mixture. After four weeks, each rat was given one weekly subcutaneous injection of DMH (50 mg/kg bw) for 10 weeks. The experiment was terminated 35 weeks after initiation of the diet regimen. The fruit–vegetable mixture added to either the low-fat or the high-fat diet induced a non-significant decrease in the number of adenomas.

The effect of a fruit–vegetable mixture on *N*-methyl-*N*-nitro-*N*-nitrosoguanidine (MNNG)-induced colon carcinogenesis was studied in male Wistar rats (Rijnkels *et al.*, 1997c). Groups of 30 five-week-old rats were fed low-fat or high-fat semi-purified diets with or without 19.5% of a fruit–vegetable mixture. After four weeks, all animals were given weekly intrarectal instillations of MNNG (6 mg/kg bw) for five weeks. After 35 weeks, all animals were killed and colon tumours were evaluated histopathologically. The fruit–vegetable mixture significantly reduced the development of colon adenocarcinomas ($p < 0.01$) when added to the high-fat diet, but not when added to the low-fat diet.

The effects of a fruit–vegetable mixture administered during the initiation and promotion stages of azoxymethane (AOM)-induced colon carcinogenesis were studied in rats (Rijnkels *et al.*, 1998). Groups of 30 five-week-old male Fischer 344 rats were fed semi-purified low-fat (20% fat energy) or high-fat (40% fat energy) diets with or without 19.5% of fruit–vegetable mixture. Four weeks after initiation of the experiment, all animals were given three weekly subcutaneous injections of AOM (15 mg/kg bw). Eight weeks after the start of the study, animals on control diets were switched to the corresponding diet supplemented with a fruit–vegetable mixture and those on the fruit–vegetable diets were switched to the corresponding control diet, in both cases until 36 weeks from the beginning of the experiment. The fruit–vegetable mixture administered during either the initiation or the post-initiation stage had no effect on AOM-induced colon carcinogenesis, irrespective of the fat content of the diet.

The effect of tomato juice on *N*-methylnitrosourea (MNU)-induced colon carcinogenesis was studied in female Fischer 344 rats (Narisawa *et al.*, 1998). Groups of 24 or 25 seven-week-old rats received intrarectal instillations of MNU at 2 mg or 4 mg three times per week for three weeks. Animals had free access to water (control group), a 17 ppm aqueous lycopene solution, or tomato juice diluted 1:2 or 1:14 and containing 17 ppm or 3.4 ppm [*sic*] lycopene, respectively. The colon tumour incidence was evaluated at week 35. After administration of 2 or 4 mg MNU, consumption of tomato juice containing 17 ppm lycopene significantly reduced colon tumour incidence compared with the other groups, and tumour multiplicity compared with controls only. The more dilute tomato juice had no effect on colon carcinogenesis.

Miyagi *et al.* (2000) studied the effect of orange juice administered during the post-initiation period of AOM-induced colon carcinogenesis in rats. Groups of 30 male Fischer 344 rats, 21 days old, were fed control diet until 36 days of age. At 22 and 29 days of age, all animals were given a subcutaneous injection of AOM (15 mg/kg bw). One week after the second dose of AOM, one group was switched from drinking water to orange juice and a modified diet, while the other group remained on the control diet. [The Working Group noted that the source of carbohydrate in the control diet was primarily corn flour, whereas the diet of the orange juice group was more sucrose-based]. The study was terminated at 33 weeks of age. There was a 22% lower colon tumour incidence

($p < 0.05$) in the animals given orange juice. [The Working Group noted that the total energy intake was not calculated, but final body weights were similar between the groups].

The effect of mandarin juice on AOM-induced colon carcinogenesis was studied in seven-week-old male Fischer 344 rats (20–29 per group) (Tanaka et al., 2000). All animals were fed control diet and were given a subcutaneous dose of AOM (20 mg/kg bw) once per week for two weeks. Beginning one week after the second dose of AOM, one group was switched from drinking water to commercial mandarin juice at night-time, while maintained on a control diet. The experiment was terminated at week 38. The incidence and multiplicity of colon adenocarcinomas were significantly decreased in animals given mandarin juice (35% versus 69% in controls, $p < 0.02$; 0.40 ± 0.58 versus 0.76 ± 0.57 tumours per rat; $p < 0.05$, respectively).

The effect of orange pulp on DMH-induced colon tumorigenesis was studied in Sprague-Dawley rats (Kossoy et al., 2001). Five week-old rats [sex unspecified] were fed control diet ($n = 30$) or experimental diet containing 15% orange pulp ($n = 42$). DMH was injected at 20 mg/kg bw once weekly for six weeks starting together with administration of experimental diet. The experiment was continued for eight months. Administration of orange pulp in the diet had no effect on the incidence of total colon adenocarcinomas, but significantly reduced the incidence of the more advanced endophytic adenocarcinomas in the colon ($p < 0.05$), while significantly increasing that of the less advanced exophytic adenocarcinomas ($p < 0.05$).

Inhibition of AOM-induced colon carcinogenesis by black raspberries (Rubus occidentalis) of the Jewel variety was studied in rats (Harris et al., 2001). Groups of 18 male Fischer 344 rats, 8–9 weeks old, were given intraperitoneal injections of AOM (15 mg/kg bw) once per week for two weeks. Control animals received an equal volume of saline only or a diet containing 5% freeze-dried black raspberries. Animals were switched to a diet containing 0, 2.5, 5 or 10% black raspberries 24 hours after the last AOM injection and were maintained on these diets throughout the experiment. The sucrose content of the berry diets was reduced to maintain the energy content of the diets. The number of aberrant crypt foci nine weeks after the last dose of AOM decreased by 34%, 25% and 21% in the groups fed 2.5, 5 and 10% black raspberry, respectively, relative to the AOM-only group. The reductions were significant compared with controls in all groups ($p < 0.01$), although there was not a significant dose–response relationship. At 33 weeks after the last dose of AOM, the remaining animals were killed and the tumours analysed. Control animals had no tumours. Total tumour multiplicity (adenomas + adenocarcinomas) was reduced by 42, 45 and 71% in the groups fed 2.5, 5 and 10% black raspberry, respectively, relative to AOM controls ($p < 0.05$ for all groups). Adenocarcinoma multiplicity decreased by 28, 35 and 80% in the same groups; only the reduction in rats fed 10% black raspberry was significant ($p < 0.01$).

Liver
Rat
Groups of male weanling Fischer 344 rats were fed a semi-purified diet containing 25% (w/w) freeze-dried ground cabbage (*Brassica oleracea* L.) or table beet (*Beta vulgaris* L.), with or without 1 ppm aflatoxin B$_1$ (Boyd et al., 1982). After 26 weeks of treatment, all animals were maintained on basal diet without aflatoxin for a further 16 weeks. Control animals had no tumours. The mean, median and maximum size, and the number of tumours exceeding 10 mm in diameter were all significantly lower ($p < 0.05$) in animals fed the cabbage diet. [The Working Group noted that the cabbage diet resulted in decreased food intake and thus decreased intake of aflatoxin B$_1$.]

Groups of 25 male Sprague-Dawley rats, two months old, were given N-nitrosodiethlamine (NDEA) in drinking water for 10 weeks (total dose 500 mg/kg bw) (Rieder et al., 1983). Animals were fed a control diet or 120 or 160 g of carrots per week without any other supplementary food. [The Working Group considered that the amount of carrots given was very high (unbalanced diet), as was the dose of carcinogen administered.] In the first study (120 or 160 g carrots per week), feeding of carrots started together with carcinogen administration; in the second study (160 g of 'biological' or 'market' carrots per week), feeding started two weeks before carcinogen administration. Carrots were given for 14 weeks. Feeding 120 g or 160 g carrots per week together with or before carcinogen treatment significantly delayed tumour occurrence and prolonged survival compared with animals on the control diet. The effects with 160 g carrots per week were significantly greater than those with 120 g carrots per week. No difference was observed between the 'biological' and 'market' carrots.

Toad
Sadek et al. (1995) assessed the effect of cabbage on DMBA-induced hepatocarcinogenesis in toads (*Bufo viridis*). DMBA (0.5 mg in 0.1 mL olive oil) was administered into dorsal lymph sacos of sexually mature male and female toads weighting 40 g, three times per week for 12 weeks. Controls received olive oil only. A solution of ground cabbage leaves was fed at 1 or 2 mL per animal per day for 12 weeks starting 3 h before carcinogen treatment or 3 h

after carcinogen treatment. Toads treated with 1 or 2 mL cabbage 3 h before DMBA treatment (initiation period) showed a significantly lower incidence of hepatocellular carcinomas compared with those treated with DMBA alone. However, feeding of cabbage after carcinogen treatment (post-initiation period) had no effect on liver tumour incidence compared with animals treated with DMBA alone.

Lung
Mouse
The ability of strawberries (*Fragaria ananassa*) of the Allstar variety to inhibit lung tumorigenesis after induction with 4-(methylnitrosamino)-1-(3-pyridyl)-1-butanone (NNK) or benzo[*a*]pyrene (B[a]P) was examined in A/J mice (Carlton et al., 2000). Groups of 20 mice were fed AIN-76A diet or a diet containing 10% freeze-dried strawberries for the entire duration of the study. The diet was modified to maintain total energy intake. One week after diet initiation, mice were treated with NNK or B[a]P over a two-week period. NNK was administered in saline by intraperitoneal injection in five doses of 0.414 mg each. B[a]P was administered in cottonseed oil by gavage in five doses of 0.2 mg each. Animals were killed 20 or 24 weeks after the first dose of NNK or B[a]P, respectively. There was no significant difference in lung tumour incidence or tumour multiplicity between the 10% strawberry groups and their respective control groups.

The effect of mandarin juice on NNK-induced pulmonary carcinogenesis was studied in male A/J mice (Kohno et al., 2001). Seven-week-old mice (20–23 per group) were given a single intraperitoneal injection of NNK (10 μmol per mouse). One week later, one group received mandarin juice in drinking water at night for 21 weeks. Administration of mandarin juice had no effect on lung tumour incidence or multiplicity or on incidence of alveolar cell hyperplasia.

Skin
Mouse
The effect of bitter gourd extract in water (*Momordica charantia*) was studied in 4–5-week-old female Swiss albino mice (Ganguly et al., 2000). One group of 25 mice received three topical applications of 1% DMBA on alternate days followed by 1% croton oil applied twice weekly for two months. The other group of 25 mice received the same treatment simultaneously with oral administration of 5% bitter gourd extract (50 μL per mouse) daily for three months. Treatment with bitter gourd extract delayed the appearance of skin papillomas and significantly reduced the incidence of papillomas at 12 weeks (control diet, 78%; bitter gourd diet, 19.5% [values read from diagram]; $p < 0.05$), but did not affect the multiplicity.

Mammary gland
Rat
The effect of Brussels sprouts (*Brassica oleracea* L.) administered during the initiation and progression stages of DMBA-induced mammary carcinogenesis was studied in Sprague-Dawley rats (Stoewsand et al., 1988). Female rats, five weeks old, were divided into groups of 15 animals. One group (I) was fed 20% freeze-dried Brussels sprouts for the first four weeks, followed by 48 weeks on basal diet. The other group (II) was fed basal diet for 17 weeks and then switched to the Brussels sprouts diet for 35 weeks, until termination of the study. All animals received a single oral dose of DMBA (60 mg/kg bw) two weeks after the beginning of the study. Administration of Brussels sprouts during the initiation period (group I) significantly reduced the incidence of DMBA-induced palpable mammary tumours 15 weeks after dosing (13% versus 77%; $p < 0.01$) and of adenocarcinomas 50 weeks after dosing ($p < 0.05$). [The Working Group noted that the study did not include appropriate controls for the progression period and that animals in group II had significantly lower body weight.] In another study with the same initiation protocol (Stoewsand et al., 1989), administration of Brussels sprouts 27 weeks after DMBA injection reduced the incidence and multiplicity of DMBA-induced papillary carcinomas and adenocarcinomas, and significantly reduced proliferation, anaplasia and invasiveness in these tumours.

Groups of 50-day old female Sprague-Dawley rats were given a single injection of MNU (50 mg/kg bw) into the tail vein. Rats were then assigned to groups (25–35 in each group) and fed a control-fat (5%) diet containing 5 or 10% dried cabbage, 3.2% cabbage residue or 5% collards, or a high-fat (24.6%) diet containing 5% cabbage or 5% collards. The study was terminated when palpable mammary tumours reached a diameter of 0.5 cm or at 24 weeks. The rats on the control-fat diet containing 5% cabbage or 3.2% cabbage residue had significantly lower incidence [25 to 38% decrease] of mammary adenocarcinomas than rats fed the control diet without cabbage. This effect was not observed in rats on the high-fat diet containing cabbage (Bresnick et al., 1990).

Liu et al. (1992) determined the efficacy of garlic powder administered during the initiation and post-initiation periods of DMBA-induced mammary carcinogenesis in rats. In an initiation study, groups of 41-day old female Sprague-Dawley rats were fed a diet containing 0, 1, 2 or 4% garlic powder for two weeks before and two weeks after a single DMBA treatment by intubation (25 mg/kg bw). In an initiation and post-initiation study, groups of female Sprague-Dawley rats were fed

2% garlic powder from two weeks before DMBA treatment until termination of the study at 24 weeks. Garlic administered during initiation (at the 4% level) and during initiation and post-initiation significantly ($p < 0.05$) reduced DMBA-induced mammary tumour incidence (35% and 40%, respectively, versus 85% in controls) and multiplicity (1.57 and 1.50 tumours per tumour-bearing rat, respectively, versus 2.41 in controls).

Three groups of 25 female Sprague-Dawley rats, 41 days of age, were fed control diet or a 2% freeze-dried milled garlic powder diet two weeks before and one week after intragastric administration of 10 mg DMBA (initiation period), or the same diet from two weeks before until 24 weeks after DMBA administration (initiation and post-initiation period), when the experiment was terminated (Ip et al., 1992). Administration of garlic powder during the initiation stage had a slight but not significant effect on mammary tumour incidence and multiplicity, whereas continuous administration of garlic powder significantly ($p < 0.05$) reduced both mammary tumour incidence (84 versus 56%) and multiplicity [2.84 versus 1.52 tumours per rat].

The effect of garlic powder on MNU-induced mammary carcinogenesis was studied in female Sprague-Dawley rats (Schaffer et al., 1996). Groups of rats, 41 days of age, were fed the control diet or experimental diet containing 2% garlic powder for 14 days (21 rats per group). All rats then received MNU intraperitoneally (15 mg/kg bw) and continued on their dietary regimen for 25 weeks. Administration of garlic powder in the diet significantly ($p < 0.05$) reduced mammary tumour incidence (by 76%) and tumour multiplicity (by 81%).

The effect of dietary Thai bitter gourd administered during the initiation stage of DMBA-induced mammary carcinogenesis was studied in female Sprague-Dawley rats (Kusamran et al., 1998a). Groups of 41-day-old animals were pair-fed on control diet or experimental diet containing 6.25 or 12.5% freeze-dried Thai bitter gourd for two weeks before and one week after a single oral dose of DMBA (50 mg/kg bw) and killed 25 weeks after dosing. Administration of Thai bitter gourd at 6.25 and 12.5% during the initiation stage significantly suppressed the multiplicity of mammary tumours [by 50%, read from diagram], but had no effect on the incidence.

Uterine cervix
Mouse
The effect of garlic on 3-methylcholanthrene (3-MC)-induced cervical carcinogenesis was evaluated in groups of random-bred 8–10-week-old virgin Swiss albino mice (Hussain et al., 1990). A sterile cotton thread impregnated with beeswax containing about 600 µg 3-MC was inserted into the canal of the uterine cervix by means of a laparotomy. Ground garlic prepared in distilled water at a level of 1% was administered orally at a dose of 400 mg/kg bw per day for two weeks before and four weeks after 3-MC thread insertion. Twelve weeks after the insertion of threads, all animals were killed and tissues were processed for histopathological examination. Administration of garlic significantly decreased the incidence of 3-MC-induced squamous-cell carcinoma of the uterine cervix (23% versus 73% in controls). However, garlic had no effect on the incidences of hyperplasia and dysplasia in the uterine cervix.

Bladder
Mouse
The effect of aged garlic extract on bladder carcinogenesis was evaluated in female C3H/HeN mice given implants of MBT2 bladder tumour cells (Riggs et al., 1997). MBT2 bladder tumours were originally induced in C3H/HeN mice by oral administration of N-[4-(5-nitro-2-furyl)-2-thiazolyl]formamide (FANFT). Tumour cells for transplantation were prepared by mincing tumours and mechanically dispersing the tissue into a single-cell suspension. Garlic extract was administered orally at doses of 5, 50 and 500 mg/100 mL drinking water. One month after initiation of garlic treatment, 1000 MBT2 cells in 0.1 mL cell culture medium were subcutaneously injected into the right thigh. The experiment was terminated 23 days after tumour cell implantation for determination of tumour incidence and after 35 days for tumour volume. Treatment with garlic led to a dose-dependent reduction in tumour incidence, which was statistically significant at the highest dose (500 mg/100 mL). In addition, animals that received 50 and 500 mg garlic extract in drinking water had significant reductions in tumour volume (2563 and 1644 mm^3, respectively, versus 4047 mm^3 in controls).

Rat
The inhibitory properties of tomato juice against urinary bladder carcinogenesis were evaluated in rats (Okajima et al., 1998). Bladder cancer was induced in six-week-old male Fischer 344 rats by 0.05% N-butyl-N-(4-hydroxybutyl)nitrosamine (BBN) given in the drinking water for eight weeks. This was followed by tap water (control) or tomato juice diluted 1:4 for 12 weeks. BBN induced simple hyperplasia, nodulopapillary hyperplasia and transitional-cell carcinomas in the urinary bladder. Tomato juice reduced the multiplicity (1.17 ± 0.9 versus 2.20 ± 1.4; $p < 0.05$) but not the incidence of transitional-cell carcinomas, and had no effect on simple or nodulopapillary hyperplasia in the bladder.

Biomarkers

Intermediary biomarkers that are potentially related to cancer risk include markers for uptake, chemical activation, deactivation and DNA-binding of carcinogens, DNA repair, cytogenetic markers and markers for oxidative damage to DNA. Other intermediary cancer biomarkers relate to cell turnover and apoptosis, to intercellular communication and to altered expression of genes involved in the cell cycle and its regulation. The following review covers studies of the effect of diets enriched with fruits and vegetables on such biomarkers in experimental animals, which have mostly used extracts prepared from single fruits and vegetables. Much research has concentrated on the effects of compounds contained in *Brassica* vegetables, *Allium* vegetables and polyphenol-rich plants or their extracts.

Effects on phase I and II enzymes
Total fruit and vegetables

Several studies have considered the effects of fruit and vegetable mixtures on enzyme induction. In a three-month feeding study on the effects of human-type diets on hepatic drug-metabolizing enzymes (Alink et al., 1988), groups of five male and five female Wistar SPF rats were fed a semi-synthetic control diet or a complete northern European (Dutch) diet without vegetables and fruit, or a complete northern European diet including 19.9% local summer vegetables and fruit (40.1% potato, 3.4% banana, 10.3% orange, 21.8% apple, 4.3% each of lettuce, tomato, cucumber and cauliflower, 2.9% each of leek and spinach, and 1.4% pepper) or lyophilized semi-synthetic diets containing 20.1% local summer vegetables plus fruit or 20.0% local winter vegetables (44.6% potato, 3.8% banana, 11.5% orange, 24.2% apple, 3.2% each of red cabbage, white cabbage, sauerkraut and beet, and 1.6% each of carrot and Brussels sprout) plus fruit. Vitamins and minerals were added to all diets to the same final content and diets were isocaloric and with similar distribution of energy from fat (40%), protein (13%) and carbohydrate (47%) by addition of semi-purified components identical to those used in the control feed. The diets were irradiated at 500 krad and analysed to ensure equal contents of vitamins and minerals in each diet and stored at −40 °C until use. All three diets containing fruits or vegetables significantly increased hepatic ethoxycoumarin-*O*-deethylase activity (ECOD) in the male rats by 33–42%, whereas only hepatic ethoxyresorufin-*O*-deethylase (EROD) activity was increased (by 96–122%) in the female group fed summer vegetables and fruit compared to the control group. The increase in the females dosed with summer vegetables based on the northern European diet also was not significant compared with the group given the corresponding diet without vegetables and fruit (12%). Aminopyrine-*N*-demethylase was not affected by any of the treatments in either sex. Total CYP enzyme activity was increased only in male rats given the northern European diet without vegetables and in the winter vegetables group (by 20%). Hepatic glutathione-*S*-transferase (GST) was only increased in the males by summer vegetables and fruits (by 81%), while UDP-glucuronosyltransferase (UGT) activity was unaffected. Microsomes from the rat livers were subsequently screened in *Salmonella typhimurium* TA98 for their ability to activate benzo[a]pyrene (B[a]P) to mutagenic products. All fruit- and vegetable-containing diets decreased the ability of subsequently prepared hepatic microsomes to activate B[a]P by 20–40% (estimated from diagram). A similar assay in *S. typhimurium* TA100 showed that all human diets, except the complete northern European diet including summer vegetables and fruit, caused a 25–50% decrease (estimated from diagram) in the activation of *N*-nitrosodimethylamine (NDMA) by subsequently prepared hepatic microsomes.

Hepatic and colonic enzyme activities induced by six weeks' feeding of a vegetable–fruit mixture (19.5% w/w) (35.1% potato, 3.0% banana, 9.0% orange, 19.1% apple, 3.75% lettuce, 1.25% green pepper, 3.75% tomato, cucumber and cauliflower, 2.5% each of spinach, leek, red cabbage, white cabbage, sauerkraut and beetroot, and 1.25% each of carrot and Brussels sprout) was investigated in groups of five male Wistar rats fed low- or high-fat diets (20 or 40% of energy) (Rijnkels & Alink, 1998). Half of the animals in each group were treated with DMH (four subcutaneous injections of 50 mg/kg bw from week 2 to 5). In the liver of control rats on the low-fat diet, the vegetable mixture increased GST, decreased NDMA-demethylase and left EROD and pentoxyresorufin-*O*-deethylase (PROD) unaffected. In low-fat DMH-treated rats, the effect was reversed and PROD was increased by the vegetable and fruit treatment. The reported changes in enzyme activities were from 1.2- to 2.1-fold. In rats fed the high-fat diet, fruit and vegetable treatments had no effect.

Studies with several individual vegetables

A few studies have been performed to compare the effects of individual vegetables on enzyme induction. Bradfield et al. (1985) fed a range of powdered vegetables (cauliflower, carrot, kale, beet, Brussels sprout, egg plant or onion), mixed individually at a 20% level into isocaloric feeds, for 10 days to groups of four or five male C57BL/6 mice. Kale, cauliflower and carrots significantly increased hepatic ECOD activity 1.3, 2.2 and 1.2-fold, respectively, whereas Brussels sprouts, cauliflower and onions similarly increased hepatic epoxide hydrolase (1.6-, 1.6-, and 2.3-fold) and GST activities (2.0-, 1.2-, and 1.8-fold), respectively.

Dried powdered preparations of cabbage (20% w/w) or Brussels sprouts (20% w/w) fed individually to groups of 5–10 female ICR/Ha mice for two weeks also significantly increased GST activity in the small intestine (2.1- and 3.1-fold, respectively) (Sparnins et al., 1982). In the liver, only Brussels sprouts increased the activity (1.8-fold). [The Working Group noted that no compensation for the vegetables was made to the control diets.]

Lyophilized vegetables were individually added (12 g per rat per day) to human-type diets (23 g per rat per day) offered for three weeks to groups of three male Fischer 344 rats and induction of phase I and II enzymes in the liver and colon was measured (O'Neill et al., 1997). [The Working Group noted that actual intakes were not recorded.] Broccoli and Brussels sprouts significantly increased hepatic GST by 24–64%, whereas broccoli decreased colonic GST by 35%. Spinach, tomato paste, peas and peppers significantly decreased GST, mainly in the liver, and changes were all below 20%. [The Working Group noted that the changes seemed too small to be truly statistically significant taking into account the small numbers in each group]. GST activity determined with either chloro-dinitrobenzene (CDNB) or dichloro-nitrobenzene (DCNB) as substrate gave highly correlated results. No effect on quinone reductase (QR) in liver or colon was reported. CYP 1A1 was increased in liver only after treatment with Brussels sprouts, whereas no effects on this enzyme or on CYP 1A2, 2B1, 2B2, 3A or 2E11 were observed in liver or colon with any other treatment.

Kusamran et al. (1998b) fed two freeze-dried preparations of vegetables commonly consumed in Thailand (Thai and Chinese bitter gourd, both at 12.5% in the diet, substituting proportional amounts of carbohydrate, fibre and protein) to groups of 10 pair-fed male Wistar rats for two weeks. Thai bitter gourd decreased hepatic aniline hydroxylase and aminopyrine-N-demethylase by 37% and 28%, respectively, increased GST by 59% and counteracted ex vivo activation by hepatic S9 preparations of aflatoxin B$_1$ and B[a]P by 30–64%.

Single fruits and vegetables
Various studies have examined the ability of a single fruit or vegetable to modify activities of phase I or II enzymes in experimental animals. Experiments with *Brassica* (broccoli, cabbage, Brussels sprout), *Allium* (garlic and onion), *Momordica* (bitter gourd) and citrus (grapefruit) species have been reported.

Groups of female ICR/Ha mice [number of animals per group not given] were given suspensions of broccoli tablets in 1% carboxymethylcellulose, 25% glycerol (1 g/kg bw) by gavage (Clapper et al., 1997). [The Working Group noted that the dose was unclear; the concentration of broccoli in the suspension was not stated.] The broccoli tablets contained 5 g of lyophilized pesticide-free broccoli. GST activity in colon tissues was higher one day after broccoli administration, but decreased by day two. GSTμ and π were significantly induced one day after the treatment and decreased almost to baseline by day 2 [the Working Group noted that the exact increase was not stated].

Groups of five female Wistar rats were fed a 10% broccoli diet for seven days or a control diet containing the same amount of carbohydrates, fibres, proteins and vitamins (Vang et al., 1991). In the liver, levels of CYP1A1, 1A2, 2B and 2E1 proteins and of total CYP1A mRNA increased, whereas mRNAs corresponding to the other proteins were unaffected. In the colon, CYP1A1, 2B and 2E1 proteins as well as CYP1A1 mRNA increased, whereas CYP2B mRNA decreased. CYP1A2 protein and mRNA were either unaffected or undetectable.

A subsequent study with a similar design examined the effects of feeding broccoli samples, varying in their contents of glucosinolates, on testicular phase I and II enzymes and antioxidant enzymes (Vang et al., 1999). The broccoli, grown with varying amounts of N and S fertilizer or organically, was fed at a level of 10% in the diet to groups of 8–10 male Wistar rats for one week. Broccoli, most prominently that grown with high levels of N fertilizer, affected GST (1.6-fold induction) and UGT (1.8-fold induction), but did not statistically significantly change the activities of epoxide hydrolase, QR, p-sulfotransferase or the anti-oxidative enzymes catalase (CAT) and glutathione peroxidase (GPX) in rat testes. CYP enzyme activities were also measured in this study (Vang et al., 2001). Dietary broccoli induced the CYP1A activities, EROD and 7 methoxy-resorufin-O-demethylase (MROD), in rat liver and weakly in colon, but not in kidney. Consistent with this finding, the hepatic metabolism of 2-amino-1-methyl-6-phenylimidazo[4,5-b]pyridine (PhIP) to the proximate carcinogen N-hydroxy-PhIP, a CYP1A-related activity, was enhanced by broccoli. PROD activity, an assay for CYP2B1/2, was weakly induced in colon and kidney but not in liver. The 2β-hydroxy- and 6β-hydroxy-testosterone hydroxylase activities were induced in liver microsomes, showing that broccoli increased CYP3A activity. The observed modulations of CYP activities depended clearly on the broccoli sample used, the Shogun cultivar giving a higher response than Emperor. Significantly different levels of enzyme induction were observed with broccoli samples grown under different conditions.

Groups of four male Wistar rats (McDanell et al., 1989) were fed *ad libitum* during six days a semi-synthetic diet with or without 25% freeze-dried Brussels sprouts, or an equivalent amount of aqueous methanolic Brussels sprouts extract, or the residue remaining after this extraction. Feeding Brussels sprouts increased EROD 2.5-, 4.9- and 4.1-fold in the liver, small and large intestine, respectively; feeding the extract also increased, although slightly, the enzymatic activity, whereas the residue was without effect. In a time-course study, groups of four male Wistar rats were fed 20 g of a single semi-synthetic meal containing 25% (dry weight) cabbage [the Working Group noted that no modification was made to the control feed] (McDanell et al., 1989). EROD activity was significantly decreased in the liver 1–2 hours after dosing and in the small intestine was significantly increased 4–6 h after dosing. No effect was observed in the large intestine.

In two dose–response studies (Bogaards et al., 1990), groups of 5–8 newly weaned male Fischer 344 rats were fed a semi-synthetic diet with 0, 2.5, 5, 10, 15, 20 or 30% Brussels sprouts added (substituting for protein and fibre) during a 28-day period, after which the liver and small intestines were analysed for GST activity (using CDNB as substrate) and content of GST subunits 1, 2, 3, 4 and 7. Casein and cellulose were given to controls, for protein and fibre compensation. A significant dose–response relationship was observed, with increases of 17% in GST activity and 15% in GST protein content in the liver after the lowest dose. The corresponding figures were 182% and 121% after the highest dose. Subunits 1, 2 and 3 appeared to be the most responsive. In the small intestine, GST activity was induced only after feeding 15% or more of Brussels sprouts. GST protein subunits 1, 2 and 4 were significantly induced after feeding 15% or 30% Brussels sprouts. Total GST protein, determined only in the second experiment, was not significantly induced after feeding 20% Brussels sprouts.

Groups of six male Wistar rats were fed 0–20% cooked Brussels sprouts in the diet for periods of 2–28 days and liver and small intestines were assayed for various phase I and phase II activities (Wortelboer et al., 1992). Hepatic microsomal EROD and PROD were increased from day 2 onwards in rats given 20% Brussels sprouts in the diet and from day 14 onwards in rats given 5%. No effect was observed at the 2.5% dietary level. In the small intestine, EROD and PROD activities were increased only at the highest dose, after 2 and 7 days, respectively. Hepatic microsomal testosterone 2β- and 6β-hydroxylase activities were increased from 7 and 14 days onwards in the highest dose group only and no effects were observed in microsomes from the small intestine. Western blots indicated dose-related increased levels of CYP1A2 in the liver and of CYP2B1/2 in the small intestine. Hepatic GST, UGT type 1 and DT-diaphorase tended to increase from day 2 at the two higher dose levels and glucuronyl transferase 1 also increased after 28 days of feeding with 2.5% Brussels sprouts. In contrast, glucuronyl transferase 2 decreased initially at the 2.5 and 5% levels, but after 28 days there was no effect at these lower dose levels, while an increase was observed in the rats fed 20% Brussels sprouts. In the small intestine, GST increased from day 2 at the 20% dose level whereas DT-diaphorase increased, on day 2 only, at both the 5% and 20% dose levels.

Groups of eight male Wistar rats were treated by gavage with Brussels sprouts extract equivalent to 7 g per day of fresh vegetable for four days and livers and kidneys were removed 6 h after the last dose to assay expression or activities of phase I and II enzymes (Sorensen et al., 2001). No change was observed in the expression of hepatic CYP1A2, CYP2B or CYP2E1. The QR activity increased by 155% in liver but not in kidney, and hepatic expression of GSTπ increased by 30%.

Liu et al. (1992) examined the influence on liver and mammary GST activity of dietary supplements of garlic powder (2 or 4%) fed to groups of five female Sprague-Dawley rats. After two weeks of treatment, garlic at 2 or 4% increased GST activity by 91 and 100%, respectively, in liver and by 42% and 47% in the mammary tissue.

In groups of 6–8 male Sprague-Dawley rats, oral treatment with 200–1000 mg/kg bw garlic oil daily for 1–3 days led to increases in GST expression (50–150%) and activity (~40%) in rat liver and decreases in CYP activities, notably inducible CYP2E1 (Kwak et al., 1995).

Groups of male Wistar rats [number of rats per group not given] were fed 0.1, 0.5 or 1% powdered garlic for four weeks before a single dose of B[a]P or 3-MC and urine was collected for 24 h (Polasa & Krishnaswamy, 1997). The animals were then killed and the liver and lungs assayed for QR and the liver for GST (CDNB substrate). Garlic dose-dependently decreased urinary mutagenicity in *S. typhimurium* TA98 after B[a]P dosing, whereas mutagenicity in TA100 or mutagenicity in both strains after 3-MC dosing was decreased to an equal extent by all three garlic dose levels. All three doses increased hepatic GST (30–43%) and QR (80–100%, read from diagram) and lung QR (40–50%, read from diagram) to similar extents.

The interaction with respect to hepatic phase I and II enzymes between dietary fat and garlic oil (200 mg/kg bw) given as three weekly intubations during seven weeks was investigated in groups of 4–5 male Sprague-Dawley rats (Sheen et al., 1999). Garlic oil increased GST activity by 38–40%, but did not significantly affect NDMA-demethylase, PROD, total CYP or total NADPH-cytochrome c reductase. Immunoblot analyses revealed increased hepatic levels of CYP2B1 and GST (placental form) and decreased CYP2E1 after intubation with garlic oil. The content of fat (5 or 20%) in the feed did not interact with garlic oil. In a subsequent study, groups of five male Sprague-Dawley rats, fed either a low- or high-fat diet, were treated with 0, 30, 80 or 200 mg/kg bw garlic oil by gavage three times per week for six weeks (Chen et al., 2001a). Garlic oil dose-dependently increased liver GST and PROD activities and CYP2B1 mRNA and protein levels. Again, the effects of garlic oil were independent of dietary fat content.

Oral administration of bitter gourd extract (5% in water) daily for three months to groups of eight Swiss albino female mice significantly increased hepatic GST in normal mice and in mice skin-painted with DMBA (Ganguly et al., 2000).

Grapefruit juice is known to have some capacity to modify the biotransformation of certain drugs (Bailey et al., 1994). The effect was investigated in groups of 6–9 male Sprague-Dawley rats given a daily oral dose of 4 or 8 mL/kg of grapefruit juice for two days, followed on the second day by a dose of pentobarbitone sodium (50 mg/kg). The juice significantly increased sleeping time in a dose-dependent manner (46% and 79%, respectively) (Sharif & Ali, 1994). Administration of 4 mL grapefruit juice per day for two days (four rats per time point) inhibited theophylline metabolism up to 90 min after administration of theophylline (10 mg/kg bw). Pure commercial grapefruit juice offered instead of drinking water to groups of three male Fischer 344 rats did not affect the plasma clearance of a subsequent dose of PhIP (60 mg/kg bw) (Miyata et al., 2002).

In summary, fruit and vegetable mixtures at levels relevant to human dietary intakes can increase both phase I and II xenobiotic-metabolizing enzyme activities. Evidence from studies with high doses of single vegetables indicates a stronger ability to induce phase II enzymes. Induction has been observed both in the liver and extrahepatically in lung, intestines and mammary tissue. In studies looking at dose–response effects, phase II enzymes were induced in a dose-related manner.

Inhibition of damage to macromolecules
Mixtures of fruit and vegetables
Groups of 4–5 female Sprague-Dawley rats were fed a standard diet, or a specially composed diet with cereals and cereal by-products, or vegetable by-products, milk and sugar, or vegetable by-products together with meat and fish by-products and vegetable oil. Blood samples were collected after four weeks to determine background levels of 4-aminobiphenyl adducts in haemoglobin (Richter et al., 2000). [The Working Group noted that no information was given on the nature of the vegetables included in the diets and that only the vegetable and milk diet was similar to the control diet in macronutrient composition]. Adduct levels were significantly decreased by 50% in animals on both diets containing vegetable by-products, whereas the cereal-based (high-fibre) diet had no effect.

Individual fruit and vegetables
The protective effect of garden cress (*Lepidium sativum*) towards genotoxic effects induced by 2-amino-3-methylimidazo[4,5-*f*]quinoline (IQ) was investigated by single-cell gel electrophoresis (SCGE) assays (Kassie et al., 2002). Pretreatment of groups of three male Fischer 344 rats with fresh garden cress juice (0.8 mL) for three consecutive days led to significant reductions ($p < 0.05$) in DNA damage induced by IQ (90 mg/kg, 0.2 mL corn oil/animal) in colon and liver cells in the range of 75–92%.

The influence of dietary supplements of garlic powder (2 or 4%), offered two weeks before and two weeks after DMBA treatment (25 mg/kg bw), significantly and dose-dependently reduced mammary DNA adduct levels (approximately 30–70%, respectively), as determined by ^{32}P-postlabelling in groups of five female Sprague-Dawley rats (Liu et al., 1992). In a subsequent study on the interaction between garlic and selenite on DMBA-induced liver and mammary DNA adducts, marked enhancement of the selenium-induced protection was observed with concomitant garlic treatment (Schaffer et al., 1997). Groups of five female Sprague-Dawley rats were fed sodium selenite (0.1, 0.5 or 1 mg/kg diet) in combination with garlic powder (0, 20 or 40 mg/kg diet) in a 3 × 3 factorial design. After two weeks of feeding, all rats were given 25 mg/kg bw DMBA in corn oil by intubation. After 24 h, total DNA adducts in mammary tissue were determined. Garlic dose-dependently decreased the adduct level in the low-selenium group (40–80%) and the effect was potentiated by dietary selenium, increasing to 50% and almost 100% in the high-selenium group (values read from diagram). A decrease in the specific *anti*-3,4-dihydrodiol-1,2-epoxide deoxyguanosine adduct accounted for almost the entire effect.

Various garlic preparations were fed to groups of six female Sprague-Dawley rats for two weeks before a single intubation of DMBA (25–50 mg/kg bw) and 24 h later, DNA adducts in breast tissue were analysed by ^{32}P-postlabelling (Amagase & Milner, 1993). Feeding fresh garlic, which was frozen before grinding, at 2% in the diet decreased DMBA–DNA binding by 33%, and subsequently extracting the ground garlic with water for 1 h at 25°C yielded an active extract, which decreased binding by 46%. Two commercial preparations based on sliced garlic decreased binding by 51% when fed at the 2% level and by 78% at the 4% level. The postlabelling spots representing different DMBA–DNA adducts all decreased to similar extents. In a second experiment with groups of five pair-fed rats, fresh garlic powder fed at 1% in the diet did not significantly decrease DMBA–DNA binding (16% decrease), but the water extract decreased binding by 44%. An overnight ethanolic extract was less active, decreasing binding by 24%. The two commercial preparations based on sliced garlic were active after pair-feeding at the 1% level and decreased DMBA-binding by 65–71%.

The interaction of garlic with other dietary factors, including casein, corn oil, retinyl acetate, selenium and methionine, in mammary DMBA–DNA binding was subsequently investigated in experiments using groups of 5–6 female Sprague-Dawley rats fed diets varying in these components for two weeks before a single dose of DMBA (Amagase et al., 1996). Garlic powder (20 g/kg diet), prepared by ethanol extraction of sliced garlic, decreased DMBA adduct levels to the same extent (32–35%) when fed with 36% or 12% casein (at the expense of corn starch and sucrose). Casein as such also decreased DMBA–DNA binding. In contrast, garlic depressed adduct formation to a greater extent in rats given 0.3 g methionine per 100 g diet than in those given 0.9 g (54% versus 26%) and also more in animals fed a 20% corn-oil diet than a 10% corn-oil diet [~60% versus ~30%, read from diagram]. Methionine itself decreased DNA binding, while lipid increased it. In animals fed only 5% corn oil, garlic did not significantly affect mammary adduct formation (corn oil was decreased while corn starch and sucrose were increased). A second experiment with adjustment for energy density while feeding corn oil at the same three dietary levels gave a similar result except that garlic decreased adduct formation only at the 20% corn-oil level. In a third experiment, DMBA–DNA binding was decreased by 35% with dietary selenite (0.5 mg/kg diet) and by 63% when the garlic extract was also fed. The corresponding decreases were 29% and 75% with dietary retinyl acetate (328 mg/kg diet) with or without garlic extract, and a combination of retinyl acetate, selenite and garlic extract gave a decrease in binding of 82%.

In groups of five female Sprague-Dawley rats, the ability of garlic to decrease (by 64%) DMBA-induced mammary gland DNA adducts was eliminated by heating the garlic with microwaves for 60 s; heating for 30 s had no effect (Song & Milner, 1999). There was no effect of heating after garlic was crushed and left to stand for 10 min, allowing the heat-sensitive alliinase to convert alliin present in garlic to active sulfur compounds.

The ability of garlic to inhibit DNA methylation adducts was investigated (Lin et al., 1994). Feeding groups of six female Sprague-Dawley rats with garlic powder at 2 or 4% for three weeks in a diet containing aminopyrine and sodium nitrite (each at 600 mg/kg diet) decreased the formation of N^7-methyl-deoxyguanosine (N^7-Me-dG) in DNA by 60 and 82%, respectively, and of O^6-methyldeoxyguanosine (O^6-Me-dG) by 54 and 82%, respectively. Pretreatment with NDMA (150 mg/kg bw) also induced liver DNA methylation, which was counteracted by 2 and 4% garlic powder treatments for two weeks (N^7-Me-dG: 45% and 57%, respectively, and O^6-Me-dG: 40 and 66%, respectively). Mammary DNA methylation after pretreatment with MNU (50 mg/kg bw) was also counteracted by feeding 2 and 4% garlic powder for two weeks (N^7-Me-dG: 57 and 69%, respectively, and O^6-Me-dG: 51 and 71%, respectively).

In a subsequent study, groups of 21 female Sprague-Dawley rats were fed 2% garlic powder in the diet for two weeks before a single dose of MNU (15 mg/kg bw) (Schaffer et al., 1996). In mammary tissue obtained 3 h later, N^7-Me-dG and O^6-Me-dG were decreased by 48 and 27%, respectively, in the garlic-fed animals compared with controls.

Groups of 24–26 male Fischer 344 rats were fed a control semi-synthetic diet or a similar diet containing 5 or 10% freeze-dried strawberries (at the expense of corn-starch) for two weeks, after which they received a single dose of NMBA (0.25–0.5 mg/kg bw) and were killed 24 h later for determination of gastric mucosal O^6-Me-dG (Stoner et al., 1999). The animals fed 5 and 10% strawberries had levels of adducts lower by 68 and 57%, respectively, indicating no dose–response relationship. A subsequent study with a similar protocol showed significant decreases (59 and 64%, respectively) also in oesophageal O^6-Me-dG in NMBA-treated rats fed 5 and 10% strawberries (Carlton et al., 2001).

In summary, four different fruit or vegetable preparations have been found to decrease carcinogen–DNA binding. The majority of studies evaluating dose–response effects found a relationship.

Oxidative damage and defence

No studies on modulation of oxidative damage or defence by treatment of experimental animals with combined fruits, vegetables or their extracts were available. Several studies with individual fruits and vegetables have been reported.

The individual effects of chloroform-extracted tomato paste, orange juice concentrate and canned carrots on erythrocyte stability, blood glutathione and erythrocyte CAT and superoxide dismutase (SOD) activities were investigated in groups of 12 male Fischer 344 rats treated with aflatoxin B$_1$ (250 μg/kg bw, daily for two periods of five days with a two-day interval). The extracts were administered by gastric intubation either daily for a 12-day period from weeks 2 to 4 after aflatoxin dosing (initiation) or every second day for a 12-week period from four weeks onwards after aflatoxin dosing (promotion) (He et al., 1997). Blood samples were collected at termination after 16 weeks in all groups. All extracts significantly increased erythrocyte stability by 33–98%, as determined as the amount of haemolysis 6 h after an ascorbate challenge. The effect was most pronounced after the 12-week treatment (49–98%) and carrot treatment had the greatest effect. An aflatoxin-induced increase in plasma glutathione was counteracted significantly by the extracts (17–45%), again most strongly with the longer treatment (33–45%) and with the carrot extract. The 12-week extract treatments also decreased erythrocyte CAT (25–29%) and SOD (34–41%).

Lyophilized apple (20% in the diet) fed for three weeks to groups of eight obese or lean Zucker rats significantly decreased urinary malondialdehyde excretion, measured as thiobarbituric acid-reactive substances (TBARS), by 45% in both strains (Aprikian et al., 2002). Levels of malondialdehyde in the heart were also significantly decreased in the obese strain (11%). Ferric-reducing capacity of plasma, a measure of one-electron reduction capacity, did not change in either strain.

The effects of raw or cooked Brussels sprouts and of a mixture of cooked green beans and endives (1:1) on spontaneous and induced oxidative DNA damage, in terms of 8-oxo-7,8-dihydro-2'-deoxyguanosine (8-oxodG) in tissue DNA or its urinary excretion, were determined in groups of 6–8 male Wistar rats (Deng et al., 1998). Excess oxidative DNA damage was induced by 2-nitropropane (100 mg/kg bw). Four days' oral administration of 3 g of cooked Brussels sprouts homogenate reduced spontaneous urinary 8-oxodG excretion by 31% ($p < 0.05$), whereas raw sprouts or green beans and endive (1:1) had no significant effect. An aqueous extract of cooked Brussels sprouts (corresponding to 6.7 g vegetable per day for four days) decreased the spontaneous 8-oxodG excretion by 43%. Pretreatment with sprout extract reduced nitropropane-induced 8-oxodG excretion by 28%. The background level of 8-oxodG in nuclear DNA from liver and bone marrow was not significantly affected by the sprout extract, whereas the level in the kidney decreased by 27%. In the liver, the sprouts extract reduced the nitropropane-induced increase in nuclear 8-oxodG by 57% at 6 h, whereas there was no significant effect at 24 h. Pretreatment with the sprout extract altogether abolished the nitropropane-induced increase in the kidneys. Similarly, in the bone marrow, the extract protected completely ($p < 0.05$) against a 4.9-fold nitropropane-induced increase in the 8-oxodG level.

Oral administration of an aqueous extract of Brussels sprouts (corresponding to 6.4 g fresh vegetable per day) for three or seven days to groups of four male Wistar rats significantly increased the level of 8-oxodG in rat liver by 20–30% (Sørensen et al., 2001). No effect on liver malondialdehyde levels was found. In a second experiment, groups of eight male Wistar rats were given Brussels sprout extract equivalent to 7 g per day of fresh vegetables by gavage for four days. No effect was observed on activity of CAT or GPX or on hepatic expression of γ-glutamylcysteine synthetase light and heavy chains in livers and kidneys removed 6 h after the last dose.

Two varieties of broccoli (Emperor and Shogun) grown under conventional or organic conditions were fed at a level of 10% in the diet to groups of 8–10 male Wistar rats during one week and hepatic, renal and colon glutathione reductase, GPX and SOD were determined (Vang et al., 1997). Feeding broccoli overall decreased the level of glutathione in the colon and reduced the activity of SOD in liver. Significant, albeit minor, differences between the two varieties and between organically and conventionally grown broccoli were noted. [The Working Group noted that details of the statistical methods were not given.]

Onion oil (100 mg/kg bw), given daily for 21 days by stomach tube to groups of 15 male Sprague-Dawley rats treated with nicotine (0.6 mg/kg bw, daily) as a pro-oxidant, significantly decreased the level of TBARS, lipid hydroperoxides and conjugated dienes in the liver, lungs and heart (Helen et al., 2000).

Groups of 4–5 male Sprague-Dawley rats fed low- or high-fat diets were given three weekly intubations of garlic oil (200 mg/kg bw) over seven weeks (Sheen et al., 1999). Garlic oil increased hepatic glutathione reductase by 20–27% and erythrocyte glutathione by 51–70%, but did not significantly affect hepatic glutathione. Hepatic SOD was increased by 14–44%, whereas hepatic GPX decreased by 27–34%. Garlic oil did not affect hepatic TBARS or α-tocopherol. The fat content (5 or 20%) in the feed did not significantly interact with the garlic oil treatment.

Lyophilized garlic fed at 2% in the diet to groups of eight male Wistar rats for three weeks decreased CAT activity and CAT protein levels in renal cortex, but did not influence CAT expression (Pedraza-Chaverri et al., 2000). Treatment of rats with the nephrotoxic drug gentamicin (75 mg/kg by subcutaneous injection every 12 hours during the last six days) led to increased urinary excretion of lipid peroxidation products, decreased activity of Mn-SOD and GPX in the renal cortex and of plasma GPX and decreased activity and expression of CAT in the renal cortex in rats given ordinary chow. Gentamicin-treated and garlic-supplemented rats only experienced a decrease in renal cortex CAT activity similar to the action of garlic alone. A subsequent study by the same group indicated that the decrease in CAT activity in the renal cortex followed a garlic-induced decrease in tissue levels of H_2O_2 (Pedraza-Chaverri et al., 2001).

Three months' daily feeding of a 5% bitter gourd extract to groups of eight female Swiss albino mice increased hepatic GPX, CAT and SOD by 110%, 100% and 57%, respectively [values read from diagram] and decreased the ex vivo susceptibility of hepatic microsomes to lipid peroxidation (>60%; read from diagram) and to lymphocyte DNA strand breakage (61%; read from diagram) (Ganguly et al., 2000). Similar effects were found in mice treated with DMBA in croton oil.

In summary, the evidence from animal studies with respect to effects of fruit and vegetables on antioxidant enzymes and direct oxidative damage to DNA is inconsistent, whereas lipid oxidation seems in many cases to be reduced by such treatments.

Effects on mutation and DNA strand breaks

Groups of six Long-Evans male rats were allowed to drink ad libitum only fresh or boiled (100°C, 15 min) vegetable juices (500 g vegetable to 1 L juice, 7–17 mL juice per day) during one week and bone marrow micronucleus formation induced by DMBA was measured (Ito et al., 1986). Fresh or boiled extracts of onion, burdock, egg plant, cabbage and Welsh onion and boiled pumpkin extract all reduced DMBA-induced clastogenicity by 40–68%. Fresh pumpkin juice increased clastogenicity, while fresh or boiled juices from lettuce, carrot, peaman (bell pepper) and celery were inactive.

Seven fruit and ten vegetable extracts, prepared with organic solvents, were tested for their ability to inhibit the clastogenic effects of cyclophosphamide and B[a]P in the mouse bone marrow micronucleus assay (Edenharder et al., 1998). Groups of four 7–12-week-old male NMRI mice were treated intraperitoneally with B[a]P (150 mg/kg bw in 200 µL corn oil) or orally with cyclophosphamide (200 mg/kg bw in saline by gastric intubation) to induce micronuclei and simultaneously by gastric intubation with 0.5m mL suspension of freeze-dried fruit or vegetable extracts. Sweet cherries, strawberries, bananas, kiwi fruit, oranges and peaches all decreased the clastogenic effects significantly (10–40% decrease); a 39% decrease caused by apples was not significant. Among the vegetables, cucumber, radish, tomato, Brussels sprouts, asparagus, red beet, yellow-red peppers and spinach (22–79% decrease) had significant activity, but cauliflower and onions did not significantly decrease clastogenicity. Further fractionation of the orange extract revealed that several fractions contained active principles, and that different fractions contained activity against each of the two clastogens tested.

The influence of five days of grapefruit juice intake on PhIP-induced DNA damage in the colon was examined by the comet assay in groups of three male Fischer 344 rats given 60 mg/kg of PhIP by gavage three hours before sacrifice. DNA damage in the colon of rats allowed free access to grapefruit juice for five days was significantly reduced to 40% of the level in control rats (Miyata et al., 2002). The effect was found to be unrelated to absorption and biotransformation of PhIP.

In summary, evidence from three studies with more than ten different fruits and vegetables points to a preventive effect of many on carcinogen-induced DNA damage and mutation.

Effects on DNA repair

No studies on modulation of DNA repair caused by treatment of experimental animals with combined fruits, vegetables or their extracts were available.

Groups of eight male Wistar rats were given an aqueous Brussels sprout extract equivalent to 7 g per day of fresh vegetable for four days by gavage and the livers and kidneys were removed 6 h after the last dose (Sørensen et al., 2001). No effect on the activity of 8-oxoguanosine DNA glycosylase (OGG1) was observed in either organ.

Intermediary markers related to the cell cycle

A range of lyophilized vegetables were individually added to human-type diets [no details were given] at a level of 12 g per day and fed to groups of three male Fischer 344 rats and the mitotic index and proliferating cell nuclear antigen (PCNA) in colon cells were measured (O'Neill et al., 1997). PCNA responded only marginally, whereas spinach, petit pois (green peas) and peppers decreased the mitotic index substantially. Only the effect of petit pois (41% decrease) was statistically significant. There was an inverse relationship between colonic mitotic index and colonic GST activities across the test groups.

Mechanisms of cancer prevention

The epidemiological evidence for a cancer-protective effect of diets rich in fruit and vegetables and the ability of many extracts from fruits or vegetables to counteract carcinogenesis in experimental animals has prompted a range of studies into mechanisms that may underlie these effects. Whole plants, extracts and subfractions have been tested, as well as certain purified plant compounds. Relatively few experimental studies have tested the effect of diets mimicking human habitual patterns of fruit and vegetable intake. Rather, most studies in humans and animals have investigated the potential of single test components to influence intermediate markers related to mechanisms of carcinogenesis.

Proposals that antioxidant vitamins (Mirvish et al., 1972; Anon., 1980), fibres (Wynder, 1985; Weisburger et al., 1993) or enzyme inducers (Wattenberg, 1975; Das et al., 1985; Prochaska & Talalay, 1988; Talalay et al., 1988) present in fruit and vegetables might be responsible for preventive effects prompted early research into these areas. Subsequently, there has been much research on plants rich in nitrosation inhibitors, antioxidants or enzyme inducers, e.g., ascorbate and polyphenols (Bartsch et al., 1988) or carotenoid-rich vegetables, garlic (Bianchini & Vainio, 2001) and cruciferous vegetables (van Poppel et al., 1999).

Several reviews have described potential mechanisms behind the cancer-protective actions of fruit and vegetables (Wattenberg et al., 1976; De Flora & Ramel, 1988; Hartman & Shankel, 1990; Dragsted et al., 1993; Potter & Steinmetz, 1996; Lampe, 1999). This section summarizes the range of mechanisms through which fruit and vegetables might influence carcinogenesis. The end-points studied experimentally are largely intermediate biomarkers for carcinogen uptake, activation, damage and later cellular effects, which theoretically are related to cancer risk. In many cases, however, the relationships of these intermediate markers (e.g., oxidative damage, DNA-adduct formation or cell proliferation) to subsequent cancer outcomes are not well established. Surrogate markers used in human studies (e.g., damage to lymphocyte DNA in place of the target tissue DNA) often have not been well validated. Furthermore, the effects of high doses of single compounds on animal models of carcinogen-induced tumours are often difficult to extrapolate to humans.

In some cases, it has been shown that interactions between several dietary components increase the preventive activity, and the growth conditions of fruits and vegetables might directly influence such synergies (Vang et al., 1999, 2001). The interactions between garlic and selenium in enzyme induction, prevention of genetic damage and cancer prevention in experimental systems illustrate the importance of many factors in the diet acting together in cancer prevention (Ip & Lisk, 1995; Amagase et al., 1996; Ip & Lisk, 1997; Schaffer et al., 1997). Therefore, whenever possible, studies on preventive mechanisms of whole fruits and vegetables or simple extracts and lyophilized preparations are used as examples in this chapter.

Inhibition of endogenous carcinogen formation

Nitrosamines, alkenes and reactive radical species are examples of potentially carcinogenic factors that are formed endogenously. Modulation of their formation might lead to an altered risk of cancer.

Inhibition of radical formation

Free radicals are formed in one-electron reactions by transition metals, ionizing radiation or endogenous enzymes such as xanthine oxidase and nitric oxide synthase. Their formation may be propagated by redox systems such as ascorbate/ferrous ion in the water phase or by transition metal-catalysed peroxide degradation in unsaturated lipids. Free radical formation may be counteracted by scavenging of radicals by antioxidants or by chelation of transition metals into less reactive complexes. Fruits and vegetables contain many natural primary (scavenging) or secondary (chelating) antioxidants that might directly prevent radical-induced damage to cellular structures, including DNA. The evidence for antioxidant actions of fruit and vegetables comes largely from studies with cell-free systems and to a lesser extent from experimental studies in animals and humans using assays of antioxidant capacity. In view of the wide range of phytochemicals with antioxidant activity and the difficulty of measuring each compound individually, several assays have been developed to assess total antioxidant activity. Serum total antioxidant capacity, determined ex vivo, can be measured by several assays: oxygen radical absorbence capacity (ORAC), ferric-reducing ability (FRAP) and Trolox equivalent antioxidant capacity (TEAC). However, these assays have been insufficiently validated (Crews et al., 2001) and the relevance of these measures to cancer risk has not been established.

Formation of radicals is an important part of several physiological processes, including inflammation and metabolism of xenobiotics, both of which have dual roles in carcinogenesis. Direct evidence of primary or secondary antioxidant activity from animal and human experimental studies is scarce; the indirect evidence of decreased oxidative damage is discussed later in this chapter. No long-term studies have investigated the relationship between markers of antioxidant capacity and cancer risk. In one small case–control study, increased serum total antioxidant status, measured by TEAC, was found to be associated with reduced breast cancer risk (Ching et al., 2002); however, the case–control design limited the conclusions that could be drawn regarding temporality. To date, there is no evidence for a relationship between increased ex vivo antioxidant capacity of plasma and feeding with whole fruits or vegetables in experimental animals; the only study identified had a negative outcome (Aprikian et al., 2002).

Inhibition of nitrosation

Some of the factors that contribute to oxidative damage and the production of reactive oxygen species can also lead to production of reactive nitrogen species. A wide range of nitrogen-containing compounds and nitrosating agents to which humans are exposed react in vivo to form potentially carcinogenic N-nitroso, C-nitroso and reactive diazo compounds. Nitrosating agents are also synthesized endogenously by bacteria and activated macrophages. High exposure to nitrate leading to increased endogenous nitrosation has been proposed as a possible risk factor for several cancers (Bartsch et al., 1992). Therefore, interventions that reduce formation of nitroso compounds may lower risk, although evidence to support this directly is lacking (Bartsch & Frank, 1996; Hughes et al., 2002).

Modulation of carcinogen bioavailability

Dietary carcinogens need to be absorbed from the gut or at least to enter the epithelial cell lining of the gastrointestinal tract in order to have an effect on cancer risk. In theory, fruit and vegetables may influence the bioavailability of carcinogens by inhibiting their uptake or by increasing their excretion. Carcinogens may adsorb to structures in fruit and vegetables such as fibres or chlorophyll or may be diluted by the increased bulk of material in the gastrointestinal tract after meals containing large amounts of fruit and vegetables.

Aflatoxins adsorb strongly to chlorophyllin (a water-soluble copper complex of chlorophyll used as a food colorant), making them less bioavailable and decreasing DNA binding and subsequent tumour development in trout (Breinholt et al., 1999; Hayashi et al., 1999). Chlorophyllin also reduces aflatoxin adduct formation in humans (Egner et al., 2001). Although chlorophyll was less potent than chlorophyllin in adsorbing aflatoxins (Dashwood et al., 1998), the ubiquitous presence of chlorophylls and other porphyrins in green fruits and green leafy vegetables suggests that such a mechanism may be relevant to cancer prevention by fruit and vegetables.

The bulking or carcinogen-adsorbing effect of plant-based fibre-rich foods, including fruit and vegetables, has been hypothesized to be important for protection against exogenous and endogenous cancer-enhancing factors, including secondary bile acids (Jacobs, 1986) and hydrophobic carcinogens (Harris et al., 1996). Certain fibres may be able to inhibit carcinogenesis by heterocyclic amines (Ferguson & Harris, 1996). In humans, supplementation with dietary fibre from vegetable and grain sources lowers faecal bile acid concentrations in a dose-dependent manner as a result of faecal bulking (Lampe et al., 1992), but there are no experimental studies to support such an effect of fruit and vegetables in general.

Modulation of enzyme systems

Many carcinogens need metabolic activation in order to elicit their effects. The oxidation (phase I) and conjugation (phase II) reactions involved in this process may be influenced by dietary fruit and vegetables. The enzyme systems responsible for these transformations also participate in steroid hormone metabolism and their modulation may therefore also affect risk of hormone-dependent cancers. The enzymes involved in antioxidative defence against reactive oxygen and nitrogen species are another group that may be modulated by dietary factors.

Phase I and II enzymes

Phase I enzymes such as the cytochrome P450-dependent monooxygenases (CYP) catalyse oxidation, hydroxylation and reduction reactions, but may also convert hydrophobic compounds to reactive electrophiles. Phase II enzymes such as UGT, sulfotransferases and GSTs catalyse conjugation reactions with water-soluble moieties to improve excretion. The balance between carcinogen activation and detoxification is potentially important for cancer risk. Both oxidation reactions and conjugation can lead to formation of either activated, DNA-reactive metabolites or less toxic metabolites. Modulation of phase I and II metabolism may therefore lead to increased or decreased risk of cancer, depending on the carcinogen in question. However, there are few examples of activation solely by conjugation and lack of ability to induce conjugating enzymes is associated with increased cancer risk in transgenic knock-out mice (Talalay & Fahey, 2001). Excessive induction of phase I enzymes has been associated with increased risk of cancer at several sites in humans (Lee et al., 1994; Landi et al., 1999; Mollerup et al., 1999; Stucker et al., 2000; Guengerich, 2001). Therefore, induction of phase II enzymes alone (monofunctional action) is regarded in general as protective, whereas the effect of simultaneously inducing both phase I and II enzymes (bifunctional action) is less clear.

In animal studies, mixtures of fruits and vegetables at 20% in the diet had relatively weak and variable effects on CYP induction (Alink et al., 1988). In contrast, potent GST induction was repeatedly observed in male rats (Alink et al., 1988; Rijnkels & Alink, 1998). Several vegetables or vegetable extracts at levels of 7–20% in the diet have been shown to induce xenobiotic-metabolizing enzymes in rodents. Brassica vegetables appear to induce both phase I and II enzymes in liver, but apparently the induction of phase II enzymes is most pronounced. GST induction takes place in extrahepatic organs, including testis, small intestine, colon and kidney (Clapper et al., 1997; Vang et al., 1999, 2001). The bifunctional indole derivatives and the monofunctional isothiocyanates, formed during cutting or chewing of the fresh vegetables, seem to be the main active principles in this group of vegetables (Verhoeven et al., 1997b).

The mode of induction by compounds from Brassica vegetables depends on their chemical structures, with indole derivatives and isothiocyanates having distinct effects. Binding of indole derivatives (e.g., diindolylmethane) to the aryl hydrocarbon receptor (AhR) leads to translocation of the AhR complex to the nucleus and interaction with xenobiotic response elements (XRE) in the Ah responsive gene promoter. Subsequent recruitment of co-activators and transcription factors results in transactivation (Safe, 2001). Induction of CYP1A, CYP1B, GSTA, NAD(P)H:quinone oxidoreductase (NQO1) and UGT is mediated through the AhR (Wolf, 2001). In contrast, isothiocyanates typically activate genes via the antioxidant or electrophile response element (ARE/EpRE) (Bonnesen et al., 2001; Kong et al., 2001). Regulation of NQO1, γ-glutamylcysteine synthase and several GSTs is mediated through the ARE/EpRE (Wolf, 2001).

Garlic preparations also increase GST and CYP2B1 activity in a dose-dependent manner in rat liver (Chen et al., 2001a) and GST in breast tissue (Liu et al., 1992) and decrease CYP activities, notably inducible CYP2E1 (Kwak et al., 1995). Allyl polysulfides are the main active principles causing enzyme induction after treatment with the Allium species (Bianchini & Vainio, 2001) and cutting or squeezing of fresh garlic is important for their formation and activity. Data on other fruits or vegetables are sparse; the importance for drug interactions of the induction of CYP3A4 by grapefruit remains controversial (Bailey et al., 1994).

Generally, induction of both phase I (e.g., XRE-driven) and phase II (e.g., ARE-driven) enzymes is thought to speed carcinogenic compounds through the metabolic pathway towards elimination, whereas agents that induce XRE-driven gene expression without stimulating ARE-driven expression are thought to enhance, rather than retard, chemical carcinogenesis (Bonnesen et al., 2001). However, the picture is complex, for not all AhR ligands promote neoplastic disease and the promoter regions of some human biotransformation enzymes (e.g., NQO1) contain both an XRE and an ARE (Bonnesen et al., 2001).

Numerous phytochemicals in fruits and vegetables, including flavonoids (Eaton et al., 1996), isothiocyanates (Hecht, 1995) and allyl sulfides (Brady et al., 1988), act as potent modulators of CYP activities in vitro; however, their effects are complex. Some have the capacity to inhibit certain enzymes at high concentrations of the compound, and to activate moderately the same enzyme at lower concentrations (Obermeier et al., 1995). Others may act as competitive CYP inhibitors; even when present at low concentrations and in combination with other compounds, their actions can be significant (Yang et al., 1994). Even slight differences in chemical structure can significantly alter activity. However, the concentrations of the individual compounds which have been shown to modulate CYP activities in vitro or in animal studies are still much higher than those likely to be achieved in humans at ordinary dietary levels of fruit and vegetables (Dragsted et al., 1997). Good evidence that habitual dietary fruit and vegetable intakes modulate CYP activities in humans is still lacking. In animal models and cell systems, certain combinations of bioactive compounds may confer protection against genotoxic agents at levels that individual compounds do not achieve alone (Bonnesen et al., 2001; Nho & Jeffery, 2001). Given that any particular Brassica species contains dozens of different glucosinolates (Fahey et al., 2001), a mixture of glucosinolate-containing vegetables might also exert synergistic effects towards a lower-risk enzyme profile in humans.

Efforts to determine the effects of fruit and vegetable constituents on biotransformation enzymes in humans in vivo are hampered by lack of access to relevant tissues. Measurements of enzyme concentrations or activities in circulation or in peripheral leukocytes or of drug metabolites provide indirect support for the capacity of various vegetables, particularly Brassica species, to alter enzyme function in humans (Bogaards et al., 1994; Nijhoff et al., 1995a; Lampe et al., 2000 a,b). Direct effects of vegetable diets on tissue levels of enzymes have been little explored, but Nijhoff et al. (1995b) showed that consumption of Brussels sprouts led to increased rectal GST-π.

Human studies of the effects of cruciferous vegetable supplementation on metabolism of carcinogens and promoting agents, such as estrogens, have also provided support for a protective effect through modulation of phase I and phase II enzymes. Watercress added to the diet of smokers significantly increased glucuronidation of nicotine and tobacco-carcinogen metabolites, but had modest effects on oxidative metabolism of these compounds (Hecht et al., 1999; Murphy et al., 2001). Similarly, broccoli and Brussels sprouts increased the metabolism (reducing the excretion) of heterocyclic aromatic amines derived from cooked meat; this implied induction of both CYP1A2 and relevant phase II enzymes (Murray et al., 2001; Knize et al., 2002).

Phase I and II enzymes that metabolize and/or are modulated by phytochemicals also contribute to inactivation of endogenous steroid hormones. They alter the potency of testosterone, estrogen and their derivatives via oxidation and hydroxylation reactions and conjugation with sulfate and glucuronide moieties (Aoyama et al., 1990). Thus, induction or inhibition of these enzyme systems in vivo can modify the biological effects of hormones. Several studies have demonstrated that high dietary levels of cruciferous vegetables can increase 2-hydroxylation of estrogens in humans, probably by inducing CYP1A2 (Bradlow et al., 1994; Kall et al., 1996).

In conclusion, some mechanisms by which constituents of certain fruits and vegetables, notably *Brassica* and *Allium* species, induce phase I and II enzymes have been identified. However, the magnitude of effects in relevant human tissues remains unclear, because of the difficulties associated with accessing these tissues. Although induction may take place after consumption of several hundred grams of certain vegetables, effects of habitual dietary intakes of fruit and vegetables have received little attention.

Antioxidant enzymes

Modulation of antioxidant enzymes is hypothesized to affect protection against reactive oxygen species, but the cancer-preventive effects are not clear. An increase might be interpreted as a response to an oxidative challenge or as an increased capacity for antioxidative defence, depending upon the experimental design.

In aflatoxin B_1-dosed rats, CAT and SOD activity in blood decreased in relation to treatment time when the rats were treated with carrot, orange or tomato juice by gavage (He et al., 1997). Since plasma glutathione levels and erythrocyte haemolysis also decreased, the simplest explanation for these results would be that the decrease in the enzymes was a response to a decreased need for degradation of hydrogen peroxide and superoxide. These reactive oxygen species were not measured in the study, however, and no feedback system is known for the regulation of antioxidant enzymes in erythrocytes, which have no capacity for *de novo* protein synthesis. In rats that were not pretreated with a carcinogen, treatment for two weeks with garlic led to a decrease in hydrogen peroxide in the renal cortex (Pedraza-Chaverri et al., 2001), which coincided with a decrease in CAT, in support of a feedback regulation. Since CAT activity and protein levels were affected but not CAT mRNA levels (Pedraza-Chaverri et al., 2000), post-translational regulation may take place. Short-term treatment with *Brassica* juices did not seem to influence GPX or CAT activity in liver (Sørensen et al., 2001) or testes (Vang et al., 1999). There is some evidence that the long-term effects of constitutive increases in GPX or SOD may be either protective against cancer (Zhao et al., 2001; Shoichet et al., 2002) or, conversely, increase cancer in transgenic animals (Lu et al., 1997; Marikovsky et al., 2002). Thus, in relation to cancer, changes in cellular antioxidant defence can have complex consequences.

In humans, expression and activities of SOD, CAT and GPX have been reported to be lower in tumours than in tumour-free adjacent tissue (Bostwick et al., 2000; Ho et al., 2001; Durak et al., 1996), as well as in conditions associated with elevated cancer risk, such as chronic pancreatitis (Cullen et al., 2003) and prostatic intraepithelial neoplasia (Bostwick et al., 2000). These data support the hypothesis that inflammation and the associated decreases in antioxidant enzyme activity create an intracellular environment that favours DNA damage and the promotion of cancer (Ho et al., 2001). This is likely to be a local tissue effect and causality remains to be established; however, antioxidant enzyme activities in blood may serve as surrogate markers of exposure and response to general oxidative stress. In healthy individuals, activities of CAT and GPX in whole blood haemolysates were significantly higher in those exposed to environmental tobacco smoke than in the unexposed, and levels of oxidative DNA damage were also higher in the exposed individuals (Howard et al., 1998). The few studies that examined effects of fruit or vegetable interventions on antioxidant enzyme activities in humans restricted their measurements to erythrocytes or plasma. The responses varied widely with the fruit or vegetable type and dose, and only a few disparate foods were tested (Castenmiller et al., 1999; Lean et al., 1999; Nielsen et al., 1999; Young et al., 1999, 2000).

Inhibition of damage to macromolecules

Many carcinogens are activated to electrophilic metabolites, which react with cellular macromolecules, including DNA, proteins and lipids (Miller & Miller, 1981). Reactive radical species have a similar pattern of activity. Fruit and vegetables contain factors that decrease the damage to macromolecular structures, determined as decreases in oxidative damage, in adducts, or in the downstream consequences of adduct formation, such as mutations or repair.

Decreased oxidative damage to lipids, proteins and DNA

Experimental evidence is consistent with the view that increased oxidative DNA damage leads to elevated cancer risk (Halliwell, 2002). The 8-hydroxylation of guanine bases in DNA is a frequent type of oxidative DNA damage that can lead to GC to TA transversions unless repairs are made before DNA replication (Cheng et al., 1992b). In vivo, when DNA is repaired by exonucleases, 8-hydroxy-2'-deoxyguanosine (8-OHdG) is subsequently excreted in the urine without further metabolism. Increased levels of urinary 8-OHdG are associated with conditions characterized by increased oxidative stress, such as smoking, whole-body irradiation and cytotoxic chemotherapy (Kasai et al., 1986; Loft et al., 1992; Tagesson et al., 1995). Urinary levels of 8-OHdG also declined in response to intervention with Brussels sprouts (Verhagen et al., 1997) or to a high-vegetable and fruit dietary intervention (Thompson et al., 1999a), but tomato sauce or fruit juice supplements had no effect (Rao & Agarwal, 1998; Dragsted et al., 2001). Raw Brussels sprouts did not affect urinary 8-OHdG excretion in rats, but cooked sprouts were effective and also significantly decreased nuclear 8-OHdG levels in bone marrow and kidneys (Deng et al., 1998). Levels in the liver were unaffected. In another study, Brussels sprouts increased 8-OHdG levels in rat liver (Sørensen et al., 2001).

As with many biomarkers associated with early events in carcinogenesis, direct and compelling evidence that 8-OHdG is a biomarker of subsequent cancer development in humans is not available. There are several explanations why elevated oxidative DNA damage may not be consistently associated with increased cancer risk (Halliwell, 2002). Measurement of 8-OHdG in urine and/or easily accessible tissues does not necessarily reflect damage in the target tissues of interest. For example, steady-state levels of 8-OHdG in rats can differ in different tissues (Devanaboyina & Gupta, 1996). The biomarker also does not adequately account for oxidative damage to RNA or to free deoxyguanosine and may be influenced by variations in DNA repair rates and by site of DNA oxidative damage. For example, unrepaired damage in genes encoding functional proteins crucial to tumour suppression such as p53 is likely to be more deleterious than damage in non-coding regions of DNA (Halliwell, 2002). Finally, another explanation for the lack of evidence from human studies may be insufficient statistical power due to the large inter-individual variation in 8-OHdG excretion levels and the relatively small sample sizes in many of the studies.

Tissue levels of oxidative damage remain difficult to measure, although recent improvements in DNA extraction have led to more reliable techniques (Ravanat et al., 2002). Oxidative damage to DNA may also be determined by single-cell gel electrophoresis (SCGE) using restriction enzymes sensitive to oxidative damage to purines or pyrimidines. Protective effects towards DNA oxidation have been observed by this technique in several human studies after dietary modulation with fruits or vegetables (Duthie et al., 1996; Pool-Zobel et al., 1997; Collins et al., 1998, 2001; Porrini et al., 2002). However, the effects are generally not strong, and, as with other markers of oxidative DNA damage, the technique shows large inter-individual variation.

Animal and human evidence points towards decreased lipid oxidation with increasing fruit and vegetable intake (Miller et al., 1998; Maskarinec et al., 1999; Aprikian et al., 2002). Lipid oxidation products have been observed to form adducts with DNA in several human organs, including oral mucosa, colon, liver and breast, leading to increased genetic damage, and have been implicated as a risk factor for human colorectal adenomas (Chaudhary et al., 1994; Wang et al., 1996; Zhang et al., 2002a; Leuratti et al., 2002). Adduct levels were similar to levels of 8-OHdG in human pancreas (Thompson et al., 1999b), underlining their potential importance. Protection against lipid oxidation may therefore contribute to cancer prevention.

In conclusion, it appears that fruit and vegetables may decrease direct or indirect (through lipid oxidation products) oxidative damage to DNA, but the evidence linking such damage to decreased cancer risk is still very limited.

Decreased carcinogen–DNA binding or increased DNA repair

Many carcinogens bind to DNA and it is generally believed that changes in the DNA code resulting from such binding are the main cause of cancer initiation, constituting the core of subsequent heritable genetic damage from early precancerous lesions up to the development of malignancy. Any decrease in carcinogen–DNA binding is therefore important for the prevention of cancer. Decreased binding may be a result of decreased absorption, decreased formation of activated carcinogen metabolites or increased detoxification and excretion. Many fruit and vegetables can influence these pathways, as discussed above. For instance, the potent inhibition of mammary DNA binding of DMBA in rats pretreated with garlic extracts (Liu *et al.*, 1992), the dependence of the effect on garlic crushing or ageing (Amagase & Milner, 1993; Song & Milner, 1999) and the synergy with selenite in eliciting this effect (Amagase *et al.*, 1996; Ip & Lisk, 1997; Schaffer *et al.*, 1997) are paralleled by similar actions of garlic and garlic constituents with respect to enzyme induction (Liu *et al.*, 1992; Ip & Lisk, 1997). This strongly implicates changes in the enzymatic activation and deactivation of DMBA in the prevention of DNA damage. Deactivation seems to be important, since urinary excretion products of polycyclic aromatic hydrocarbons have been observed to be less mutagenic after garlic supplementation in rats (Polasa & Krishnaswamy, 1997). Garlic preparations also decrease the activity of hepatic CYP2E1 (Kwak *et al.*, 1995), which is likely to account for the observed decrease in alkylation of DNA by nitrosamines and nitrosoureas (Lin *et al.*, 1994). Examples exist of bioactive components in fruits and vegetables which are able directly to scavenge electrophilic metabolites (Wang *et al.*, 1989; Athar *et al.*, 1989) or to shield sensitive sites in DNA (Teel, 1986; Barch & Fox, 1988). Such actions or other as yet unknown mechanisms may contribute to prevention of adduct formation by fruits and vegetables.

The evidence for a link between decreased carcinogen–DNA adduct formation and dietary fruit and vegetable intake in humans is very limited. In a cross-sectional study among 104 healthy Japanese men, no relationship was observed between total bulky adducts in human lymphocytes and plasma β-carotene, a marker of vegetable intake (Wang *et al.*, 1997). Evidence from human studies of polymorphisms in drug-metabolizing enzymes supports a link between carcinogen activation, adduct formation and cancer risk at several sites (Li *et al.*, 1996; Poirier, 1997; Peluso *et al.*, 1998; Li *et al.*, 2002; Chen *et al.*, 2002c), but clear evidence that dietary fruit and vegetables may reduce the risk of cancers specifically through this mechanism is still lacking.

Measurements of DNA binding reflect the balance between adduct formation and removal. Alterations in DNA repair will also influence this balance, and defects or polymorphisms in DNA-repair genes are known to affect cancer risk (Cheng *et al.*, 2000b; Matullo *et al.*, 2001; Bohr, 2002; Ito *et al.*, 2002; Tang *et al.*, 2002). However, there are no data indicating that fruit and vegetables enhance DNA repair. Thus, hepatic or renal expression of the DNA-repair enzyme OGG1 was not affected in rats after dosing with extracts of Brussels sprouts (Sørensen *et al.*, 2001). In a human study with complete dietary control, a 25-day intervention with 600 g of fruit and vegetables had no effect on expression of the repair enzymes OGG1 and ERCC1 in lymphocytes (Vogel *et al.*, 2002).

Decreased mutation or cytogenetic damage

Interaction of electrophilic compounds, including reactive oxygen or nitrogen species, with DNA bases can result in formation of DNA adducts or cross-links, which, during the course of attempted repair or replication, can lead to gene mutations, DNA strand breaks and other structural changes in DNA. Accumulation of genetic damage in crucial genes may contribute to the development of neoplastic cells. In animal studies, the majority of the twenty-odd different fruit and vegetable juices that have been tested counteracted cytogenetic damage to mouse bone marrow (Ito *et al.*, 1986; Edenharder *et al.*, 1998). The observation that inhibitory activity was found with the majority of preparations suggests that this effect may be important for the preventive effects of fruit and vegetables. Mutagenicity *in vivo* is generally regarded as a strong predictor of carcinogenicity in animal tests and decreased chromosomal damage may similarly be a predictor of protection against tumorigenicity. As already discussed, adduct levels seem to correlate closely with treatments which cause a decrease in carcinogen activation, and it is possible that the ability of many fruits and vegetables to influence drug-metabolizing enzymes underlies the surprisingly common ability of these foods to decrease cytogenetic damage in animals. In contrast, the effect of grapefruit juice on phase I enzymes does not seem to lead to any alteration of the metabolism of the heterocyclic aromatic amine PhIP. Neither does the juice cause changes in the bioavailability of PhIP, so the inhibition of PhIP-induced strand breakage in colon DNA by grapefruit juice must involve other mechanisms (Miyata *et al.*, 2002). Thus, links between the influence of dietary fruit and vegetables on carcinogen metabolism, adduct formation and decreased mutagenic or clastogenic effects in humans or in animals are still not clearly established.

Human studies give an equivocal picture of the ability of fruits or vegetables to decrease DNA strand breaks or micronuclei. Four studies used the comet assay without restriction enzymes or *ex vivo* oxidative challenge and one of them observed a decreased level of strand breaks after intervention with tomato and carrot juice or spinach powder (Pool-Zobel *et al.*, 1997). The others failed to show such an effect after intervention with onion, kiwi fruit or a mixed-vegetable burger (Boyle et al., 2000; van den Berg et al., 2001; Collins et al., 2001). Vegetable intake was negatively correlated with micronucleus formation in peripheral blood lymphocytes in a cross-sectional study in Hungary, whereas no effect of fresh fruit intake on micronucleated cells in the oesophageal mucosa was observed in young Chinese men and women (Chang-Claude et al., 1992; Pastor et al., 2002).

In humans, there seems to be a strong link between chromosomal aberrations and subsequent cancer risk (Hagmar et al., 1998; Bonassi et al., 2000), but no studies have provided a strong link between the other cytogenetic end-points and cancer risk.

In conclusion, there is good evidence from animal studies that fruit and vegetables decrease cytogenetic damage, but the human evidence is weak.

Post-initiation effects

The biokinetics of cell turnover are of central importance to cancer prevention, since a hallmark of cancer is dysregulation of the cell cycle. Effects on cell turnover are important early as well as late in the development of cancer. Toxic effects leading to enhanced proliferation increase the efficiency of cancer initiation. Many experimental co-carcinogens are irritants or agents causing inflammation. The same is true for many substances that act as promoters in two-stage carcinogenesis experiments and for factors that enhance human cancer but lack a potential to cause direct DNA damage. Inhibition of excess cell proliferation or increased apoptosis would consequently be expected to prevent cancer; however the picture is complex and it is necessary to gain better understanding of the underlying processes before generalizing from specific effects affecting the cell cycle to subsequent cancer prevention. Many specific compounds derived from plant foods affect cell turnover in cell culture or in animal studies, but relatively few studies have examined the effects of increased intake of preparations made from whole fruits or vegetables on cell turnover and they are all concerned with markers of cell proliferation, mitosis or apoptosis.

Fruit and vegetable preparations given after treatment with an initiator have been observed to inhibit tumour development and growth and to delay cancer onset in some experimental studies, but the evidence is equivocal. Garlic preparations had preventive activity against breast cancer when dosed after an initiator (Ip & Lisk, 1995). Lyophilized strawberries or black raspberries in the diet inhibited rat oesophageal tumorigenicity when given after initiation with NMBA (Carlton et al., 2001; Kresty et al., 2001). Feeding cabbage after initiation inhibited tumour development in the mouse colon in one of two similar studies (Temple & Basu, 1987; Temple & el-Khatib, 1987), but in a third study, feeding a fruit and vegetable mixture after azoxymethane treatment had only marginal effects on rat colon carcinogenesis (Rijnkels et al., 1998). Likewise, pure mandarin juice did not significantly affect lung tumorigenesis when given to mice after initiation with NNK (Kohno et al., 2001) and the post-initiation effects of Brussels sprouts or garlic powder on DMBA-induced rat breast cancer were also much weaker than dosing before and during initiation (Stoewsand et al., 1988; Ip et al., 1992). In adenomatous polyp patients, intervention with a diet low in fat and high in fibre, fruits and vegetables did not reduce the risk for recurrence of colorectal adenomas (Schatzkin et al., 2000).

Modulation of cell proliferation or apoptosis

A range of different lyophilized vegetables decreased the mitotic index in the rat colon without affecting proliferating cell nuclear antigen (PCNA) (O'Neill et al., 1997). However, in rats initiated with NMBA, feeding lyophilized raspberries decreased oesophageal levels of PCNA (Kresty et al., 2001). Citrus products have been observed to enhance cyclin D1, apoptosis and activity of T killer cells in the colon and to decrease mucosal PCNA and the proliferation zone, but the effect was not consistently associated with decreased tumour incidence (Miyagi et al., 2000; Tanaka et al., 2000; Kossoy et al., 2001).

There is no direct evidence for an effect of fruit and vegetable consumption on cell proliferation in humans. Although constituents of fruit and vegetables can affect indices of cell proliferation and turnover in vitro, there is little evidence from experiments with dietary change or from feeding studies with whole fruits or vegetable preparations.

In summary, the evidence for a post-initiation effect of fruit and vegetables is relatively weak.

Immune function

In vitro and in vivo studies suggest a possible role of immunological defence against cancer and its metastasis (outlined in Imai et al., 2000). The mechanism of immunosurveillance (Burnet, 1970) is hypothesized to be non-specific, with natural killer cells, activated macrophages, K cells and NKT cells playing key roles (Kubena & McMurray, 1996). Although immune-compromised individuals are at higher risk for certain cancers such as Kaposi sarcoma, data on cancer risk in relation to immune function in the general population are sparse. One cohort study in Japan found that medium and high cytotoxic activity of peripheral lymphocytes at study entry was associated with reduced risk of cancer (all sites combined) and that low activity was associated with increased risk of cancer at 11-year follow-up (Imai *et al.*, 2000). The relationship of single nutrients to immune function (Chandra & Sarchielli, 1993), as well as the effect of nutrient–nutrient interactions (Kubena & McMurray, 1996) in humans and in animal models support a role for fruits and vegetables in maintaining immune function, but the effects of whole fruits and vegetables and their constituents on cancer-related immune function parameters have been little studied.

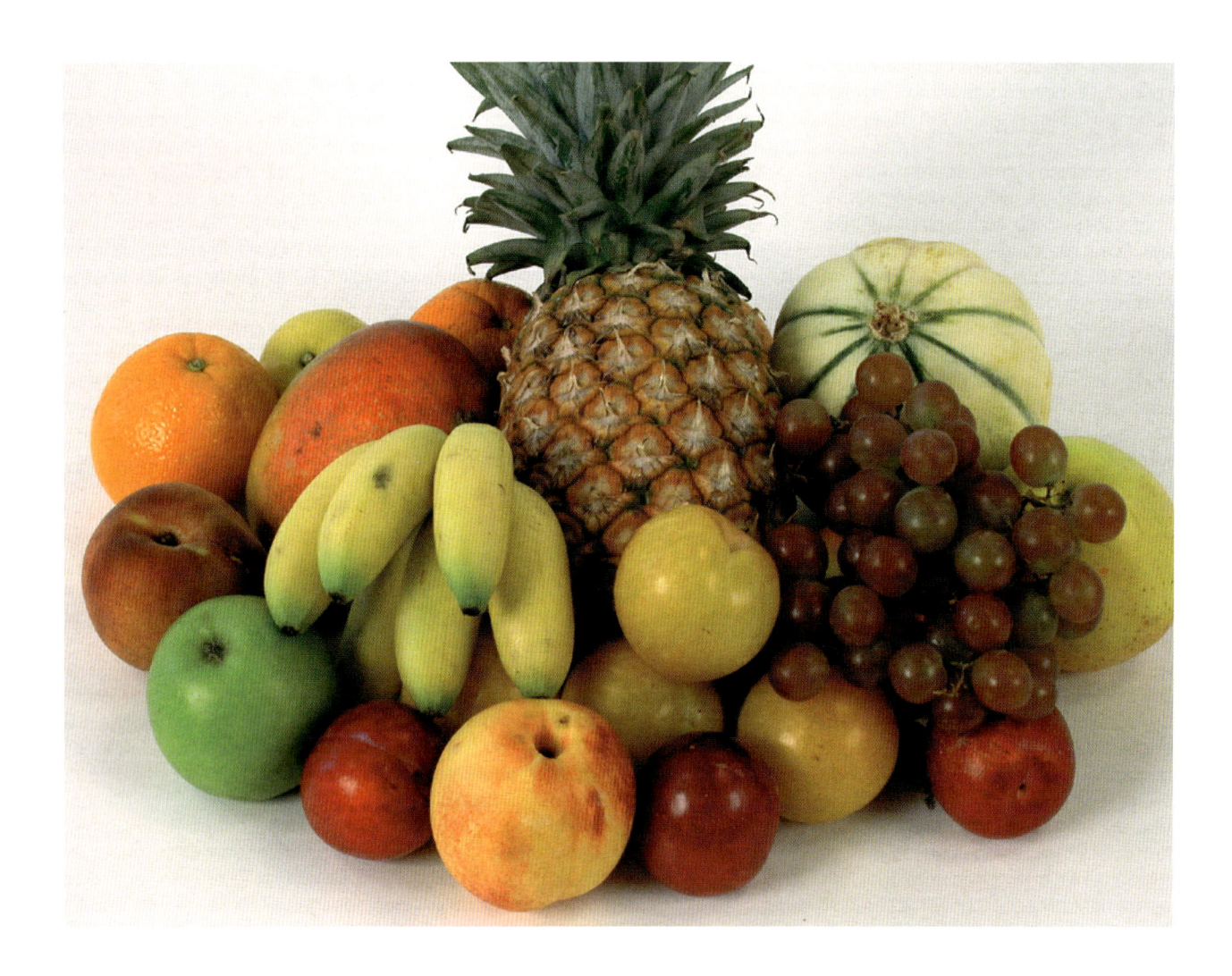

Chapter 5
Associations with diseases other than cancer

This chapter briefly reviews associations between fruit and vegetable intake and chronic diseases other than cancer, summarizing findings from the main epidemiological studies that have assessed fruit and vegetables directly or through an indicator of fruit and vegetable intake. The relationship between fruit and vegetables in the diet and chronic diseases has been reviewed recently by a joint FAO/WHO Expert Consultation panel (WHO, 2003), which rated the evidence to be convincing for a protective effect of fruit and vegetables against cardiovascular diseases (the panel defined convincing as epidemiological studies showing consistent associations between exposure and disease, with little or no evidence to the contrary).

The beneficial effects of dietary fruit and vegetables are clearly demonstrated by scurvy, a well documented, dramatic consequence of a dietary deficiency in these foods (Passmore & Eastwood, 1986). Two main lines of research have drawn increasing attention to other long-term beneficial effects of fruit and vegetables. One line of research is based on knowledge, derived from the study of clinical deficiency conditions, of the physiological functions of specific components of fruit and vegetables, such as individual vitamins. The antioxidant, free radical-scavenging properties of fruit and vegetables have prompted investigations of cardiovascular diseases in relation to intake of single vitamins, and, more recently, of fruit and vege-tables as complex mixtures of naturally occurring chemicals that may have beneficial effects because of the simultaneous presence of several active components. A second line of research has developed from the "Seven Countries" investigation of coronary heart disease (Keys, 1983). The observation of the rarity of myocardial infarction cases in the late 1940s in areas of southern Italy, Spain and Greece led to the idea that diets low in saturated fat and rich in vegetables were cardio-protective (Keys, 1980). While this line of research focused mainly on the adverse role of saturated fats, it also provided the basis for more recent work on the possible protective role of omega-3 fatty acids of vegetable or marine-fish origin. It has in fact been hypothesized that the markedly low rate of coronary heart disease in the Greek island of Crete (Renaud et al., 1995) could be mainly due to a diet rich in the omega-3 α-linolenic acid of vegetable origin, a conjecture that has received some recent support (Renaud & Lanzmann-Petithory, 2002).

These different lines of investigation are now converging in studies of how fruit and vegetables, with their micronutrient components, may influence not only the different pathogenetic steps of cardiovascular disease but also steps in the development of other chronic diseases.

Cardiovascular diseases

A number of ecological studies (Ness & Powles, 1997) have reported inverse correlations between mortality rates for coronary heart disease or stroke and the consumption of fruit and vegetables, assessed through food balance sheets or household surveys. This suggestive evidence is reinforced by the results of analytical studies of individuals. Several methodological considerations are relevant to the evaluation of such studies. Case–control studies of cardiovascular disease are few in number, while cohort studies often use only cursory measures of diet. Biomarkers of cardiovascular disease risk are also amenable to study: hypertension, hypercholesterolaemia and obesity can be regarded as intermediate steps linking diet to cardiovascular disease. Behavioural factors such as alcohol and tobacco use should be taken into account as confounding factors.

Tables 121 and 122 summarize the key findings of case–control and cohort studies on the association between fruit and vegetables (or dietary indices closely related to fruit and vegetables) and coronary heart disease; Tables 123 and 124 summarize the studies for stroke; and Table 125 summarizes the studies for total cardiovascular disease. Overall the results of these studies, on either coronary heart disease or stroke, are not entirely consistent. However, the inverse associations found in the larger studies, with better control for confounding factors, provide evidence supporting a protective effect.

Blood pressure was significantly reduced in both normotensive and hypertensive subjects in two randomized controlled trials of vegetarian diets, in which animal products were replaced with vegetable products. In an eight-week randomized controlled trial on adults with mild hypertension, a diet enriched with fruit and vegetables (and less snacks and sweets) reduced both systolic and diastolic blood pressure (Appel *et al.*, 1997). In another six-month trial, participants randomly assigned to an intervention to increase consumption of fruit and vegetables up to at least five daily portions showed a greater reduction in systolic and diastolic blood pressure than the control group (John *et al.*, 2002). These studies indicate the potential effectiveness of a diet rich in fruit and vegetables in lowering blood pressure over intervals of weeks and months. In contrast, however, increasing fruit and vegetable consumption up to at least eight servings per day over one year in subjects with a recent history of adenomas did not reduce blood pressure or body weight, despite a modest reduction in serum cholesterol level (Smith-Warner *et al.*, 2000).

Other diseases

Two recent randomized trials (Tuomilehto *et al.*, 2001; Lindstrom *et al.*, 2003) have shown that lifestyle and diet changes, including substitution of energy-dense dietary fats with fruit and vegetables, can improve glucose tolerance and prevent the onset of type II diabetes. Although these trials featured increased intake of fruit and vegetables, they were not designed to assess the independence of these changes from the effects of other factors, including physical activity and weight loss. Virtually all diets that aim at avoiding excess weight, an established risk factor for diabetes as well as coronary heart disease, involve replacing high-fat foods with low-energy density foods, such as fruit and vegetables. Higher intake of some fruits and vegetables rich in carotenoids, or a higher estimated level of dietary carotenoids, has been associated with decreased risk of cataracts in some studies, in particular two large prospective studies (Hankinsson *et al.*, 1992; Brown *et al.*, 1999). Less data are available on associations of fruit and vegetable consumption with other chronic conditions such as osteoporosis, senile macular degeneration, Alzheimer disease and Parkinson disease.

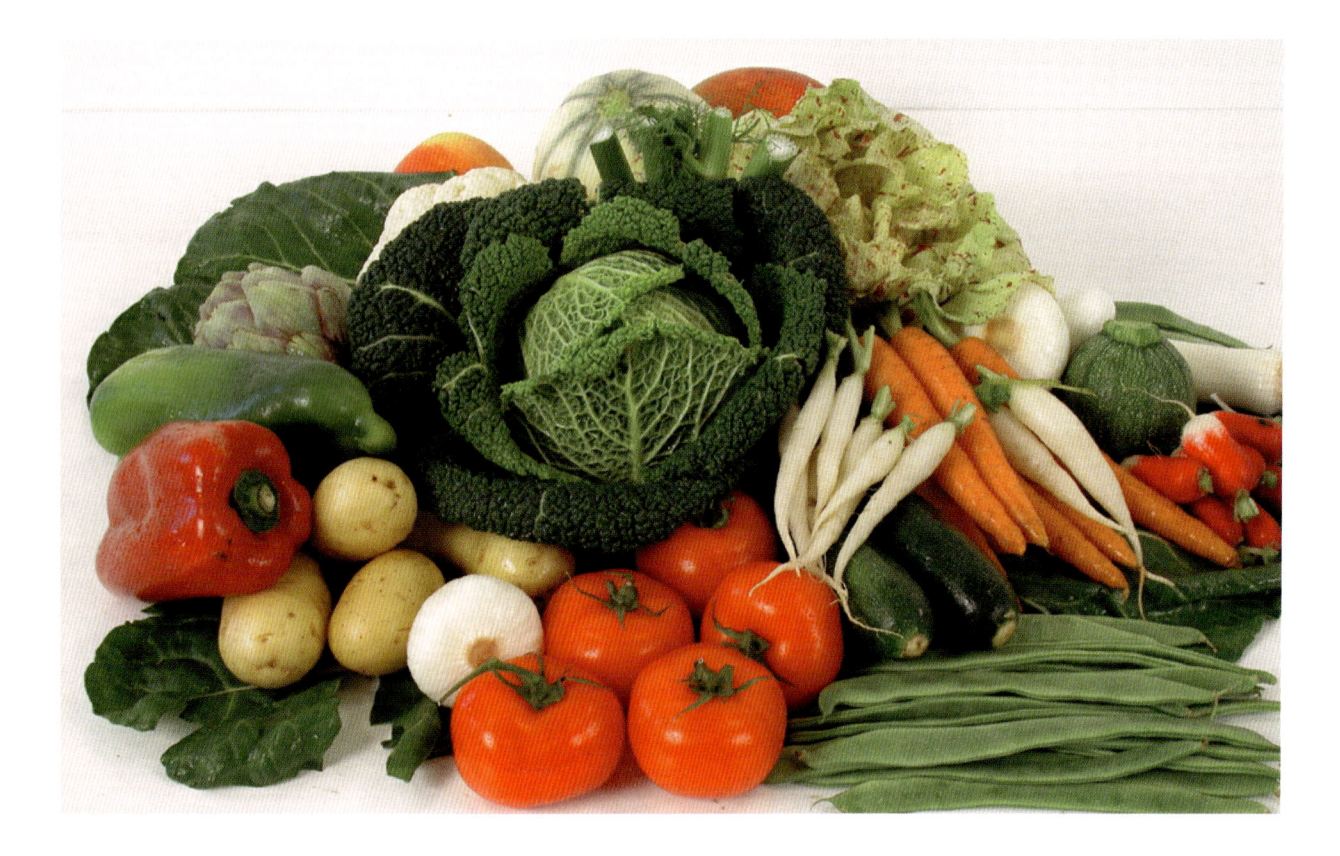

Table 121. Case-control studies reporting measures of association between intake of fruit and vegetables and coronary heart disease

Author, year country	Cases/controls, gender	Exposure assessment (no. of items)	Range contrast (no. of categories)	Relative risk (95% CI)	Stat. sign.*	Adjustment for confounding	Comments
Gramenzi et al., 1990, Italy	287 Acute MI/649 hospital controls, F	FFQ (10)	Carrots: > 1 vs < 1 portion/wk (3)	0.5	p < 0.01	Age, education, area of residence, smoking, CHD risk factors, other foods	Crude dietary measure
			Green veg.: > 7 vs < 7 portion/w (3)	0.7	NS		
			Fresh fruit: > 13 vs < 7 portion/w (3)	0.6	NS		
Tzonou et al., 1993, Greece	329 first MI or positive angiogram/570 hospital controls, M, F	FFQ (110)	Estimated vitamin C: highest vs lowest (5)	1.14 (0.67–1.95)		Gender, age, interviewer, education, BMI, exercise, siesta, smoking, alcohol, coffee, energy	No food-based analyses

*p for trend when applicable

BMI, body mass index; CHD, coronary heart disease; FFQ, food frequency questionnaire, MI, myocardial infarction; NS not significant.
Adapted and updated from Ness & Powles, 1997

Table 122. Cohort studies reporting measures of association between intake of fruit and vegetables and coronorary heart disease

Author, year country	Cases/cohort size, gender (years follow-up)	Exposure assessment (no. of items)	Range contrast (no. of categories)	Relative risk (95% CI)	Stat. sign.*	Adjustment for confounding	Comments
Morris et al., 1977, UK	45 cases of CHD (26 CHD deaths)/337, M (10–20y)	7-day weighed diary		No association with fibre from fruit, nuts, pulses, veg.		Age, occupation, follow-up	High energy intake cereal fibre protective
Vollset & Bjelke, 1983, Norway	No. ischaemic heart disease not reported/ 16 713, M, F (11.5y)	Postal dietary survey (20)	Estimated vitamin C index	No association		Age, sex, region, urbanization	Three subcohorts

Table 122 (contd)

Author, year country	Cases/cohort size, gender (years follow-up)	Exposure assessment (no. of items)	Range contrast (no. of categories)	Relative risk (95% CI)	Stat. sign.*	Adjustment for confounding	Comments
Hirayama, 1990, Japan	Deaths – numbers not given/ 265 118, M, F (17 y)	FFQ (7)	Green and yellow veg.: daily vs not (2)	No association			Census-based cohort Crude diet measure
Lapidus et al., 1986, Sweden	23 MI (8 fatal; 15 non-fatal)/ 1462 F (12 y)	24-h recall	Estimated vitamin C	No association		Age, obesity, smoking, CHD risk factors, exercise	Energy negatively associated with MI
Fraser et al., 1992, USA	134 non-fatal MI, 260 fatal CHD/26 473 M, F (6 y)	FFQ (65)	Fruit index: > 2 vs < 1/d (3)	Non-fatal MI: 1.07 (0.58–1.96) Fatal CHD: 1.08 (0.67–1.75)		Age, sex, smoking, exercise, weight, blood pressure	Seventh-Day Adventists Low-risk cohort High fruit intake not well discriminated
Manson et al., 1992, USA	437 non-fatal MI, 115 CHD deaths/87 245, F (8 y)	FFQ	Estimated vitamin C: Highest vs lowest (5)	0.80 (0.58–1.10)		Age, smoking, CHD risk factors, vitamin supplements	Nurses' Health Study Only reported as abstract
Fehily et al., 1993, Wales	148 CHD events/2423, M (5 y)	FFQ	Estimated vitamin C: ≥ 66.5 vs ≤ 34.7 mg/d (5)	[0.63]	NS	Age, BMI, smoking, CHD at baseline	25% had CHD at baseline
Rimm et al., 1993, USA	667 CHD/ 39 910, M (4 y)	FFQ (131)	Estimated vitamin C (median values: 1162 vs 92 mg/day) (5) Estimated β-carotene (median values: 190.34 vs 3969 mg/day) (5)	1.25 (0.91–1.71) Smokers: 0.30 (0.11–0.82) Former smokers: 0.60 (0.38–0.94) Non-smokers: 1.09 (0.66–1.79)	$p = 0.98$ $p = 0.02$ $p = 0.04$ $p = 0.64$	Age, smoking, diet, aspirin, exercise, BMI, energy, fibre, alcohol, parental history of MI, other antioxidants	Health professionals study Main finding was for vitamin E High vitamin C ranges

Associations with diseases other than cancer

Table 122 (contd)

Author, year country	Cases/cohort size, gender (years follow-up)	Exposure assessment (no. of items)	Range contrast (no. of categories)	Relative risk (95% CI)	Stat. sign.*	Adjustment for confounding	Comments
Hertog et al., 1993, Netherlands	43 CHD deaths/805 M (5 y)	Cross-check diet history interview	Apples: ≥110 vs <18 g/d (3)	0.51 (0.23–1.16)	p = 0.12	Age, diet, BMI, exercise, CHD risk factors, energy, saturated fatty acids, smoking, history of MI	Main focus on flavonoids
Knekt et al., 1994, Finland	244 CHD deaths/5133, M, F (14 y)	Diet history interview	Fruit: > 159 vs ≤ 75 g/d (M) and > 137 vs ≤ 77 g/d (F) (3)	M: 0.77 (0.52–1.12)	p = 0.28	Age, smoking, CHD risk factors, BMI, energy	Main focus on antioxidants. Similar effects in F but NS
			Veg.: > 117 vs ≤ 61 g/d (M) and > 137 vs ≤ 77 (F) (3)	M: 0.66 (0.46–0.96)	p=0.02		
Gaziano et al., 1995, USA	48 fatal MI/ 1299, M, F (4.75 y)	FFQ (43)	Estimated β-carotene index	0.27 (0.10–0.74)	p =0.005	Age, sex, smoking, cholesterol intake, alcohol, activities of daily living	Cause of death not confirmed in 15%
Gale et al., 1995, UK	182 CHD deaths/730, M, F (20 y)	7-day weighed record	Estimated vitamin C: > 44.9 vs ≤ 27.9 mg/d (3)	0.8 (0.6–1.2)	p = 0.595	Age, sex	Low vitamin C intake and infrequent supplement use. No food-based analyses
Gillman et al., 1995, USA	CHD numbers. not reported/ 832 M (20 y)	24-h recall		CHD no association		CHD risk factors, left ventricular hypertrophy, BMI, energy, alcohol, exercise	Potatoes included as fruit and veg. Poor exposure measure
Pandey et al., 1995, USA	231 CHD deaths/1556, M (24 y)	Diet history (twice, 1 year apart)	Increment of 19 points in estimated vitamin C + β-carotene index (highest/lowest: vitamin C 138/66, β-carotene 5.3/2.3)	0.70 (0.49–0.98)		Age, family history, CHD risk factors, smoking, BMI, energy, fats, iron, education, alcohol, cholesterol intake	Few supplement takers

Table 122 (contd)

Author, year country	Cases/cohort size, gender (years follow-up)	Exposure assessment (no. of items)	Range contrast (no. of categories)	Relative risk (95% CI)	Stat. sign.*	Adjustment for confounding	Comments
Knekt et al., 1996, Finland	473 CHD deaths/5133 M, F (26 y)	Diet history interview	Highest vs lowest (4)	RR between 0.50–0.89 for apples, berries (only in women), other fruit, onions and veg.		Age, smoking, CHD risk factors, BMI	Main focus on flavonoids
Kushi et al., 1996, USA	242 CHD deaths/34 486, F (post-menopausal) (7 y)	FFQ (127)	Vitamin C from food and supplements: ≥ 391 vs ≤ 112.3 mg/d (5)	1.49 (0.96–2.30)	p = 0.02	Age, energy, BMI, WHR, smoking, hypertension, diabetes, HRT, contraceptive use, physical activity, alcohol, marital status, education	No analysis for fruits and veg. Intake of vitamin C from foods and supplements high Result similar in non supplement takers
			Carotenoids from food and supplements: ≥ 13 465 vs ≤ 4421 IU/d (5)	1.03 (0.63–1.70)	p = 0.71		
Liu et al., 2000, USA	126 MI/ 39 127, F (6 y)	FFQ, (131)	Fruit and veg.: highest vs lowest (5) (median values: 10.2 vs 2.6 servings/d)	0.63 (0.38–1.17)	p = 0.21	Age, smoking, physical activity, alcohol, meno-pausal status, HRT use, BMI, vitamin supplement use, parental history MI, history of MI, diabetes, hypertension, hypercholes-terolaemia	Women's Health Study
Liu et al., 2001, USA	1148 incident CHD/15 220, M (12 y)	FFQ (8 veg.)	Veg.: > 2.5 vs < 1 serving/d (5)	0.77 (0.60–0.98)	p = 0.03	Age, randomization assigment, BMI, smoking, alcohol, physical activity, history of hypercholes-terolaemia, hypertension and diabetes, multivitamin supplements	Physicians' Health Study end-points: MI plus coronary artery bypass grafting plus percutaneous transluminal angioplasty

Table 122 (contd)

Author, year country	Cases/cohort size, gender (years follow-up)	Exposure assessment (no. of items)	Range contrast (no. of categories)	Relative risk (95% CI)	Stat. sign.*	Adjustment for confounding	Comments
Joshipura et al., 2001, USA	CHD 1063 M, 1127 F (fatal and non-fatal)/ 42 148 M, 84 251 F (M: 8 y F: 14 y)	FFQ (126, 15 fruits, 28 veg.)	Fruit and veg.: highest vs lowest (5) (median values: 9.15 vs 2.54 servings/d)	0.80 (0.69–0.93)		Age, smoking, alcohol, family history of MI, BMI, energy, multi-vitamins and vitamin E supplements, aspirin, physical activity, HRT, hypertension, hypercholesterolaemia	Nurses' and Health Professionals' studies. Main contributors: green leafy veg. and vitamin C-rich fruits and veg.
Bazzano et al., 2002, USA	1786 CHD (639 deaths)/ 9608, M, F (19 y)	FFQ (13, 3 fruits and veg.)	Fruit and veg.: > 3 vs < 1 times/d (4)	Mortality 0.76 (0.56–1.03) Incidence: 1.01 (0.84–1.21)	$p = 0.07$ $p = 0.8$	Age, sex, race, education, physical activity, alcohol, smoking, history of diabetes, energy, vitamin supplements	National Health and Nutrition Examination Survey Study
Michels & Wolk, 2002, Sweden	1558 CHD deaths/ 59 038, F (9.9 y)	FFQ (60) Creation of categories of 'good' diet or RFS (recommended foods score) and 'bad; or NRFS (non-recommended foods score)	RFS: highest vs lowest (5)	0.47 (0.33–0.68)	$p < 0.0001$	Age, height, BMI, parity, age at first birth, education, marital status, alcohol, energy	Mammography cohort. No association with NRFS

*p for trend when applicable

BMI, body mass index; CHD, coronary heart disease; FFQ, food frequency questionnaire; HRT, hormone replacement therapy; MI, myocardial infarction; NS, not significant; WHR, waist-to-hip ratio

Adapted and updated from Ness & Powles, 1997

Table 123. Case–control study reporting measures of association between intake of fruit and vegetables and stroke

Author, year country	Cases/ controls, gender	Exposure assessment (no. of items)	Range contrast (no. of categories)	Relative risk (95% CI)	Stat. sign.*	Adjustment for confounding	Comments
Barer et al., 1989, UK	63 thrombotic stroke/91, M, F	Questionnaire	Estimated vitamin C index	No association		Age, sex, socio-economic status, smoking, alcohol, non-steroidal anti-inflammatory drugs, build	Hospital cases and controls Crude measure of habitual diet

*p for trend when applicable
Adapted and updated from Ness & Powles, 1997

Table 124. Cohort studies reporting measures of association between intake of fruit and vegetables and stroke

Author, year country	Cases/cohort-size, gender, (years follow-up)	Exposure assessment (no. of items)	Range contrast (no. of categories)	Relative risk (95% CI)	Stat. sign.*	Adjustment for confounding	Comments
Vollset & Bjelke, 1983, Norway	438 cerebrovascular deaths/16 713, M, F (11.5 y)	Postal dietary survey (20)	Estimated vitamin C index: highest vs lowest (3)	0.67 (0.52–0.87)	$p = 0.0005$	Age, sex, region, urbanization	3 subcohorts Negative association with fruit and veg.
Hirayama, 1990, Japan	Deaths – numbers not given/ 265 118, M, F (17 y)	FFQ (7)	Green and yellow veg.: daily vs not (2)	No association			Census-based cohort Crude diet measure
Lapidus et al., 1986, Sweden	13 strokes/ 1462 F (12 y)	24-h recall	Estimated vitamin C	No association		Age, obesity, smoking, CHD risk factors, exercise	
Manson et al., 1994, USA	345 stroke cases/ 87 245, F (8 y)	FFQ	Veg. score: highest vs lowest (5) Carrots, spinach ≥ 5/wk vs < 1/mo	0.74 Carrots: 0.32 Spinach: 0.57	$p = 0.03$	Age, smoking	Nurses' Health Study No association for fruit
Gale et al., 1995, UK	124 stroke deaths/730, M, F (20) y	7-day weighed diet record	Estimated vitamin C: > 44.9 vs ≤ 27.9 mg/d (3)	0.5 (0.3–0.8)	$p = 0.003$	Age, sex, CHD risk factors	Low vitamin C intake and infrequent supplement use No food-based analyses

Associations with diseases other than cancer

Table 124 (contd)

Author, year country	Cases/cohort size, gender (years follow-up)	Exposure assessment (no. of items)	Range contrast (no. of categories)	Relative risk (95% CI)	Stat. sign.*	Adjustment for confounding	Comments
Gillman et al., 1995, USA	97 strokes (14 deaths)/832 M (20 y)	24-h recall	Fruit and veg.: increment of 3 servings/d	0.77 (0.60–0.98)		Age, CHD risk factors, BMI, exercise, left ventricular hypertrophy, energy, fat, alcohol	Potatoes included in fruit and vegetables. Poor exposure measure. Same association for mortality
Joshipura et al., 1999, USA	Ischaemic stroke: 204 (M), 366 (F)/38 683 (M), 75 596 (F) (M: 8 y F: 14 y)	FFQ (116, 15 fruits, 28 veg.)	Fruit and veg.: highest vs lowest (5) (median values: 9.15 vs 2.54 servings/d)	0.69 (0.52–0.92)		Age, smoking, alcohol, family history of MI, BMI, energy, multivitamin and vitamin E supplements, aspirin use, physical activity, HRT, hypertension, hypercholesterolaemia	Nurses' and Health Professionals' Studies. Most contribution from cruciferous veg., green leafy veg., citrus fruits, including juice
Bazzano et al., 2002, USA	888 stroke, 218 fatal/9608, M, F (19 y)	FFQ (13, 3 fruits and veg.)	Fruit and veg.: > 3 vs < 1 time/d (4)	Mortality: 0.58 (0.33–1.02) Incidence: 0.73 (0.57–0.95)	$p = 0.05$ $p = 0.01$	Age, sex, race, education, physical activity, history of diabetes, alcohol, smoking, energy, vitamin supplements	National Health and Nutrition Examination Survey Study
Michels & Wolk, 2002, Sweden	684 stroke/59 038, F (9.9 y)	FFQ (60) Creation of categories of 'good' diet or RFS (recommended foods score) and 'Bad' or NRFS (non-recommended foods score)	RFS: highest vs lowest (5)	0.40 (0.22–0.73)	$p = 0.007$	Age, height, BMI, parity, age first birth, education, marital status, alcohol, energy	Mammography cohort. No association with NRFS

*p for trend when applicable

BMI, body mass index, CHD, coronary heart disease; FFQ, food frequency questionnaire; HRT, hormone replacement therapy; MI, myocardial infarction

Adapted and updated from Ness & Powles, 1997

Table 125. Cohort studies reporting measures of association between intake of fruit and vegetables and total circulatory disease

Author, year country	Cases/cohort size, gender (years follow-up)	Exposure assessment (no. of items)	Range contrast (no. of categories)	Relative risk (95% CI)	Stat. sign.*	Adjustment for confounding	Comments
Enstrom et al., 1992, USA	929 cardiovascular disease deaths/11 348, M, F (10 y)	24-h recall and FFQ	Estimated vitamin C index: ≥ 50 vs < 50 mg/d (2)	SMR (relative to US whites): No regular supplement: 0.90 (0.82–0.99) Regular supplements: 0.66 (0.53–0.82)		Age, sex, smoking, education, race, disease, exercise, alcohol, energy, nutrients	National Health and Nutrition Examination Survey
Gaziano et al., 1995, USA	161 fatal cardiovascular disease/1299, M, F (4.75 y)	FFQ (43)	≥ 1 vs < 1/d	Carrots: 0.40 (0.17–0.98) Salads: 0.49 (0.31–0.77)		Age, sex	Cause of death not confirmed in 15%. Significant inverse association with estimated β-carotene index
Cox et al., 2000, UK	392 cardiovascular events (162 fatal)/3389, M, F (7 y)	FFQ (31, considering seasons)	Daily vs never (5)	Salads: inverse association (consumption either in winter and summer for F; only in winter for M). Fruit: inverse association (consumption either in winter and summer only in F)	$p < 0.001$	Age, smoking, socioeconomic status	
Strandhagen et al., 2000, Sweden	209 non-fatal cardio-vascular events, 226 deaths/730 M (26 y)	FFQ	6–7 vs 0–1 times/wk (4)	Fruit (M) 16 y follow-up: 0.87 (0.76–0.96) 26 y follow-up: 0.92 (0.84–1.00) Veg.: no association	$p = 0.051$	Smoking, hypertension, serum cholesterol (no age control, since all men were born same year)	
Rissanen et al., 2003, Finland	115 cardiovascular disease deaths/ 1950, M (12.8 y)	Food record	Fruits, berries and vegetables: > 408 vs < 133 g/d (5)	0.66 (0.28–1.55)	$p = 0.13$	Age, examination year, BMI, CHD risk factors, energy, intake of vitamins C and E, β-carotene, lycopene, folate, fibre	

*p for trend when applicable
BMI, body mass index; CHD, coronary heart disease; FFQ, food frequency questionnaire
Adapted and updated from Ness & Powles, 1997

Chapter 6
Carcinogenic effects

Human studies

Chapter 4 reviewed epidemiological studies of cancer, in a few of which the reported relative risks for high versus low consumption of either fruit or vegetables were significantly greater than 1.0 (for example, some studies of cancer of the colorectum, breast and prostate). In general, these were extreme examples of estimates that overall tended to centre close to the null. None of these results were evaluated by the Working Group as evidence of carcinogenicity in humans.

For some specific food constituents, such as β-carotene (IARC, 1998) and some vegetables (e.g., bracken fern; IARC, 1986), there is some evidence of carcinogenicity to humans, but this does not affect the evaluations of the overall cancer preventive activity of total fruit or total vegetables.

Fruit and vegetables have sometimes been regarded as a possible vehicle for carcinogens, either intrinsic to the plant itself or as external contaminants (e.g., pesticides and herbicides) (Ames et al., 1990).

Pickled vegetables, as prepared traditionally in parts of China, Japan and Korea by fermentation of local vegetables, have been found to be associated with cancers of the stomach, oesophagus and nasopharynx (IARC, 1993). High levels of aflatoxin contamination have been found in groundnuts and maize in regions of Africa, south-east Asia and southern China, where these foods are dietary staples (IARC, 2002). Lower levels have been observed in other grains, cereal products and nuts. Exposures in other countries arise as a result of importing foods from areas where aflatoxin contamination is high, but at lower levels than in the hot humid areas where aflatoxin-producing *Aspergillus* species are present. Exposure to aflatoxin B_1 is consistently associated with hepatocellular carcinoma.

Animal studies

A few studies in experimental animals have found increased tumour yields after administration of fruit and vegetables in the diet.

Only one study was conducted on spontaneous tumours. Groups of 50 male and 50 female Wistar rats were fed one of the following diets: a semi-purified animal diet (A, control); diet A in which fruit and vegetables replaced macro- and micronutrients (B); an uncooked human diet (meat, bread and eggs) supplemented with semi-purified micronutrients (C); diet C with fried or baked products (D); or a complete human diet consisting of cooked products, fruit and vegetables (E). Diets B, C, D and E were prepared according to mean dietary composition figures for the Netherlands. The animal diets contained 21.6% energy fat and the human diets contained 40.6% energy fat. Rats were fed *ad libitum* for 142 weeks. Male but not female rats fed the human diets (C, D or E) had a significantly higher incidence of epithelial tumours than those fed the animal diet, mainly accounted for by tumours of the pituitary and thyroid glands. Compared to the uncooked human diet, addition of fruit and vegetables (diet E) induced minor non-significant differences in tumour incidence (Alink et al., 1989).

Out of a total of 30 experiments that examined the effects of high quantities of 13 different individual fruit or vegetables on chemically induced carcinogenesis, none reported adverse tumorigenic effects. Six experiments evaluated the effects of low amounts of a mixture of fruits and vegetables on colon cancer. Four of these showed preventive effects (Rijnkels et al., 1997a,b,c; Rijnkels & Alink, 1998; see Chapter 4) and two showed evidence of an adverse effect, as detailed below.

The effect of addition of fruit and vegetables to a simulated human diet or a rodent diet on 1,2-dimethyl-hydrazine (DMH)-induced colon carcinogenesis was evaluated by Alink et al. (1993). Groups of four-week-old male Wistar rats (36–43 rats/group) were fed a rodent diet or a European human diet (21.6 and 40.6% fat energy, respectively) with or without 19.5% fruit and vegetables replacing potato starch. After four weeks, all rats were given subcutaneous injections of 50 mg/kg bw DMH once per week for 10 weeks. The experiment was terminated 28 weeks after the first DMH dose. The multiplicity of colon adenocarcinomas was significantly higher ($p < 0.05$) in animals fed the human diet containing fruit and vegetables than in those fed the control human diet.

Another study evaluated the effects of dietary fat and a fruit–vegetable mixture on intestinal tumorigenesis in *APC*^{Min} mice (van Kranen *et al.*, 1998). Female and male *Apc*^{Min} mice were fed during the mating period a low-fat (20% fat energy) or high-fat (40% fat energy) diet with or without 19.5% fruit–vegetable mixture substituting for total carbohydrates. Both male and female mice born to these mice were weaned to their respective low- and high-fat diets with or without the fruit–vegetable mixture and were continued on these diets until 90 days of age. The fruit–vegetable mixture added to the high-fat diet significantly increased the multiplicity of small intestinal tumours in male mice (27.7 versus 17.1 tumours per tumour-bearing mouse) and in female mice (25.8 versus 16.0 tumours per tumour-bearing mouse) compared with those fed the high-fat control diet.

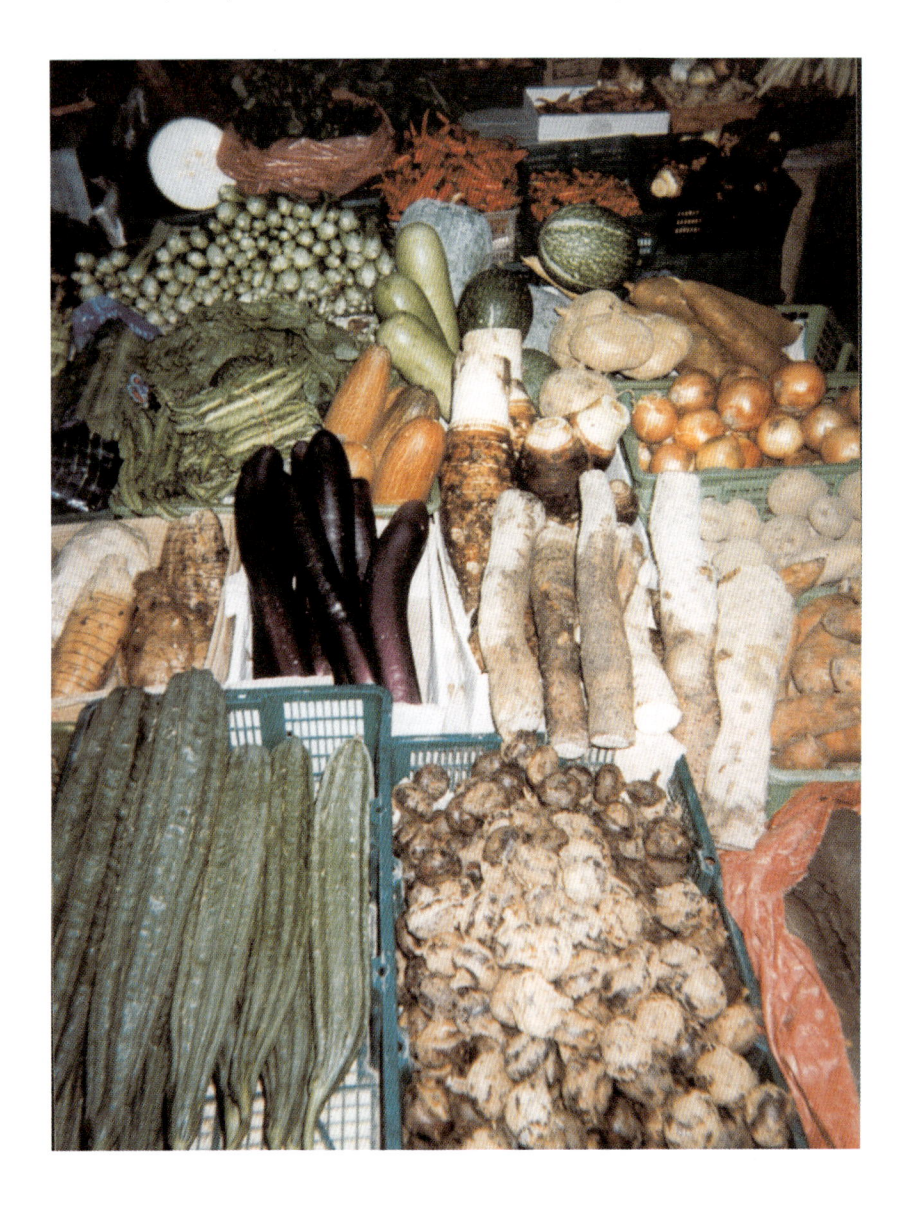

Chapter 7
Toxic effects

Human studies

Potential adverse effects of fruit and vegetable consumption have been investigated in relation to nitrates (Steinmetz & Potter, 1991), pickled vegetables, as prepared traditionally in Asia (IARC, 1993), goitrogens in cruciferous vegetables (Steinmetz & Potter, 1991), aflatoxins in dietary staples including dried fruit particularly in Africa, south-west Asia, southern China and episodically in the USA (IARC, 1993), other contaminants, e.g. cyclosporiasis (Osterholm, 1997), pesticides and herbicides (Steinmetz & Potter, 1991) and Alar, a growth regulator used to treat apples (Steinmetz & Potter, 1991). There appears to be little evidence that exposure to these factors as a result of dietary intake of fruit and vegetables leads to adverse effects.

Undesirable effects from consumption of fruit and vegetables that can occur range from bloating, flatulence and cramps to immunoallergic reactions. Allergic reactions have been associated with tomatoes, kiwi fruit, bananas and other fruit (Wagner & Breiteneder, 2002). A vegetable which may cause allergic reactions is celery. Celery root is often consumed in a processed form as a cooked vegetable or as a spice. Ballmer-Weber et al. (2002) studied the allergenicity of processed celery in celery-allergic patients. In 12 patients with a history of allergic reactivity to raw or cooked celery, double-blind placebo-controlled food challenges with raw celery, cooked celery and celery spice were performed. Six patients showed a positive reaction to cooked celery. The conclusion was that celery remains allergenic even after extended thermal treatment.

Animal studies

Many toxicants occur in plants consumed by humans, but the majority of these do not occur in cultivated fruits or vegetables. A few animal studies have been conducted to test for toxic effects due to feeding of fruit or vegetables, as summarized below.

Cruciferous crops (goitre)
Glucosinolates predominantly occur in the family of the Cruciferae, in particular in the Brassica species. These include cabbage species, radish, cress and rapeseed. Thioglucosidases hydrolyse the glucosinolate into glucose, sulfate ions and the aglycone (organic isothiocyanates or mustard oil). The aglycones inhibit thyroid function and therefore are also called goitrogens.

The first harmful effect in animals fed Brassica vegetables was reported 75 years ago, when relatively large amounts of cabbage fed to rabbits caused goitre development (Chesney et al., 1928). Fifteen years later, it was shown that the thiocyanate product of the indolyl glucosinolate (GS) caused goitre in animals with a dietary iodine deficiency (Astwood, 1943). Growth retardation, liver lesions or necrosis and thyroid hypertrophy or hyperplasia occur in most animals when the diet contains approximately 2–5 mg GS/g diet (Fenwick et al., 1989). Mink have been adversely affected by diets containing GS levels of only 0.5 mg/g diet (Belzile et al., 1974). Cattle fed large quantities of kale developed severe haemolytic anaemia (Rosenberger, 1939). After 1–3 weeks of kale feeding, most ruminant animals produced the first signs of the disease: the appearance of stainable granules within the red blood cells known as Heinz–Ehrlich bodies. These bodies are formed by dimethyl disulfide, a product of S-methylcysteine sulfoxide (SMCSO). SMCSO intake in goats at 15–19 g/100 g bw elicits this haemolytic response (Smith, 1978). Rats fed SMCSO at 2% in the diet showed growth depression, anaemia and splenic hypertrophy (Uchino & Itokawa, 1972; Uchino & Otokami, 1972). SMCSO occurs in plant tissue in variable amounts up to 4%. Besides Brassica vegetables, SMCSO has been shown to be present in various beans, Allium (onion, garlic, chives), radish and cowpea. It is obtained by conversion of S-methylcysteine formed by methylation of cysteine by methionine (Stoewsand, 1995).

Umbelliferous crops (phototoxicity)
Furocoumarins present in certain food plants may give rise to phototoxicity. In

particular, umbelliferous crop plants, such as the parsnip (*Pastinaca sativa* L.) elaborate enhanced levels of furocoumarins, including psoralens, when subjected to biotic or abiotic stress. Young male mice were fed for 30 days diets containing 32.5% dried healthy, 32.5% apparently healthy or 32.5% fungicide-treated and 8, 16 or 32.5% dried diseased (*Phoma complanata*-infected) parsnip root tissue (Mongeau *et al.*, 1994). Dried healthy parsnip, compared with controls, did not significantly affect cellular proliferation or histopathological parameters. No histopathological changes were observed in the oesophagus and forestomach with any of the diets. In the liver, only the highest level of dried diseased parsnip led to swelling of cells in hepatic lobules. Using [^{3}H]thymidine, a dose-related increase in cell labelling with the level of diseased parsnip was seen in the liver; a slight, not significant, increase was noted with fungicide-treated parsnip. Increased [^{3}H]-thymidine labelling with feeding diseased parsnip was also found in the forestomach but not in the oesophagus.

Celery (allergenic compounds)

Although for humans some fruit and vegetables are known to be allergic, almost no animal studies have been performed in which fruit or vegetables have been tested for allergenicity.

Celery, which is allergic for humans, has been tested for allergenicity in mice (Ballmer-Weber *et al.*, 2002). Intraperitoneal immunization of mice followed by a rat basophil leukaemia cell mediator release assay was used to assess the allergenicity of processed celery. The murine model reflected the allergenicity observed in humans.

Bitter gourd (general toxicity)

Momordica charantia (bitter gourd) 5% aqueous extracts were tested orally in mice at doses of 50 and 100 μL/mouse per day for three months (Ganguly *et al.*, 2000). The dose of 50 μL was well tolerated but, at the higher dose, food intake was severely reduced and the animals had rapid loss in body weight, fall in blood glucose level and high mortality.

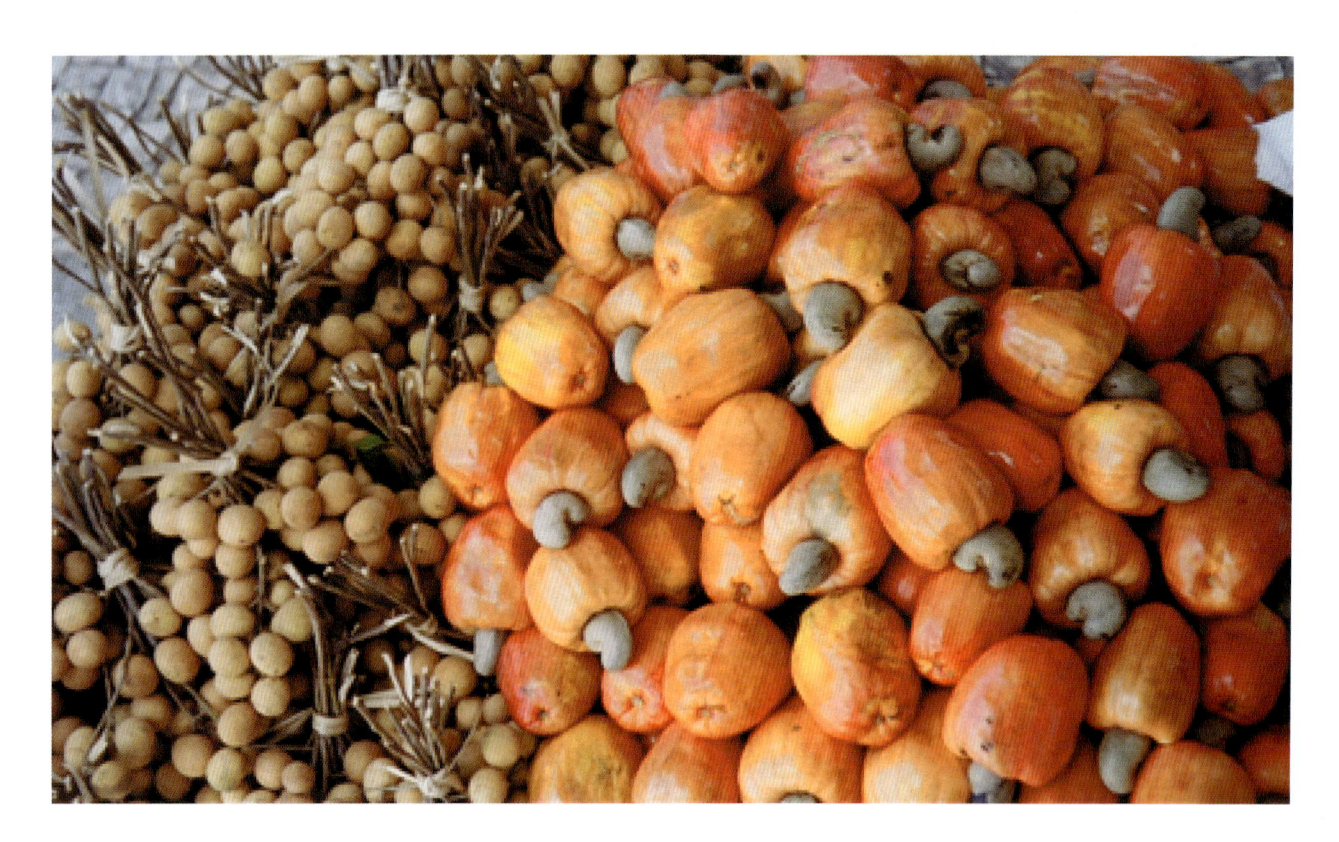

Chapter 8
Summary of data

Definitions and classifications for fruit and vegetables

Although botanical definitions for fruit and vegetables are more precise than culinary definitions, the latter are based on cultural uses of foods and are more commonly used by researchers and understood by participants in epidemiological studies. The culinary term *fruit and vegetables* generally refers to edible plant foods with the exclusion of cereal grains, nuts, and seeds. Also excluded are plant parts used to make liquid infusions (tea leaves and coffee and cacao beans) and plant parts used as herbs or spices. The culinary term *fruit* refers to the part of a plant that contains the seeds and pulpy surrounding tissue and has a sweet or tart taste. Fruits are most often used as breakfast beverages, breakfast or lunch side-dishes, snacks or desserts. Plant parts used as *vegetables* include stems and stalks, roots, tubers, bulbs, leaves, flowers, some fruits, and pulses. Vegetables are consumed raw or cooked with a main dish, in a mixed dish, as an appetizer or in a salad.

Subgroup classifications for fruit and vegetables relate to growing conditions, fruit development from flowers, classes used for national food supply or consumption data, botanical families, plant parts and colour. Some aspects of the latter three types of classification have been used to collect and report information in epidemiological studies. Examples of these types of grouping include dark green leafy vegetables (spinach); cruciferous vegetables (cabbage, broccoli); citrus family fruits (orange, tangerine); and *Allium* family bulbs (garlic, onion). The definitions and classification of fruit and vegetables are not precise and differ between dietary assessment instruments (e.g., potatoes or mushrooms may or may not be included), depending on the purposes of the study and the dietary patterns of the population being evaluated.

Measuring intake of fruit and vegetables

Methods for estimating dietary intake of fruit and vegetables include household measures of food availability, questionnaire measures of usual intake and methods for recording actual intake. These methods are used for various purposes including nutritional surveillance, epidemiological research and methodological research for validation of other dietary methods as well as clinical assessment and programme evaluation.

Household measures are used to estimate intake for nutritional surveillance and monitoring and provide data on the availability and per capita consumption of fruit and vegetable intake. Questionnaire methods – food frequency questionnaires (FFQ), and the diet history (DH) – have been the most commonly used methods to assess usual dietary intake at the individual level in cancer epidemiology cohort and case–control studies. Recording methods, 24-h recalls and food records are used in research studies and in national nutrition monitoring and to validate questionnaire methods.

Because of the large intra-individual variation in daily food intake, accurate quantification and classification of individual exposure is complex and susceptible to measurement error. The FFQ and DH are designed to estimate usual intake, to minimize the effect of intra-individual variation and provide a means to rank individuals in epidemiological analyses. In cohort studies, the aim is to assess recent habitual diet. In case–control studies, the aim is to assess habitual diet during a reference period before the onset of disease. There are large differences between epidemiological studies in the FFQ and DH used to estimate fruit and vegetable intake, in terms of (1) the fruits and vegetables included on the questionnaire, (2) how the instrument is structured, (3) the number of questions, (4) the method used to address portion sizes, and (5) the fruit and vegetable categories used in analysis.

Consumption of fruit and vegetables and relevant policies

There is a remarkable scarcity of nationally representative data on fruit and vegetable consumption, especially for developing countries. Also, the data are very diverse in quality regarding the level of representativity of the study groups, the methods used to assess intake and the format of the available data, both in terms of the age groupings and the food categories. Confusion also exists in the classification of the individual food items and the time frames of the surveys are very diverse.

It is clear nevertheless that there is remarkable diversity in the overall amounts consumed and in the proportions of fruit to vegetables. The diversity is at all levels, between individuals, between socio-cultural-economic groups within a given country, and most of all between countries. Some of the most affluent developed countries have relatively low overall intake of fruit and vegetables, such as the European Nordic countries and the USA. An age-associated positive trend in fruit and vegetable consumption seems to exist, but is not seen consistently. There are associations between fruit and vegetable intake and income, as well as with work category, attained level of education and ethnic group. These stratifying parameters are, of course, interrelated, and therefore may confound or magnify relationships to a variable extent.

Information for developed countries derives mainly from the FAO food balance sheets, with additional data from national surveys in a few countries. In general, levels of consumption are strikingly low in sub-Saharan Africa – where a large part of the fruit category is represented by bananas – and in Asia, intermediate in Central and South America, while in North Africa and the Near East, consumption of fruit and vegetables is close to that of the western, industrial areas of the world. The trend in availability of fruit and vegetables over the period 1961 to 2000 shows little change or even a decline in most of sub-Saharan Africa, while elsewhere there have been increases of variable degree.

Nutrition and health research, food policies and nutrition programmes have changed focus in the last hundred years. The early 1900s focused on identifying and preventing nutrient deficiency diseases and determining nutrient requirements. More recently, investigations have turned to the role of diet in maintaining health and reducing cancer, heart disease, osteoporosis and other noncommunicable diseases. During the past 25 years, international and national health agencies have established priorities for diet and cancer research and prevention efforts. These in turn influenced development of international and national recommendations for dietary intake and dietary guidance. The World Health Organization recently concluded that fruit and vegetables are important in health maintenance and nutrition security and recommended for adults an intake of at least 400 grams of fruit and vegetables per day. Concordant recommendations for fruit and vegetable intake have been published by several organizations recommending that at least five servings or 400 grams of fruit and vegetables be consumed per day.

National and regional health organizations have translated these international policy statements into food-based dietary guidelines that reflect the cultural food patterns and the prevalence of noncommunicable diseases in individual populations. Food guidance recommendations have led to policies and programmes for public education, nutritional surveillance, nutrition campaigns, labelling of foods and food safety. Globally there have been many campaigns and initiatives aimed at increasing fruit and vegetable intake. Some 200 nations have established food and nutrition plans and many have food-based dietary guidelines that include recommendations for fruit and vegetable intake. Strategies for increasing fruit and vegetable intake include efforts at the levels of health facilities, schools, workplaces and commercial activities.

Cancer-preventive effects

Human studies

Studies were included in the evaluation if the reports provided estimates of risk for total fruit or for total vegetable consumption, and 95% confidence intervals were available; measurement error, confounding, and selection and recall bias in case–control studies were also considered. Ecological studies were not considered in the evaluation as they were deemed to be insufficiently informative.

Estimates of a weighted mean of the reported relative risks are provided. If a study report included estimates for different sub-groups, e.g., males and females, these were both included. These weighted means must be interpreted recognizing that they do not represent the result of a formal meta-analysis, and that the contrasts of high versus low consumption are not consistent between studies.

A minority of the epidemiological studies also investigated associations between combined fruit and vegetable intake in relation to cancer risk. Overall, this did not alter the conclusions.

Oral cavity and pharynx

Most studies conducted on oropharyngeal cancer risk in relation to fruit and vegetable consumption have been hospital-based case–control studies. For the 10 evaluable case–control studies of fruit consumption, the mean relative risk for high versus low consumption was 0.45 and the range 0.10–0.70. Despite the relatively good agreement between the results, doubt remains as to whether residual confounding due to smoking habits and alcohol drinking or socioeconomic factors, recall bias among the cases, and selection bias in the control group might account for these findings.

Vegetable intake was also consistently inversely associated with risk of oropharyngeal cancer. For the seven evaluable case–control studies of vegetable consumption, the mean relative risk for high versus low consumption was 0.49 and the range 0.19–0.80. As for fruit, the possibility remains that these results are due to residual confounding by smoking and alcohol drinking as well as socioeconomic status, or to recall or selection bias.

There are no consistent findings of an inverse association of salivary gland and nasopharynx cancer with fruit or vegetable consumption.

Oesophagus

In one cohort study, an inverse association between fruit consumption and mortality from oesophageal cancer was reported. Among 16 evaluable case–control studies of fruit consumption, the mean relative risk for high versus low consumption was 0.54 and the range 0.14–1.50.

Vegetable intake was also often significantly inversely related to risk for this cancer site. For 10 evaluable case–control studies of vegetable consumption, the mean relative risk for high versus low consumption was 0.64 and the range 0.10–0.97.

A recent meta-analysis also found inverse associations for fruit and for vegetables. The set of studies used in the meta-analysis was not completely identical with the studies evaluated here.

The studies did not indicate gender-specific effects of fruit or vegetable consumption. The studies used for evaluation were underpowered to detect effect modification by strata of smoking and alcohol consumption. Thus specific effects on smokers or alcohol drinkers could not be evaluated.

It remains possible that some or all of the observed associations resulted from selection bias, recall bias or residual confounding due to insufficient control for smoking history, history of alcohol drinking, or other factors associated with the occurrence of oesophageal cancer.

Stomach

The association between intake of total fruit and risk of gastric cancer was evaluable in 10 cohort and 28 case–control studies. The mean relative risk for high versus low consumption was 0.85 and the range 0.55–1.92 in cohort studies and 0.63, range 0.31–1.39, in case–control studies.

In 25 studies (five cohort and 20 case–control), the association between intake of total vegetables and risk of gastric cancer was evaluable. The mean relative risk for high versus low consumption was 0.94 and the range 0.70–1.25 for cohort studies and 0.66 (range 0.30–1.70) for case–control studies. Most of the case–control studies adjusted for more potential confounders than the cohort studies, but many did not provide data on total fruit and total vegetable consumption.

The reason why case–control studies were more likely to show inverse associations is not clear. Case–control studies may be affected by recall bias; further, people with preclinical symptoms of stomach carcinoma or stomach disorders may have changed their dietary habits before the diagnosis.

Colon and rectum

For the 11 evaluable cohort studies of fruit consumption, the mean relative risk for high versus low consumption was 1.00 and the range 0.50–1.60. For the nine evaluable case–control studies, the mean relative risk for high versus low consumption was 0.87 and the range 0.30–1.74. A recent meta-analysis showed a small statistically significant reduction in risk across case–control studies and a small non-significant reduction across cohort studies. Among the cohort studies, the small reduction in risk was restricted to women.

For the 10 evaluable cohort studies of vegetable consumption, the mean relative risk for high versus low consumption was 0.94 and the range 0.72–1.78. For the 13 evaluable case–control studies, the mean relative risk for high versus low consumption was 0.63 and the range 0.18–1.29. A recent meta-analysis showed a substantial reduction in risk across case–control studies, but only a small non-significant reduction in risk across cohort studies.

It is not possible to rule out the possibility that bias affects the results in two ways. Recall and selection bias in the case–control studies and confounding in both cohort and case–control studies could be producing artefactual inverse associations.

Liver

One cohort study in Japan considered liver cancer mortality and fruit consumption and found no evidence of an inverse association. Only one case–control study was evaluable and showed no effect.

The only evaluable cohort study on vegetable consumption and risk of liver cancer found significant inverse associations. The evaluable case–control study showed no association. One case–control study found a significant inverse association for fruit and vegetables combined.

Biliary tract
One cohort study showed no significant effect of fruit consumption on risk of gallbladder cancer. One case–control study showed a significant association between fruit and vegetable consumption and risk of gallbladder cancer.

Pancreas
In all three evaluable cohort studies of fruit consumption, inverse associations were found, but none were significant. For six evaluable case–control studies, the mean relative risk for high versus low consumption was 0.72 and the range 0.07–0.92.

In two evaluable cohort studies of vegetable consumption, non-significant inverse associations were found. For five evaluable case–control studies, the mean relative risk for high versus low consumption was 0.80 and the range 0.32–1.03.

There is concern over studies in which large numbers of proxies of cases were interviewed, as well as those that excluded deceased cases. Further, many of the inverse associations were found in studies where the response rate for controls was low.

Larynx
Studies on larynx cancer were conducted in Europe, Asia and South America. For four evaluable case–control studies on fruit consumption, the mean relative risk for high versus low consumption was 0.63 and the range 0.38–0.80. For six evaluable case–control studies of vegetable consumption, the mean relative risk for high versus low consumption was 0.49 and the range 0.17–1.1.

The majority of the studies were hospital-based, but there was one large population-based case–control study. Control for smoking was rather crude and incomplete in the early studies; more recent studies have used more elaborate models and also observed inverse associations with fruit and vegetable intake. Only one study addressed associations between fruit and vegetables and larynx cancer in subgroups of smoking and alcohol intake. Odds ratios for fruit became weaker in these subgroups, which might indicate residual confounding by smoking and alcohol. The possibility of recall and selection bias in these case–control studies cannot be excluded.

Lung
Studies were conducted in North America, Europe, Australasia, Japan and South America. For 13 evaluable cohort studies of fruit consumption, the mean relative risk for high versus low consumption was 0.77 and the range 0.26–1.22. For 21 evaluable case–control studies, the mean relative risk for high versus low consumption was 0.70 and the range 0.33–2.04.

For 11 evaluable cohort studies of vegetable consumption, the mean relative risk for high versus low consumption was 0.80 and the range 0.47–1.37. For 18 evaluable case–control studies, the mean relative risk for high versus low consumption was 0.69 and the range 0.30–1.49.

The latest results from cohort studies and a recent meta-analysis suggest that the inverse association is stronger for fruit than for vegetables. Studies vary in the number of items included in the 'total' fruit or vegetable group. There was no clear difference in results between men and women, between hospital- and population-based case–control studies, nor between morphological categories of lung cancer. The strength of the association was smaller for cohort studies than for case–control studies, leaving the possibility of recall and selection bias in the case–control studies.

Because smoking is a strong risk factor for lung cancer, and smoking and fruit (and, to a lesser extent, vegetable) consumption are inversely associated, appropriate control for confounding by smoking is crucial. While the newer cohort studies have attempted to control for confounding by smoking much better than earlier cohort studies, residual confounding by smoking cannot be excluded and cohort studies often fail to capture changes in smoking and diet after the baseline measurement. Subgroup analyses among categories of smoking showed inverse associations in never-smokers (often non-significant) in the cohort studies. However, case–control studies among never- or non-smokers were not entirely consistent in showing an inverse association with fruits or vegetables.

Breast
About 30 epidemiological studies have examined the association between total fruit and total vegetable consumption during adulthood and the risk of breast cancer in women.

For six evaluable cohort studies of fruit consumption, the mean relative risk for high versus low consumption was 0.82 and the range 0.74–1.08. For 12 evaluable case–control studies, the mean relative risk for high versus low consumption was 0.99 and the range 0.57–1.82.

For five evaluable cohort studies of vegetable consumption, the mean relative risk for high versus low consumption was 0.94 and the range 0.64–1.43. For 12 evaluable case–control studies, the mean relative risk for high versus low consumption was 0.66 and the range 0.09–1.40.

A pooled analysis of eight cohort studies which included some of the

Summary of data

studies considered above found non-significant weak inverse associations between either fruit or vegetable consumption and the risk of breast cancer. In contrast, two meta-analyses of case–control studies (some studies were included in both meta-analyses) found approximately 10–20% reductions in the risk of breast cancer with increasing vegetable consumption; however, in both meta-analyses there was significant heterogeneity across the studies. There was little suggestion that associations differed by menopausal status. Because positive associations have been reported rarely for high fruit and vegetable consumption, and fruit and vegetable consumption is measured with error in epidemiological studies, the Working Group could not exclude the possibility that fruit and vegetable consumption may be associated with a slight decrease in risk of breast cancer. In addition, few studies have evaluated the influence of fruit and vegetable consumption during childhood and adolescence on the subsequent risk of developing breast cancer and of effect modification by other risk factors.

Associations between fruit or vegetable consumption and the risk of breast cancer in men have rarely been examined.

Cervix

There have been no cohort studies of fruit and vegetable consumption and risk of cervix cancer.

The case–control studies were not completely consistent and there is little evidence for a strong effect of either fruit or vegetable consumption.

Because of the strong relationship of human papillomavirus (HPV) with risk for this disease, there is concern about appropriate control for possible confounding or modifying effects of this infection. Only one study has examined risk restricted to women who were HPV-positive; results were similar when both HPV-positive and -negative controls were included or when controls were limited to women with HPV infections.

Endometrium

The associations between intake of fruit and vegetables and risk of endometrium cancer have been studied only in case–control studies.

For seven evaluable case–control studies of fruit consumption, the mean relative risk for high versus low consumption was 1.03 and the range 0.67–1.97. For five evaluable case–control studies of vegetable consumption, the mean relative risk for high versus low consumption was 0.75 and the range 0.65–1.00.

Fruit and vegetable intake combined was inversely associated in one cohort study, and in three case–control studies. Body mass index is an important known risk factor for endometrial cancer which was adjusted for in most, but not all, studies.

Ovary

The number of studies available on fruit consumption was limited and the results were inconsistent.

For vegetable consumption, an inverse association was found in two cohort studies and in five (three of which significant) out of six case–control studies.

In one case–control study, there was an inverse association with combined fruit and vegetable intake.

Prostate

For this site, there are no established risk factors other than age, family history and ethnic group. Hence generally confounding by non-dietary factors is not an issue. There is a possibility of detection bias, due to the use of PSA testing, but this would not have affected the majority of the studies reviewed.

For eight evaluable cohort studies of fruit consumption, the mean relative risk for high versus low consumption was 1.11 and the range 0.84–1.57. For nine evaluable case–control studies, the mean relative risk for high versus low consumption was 1.08 and the range 0.40–1.70.

For six evaluable cohort studies of vegetable consumption, the mean relative risk for high versus low consumption was 0.95 and the range 0.7–1.04. For nine evaluable case–control studies, the mean relative risk for high versus low consumption was 0.90 and the range 0.6–1.39.

The results for fruit are consistent and suggest that high fruit consumption does not reduce prostate cancer risk. The increased risk seen in some studies could be due to bias associated with detection in health-conscious men. For vegetables, the majority of studies have reported a slight, not significant lower risk for high consumption; vegetable consumption is measured with substantial error in epidemiological studies, so the Working Group could not exclude the possibility that vegetable consumption may be associated with a slight decrease in the risk of prostate cancer.

Testis

There were no cohort studies of testis cancer, and the two available case–control studies did not show significant associations.

Bladder

For five evaluable cohort studies of fruit consumption, the mean relative risk for high versus low consumption was 0.87 and the range 0.63–1.12. For four evaluable case–control studies, the mean relative risk for high versus low consumption was 0.74 and the range 0.53–0.95.

For three evaluable cohort studies of vegetable consumption, the mean relative risk for high versus low consumption was 0.94 and the range 0.72–1.16. For the three evaluable case–control studies, the mean relative risk for high versus low consumption was 0.89 and the range 0.66–1.04.

Most studies appropriately adjusted for potential confounding by age, gender, energy intake and smoking. In one cohort study, the estimates were stratified by smoking habits and an inverse association was found, mainly in current heavy smokers.

Kidney

One of the two cohort studies did not show an association with total fruit or vegetable intake. The other, although indicating an inverse association with total fruit, had too few cases to be informative.

For seven evaluable case–control studies of fruit consumption, the mean relative risk for high versus low consumption was 0.76 and the range 0.20–1.20.

For four evaluable case–control studies of vegetable consumption, the mean relative risk for high versus low consumption was 0.86 and the range 0.30–1.60.

The case–control studies were conducted in Australia, China, Europe and the USA and all cases were histologically confirmed. Most studies used population controls and response rates were relatively high. Potential confounding by body mass index and smoking was addressed in all analyses. However, recall bias cannot be excluded as an explanation of the results.

Brain

Three case–control studies of adult and five of childhood brain cancers have considered fruit and vegetable consumption, usually as a part of studies with other primary dietary hypotheses. All studies in adults and three studies in children showed inverse associations with fruit and/or vegetable consumption.

Thyroid

There were no cohort studies of thyroid cancer, and none of the three available case–control studies found a significant association with total fruit and vegetable consumption.

Non-Hodgkin lymphoma

In both of two cohort studies of fruit consumption, a non-significant inverse association was found. There was only one casecontrol study, which showed no evidence of an inverse association.

Among three cohort studies of vegetable consumption, a significant inverse association was seen in one. There was only one case–control study, which showed no evidence of an inverse association.

Leukaemia

Only one cohort study that considered green-yellow vegetables but not fruit consumption was available. No inverse association with risk was found.

Preventable fraction

The Working Group estimated that the preventable fraction for low fruit and vegetable intake would fall into the range of 5–12%. This is only a crude range of estimates and the proportion of cancers that might be preventable by increasing fruit and vegetable intake may vary beyond this range for specific cancer sites and across different regions of the world.

Intermediate markers of cancer

In experimental dietary studies in humans relying on intermediate endpoints related to disease risk, individual fruits and vegetables have been shown to modulate biological processes relevant to cancer, including biotransformation enzymes, antioxidant enzymes, oxidative damage to macromolecules, DNA adducts. Results are sometimes inconsistent, depending on the fruit or vegetable consumed, and the type of intervention which may differ greatly in duration, sample size and study design.

Experimental studies
Cancer and pre-malignant lesions

A study in rats with complete pathological examination showed that mixed fruits and vegetables did not significantly affect the spontaneous rates of total cancer or of cancer in any organ. A few well controlled rodent studies have provided evidence for preventive effects on carcinogen-induced colon cancer or adenomas of mixed fruits and vegetables at levels relevant to human dietary intake. In an additional study using tumour-prone transgenic mice, mixed fruits and vegetables also decreased the multiplicity of intestinal polyps in males fed a low-fat diet.

Other animal experiments have evaluated the efficacy of individual fruits or vegetables in decreasing cancer risk. These experiments have generally been performed with doses of fruits or vegetables that were high compared with human dietary intakes. Most of the 30 studies conducted in four different animal species and in different organs provided good evidence that high doses of individual fruit and vegetables can decrease tumour yield after a challenge by chemical carcinogens. The majority of the tumour-preventive effects have been observed in the colon, mammary gland or oesophagus. Some evidence also points to the potential of individual fruits and vegetables at high doses to decrease incidence of cancers of the bladder, liver, oral cavity and skin.

The evidence for antitumorigenic effects during the initiation phase is strong, whereas the evidence for late effects in carcinogenesis by fruit and vegetables is weaker, with mostly negative results from animal studies.

Summary of data

Intermediate markers of cancer

Mixed fruits and vegetables at levels relevant to human dietary intakes increased the activity of both phase I and phase II xenobiotic-metabolizing enzymes in rat liver. High doses of individual fruits or vegetables, including broccoli, Brussel sprouts and garlic, mainly induced phase II enzymes. An increase in phase II enzyme activities and a decrease in DNA damage were observed to parallel decreased tumour yields in a dose-dependent manner in a few studies. Some effects have been observed on other potential early risk factors for cancer, including carcinogen–DNA binding, lipid oxidation, DNA damage and mutation.

Mechanisms of cancer prevention

Extensive study of fruit and vegetables in human intervention studies and in animal models has provided a wealth of information on the variety of mechanisms by which a diet high in fruit and vegetables may contribute to reduced cancer risk.

Fruit and vegetables, at moderate intake levels, can modulate phase I and phase II enzymes in both animals and humans. Statistically significant phase II enzyme induction has been observed in human volunteers consuming single vegetables (most experiments were performed with *Brassica* vegetables). It is therefore likely that modulation of xenobiotic-metabolizing enzymes, in particular phase II enzymes, could contribute to prevention of human cancer. Enzyme induction is dose-dependently linked in animal studies with a decrease in genetic damage and tumorigenesis.

While the evidence is inconsistent that fruit and vegetables decrease direct oxidative DNA damage, evidence is more consistent for a decrease in lipid oxidation, a source of indirect oxidative damage to DNA. Nonetheless, the evidence linking direct or indirect oxidative DNA damage with risk of cancer is weak. The evidence for other mechanisms, including inhibition of endogenous formation of carcinogens, carcinogen–DNA binding, cytogenetic damage and post-initiation effects, by fruits and vegetables is weak.

In conclusion, the best, but still tentative, evidence for a mechanism of cancer prevention by fruit and vegetables is related to xenobiotic-metabolizing enzyme modulation, while antioxidant mechanisms are less well substantiated.

Associations with diseases other than cancer

Following a number of earlier ecological studies, analytical observational investigations, in particular several cohort studies, have shown inverse associations between consumption of fruit and vegetables and risk of coronary heart disease or stroke. The results of these studies are not entirely consistent; however the inverse associations found in the large cohorts, better controlled for confounding factors, provide evidence supporting a protective effect. Results from randomized clinical trials of diets rich in fruit and vegetables indicate the efficacy of such diets in lowering systolic and diastolic blood pressure over periods of weeks and months.

Two recent randomized trials show that lifestyle and diet changes, including the substitution of energy-dense dietary fats with fruit and vegetables, improve glucose tolerance and prevent occurrence of type 2 diabetes. In two large prospective studies, frequent intake of fruit and vegetables has been associated with decreased risk of senile cataract. Less data suggesting associations with fruit and vegetables are available for other chronic conditions such as osteoporosis, senile macular degeneration, Alzheimer disease and Parkinson disease.

Carcinogenic effects

There is no evidence from human studies of carcinogenicity of consumption of fruit and vegetables as a class. In one study in rats, a fruit and vegetable mixture fed at dietary levels relevant to humans did not affect spontaneous cancer incidence in any organ, after complete pathological examination. As a part of western-type diets, mixed fruit and vegetables at dose levels relevant to human exposures had the ability to increase intestinal tumours in one rat experiment and in one transgenic mouse experiment. There is no published evidence for a net increase in tumours after dosing with any individual fruit or vegetable at high doses in rodents.

Toxic effects

The relatively few adverse effects reported for individual fruits and vegetables were caused by specific components in a few kinds of fruit and vegetables and cannot be regarded as a general adverse effect of these classes of food.

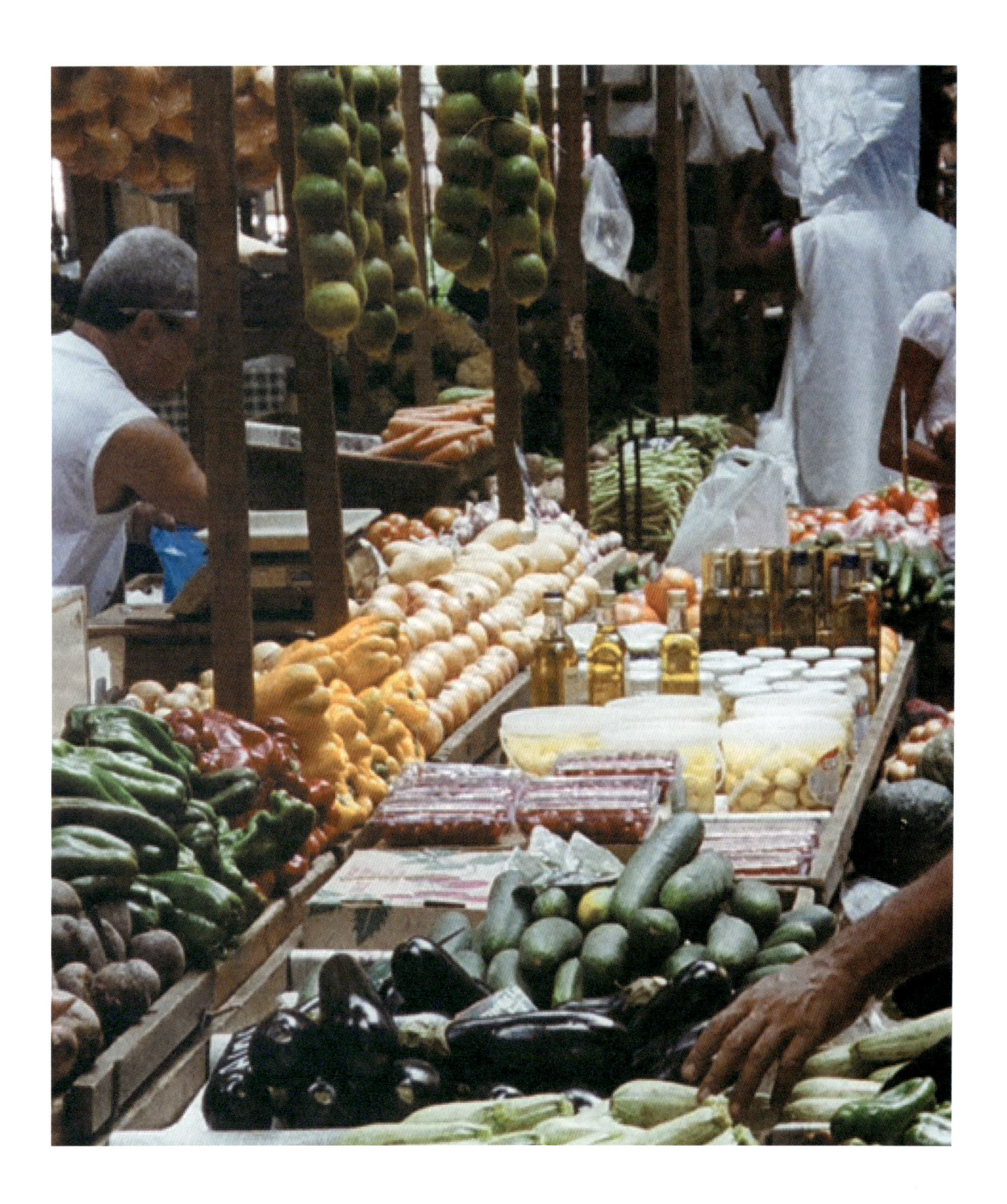

Chapter 9
Evaluation*

Cancer-preventive activity

Humans
There is *limited evidence* for a cancer-preventive effect of consumption of fruit and of vegetables for cancers of the mouth and pharynx, oesophagus, stomach, colon-rectum, larynx, lung, ovary (vegetables only), bladder (fruit only) and kidney.

There is *inadequate evidence* for a cancer-preventive effect of consumption of fruit and of vegetables for all other sites.

Experimental animals
Based on evidence obtained in relation to chemically induced cancers, especially of the colon, oesophagus and mammary gland in rodent models, there is *sufficient evidence* for a cancer-preventive effect of fruit and vegetables.

For chemically induced cancers of the bladder and oral cavity, the evidence is *limited*.

For other sites, the evidence is *inadequate*.

For spontaneous tumours, the evidence is *inadequate* for all cancer sites.

Overall evaluation

Fruit and vegetables have always been a major component of the human diet in most, though not all, parts of the world. Broadly defined, fruit and vegetables are those plant foods consumed by humans, excluding cereal grains, seeds and nuts. Some studies have excluded certain other categories such as pulses, mushrooms and high-starch foods (e.g., potatoes and plantains). Fruit and vegetables contain many nutrients; they also contain other bioactive compounds that may influence many aspects of human biology and related disease processes.

There is much diversity, between and within countries, both in the total amount of fruit and vegetables consumed and in the relative amounts of these two categories. In general, consumption is higher in more affluent, better educated, urban-dwelling populations. In recent decades, there has been a steady, worldwide, increase in availability of fruit and vegetables, and in year-round availability, although some regions have lagged behind.

In much of the published epidemiological literature and in this evaluation, fruit and vegetables have been categorized as two separate food groups – i.e., total fruit and total vegetables. For both of these two groupings, many bioactive components may act in concert in influencing carcinogenesis. Further, there is difficulty in specifying, and (in humans) in measuring, particular components of either fruit or vegetables that may especially affect cancer risk.

Review of the published scientific literature shows the following:

- The evidence from both epidemiological and animal experimental studies, along with the results of biomarker and mechanistic studies, indicates that a higher dietary intake of fruit and vegetables is associated with a lower risk of various types of cancer.
- More specifically, this evidence indicates that higher intake of fruit *probably* lowers the risk of cancers of the oesophagus, stomach and lung, while higher intake of vegetables *probably* lowers the risk of cancers of the oesophagus and colon-rectum.
- Likewise, a higher intake of fruit *possibly* reduces the risk of cancers of the mouth, pharynx, colon-rectum, larynx, kidney and urinary bladder. An increase in consumption of vegetables *possibly* reduces the risk of cancers of the mouth, pharynx, stomach, larynx, lung, ovary and kidney.

---

*Note that the evaluations refer to fruit and vegetables as whole classes, without consideration of separate sub-categories.

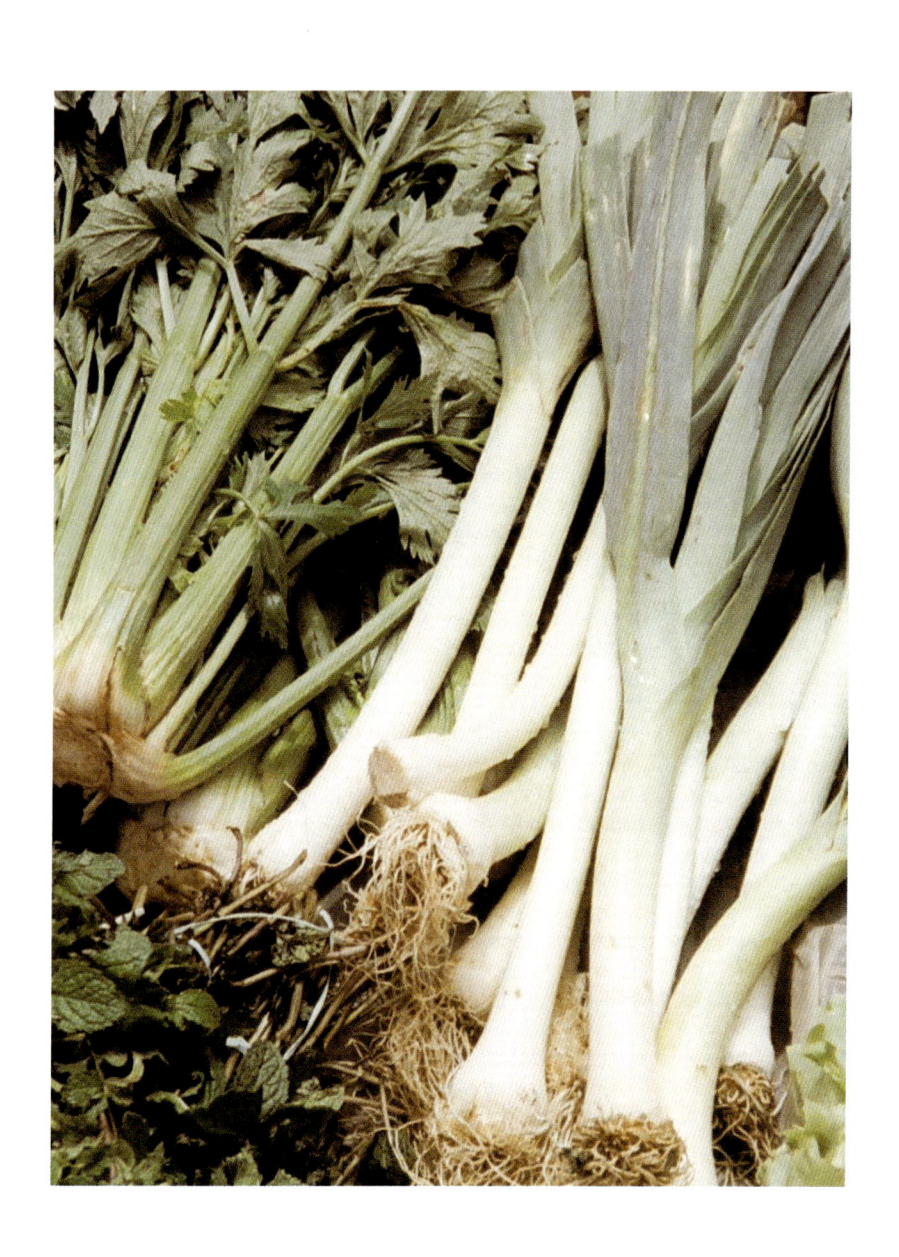

Chapter 10
Recommendations

Research recommendations

Research conducted to date suggests that many aspects of nutrition, including fruit and vegetable intake, are important factors in cancer prevention, but there remain many areas of uncertainty. Governments, voluntary organizations and the private sector should continue to invest in research on nutrition and cancer to better understand these relationships. Specific research needs and opportunities are listed below (not in any order of priority).

1. **Improve understanding of biological mechanisms linking fruit and vegetable intake to cancer risk**
- Develop and validate intermediate biomarkers of cancer risk against subsequent cancer outcomes in long-term animal and human studies to enable the assessment of effects of fruit and vegetables on intermediate steps in the cancer process.
- Conduct animal experiments to elucidate biological mechanisms, particularly experiments that test the effects of nutritional-level doses of whole foods in model systems with direct relevance to human cancers.
- Conduct research on the mechanisms of alteration of cancers by fruit and vegetable constituents across the entire lifespan, from intra-uterine life to the stages of cancer survivorship.
- Better define the biological interactions between genetic polymorphisms, cancer risk and variations in intake of fruit and vegetables. This can be done by stratified analyses and/or by analyses of genetic associations alone for genes known to affect important metabolic pathways of relevance to fruit and vegetables.

2. **Improve dietary assessment**
The interpretation of the weak associations often observed between fruit and vegetable intake and cancer risk is currently complicated by uncertainty as to whether they reflect stronger associations that have been diluted by measurement error. Considerable misclassification may result from the use of dietary assessment questionnaires derived from food frequency methods, which may be inadequate for measuring the small to modest levels of increased risk associated with common dietary exposures, that could have large public health importance. There is a need to:

- Develop and validate biomarkers of fruit and vegetable intake and include assessment of those biomarkers in future studies. Biological sample banks in cohort studies are a useful resource for this purpose.
- Develop standardized and validated methods that can be used in different populations to estimate the usual intake of fruit and vegetables by individuals. To estimate food intake in cohort studies with more accuracy, there may be a need for alternatives to current food frequency questionnaires, such as multiple dietary recalls or food records, which have traditionally been used only for food frequency validation or calibration purposes.
- Develop better ways to classify fruits and vegetables as to their cancer risk. Both empirical and theoretical approaches are needed to explore the relative advantages and limitations of alternative food classification methods, such as considering fruit and vegetables as a single class of foods, as two distinct classes and/or as various sub-classes defined by their food chemistry.
- Better assess the effects on cancer risk related to food-processing and cooking.

3. **Extend epidemiological research to explore new aspects**
- Conduct human intervention studies of the effects of fruit and vegetables on intermediate markers of cancer risk, such as cell-cycle control, early genetic changes, genetic factors, enzyme levels, immune function and infections of relevance to cancer, such as *Helicobacter pylori*.
- Conduct more epidemiological studies in developing countries. Such studies offer advantages of assessing associations between diet and cancer across a wider range of diets and cancers and with a different profile of confounding

factors. They would best be conducted in a coordinated way to allow cross-national comparisons and pooled analyses. Opportunities to add nutritional assessments into other large-scale studies in developing countries should be sought as a time-efficient and cost-efficient strategy.
- Conduct more research on the relationship between nutrition after the diagnosis of cancer and cancer outcomes and survival.
- Conduct more research on the behavioural and policy factors such as access to fruit and vegetables, and barriers to adequate consumption, that will be needed to increase consumption of fruit and vegetables in the populations of the world.
- Continue to conduct selected ecological studies to document any changes in cancer incidence that accompany dietary changes coincident with migration or special circumstances that arise in specific populations. Studies of special populations and unusual circumstances can help in assessing the effects on cancer of sudden or extreme diet changes.

4. Improve study designs

Improvements are needed in the design of future studies, both those conducted in experimental animals and in humans. In particular, there is a need to:
- Design studies to enable their pooling into joint analyses, so that a wider range of fruit and vegetable intakes as well as larger sample sizes will be available to allow assessment of associations with uncommon cancers as well as the investigation of interactions between fruit and vegetables and other factors.
- Develop methods to assess the impact of diet over longer periods of life, to capture potentially important relationships between cancer risk and diet *in utero*, in childhood or in early adulthood.
- More consistently employ animal cancer model systems to enable their findings to be better compared both with each other and with human cancer studies. When possible, excessive carcinogen loads should be avoided, and the nutritional exposures that are studied should emulate human diets.
- Develop methods to better assess the impact of selection bias and recall bias in case–control studies. Uncertainties about such biases greatly weakens confidence in the results of reported case–control studies.

5. Improve the reporting and analysis of data in nutritional epidemiological studies
- Better describe the foods included in categories of "fruit and vegetables" in study reports. A full description would list all foods included in groupings, describing how mixed dishes were analysed, and how food frequency measures were translated into amounts.
- Incorporate adjustments for measurement error in epidemiological studies. Such adjustments can be accurately made only when well conducted validation studies are incorporated into studies.
- Conduct more analyses of interactions between fruit and vegetable intake and other cancer risk factors, especially tobacco use, alcohol drinking, genetic predisposition, body weight, and physical activity.
- Conduct analyses to explore the complexity of the relationships between fruit and vegetables and many other aspects of diet. Methods of diet pattern recognition should be explored to determine whether they might add understanding of the relationship between fruit and vegetables within the diet and cancer risk reduction.
- Examine the reasons for inconsistencies in findings across different types of study, different time periods and different countries, with the aim of explaining the considerable heterogeneity of findings across studies rather than simply ignoring it or reducing it by exclusion or adjustment. Those reasons might themselves clarify the relationships being studied, as well as the public health implications of the body of evidence.

Public health recommendations

Governments, non-governmental organizations and other organizations (e.g., worksites, schools and health-care systems) should include the promotion of fruit and vegetables in the diet as an important aspect of their food policy and nutrition education. In addition to the universal importance of tobacco regulations in cancer control, governments have a special responsibility to assure the availability of fruit and vegetables as objectives of policies in agriculture, economics and trade. As research continues to better define the relationships between fruit and vegetable intake and cancer risk, it is important to remember that a diet high in fruit and vegetables also offers many health advantages in addition to cancer prevention, including lowering the risk of other chronic diseases (WHO, 2003). Therefore all organizations as well as governments should continue efforts to increase or maintain fruit and vegetable intake as an important objective of programmes to improve nutrition in order to reduce the burden of cancer and other chronic diseases.

References

Abbey, M., Noakes, M. & Nestel, P.J. (1995) Dietary supplementation with orange and carrot juice in cigarette smokers lowers oxidation products in copper-oxidized low-density lipoproteins. *J. Am. Diet. Assoc.*, **95,** 671–675

Agarwal, S. & Rao, A.V. (1998) Tomato lycopene and low density lipoprotein oxidation: a human dietary intervention study. *Lipids*, **33,** 981–984

Agudo, A. & Pera, G. (1999) Vegetable and fruit consumption associated with anthropometric, dietary and lifestyle factors in Spain. *Public Health Nutr.*, **2,** 263–271

Agudo, A., Estève, M.G., Pallares, C., Martinez-Ballarin, I., Fabregat, X., Malats, N., Machengs, I., Badia, A. & Gonzalez, C.A. (1997) Vegetable and fruit intake and the risk of lung cancer in women in Barcelona, Spain. *Eur. J. Cancer*, **33**, 1256–1261

Agudo, A., Slimani, N., Ocké, M.C., Naska, A., Miller, A.B., Kroke, A., Bamia, C., Karalis, D., Vineis, P., Palli, D., Bueno-de-Mesquita, H.B., Peeters, P.H.M., Engeset, D., Hjartåker, A., Navarro, C., Martínez Garcia, C., Wallström, P., Zhang, J.X., Welch, A.A., Spencer, E., Stripp, C., Overvad, K., Clavel-Chapelon, F., Casagrande, C. & Riboli, E. (2002) Consumption of vegetables, fruit and other plantfoods in the European Prospective Investigation into Cancer and Nutrition (EPIC) cohorts from 10 European countries. *Public Health Nutr.*, **5**, 1179–1196

Airoldi, L., Orsi, F., Magagnotti, C., Doca, R., Randone, D., Casetta, G., Peluso, M., Hautefeuille, A., Malaveille, C. & Vineis, P. (2002) Determinants of 4-aminobiphenyl–DNA adducts in bladder cancer biopsies. *Carcinogenesis*, **23**, 861–866

Alavanja, M.C., Brown, C.C., Swanson, C. & Brownson, R.C. (1993) Saturated fat intake and lung cancer risk among nonsmoking women in Missouri. *J. Natl Cancer Inst.*, **85**, 1906–1916

Alavanja, M.C., Field, R.W., Sinha, R., Brus, C.P., Shavers, V.L., Fisher, E.L., Curtain, J. & Lynch, C.F. (2001) Lung cancer risk and red meat consumption among Iowa women. *Lung Cancer*, **34**, 37–46

Alink, G.M., Reijven, P.L., Sijtsma, S.R., Jongen, W.M., Topp, R.J., Kuiper, H.A. & Koeman, J.H. (1988) Effects of human diets on biotransformation enzyme activity and metabolic activation of carcinogens in rat liver. *Food Chem. Toxicol.*, **26**, 883–891

Alink, G.M., Kuiper, H.A., Beems, R.B. & Koeman, J.H. (1989) A study on the carcinogenicity of human diets in rats: the influence of heating and the addition of vegetables and fruit. *Food Chem. Toxicol.*, **27**, 427–436

Alink, G.M., Kuiper, H.A., Hollanders, V.M.H. & Koeman, J.H. (1993) Effect of heat processing and of vegetables and fruit in human diets on 1,2-dimethylhydrazine-induced colon carcinogenesis in rats. *Carcinogenesis*, **14**, 519–524

Almendingen, K., Hofstad, B., Trygg, K., Hoff, G., Hussain, A. & Vatn, M. (2001) Current diet and colorectal adenomas: a case–control study including different sets of traditionally chosen control groups. *Eur. J. Cancer Prev.*, **10**, 395–406

Amagase, H. & Milner, J.A. (1993) Impact of various sources of garlic and their constituents on 7,12-dimethylbenz[*a*]anthracene binding to mammary cell DNA. *Carcinogenesis*, **14,** 1627–1631

Amagase, H., Schaffer, E.M. & Milner, J.A. (1996) Dietary components modify the ability of garlic to suppress 7,12-dimethylbenz(a)anthracene-induced mammary DNA adducts. *J. Nutr.*, **126,** 817–824

Ames, B.N., McCann, J. & Yamasaki, E. (1975) Methods for detecting carcinogens and mutagens with the *Salmonella*/mammalian-microsome mutagenicity test. *Mutat. Res.*, **31**, 347–364

Ames, B.N., Profet, M. & Gold, L.S. (1990) Dietary pesticides. *Proc. Natl Acad. Sci. USA*, **87**, 7777–7781

Anon. (1980) Vitamin A, retinol, carotene, and cancer prevention. *Br. Med. J.*, **281,** 957–958

Aoyama, T., Korzekwa, K., Nagata, K., Gillette, J., Gelboin, H.V. & Gonzalez, F.J. (1990) Estradiol metabolism by complementary deoxyribonucleic acid-expressed human cytochrome P450s. *Endocrinology*, **126,** 3101–3106

Appel, L.J., Moore, T.J., Obarzanek, E., Vollmer, W.M., Svetkey, L.P., Sacks, F.M., Bray, G.A., Vogt, T.M., Cutler, J.A., Windhauser, M.M., Lin, P.H. & Karanja, N. (1997) A clinical trial of the effects of dietary patterns on blood pressure. DASH Collaborative Research Group. *New Engl. J. Med.*, **336,** 1117–1124

Appleby, P.N., Key, T.J., Burr, M.L. & Thorogood, M. (2002) Mortality and fresh fruit consumption. In: Riboli, E. & Lambert, R., *Nutrition and Lifestyle: Opportunities for Cancer Prevention* (IARC Scientific Publications No. 156), Lyon, IARCPress, pp. 131–133

Aprikian, O., Busserolles, J., Manach, C., Mazur, A., Morand, C., Davicco, M.J., Besson, C., Rayssiguier, Y., Rémésy, C. & Demigne, C. (2002) Lyophilized apple counteracts the development of hypercholesterolemia, oxidative stress, and renal dysfunction in obese Zucker rats. *J. Nutr.*, **132,** 1969–1976

Armstrong, B. & Doll, R. (1975) Environmental factors and cancer incidence and mortality in different countries, with special reference to dietary practices. *Int. J. Cancer*, **15**, 617–631

Armstrong, R.W., Imrey, P.B., Lye, M.S., Armstrong, M.J., Yu, M.C. & Sani, S. (1998) Nasopharyngeal carcinoma in Malaysian Chinese: salted fish and other dietary exposures. *Int. J. Cancer*, **77**, 228–235

Assembly of Life Sciences (1982) *Diet, Nutrition, and Cancer,* Washington, DC, National Academy Press

Astwood, E.B. (1943) The chemical nature of compounds which inhibit function of the thyroid gland. *J. Pharmacol. Exp. Ther.*, **78**, 79–89

Athar, M., Khan, W.A. & Mukhtar, H. (1989) Effect of dietary tannic acid on epidermal, lung, and forestomach polycyclic aromatic hydrocarbon metabolism and tumorigenicity in Sencar mice. *Cancer Res.*, **49**, 5784–5788

Aviram, M., Dornfeld, L., Rosenblat, M., Volkova, N., Kaplan, M., Coleman, R., Hayek, T., Presser, D. & Fuhrman, B. (2000) Pomegranate juice consumption reduces oxidative stress, atherogenic modifications to LDL, and platelet aggregation: studies in humans and in atherosclerotic apolipoprotein E-deficient mice. *Am. J. Clin. Nutr.*, **71**, 1062–1076

Axelsson, G., Liljeqvist, T., Andersson, L., Bergman, B. & Rylander, R. (1996) Dietary factors and lung cancer among men in west Sweden. *Int. J. Epidemiol.*, **25**, 32–39

Aydin, A., Ersöz, G., Tuncyürek, M., Tekesin, O. & Akçiçek, E. (1997) Does garlic oil have a role in the treatment of *Helicobacter pylori* infection? *Turk. J. Gastroenterol.*, **8**, 181–184

Azevedo, L.F., Salgueiro, L.F., Claro, R., Teixeira-Pinto, A. & Costa-Pereira, A. (1999) Diet and gastric cancer in Portugal—a multivariate model. *Eur. J. Cancer Prev.*, **8**, 41–48

Aziz, R.M., Nines, R., Rodrigo, K., Harris, K., Hudson, T., Gupta, A., Morse, M., Carlton, P. & Stoner, G.D. (2002) The effect of freeze-dried blueberries on N-nitrosomethylbenzylamine tumorigenesis in the rat esophagus. *Pharmaceutical Biol.*, **40**, 43S–49S

Baghurst, P.A., McMichael, A.J., Slavotinek, A.H., Baghurst, K.I., Boyle, P. & Walker, A.M. (1991) A case–control study of diet and cancer of the pancreas. *Am. J. Epidemiol.*, **134**, 167–179

Bailey, D.G., Arnold, J.M. & Spence, J.D. (1994) Grapefruit and drugs. How significant is the interaction? *Clin. Pharmacokinet.*, **26**, 91–98

Balbi, J.C., Larrinaga, M.T., De Stefani, E., Mendilaharsu, M., Ronco, A.L., Boffetta, P. & Brennan, P. (2001) Foods and risk of bladder cancer: a case–control study in Uruguay. *Eur. J. Cancer Prev.*, **10**, 453–458

Ballmer-Weber, B.K., Hoffmann, A., Wuthrich, B., Luttkopf, D., Pompei, C., Wangorsch, A., Kastner, M. & Vieths, S. (2002) Influence of food processing on the allergenicity of celery: DBPCFC with celery spice and cooked celery in patients with celery allergy. *Allergy*, **57**, 228–235

Bandera, E.V., Freudenheim, J.L., Marshall, J.R., Priore, R.L., Brasure, J., Baptiste, M. & Graham, S. (2002) Impact of losses to follow-up on diet/alcohol and lung cancer analyses in the New York State Cohort. *Nutr. Cancer*, **42**, 41–47

Barch, D.H. & Fox, C.C. (1988) Selective inhibition of methylbenzylnitrosamine-induced formation of esophageal O^6-methylguanine by dietary ellagic acid in rats. *Cancer Res.*, **48**, 7088–7092

Barer, D., Leibowitz, R., Ebrahim, S., Pengally, D. & Neale, R. (1989) Vitamin C status and other nutritional indices in patients with stroke and other acute illnesses: a case–control study. *J. Clin. Epidemiol.*, **42**, 625–631

Barratt-Fornell, A. & Drewnowski, A. (2002) The taste of health: nature's bitter gifts. *Nutr. Today*, **37**, 144–150

Bartsch, H. & Frank, N. (1996) Blocking the endogenous formation of N-nitroso compounds and related carcinogens. In: Stewart, B.W., McGregor, D. & Kleihues, P., eds, *Principles of Chemoprevention* (IARC Scientific Publications No. 139), Lyon, International Agency for Research on Cancer, pp. 189–201

Bartsch, H., Ohshima, H. & Pignatelli, B. (1988) Inhibitors of endogenous nitrosation. Mechanisms and implications in human cancer prevention. *Mutat. Res.*, **202**, 307–324

Bartsch, H., Ohshima, H., Pignatelli, B. & Calmels S. (1992) Endogenously formed N-nitroso compounds and nitrosating agents in human cancer etiology. *Pharmacogenetics*, **2**, 272–277

Bathalon, G.P., Tucker, K.L., Hays, N.P., Vinken, A.G., Greenberg, A.S., McCrory, M.A. & Roberts, S.B. (2000) Psychological measures of eating behavior and the accuracy of 3 common dietary assessment methods in healthy postmenopausal women. *Am. J. Clin. Nutr.*, **71**, 739–745

Bazzano, L.A., He, J., Ogden, L.G., Loria, C.M., Vupputuri, S., Myers, L. & Whelton, P.K. (2002) Fruit and vegetable intake and risk of cardiovascular disease in US adults: the first National Health and Nutrition Examination Survey Epidemiologic Follow-up Study. *Am. J. Clin. Nutr.*, **76**, 93–99

Beaton, G.H., Milner, J., Corey, P., McGuire, V., Cousins, M., Stewart, E., de Ramos, M., Hewitt, D., Grambsch, P.V., Kassim, N. & Little, J.A. (1979) Sources of variance in 24-hour dietary recall data: implications for nutrition study design and interpretation. *Am. J. Clin. Nutr.*, **32**, 2546–2549

Beaton, G.H., Milner, J., McGuire, V., Feather, T.E. & Little, J.A. (1983) Source of variance in 24-hour dietary recall data: implications for nutrition study design and interpretation. Carbohydrate sources, vitamins, and minerals. *Am. J. Clin. Nutr.*, **37**, 986–995

Beatty, E.R., O'Reilly, J.D., England, T.G., McAnlis, G.T., Young, I.S., Geissler, C.A., Sanders, T.A. & Wiseman, H. (2000) Effect of dietary quercetin on oxidative DNA damage in healthy human subjects. *Br. J. Nutr.*, **84**, 919–925

References

Becker, W. (1999) Dietary guidelines and patterns of food and nutrient intake in Sweden. *Br. J. Nutr.,* **81 Suppl. 2,** S113–S117

Becker, W. (2001) Comparability of household and individual food consumption data – evidence from Sweden. *Public Health Nutr.,* **4,** 1177–1182

Bellach, B. & Kohlmeier, L. (1998) Energy adjustment does not control for differential recall bias in nutritional epidemiology. *J. Clin. Epidemiol.,* **51,** 393–398

Belzile, R.J., Poliquin, L.SA. & Jones, J.D. (1974) Nutritive value of rapeseed flour for mink: effects on live performance, nutrient utilisation, thyroid function and pelt quality. *Can. J. Animal Sci.,* **54,** 639–644

Benito, E., Obrador, A., Stiggelbout, A., Bosch, F.X., Mulet, M., Muñoz, N. & Kaldor, J. (1990) A population-based case–control study of colorectal cancer in Majorca. I. Dietary factors. *Int. J. Cancer,* **45,** 69–76

Bergmann, M.M. & Boeing, H. (2002) Behavioral changes in observational and intervention studies. *J. Nutr.,* **132,** 3530S–3533S

Berlin, J.A. & Colditz, G.A. (1990) A meta-analysis of physical activity in the prevention of coronary heart disease. *Am. J. Epidemiol.,* **132,** 612–628

Bernstein, L. & Wu, A.H. (1998) Colon and rectal cancer among Asian Americans and Pacific Islanders. *Asian Am. Pac. Isl. J. Health,* **6,** 184–200

Bianchini, F. & Vainio, H. (2001) Allium vegetables and organosulfur compounds: do they help prevent cancer? *Environ. Health Perspect.,* **109,** 893–902

Bidoli, E., Franceschi, S., Talamini, R., Barra, S. & La Vecchia, C. (1992) Food consumption and cancer of the colon and rectum in north-eastern Italy. *Int. J. Cancer,* **50,** 223–229

Billson, H., Pryer, J.A. & Nichols, R. (1999) Variation in fruit and vegetable consumption among adults in Britain. An analysis from the dietary and nutritional survey of British adults. *Eur. J. Clin. Nutr.,* **53,** 946–952

Bingham, S., Williams, D.R., Cole, T.J. & James, W.P. (1979) Dietary fibre and regional large-bowel cancer mortality in Britain. *Br. J. Cancer,* **40,** 456–463

Bingham, S.A., Gill, C., Welch, A., Cassidy, A., Runswick, S.A., Oakes, S., Lubin, R., Thurnham, D.I., Key, T.J., Roe, L., Khaw, K.T. & Day, N.E. (1997) Validation of dietary assessment methods in the UK arm of EPIC using weighed records, and 24-hour urinary nitrogen and potassium and serum vitamin C and carotenoids as biomarkers. *Int. J. Epidemiol.,* **26 Suppl 1,** S137–S151

Black, A.E. & Cole, T.J. (2001) Biased over- or under-reporting is characteristic of individuals whether over time or by different assessment methods. *J. Am. Diet. Assoc.,* **101,** 70–80

Blake, A.J., Guthrie, H.A. & Smiciklas-Wright, H. (1989) Accuracy of food portion estimation by overweight and normal-weight subjects. *J. Am. Diet. Assoc.,* **89,** 962–964

Block, G. (1992) Dietary assessment issues related to cancer for NHANES III. *Dietary Methodology Workshop for the Third National Health and Nutrition Examination Survey,* Hyattsville, MD, US Department of Health and Human Services, pp. 24–31

Block, G. (2001) Invited commentary: another perspective on food frequency questionnaires. *Am. J. Epidemiol.,* **154,** 1103–1104

Block, G., Hartman, A.M. & Naughton, D. (1990) A reduced dietary questionnaire: development and validation. *Epidemiology,* **1,** 58–64

Block, G., Gillespie, C., Rosenbaum, E.H. & Jenson, C. (2000) A rapid food screener to assess fat and fruit and vegetable intake. *Am. J. Prev. Med.,* **18,** 284–288

Boeing, H. (2002) Alcohol and risk of cancer of the upper GI tract: first analysis of the EPIC data. In: Riboli, E. & Lambert, R., eds, *Nutrition and Lifestyle: Opportunities for Cancer Prevention* (IARC Scientific Publications No. 156), Lyon, IARCPress, pp. 151–154

Boeing, H., Frentzel-Beyme, R., Berger, M., Berndt, V., Göres, W., Körner, M., Lohmeier, R., Menarcher, A., Männl, H.F., Meinhardt, M., Müller, R., Ostermeier, H., Paul, F., Schwemmle, K., Wagner, K.H. & Wahrendorf, J. (1991a) Case–control study on stomach cancer in Germany. *Int. J. Cancer,* **47,** 858–864

Boeing, H., Jedrychowski, W., Wahrendorf, J., Popiela, T., Tobiasz-Adamczyk, B. & Kulig, A. (1991b) Dietary risk factors in intestinal and diffuse types of stomach cancer: a multicenter case–control study in Poland. *Cancer Causes Control,* **2,** 227–233

Boeing, H., Schlehofer, B. & Wahrendorf, J. (1997) Diet, obesity and risk for renal cell carcinoma: results from a case control-study in Germany. *Z. Ernährungswiss.,* **36,** 3–11

Bogaards, J.J., van Ommen, B., Falke, H.E., Willems, M.I. & van Bladeren, P.J. (1990) Glutathione S-transferase subunit induction patterns of Brussels sprouts, allyl isothiocyanate and goitrin in rat liver and small intestinal mucosa: a new approach for the identification of inducing xenobiotics. *Food Chem. Toxicol.,* **28,** 81–88

Bogaards, J.J., Verhagen, H., Willems, M.I., van Poppel, G. & van Bladeren, P.J. (1994) Consumption of Brussels sprouts results in elevated alpha-class glutathione S-transferase levels in human blood plasma. *Carcinogenesis,* **15,** 1073–1075

Bohlscheid-Thomas, S., Hoting, I., Boeing, H. & Wahrendorf, J. (1997) Reproducibility and relative validity of food group intake in a food frequency questionnaire developed for the German part of the EPIC project. European Prospective Investigation into Cancer and Nutrition. *Int. J. Epidemiol.,* **26 Suppl. 1,** S59–S70

Böhm, F., Edge, R., Burke, M. & Truscott, T.G. (2001) Dietary uptake of lycopene protects human cells from singlet oxygen and nitrogen dioxide – ROS components from cigarette smoke. *J. Photochem. Photobiol. B,* **64,** 176–178

Bohr, V.A. (2002) DNA damage and its processing in relation to human disease. *J. Inherit. Metab. Dis.*, **25,** 215–222

Boker, L.K., Van der Schouw, Y.T., De Kleijn, M.J., Jacques, P.F., Grobbee, D.E. & Peeters, P.H. (2002) Intake of dietary phytoestrogens by Dutch women. *J. Nutr.*, **132,** 1319–1328

Bolland, J.E., Yuhas, J.A. & Bolland, T.W. (1988) Estimation of food portion sizes: effectiveness of training. *J. Am. Diet. Assoc.*, **88**, 817–821

Bonassi, S., Hagmar, L., Strömberg, U., Montagud, A.H., Tinnerberg, H., Forni, A., Heikkilä, P., Wanders, S., Wilhardt, P., Hansteen, I.L., Knudsen, L.E. & Norppa, H. (2000) Chromosomal aberrations in lymphocytes predict human cancer independently of exposure to carcinogens. European Study Group on Cytogenetic Biomarkers and Health. *Cancer Res.*, **60,** 1619–1625

Bonnesen, C., Eggleston, I.M. & Hayes, J.D. (2001) Dietary indoles and isothiocyanates that are generated from cruciferous vegetables can both stimulate apoptosis and confer protection against DNA damage in human colon cell lines. *Cancer Res.*, **61,** 6120–6130

Bosetti, C., La Vecchia, C., Talamini, R., Simonato, L., Zambon, P., Negri, E., Trichopoulos, D., Lagiou, P., Bardini, R. & Franceschi, S. (2000a) Food groups and risk of squamous cell esophageal cancer in northern Italy. *Int. J. Cancer*, **87**, 289–294

Bosetti, C., Negri, E., Franceschi, S., Conti, E., Levi, F., Tomei, F. & La Vecchia, C. (2000b) Risk factors for oral and pharyngeal cancer in women: a study from Italy and Switzerland. *Br. J. Cancer*, **82**, 204–207

Bosetti, C., Negri, E., Franceschi, S., Pelucchi, C., Talamini, R., Montella, M., Conti, E. & La Vecchia, C. (2001) Diet and ovarian cancer risk: a case–control study in Italy. *Int. J. Cancer*, **93**, 911–915

Bosetti, C., La Vecchia, C., Talamini, R., Negri, E., Levi, F., Dal Maso, L. & Franceschi, S. (2002a) Food groups and laryngeal cancer risk: a case–control study from Italy and Switzerland. *Int. J. Cancer*, **100**, 355–360

Bosetti, C., Negri, E., Kolonel, L., Ron, E., Franceschi, S., Preston-Martin, S., McTiernan, A., Dal Maso, L., Mark, S.D., Mabuchi, K., Land, C., Jin, F., Wingren, G., Galanti, M.R., Hallquist, A., Glattre, E., Lund, E., Levi, F., Linos, D. & La Vecchia, C. (2002b) A pooled analysis of case–control studies of thyroid cancer. VII. Cruciferous and other vegetables (international). *Cancer Causes Control*, **13**, 765–775

Bostwick, D.G., Alexander, E.E., Singh, R., Shan, A., Qian, J., Santella, R.M., Oberley, L.W., Yan, T., Zhong, W., Jiang, X. & Oberley, T.D. (2000) Antioxidant enzyme expression and reactive oxygen species damage in prostatic intraepithelial neoplasia and cancer. *Cancer*, **89**, 123–134

Botterweck, A.A., van den Brandt, P.A. & Goldbohm, R.A. (1998) A prospective cohort study on vegetable and fruit consumption and stomach cancer risk in The Netherlands. *Am. J. Epidemiol.*, **148**, 842–853

Boutron, M.C., Faivre, J., Milan, C., Lorcerie, B. & Estève, J. (1989) A comparison of two diet history questionnaires that measure usual food intake. *Nutr. Cancer*, **12**, 83–91

Boutron-Ruault, M.C., Senesse, P., Faivre, J., Chatelain, N., Belghiti, C. & Meance, S. (1999) Foods as risk factors for colorectal cancer: a case–control study in Burgundy (France). *Eur. J. Cancer Prev.*, **8**, 229–235

Bowen, D., Raczynski, J., George, V., Feng, Z. & Fouad, M. (2000) The role of participation in the women's health trial: feasibility study in minority populations. *Prev. Med.*, **31,** 474–480

Boyd, J.N., Babish, J.G. & Stoewsand, G.S. (1982) Modification by beet and cabbage diets of aflatoxin B$_1$-induced rat plasma α-foetoprotein elevation, hepatic tumorigenesis, and mutagenicity of urine. *Food Chem. Toxicol.,* **20,** 47–52

Boyle, S.P., Dobson, V.L., Duthie, S.J., Kyle, J.A. & Collins, A.R. (2000) Absorption and DNA protective effects of flavonoid glycosides from an onion meal. *Eur. J. Nutr.*, **39,** 213–223

Bradfield, C.A., Chang, Y. & Bjeldanes, L.F. (1985) Effects of commonly consumed vegetables on hepatic xenobiotic-metabolizing enzymes in the mouse. *Food Chem. Toxicol.*, **23**, 899–904

Bradlow, H.L., Hershcopf, R.E. & Fishman, J.F. (1986) Oestradiol 16 alpha-hydroxylase: a risk marker for breast cancer. *Cancer Surveys*, **5**, 573–583

Bradlow, H.L., Michnovicz, J.J., Halper, M., Miller, D.G., Wong, G.Y. & Osborne, M.P. (1994) Long-term responses of women to indole-3-carbinol or a high fiber diet. *Cancer Epidemiol. Biomarkers Prev.*, **3,** 591–595

Brady, J.F., Li, D.C., Ishizaki, H. & Yang, C.S. (1988) Effect of diallyl sulfide on rat liver microsomal nitrosamine metabolism and other monooxygenase activities. *Cancer Res.*, **48,** 5937–5940

Braga, C., La Vecchia, C., Negri, E. & Franceschi, S. (1997a) Attributable risks for hepatocellular carcinoma in northern Italy. *Eur. J. Cancer*, **33**, 629–634

Braga, C., La Vecchia, C., Negri, E., Franceschi, S. & Parpinel, M. (1997b) Intake of selected foods and nutrients and breast cancer risk: an age- and menopause-specific analysis. *Nutr. Cancer*, **28**, 258–263

Brauch, H., Weirich, G., Brieger, J., Glavac, D., Rodl, H., Eichinger, M., Feurer, M., Weidt, E., Puranakanitstha, C., Neuhaus, C., Pomer, S., Brenner, W., Schirmacher, P., Storkel, S., Rotter, M., Masera, A., Gugeler, N. & Decker, H.F. (2000) VHL alterations in human clear cell renal cell carcinoma: association with advanced tumor stage and a novel hot spot mutation. *Cancer Res.*, **60**, 1942–1948

Breinholt, V., Arbogast, D., Loveland, P., Pereira, C., Dashwood, R., Hendricks, J. & Bailey, G. (1999) Chlorophyllin chemoprevention in trout initiated by aflatoxin B(1) bath treatment: An evaluation of reduced bioavailability vs. target organ protective mechanisms. *Toxicol. Appl. Pharmacol.*, **158,** 141–151

References

Brennan, P., Fortes, C., Butler, J., Agudo, A., Benhamou, S., Darby, S., Gerken, M., Jokel, K.H., Kreuzer, M., Mallone, S., Nyberg, F., Pohlabeln, H., Ferro, G. & Boffetta, P. (2000) A multicenter case–control study of diet and lung cancer among non-smokers. *Cancer Causes Control*, **11**, 49–58

Breslow, R.A., Graubard, B.I., Sinha, R. & Subar, A.F. (2000) Diet and lung cancer mortality: a 1987 National Health Interview Survey cohort study. *Cancer Causes Control*, **11**, 419–431

Bresnick, E., Birt, D.F., Wolterman, K., Wheeler, M. & Markin, R.S. (1990) Reduction in mammary tumorigenesis in the rat by cabbage and cabbage residue. *Carcinogenesis*, **11**, 1159–1163

Briss, P.A., Zaza, S., Pappaioanou, M., Fielding, J., Wright-De Aguero, L., Truman, B.I., Hopkins, D.P., Mullen, P.D., Thompson, R.S., Woolf, S.H., Carande-Kulis, V.G., Anderson, L., Hinman, A.R., McQueen, D.V., Teutsch, S.M. & Harris, J.R. (2000) Developing an evidence-based *Guide to Community Preventive Services* - Methods. *Am. J. Prev. Med.*, **18**, 35S–43S

Britton, A., McKee, M., Black, N., McPherson, K., Sanderson, C. & Bain, C. (1998) Choosing between randomised and non-randomised studies: a systematic review. *Health Technol. Assessment*, **2** (13)

Brown, L.M., Blot, W.J., Schuman, S.H., Smith, V.M., Ershow, A.G., Marks, R.D. & Fraumeni, J.F., Jr (1988) Environmental factors and high risk of esophageal cancer among men in coastal South Carolina. *J. Natl Cancer Inst.*, **80**, 1620–1625

Brown, L.M., Swanson, C.A., Gridley, G., Swanson, G.M., Schoenberg, J.B., Greenberg, R.S., Silverman, D.T., Pottern, L.M., Hayes, R.B. & Schwartz, A.G. (1995) Adenocarcinoma of the esophagus: role of obesity and diet. *J. Natl Cancer Inst.*, **87**, 104–109

Brown, L.M., Swanson, C.A., Gridley, G., Swanson, G.M., Silverman, D.T., Greenberg, R.S., Hayes, R.B., Schoenberg, J.B., Pottern, L.M., Schwartz, A.G., Liff, J.M., Hoover, R. & Fraumeni, J.F., Jr (1998) Dietary factors and the risk of squamous cell esophageal cancer among black and white men in the United States. *Cancer Causes Control*, **9**, 467–474

Brown, L., Rimm, E.B., Seddon, J.M., Giovannucci, E.L., Chasan-Taber, L., Spiegelman, D., Willett, W.C. & Hankinson, S.E. (1999) A prospective study of carotenoid intake and risk of cataract extraction in US men. *Am. J. Clin. Nutr.*, **70**, 517–524

Brown, L.M., Hoover, R., Silverman, D., Baris, D., Hayes, R., Swanson, G.M., Schoenberg, J., Greenberg, R., Liff, J., Schwartz, A., Dosemeci, M., Pottern, L. & Fraumeni, J.F., Jr (2001) Excess incidence of squamous cell esophageal cancer among US Black men: role of social class and other risk factors. *Am. J. Epidemiol.*, **153**, 114–122

Bruemmer, B., White, E., Vaughan, T.L. & Cheney, C.L. (1996) Nutrient intake in relation to bladder cancer among middle-aged men and women. *Am. J. Epidemiol.*, **144**, 485–495

Bub, A., Watzl, B., Abrahamse, L., Delincee, H., Adam, S., Wever, J., Müller, H. & Rechkemmer, G. (2000) Moderate intervention with carotenoid-rich vegetable products reduces lipid peroxidation in men. *J. Nutr.*, **130**, 2200–2206

Bueno de Mesquita, H.B., Maisonneuve, P., Runia, S. & Moerman, C.J. (1991) Intake of foods and nutrients and cancer of the exocrine pancreas: a population-based case–control study in The Netherlands. *Int. J. Cancer*, **48**, 540–549

Bueno de Mesquita, H.B., Ferrari, P. & Riboli, E. (2002) Plant foods and the risk of colorectal cancer in Europe: preliminary findings In: Riboli, E. & Lambert, R., eds, *Nutrition and Lifestyle: Opportunities for Cancer Prevention* (IARC Scientific Publications No. 156), Lyon, IARCPress, pp. 89–96

Buiatti, E., Palli, D., Decarli, A., Amadori, D., Avellini, C., Bianchi, S., Biserni, R., Cipriani, F., Cocco, P., Giacosa, A., Marubini, E., Puntoni, R., Vindigni, C., Fraumeni, J., Jr & Blot, W. (1989) A case–control study of gastric cancer and diet in Italy. *Int. J. Cancer*, **44**, 611–616

Bunin, G.R., Kuijten, R.R., Buckley, J.D., Rorke, L.B. & Meadows, A.T. (1993). Relation between maternal diet and subsequent primitive neuroectodermal brain tumours in young children. *New Engl. J. Med.*, **329**, 536–541

Burke, B. (1947) Dietary history as a tool in research. *J. Am. Diet. Assoc.*, 1041–1046

Burke, M.C. & Pao, E.M. (1976) *Methodology for Large-scale Surveys of Household and Individual Diets* (Home Economics Research Report No. 40), Washington, DC, US Department of Agriculture, Agriculture Research Service

Burnet, F.M. (1970) The concept of immunological surveillance. *Progr. Exp. Tumor Res.*, **13**, 1–27

Byers, T. (2001) Food frequency dietary assessment: how bad is good enough? *Am. J. Epidemiol.*, **154**, 1087–1088

Byers, T., Nestle, M., McTiernan, A., Doyle, C., Currie-Williams, A., Gansler, T. & Thun, M. (2002) American Cancer Society guidelines on nutrition and physical activity for cancer prevention: reducing the risk of cancer with healthy food choices and physical activity. *CA Cancer J. Clin.*, **52**, 92–119

Byrne, C., Ursin, G. & Ziegler, R.G. (1996) A comparison of food habit and food frequency data as predictors of breast cancer in the NHANES I/NHEFS cohort. *J. Nutr.*, **126**, 2757–2764

Caccetta, R.A.-A., Croft, K.D., Beilin, L.J. & Puddey, I.B. (2000) Ingestion of red wine significantly increases plasma phenolic acid concentrations but does not acutely affect ex vivo lipoprotein oxidizability. *Am. J. Clin. Nutr.*, **71**, 67–74

Candelora, E.C., Stockwell, H.G., Armstrong, A.W. & Pinkham, P.A. (1992) Dietary intake and risk of lung cancer in women who never smoked. *Nutr. Cancer*, **17**, 263–270

Cao, G., Sofic, E. & Prior, R.L. (1996) Antioxidant capacity of tea and common vegetables. *J. Agric. Food Chem.*, **44**, 3426–3431

Cao, G., Russell, R.M., Lischner, N. & Prior, R.L. (1998a) Serum antioxidant capacity is increased by consumption of strawberries, spinach, red wine or vitamin C in elderly women. *J. Nutr.*, **128**, 2383–2390

Cao, G., Booth, S.L., Sadowski, J.A. & Prior, R.L. (1998b) Increases in human plasma antioxidant capacity after consumption of controlled diets high in fruit and vegetables. *Am. J. Clin. Nutr.*, **68**, 1081–1087

Caporaso, N., Whitehouse, J., Monkman, S., Boustead, C., Issaq, H., Fox, S., Morse, M.A., Idle, J.R. & Chung, F.L. (1994) In vitro but not in vivo inhibition of CYP2D6 by phenethyl isothiocyanate (PEITC), a constituent of watercress. *Pharmacogenetics*, **4**, 275–280

Carlton, P.S., Kresty, L.A. & Stoner, G.D. (2000) Failure of dietary lyophilized strawberries to inhibit 4-(methylnitrosamino)-1-(3-pyridyl)-1-butanone and benzo[a]pyrene-induced lung tumorigenesis in strain A/J mice. *Cancer Lett.*, **159**, 113–117

Carlton, P.S., Kresty, L.A., Siglin, J.C., Morse, M.A., Lu, J., Morgan, C. & Stoner, G.D. (2001) Inhibition of N-nitrosomethylbenzylamine-induced tumorigenesis in the rat esophagus by dietary freeze-dried strawberries. *Carcinogenesis*, **22**, 441–446

Castelletto, R., Castellsague, X., Muñoz, N., Iscovich, J., Chopita, N. & Jmelnitsky, A. (1994) Alcohol, tobacco, diet, mate drinking, and esophageal cancer in Argentina. *Cancer Epidemiol. Biomarkers Prev.*, **3**, 557–564

Castellsague, X., Muñoz, N., De Stefani, E., Victora, C.G., Castelletto, R. & Rolon, P.A. (2000) Influence of mate drinking, hot beverages and diet on esophageal cancer risk in South America. *Int. J. Cancer*, **88**, 658–664

Castenmiller, J.J., Lauridsen, S.T., Dragsted, L.O., het Hof, K.H., Linssen, J.P. & West, C.E. (1999) β-Carotene does not change markers of enzymatic and nonenzymatic antioxidant activity in human blood. *J. Nutr.*, **129**, 2162–2169

Casto, B.C, Kresty, L.A., Kraly, C.L., Pearl, D.K., Knobloch, T.J., Schut, H.A., Stoner, G.D., Mallery, S.R. & Weghorst, C.M. (2002) Chemoprevention of oral cancer by black raspberries. *Anticancer Res.*, **22**, 4005–4016

Centonze, S., Boeing, H., Leoci, C., Guerra, V. & Misciagna, G. (1994) Dietary habits and colorectal cancer in a low-risk area. Results from a population-based case–control study in southern Italy. *Nutr. Cancer*, **21**, 233–246

Chan, J.M., Pietinen, P., Virtanen, M., Malila, N., Tangrea, J., Albanes, D. & Virtamo, J. (2000) Diet and prostate cancer risk in a cohort of smokers, with a specific focus on calcium and phosphorus (Finland). *Cancer Causes Control*, **11**, 859–867

Chandra, R.K. & Sarchielli, P. (1993) Nutritional status and immune responses. *Clin. Lab. Med.*, **13**, 455–461

Chang-Claude, J.C., Wahrendorf, J., Liang, Q.S., Rei, Y.G., Muñoz, N., Crespi, M., Raedsch, R., Thurnham, D.I. & Correa, P. (1990) An epidemiological study of precursor lesions of esophageal cancer among young persons in a high-risk population in Huixian, China. *Cancer Res.*, **50**, 2268–2274

Chang-Claude, J., Shimada, H., Muñoz, N., Wahrendorf, J., Liang, Q.S., Rei, Y.G., Crespi, M., Raedsch, R. & Correa, P. (1992) Micronuclei in esophageal cells of Chinese youths in a high-incidence area for esophageal cancer in China. *Cancer Epidemiol. Biomarkers Prev.*, **1**, 463–466

Chaudhary, A.K., Nokubo, M., Reddy, G.R., Yeola, S.N., Morrow, J.D., Blair, I.A. & Marnett, L.J. (1994) Detection of endogenous malondialdehyde-deoxyguanosine adducts in human liver. *Science*, **265**, 1580–1582

Chen, J., Campbell, T.C., Junyao, L. & Peto, R., eds (1990) *Diet, Life-style, and Mortality in China: A Study of the Characteristics of 65 Chinese Counties*, Oxford, Ithaca, Beijing, Oxford University Press, Cornell University Press, People's Medical Publishing House

Chen, L., Mohr, S.N. & Yang, C.S. (1996) Decrease of plasma and urinary oxidative metabolites of acetaminophen after consumption of watercress by human volunteers. *Clin. Pharmacol. Ther.*, **60**, 651–660

Chen, H.W., Yang, J.J., Tsai, C.W., Wu, J.J., Sheen, L.Y., Ou, C.C. & Lii, C.K. (2001a) Dietary fat and garlic oil independently regulate hepatic cytochrome P_{450} 2B1 and the placental form of glutathione S-transferase expression in rats. *J. Nutr.*, **131**, 1438–1443

Chen, L., Stacewicz-Sapuntzakis, M., Duncan, C., Sharifi, R., Ghosh, L., van Breemen, R., Ashton, D. & Bowen, P.E. (2001b) Oxidative DNA damage in prostate cancer patients consuming tomato sauce-based entrees as a whole-food intervention. *J. Natl Cancer Inst.*, **93**, 1872–1879

Chen, H., Ward, M.H., Graubard, B.I., Heineman, E.F., Markin, R.M., Potischman, N.A., Russell, R.M., Weisenburger, D.D. & Tucker, K.L. (2002a) Dietary patterns and adenocarcinoma of the esophagus and distal stomach. *Am. J. Clin. Nutr.*, **75**, 137–144

Chen, H., Ward, M.H., Tucker, K.L., Graubard, B.I., McComb, R.D., Potischman, N.A., Weisenburger, D.D. & Heinemann, E.F. (2002b) Diet and risk of adult glioma in eastern Nebraska, United States. *Cancer Causes Control*, **13**, 647–655

Chen, S.Y., Wang, L.Y., Lunn, R.M., Tsai, W.Y., Lee, P.H., Lee, C.S., Ahsan, H., Zhang, Y.J., Chen, C.J. & Santella, R.M. (2002c) Polycyclic aromatic hydrocarbon–DNA adducts in liver tissues of hepatocellular carcinoma patients and controls. *Int. J. Cancer*, **99**, 14–21

Cheng, K.K., Day, N.E., Duffy, S.W., Lam, T.H., Fok, M. & Wong, J. (1992a) Pickled vegetables in the aetiology of oesophageal cancer in Hong Kong Chinese. *Lancet*, **339**, 1314–1318

Cheng, K.C., Cahill, D.S., Kasai, H., Nishimura, S. & Loeb, L.A. (1992b) 8-Hydroxyguanine, an abundant form of oxidative DNA damage, causes G→T and A→C substitutions. *J. Biol. Chem.*, **267**, 166–172

References

Cheng, K.K., Duffy, S.W., Day, N.E. & Lam, T.H. (1995) Oesophageal cancer in never-smokers and never-drinkers. *Int. J. Cancer*, **60**, 820–822

Cheng, K.K., Sharp, L., McKinney, P.A., Logan, R.F., Chilvers, C.E., Cook-Mozaffari, P., Ahmed, A. & Day, N.E. (2000a) A case–control study of oesophageal adenocarcinoma in women: a preventable disease. *Br. J. Cancer*, **83**, 127–132

Cheng, L., Spitz, M.R., Hong, W.K. & Wei, Q. (2000b) Reduced expression levels of nucleotide excision repair genes in lung cancer: a case–control analysis. *Carcinogenesis*, **21**, 1527–1530

Chesney, A.M., Clawson, T.A. & Webster, B. (1928) Endemic goitre in rabbits. I. Incidence and characteristics. *Bull. Johns Hopkins Hosp.*, **43**, 261–277

Chinese Nutrition Society (2000) Dietary guidelines and the Food Guide Pagoda. *J. Am. Diet. Assoc.*, **100**, 886–887

Ching, S., Ingram, D., Hahnel, R., Beilby, J. & Rossi, E. (2002) Serum levels of micronutrients, antioxidants and total antioxidant status predict risk of breast cancer in a case control study. *J. Nutr.*, **132**, 303–306

Chiu, B.C., Cerhan, J.R., Folsom, A.R., Sellers, T.A., Kushi, L.H., Wallace, R.B., Zheng, W. & Potter, J.D. (1996) Diet and risk of non-Hodgkin lymphoma in older women. *JAMA*, **275**, 1315–1321

Chopra, M., O'Neill, M.E., Keogh, N., Wortley, G., Southon, S. & Thurnham, D.I. (2000) Influence of increased fruit and vegetable intake on plasma and lipoprotein carotenoids and LDL oxidation in smokers and nonsmokers. *Clin. Chem.*, **46**, 1818–1829

Chouinard, E. & Walter, S. (1995) Recall bias in case-control studies: an empirical analysis and theoretical framework. *J. Clin. Epidemiol.*, **48**, 245–254

Chow, W.H., Schuman, L.M., McLaughlin, J.K., Bjelke, E., Gridley, G., Wacholder, S., Chien, H.T. & Blot, W.J. (1992) A cohort study of tobacco use, diet, occupation, and lung cancer mortality. *Cancer Causes Control*, **3**, 247–254

Chow, W.H., Gridley, G., McLaughlin, J.K., Mandel, J.S., Wacholder, S., Blot, W.J., Niwa, S. & Fraumeni, J.F., Jr (1994) Protein intake and risk of renal cell cancer. *J. Natl Cancer Inst.*, **86**, 1131–1139

Chung, M.J., Lee, S.H. & Sung, N.J. (2002) Inhibitory effect of whole strawberries, garlic juice or kale juice on endogenous formation of N-nitrosodimethylamine in humans. *Cancer Lett.*, **182**, 1–10

Chyou, P.H., Nomura, A.M., Hankin, J.H. & Stemmermann, G.N. (1990) A case–cohort study of diet and stomach cancer. *Cancer Res.*, **50**, 7501–7504

Chyou, P.H., Nomura, A.M. & Stemmermann, G.N. (1993) A prospective study of diet, smoking, and lower urinary tract cancer. *Ann. Epidemiol.*, **3**, 211–216

Clapp, J.A., McPherson, R.S., Reed, D.B. & Hsi, B.P. (1991) Comparison of a food frequency questionnaire using reported vs standard portion sizes for classifying individuals according to nutrient intake. *J. Am. Diet. Assoc.*, **91**, 316–320

Clapper, M.L., Szarka, C.E., Pfeiffer, G.R., Graham, T.A., Balshem, A.M., Litwin, S., Goosenberg, E.B., Frucht, H. & Engstrom, P.F. (1997) Preclinical and clinical evaluation of broccoli supplements as inducers of glutathione S-transferase activity. *Clin. Cancer Res.*, **3**, 25–30

Claude, J., Kunze, E., Frentzel-Beyme, R., Paczkowski, K., Schneider, J. & Schubert, H. (1986) Life-style and occupational risk factors in cancer of the lower urinary tract. *Am. J. Epidemiol.*, **124**, 578–589

Clayton, D. & Hills, M., eds (1993) *Statistical Models in Epidemiology*, Oxford, Oxford University Press

Coggon, D., Barker, D.J., Cole, R.B. & Nelson, M. (1989) Stomach cancer and food storage. *J. Natl Cancer Inst.*, **81**, 1178–1182

Cohen, J.H., Kristal, A.R. & Stanford, J.L. (2000) Fruit and vegetable intakes and prostate cancer risk. *J. Natl Cancer Inst.*, **92**, 61–68

Colditz, G.A., Martin, P., Stampfer, M.J., Willett, W.C., Sampson, L., Rosner, B., Hennekens, C.H. & Speizer, F.E. (1986) Validation of questionnaire information on risk factors and disease outcomes in a prospective cohort study of women. *Am. J. Epidemiol.*, **123**, 894–900

Collins, A.R., Olmedilla, B., Southon, S., Granado, F. & Duthie, S.J. (1998) Serum carotenoids and oxidative DNA damage in human lymphocytes. *Carcinogenesis*, **19**, 2159–2162

Collins, B.H., Horska, A., Hotten, P.M., Riddoch, C. & Collins, A.R. (2001) Kiwifruit protects against oxidative DNA damage in human cells and *in vitro*. *Nutr. Cancer*, **39**, 148–153

Cook-Mozaffari, P.J., Azordegan, F., Day, N.E., Ressicaud, A., Sabai, C. & Aramesh, B. (1979) Oesophageal cancer studies in the Caspian littoral of Iran: results of a case–control study. *Br. J. Cancer*, **39**, 293–309

Cordier, S., Iglesias, M.-J., Le Goaster, C., Guyot, M.-M., Mandereau, L. & Hemon, D. (1994) Incidence and risk factors for childhood brain tumors in the Ile de France. *Int. J. Cancer*, **59**, 776–782

Corella, D., Cortina, P., Guillen, M. & Gonzalez, J.I. (1996) Dietary habits and geographic variation in stomach cancer mortality in Spain. *Eur. J. Cancer Prev.*, **5**, 249–257

Cornée, J., Pobel, D., Riboli, E., Guyader, M. & Hémon, B. (1995) A case–control study of gastric cancer and nutritional factors in Marseille, France. *Eur. J. Epidemiol.*, **11**, 55–65

Correa, P., Fontham, E., Pickle, L.W., Chen, V., Lin, Y.P. & Haenszel, W. (1985) Dietary determinants of gastric cancer in south Louisiana inhabitants. *J. Natl Cancer Inst.*, **75**, 645–654

Coughlin, S.S. (1990) Recall bias in epidemiologic studies. *J. Clin. Epidemiol.*, **43**, 87–91

Coward, L., Barnes, N.C., Setchell, K.D. & Barnes, S. (1993) Genistein, diadzein and their β-glycoside conjugates: antitumor isoflavones in soybean foods from American and Asian diets. *J. Agric. Food Chem.*, **41**, 1961–1967

Cox, B.D., Whichelow, M.J. & Prevost, A.T. (2000) Seasonal consumption of salad vegetables and fresh fruit in relation to the development of cardiovascular disease and cancer. *Public Health Nutr.*, **3,** 19–29

Cresta, M., Ledermann, S., Garnier, A., Lombardo, E. & Lacourly, G., eds (1969) *Etude des consommations alimentaires des populations de onze régions de la Communauté Européenne en vue de la détermination des niveaux de contamination radioactive. Rapport établi au Centre d'Etude Nucléaire de Fontenay-aux-Roses, France,* Brussels, EURATOM

Crews, H., Alink, G., Andersen, R., Braesco, V., Holst, B., Maiani, G., Ovesen, L., Scotter, M., Solfrizzo, M., van den Berg, R., Verhagen, H. & Williamson, G. (2001) A critical assessment of some biomarker approaches linked with dietary intake. *Br. J. Nutr.*, **86 Suppl. 1,** S5–35

Cronin, F.J., Shaw, A.M., Krebs-Smith, S.M. & Marsland, P.M. (1987) Developing a food guidance system to implement the dietary guidelines. *J. Nutr. Educ.*, **19,** 281–302

Cullen, J.J., Mitros, F.A. & Oberley, L.W. (2003) Expression of antioxidant enzymes in diseases of the human pancreas: another link between chronic pancreatitis and pancreatic cancer. *Pancreas,* **26,** 23–27

Cuzick, J., Sasieni, P. & Singer, A. (1996) Risk factors for invasive cervix cancer in young women. *Eur. J. Cancer*, **32A,** 836–841

Das, M., Bickers, D.R. & Mukhtar, H. (1985) Effect of ellagic acid on hepatic and pulmonary xenobiotic metabolism in mice: studies on the mechanism of its anticarcinogenic action. *Carcinogenesis,* **6,** 1409–1413

Dashwood, R., Negishi, T., Hayatsu, H., Breinholt, V., Hendricks, J. & Bailey, G. (1998) Chemopreventive properties of chlorophylls towards aflatoxin B1: a review of the antimutagenicity and anticarcinogenicity data in rainbow trout. *Mutat. Res.*, **399,** 245–253

D'Avanzo, B., La Vecchia, C., Braga, C., Franceschi, S., Negri, E. & Parpinel, M. (1997) Nutrient intake according to education, smoking, and alcohol in Italian women. *Nutr. Cancer,* **28,** 46–51

Davies, T.W., Palmer, C.R., Ruja, E. & Lipscombe, J.M. (1996) Adolescent milk, dairy product and fruit consumption and testicular cancer. *Br. J. Cancer*, **74,** 657–660

Day, N. (2002) Author's response. *Int. J. Epidemiol.,* **31,** 692–693

Day, N.E. & Ferrari, P. (2002) Some methodological issues in nutritional epidemiology In: Riboli, E. & Lambert, R., eds, *Nutrition and Lifestyle: Opportunities for Cancer Prevention,* Lyon, IARCPress, pp. 5–10

Day, G.L., Blot, W.J., Austin, D.F., Bernstein, L., Greenberg, R.S., Preston-Martin, S., Schoenberg, J.B., Winn, D.M., McLaughlin, J.K. & Fraumeni, J.F., Jr (1993) Racial differences in risk of oral and pharyngeal cancer: alcohol, tobacco, and other determinants. *J. Natl Cancer Inst.*, **85,** 465–473

Day, A.P., Kemp, H.J., Bolton, C., Hartog, M. & Stansbie, D. (1997) Effect of concentrated red grape juice consumption on serum antioxidant capacity and low-density lipoprotein oxidation. *Ann. Nutr. Metab.*, **41,** 353–357

Day, N.E., McKeown, N., Wong, M., Welch, A. & Bingham, S. (2001) Epidemiological assessment of diet: a comparison of a 7-day diary with a food frequency questionnaire using urinary markers of nitrogen, potassium and sodium. *Int. J. Epidemiol.,* **30,** 309–317

De Flora, S. & Ramel, C. (1988) Mechanisms of inhibitors of mutagenesis and carcinogenesis. Classification and overview. *Mutat. Res.*, **202,** 285–306

Deng, X.S., Tuo, J., Poulsen, H.E. & Loft, S. (1998) Prevention of oxidative DNA damage in rats by brussels sprouts. *Free Radic. Res.*, **28,** 323–333

De Jong, U.W., Breslow, N., Hong, J.G., Sridharan, M. & Shanmugaratnam, K. (1974) Aetiological factors in oesophageal cancer in Singapore Chinese. *Int. J. Cancer*, **13,** 291–303

de Klerk, N.H., English, D.R. & Armstrong, B.K. (1989) A review of the effects of random measurement error on relative risk estimates in epidemiological studies. *Int. J. Epidemiol.*, **18,** 705–712

De Stefani, E., Correa, P., Oreggia, F., Leiva, J., Rivero, S., Fernandez, G., Deneo-Pellegrini, H., Zavala, D. & Fontham, E. (1987) Risk factors for laryngeal cancer. *Cancer*, **60,** 3087–3091

De Stefani, E., Correa, P., Fierro, L., Carzoglio, J., Deneo-Pellegrini, H. & Zavala, D. (1990a) Alcohol drinking and tobacco smoking in gastric cancer. A case–control study. *Rev. Epidemiol. Santé Publ.*, **38,** 297–307

De Stefani, E., Muñoz, N., Estève, J., Vasallo, A., Victora, C.G. & Teuchmann, S. (1990b) Mate drinking, alcohol, tobacco, diet, and esophageal cancer in Uruguay. *Cancer Res.*, **50,** 426–431

De Stefani, E., Correa, P., Fierro, L., Fontham, E., Chen, V. & Zavala, D. (1991) Black tobacco, mate, and bladder cancer. A case–control study from Uruguay. *Cancer*, **67,** 536–540

De Stefani, E., Fierro, L., Barrios, E. & Ronco, A. (1995) Tobacco, alcohol, diet and risk of prostate cancer. *Tumori*, **81,** 315–320

De Stefani, E., Deneo-Pellegrini, H., Mendilaharsu, M. & Ronco, A. (1999) Diet and risk of cancer of the upper aerodigestive tract – I. Foods. *Oral Oncol.*, **35,** 17–21

De Stefani, E., Boffetta, P., Oreggia, F., Brennan, P., Ronco, A., Deneo-Pellegrini, H. & Mendilaharsu, M. (2000a) Plant foods and risk of laryngeal cancer: A case–control study in Uruguay. *Int. J. Cancer*, **87,** 129–132

De Stefani, E., Brennan, P., Boffetta, P., Ronco, A.L., Mendilaharsu, M. & Deneo-Pellegrini, H. (2000b) Vegetables, fruits, related dietary antioxidants, and risk of squamous cell carcinoma of the esophagus: a case–control study in Uruguay. *Nutr. Cancer*, **38,** 23–29

References

De Stefani, E., Correa, P., Boffetta, P., Ronco, A., Brennan, P., Deneo-Pellegrini, H. & Mendilaharsu, M. (2001) Plant foods and risk of gastric cancer: a case–control study in Uruguay. *Eur. J. Cancer Prev.*, **10**, 357–364

De Stefani, E., Brennan, P., Ronco, A., Fierro, L., Correa, P., Boffetta, P., Deneo-Pellegrini, H. & Barrios, E. (2002) Food groups and risk of lung cancer in Uruguay. *Lung Cancer*, **38**, 1–7

Devanaboyina, U. & Gupta, R.C. (1996) Sensitive detection of 8-hydroxy-2'-deoxyguanosine in DNA by ^{32}P-postlabeling assay and the basal levels in rat tissues. *Carcinogenesis*, **17**, 917–924

de Vet, H.C., Knipschild, P.G., Grol, M.E., Schouten, H.J. & Sturmans, F. (1991) The role of beta-carotene and other dietary factors in the aetiology of cervical dysplasia: results of a case–control study. *Int. J. Epidemiol.*, **20**, 603–610

Decarli, A., Liati, P., Negri, E., Franceschi, S. & La Vecchia, C. (1987) Vitamin A and other dietary factors in the etiology of esophageal cancer. *Nutr. Cancer*, **10**, 29–37

Deeg, D.J., van Tilburg, T., Smit, J.H. & de Leeuw, E.D. (2002) Attrition in the Longitudinal Aging Study Amsterdam. The effect of differential inclusion in side studies. *J. Clin. Epidemiol.*, **55**, 319–328

DeMarini, D.M., Hastings, S.B., Brooks, L.R., Eischen, B.T., Bell, D.A., Watson, M.A., Felton, J.S., Sandler, R. & Kohlmeier, L. (1997) Pilot study of free and conjugated urinary mutagenicity during consumption of pan-fried meats: possible modulation by cruciferous vegetables, glutathione S-transferase-M1, and N-acetyltransferase-2. *Mutat. Res.*, **381**, 83–96

Demissie, S., LaValley, M.P., Horton, N.J., Glynn, R.J. & Cupples, L.A. (2003) Bias due to missing exposure data using complete-case analysis in the proportional hazards regression model. *Stat. Med.*, **22**, 545–557

Deng, X.S., Tuo, J., Poulsen, H.E. & Loft, S. (1998) Prevention of oxidative DNA damage in rats by brussels sprouts. *Free Radic. Res.*, **28**, 323–333

Deneo-Pellegrini, H., De Stefani, E., Ronco, A. & Mendilaharsu, M. (1999) Foods, nutrients and prostate cancer: a case–control study in Uruguay. *Br. J. Cancer*, **80**, 591–597

Deneo-Pellegrini, H., Boffetta, P., De Stefani, E., Ronco, A., Brennan, P. & Mendilaharsu, M. (2002) Plant foods and differences between colon and rectal cancers. *Eur. J. Cancer Prev.*, **11**, 369–375

Department of Women & Child Development (1998) India Nutrition Profile In: *Ministry of Human Resource Development*, New Delhi, Government of India Press, Chapter 3, pp. 10–11

Devine, C.M., Wolfe, W.S., Frongillo, E.A., Jr, Bisogni, C.A. (1999) Life-course events and experiences: association with fruit and vegetable consumption in 3 ethnic groups. *J. Am. Diet. Assoc.*, **99**, 309–314

Dixon, H., Borland, R., Segan, C., Stafford, H. & Sindall, C. (1998) Public reaction to Victoria's "2 Fruit 'n' 5 Veg Every Day" campaign and reported consumption of fruit and vegetables. *Prev. Med.*, **27**, 572–582

Doll, R. & Peto, R. (1981) The causes of cancer. Quantitative estimates of avoidable risks of cancer in the United States today. *J. Natl Cancer Inst.*, **66**, 1191–1308

Domel, S.B., Baranowski, T., Davis, H., Leonard, S.B., Riley, P. & Baranowski, J. (1993a) Measuring fruit and vegetable preferences among 4th- and 5th-grade students. *Prev. Med.*, **22**, 866–879

Domel, S.B., Leonard, S.B., Baranowski, T. & Baranowski, J. (1993) "To be or not to be..." fruits and vegetables. *J. Nutr. Educ.*, **25**, 352–358

Dorgan, J.F., Ziegler, R.G., Schoenberg, J.B., Hartge, P., McAdams, M.J., Falk, R.T. , Wilcox, H.B. & Shaw, G.L. (1993) Race and sex differences in associations of vegetables, fruits, and carotenoids with lung cancer risk in New Jersey (United States). *Cancer Causes Control*, **4**, 273–281

Dos Santos Silva, I., Mangtani, P., McCormack, V., Bhakta, D., Sevak, L. & McMichael, A.J. (2002) Lifelong vegetarianism and risk of breast cancer: a population-based case–control study among South Asian migrant women living in England. *Int. J. Cancer*, **99**, 238–244

Dragsted, L.O., Strube, M. & Larsen, J.C. (1993) Cancer-protective factors in fruits and vegetables: biochemical and biological background. *Pharmacol. Toxicol.*, **72 Suppl. 1**, 116–135

Dragsted, L.O., Strube, M. & Leth, T. (1997) Dietary levels of plant phenols and other non-nutritive components: could they prevent cancer? *Eur. J. Cancer Prev.*, **6**, 522–528

Dragsted, L.O., Young, J.F., Loft, S.& Sandström, B. (2001) Biomarkers of oxidative stress and of antioxidative defense: relationship to intervention with antioxidant-rich foods. In: Nesaretnam, K. & Packer, L., eds, *Micronutrients and Health: Molecular Biological Mechanisms*, Champaign, IL, AOCS Press, pp. 272–278

Drews, C.D. & Greeland, S. (1990) The impact of differential recall on the results of case-control studies. *Int. J. Epidemiol.*, **19**, 1107–1112

Durak, I., Bayram, F., Kavutcu, M., Canbolat, O. & Ozturk, H.S. (1996) Impaired enzymatic antioxidant defense mechanism in cancerous human thyroid tissues. *J. Endocrinol. Invest.*, **19**, 312–315

Duthie, S.J., Ma, A., Ross, M.A. & Collins, A.R. (1996) Antioxidant supplementation decreases oxidative DNA damage in human lymphocytes. *Cancer Res.*, **56**, 1291–1295

Eaton, E.A., Walle, U.K., Lewis, A.J., Hudson, T., Wilson, A.A. & Walle, T. (1996) Flavonoids, potent inhibitors of the human P-form phenolsulfotransferase. Potential role in drug metabolism and chemoprevention. *Drug Metab. Dispos.*, **24**, 232–237

Eccleston, C., Baoru, Y., Tahvonen, R., Kallio, H., Rimbach, G.H. & Minihane, A.M. (2002) Effects of an antioxidant-rich juice (sea buckthorn) on risk factors for coronary heart disease in humans. *J. Nutr. Biochem.*, **13,** 346–354

Edenharder, R., Frangart, J., Hager, M., Hofmann, P. & Rauscher, R. (1998) Protective effects of fruits and vegetables against *in vivo* clastogenicity of cyclosphosphamide or benzo[*a*]pyrene in mice. *Food Chem. Toxicol.*, **36,** 637–645

Egner, P.A., Wang, J.B., Zhu, Y.R., Zhang, B.C., Wu, Y., Zhang, Q.N., Qian, G.S., Kuang, S.Y., Gange, S.J., Jacobson, L.P., Helzlsouer, K.J., Bailey, G.S., Groopman, J.D. & Kensler, T.W. (2001) Chlorophyllin intervention reduces aflatoxin-DNA adducts in individuals at high risk for liver cancer. *Proc. Natl Acad. Sci. USA*, **98,** 14601–14606

Ekström, A.M., Serafini, M., Nyrén, O., Hansson, L.E., Ye, W. & Wolk, A. (2000) Dietary antioxidant intake and the risk of cardia cancer and noncardia cancer of the intestinal and diffuse types: a population-based case–control study in Sweden. *Int. J. Cancer*, **87,** 133–140

El Sohemy, A., Baylin, A., Kabagambe, E., Ascherio, A., Spiegelman, D. & Campos, H. (2002) Individual carotenoid concentrations in adipose tissue and plasma as biomarkers of dietary intake. *Am. J. Clin. Nutr.*, **76,** 172–179

Encyclopedia Britannica (1974) *Macropedia*, Vol. 1, Chicago, Hemingway Benton

Enstrom, J.E., Kanim, L.E. & Klein, M.A. (1992) Vitamin C intake and mortality among a sample of the United States population. *Epidemiology,* **3,** 194–202

EPIC Group of Spain (1997) Relative validity and reproducibility of a diet history questionnaire in Spain. I. Foods. EPIC Group of Spain. European Prospective Investigation into Cancer and Nutrition. *Int. J. Epidemiol.*, **26 Suppl. 1,** S91–S99

Eriksen, K., Haraldsdottir, J., Pederson, R. & Flyger, H.V. (2003) Effect of a fruit and vegetable subscription in Danish schools. *Public Health Nutr.*, **6,** 57–63

Estève, J., Riboli, E., Péquignot, G., Terracini, B., Merletti, F., Crosignani, P., Ascunce, N., Zubiri, L., Blanchet, F., Raymond, L., Repetto, F. & Tuyns, A.J. (1996) Diet and cancers of the larynx and hypopharynx: the IARC multi-center study in southwestern Europe. *Cancer Causes Control*, **7,** 240–252

Ewertz, M. & Gill, C. (1990) Dietary factors and breast-cancer risk in Denmark. *Int. J. Cancer*, **46,** 779–784

Faggiano, F., Vineis, P., Cravanzola, D., Pisani, P., Xompero, G., Riboli, E. & Kaaks, R. (1992) Validation of a method for the estimation of food portion size. *Epidemiology* , **3**, 379–382

Fagt, S., Matthiessen, J., Trolle, E., Lyhne, N., Christensen, T., Hinsch, H.J., Hartkopp, H.B., Biltoft-Jensen, A., Moller, A. & Daase, A.S., eds (2002) *2. Danskernes kostvaner 2000–2001: Udviklingen i danskernes kost - forbrug, indkøb og vaner*, Søborg, Fødevaredirektoratet (Fødevare Rapport 2002:10), available at http://foedevaredirektoratet.dk/FDir/Publications/2002010/Rapport.pdf

Fahey, J.W., Zalcmann, A.T. & Talalay, P. (2001) The chemical diversity and distribution of glucosinolates and isothiocyanates among plants. *Phytochemistry*, **56,** 5–51

Fairfield, K.M., Hankinson, S.E., Rosner, B.A., Hunter, D.J., Colditz, G.A. & Willett, W.C. (2001) Risk of ovarian carcinoma and consumption of vitamins A, C, and E and specific carotenoids: a prospective analysis. *Cancer*, **92,** 2318–2326

Falk, R.T., Pickle, L.W., Fontham, E.T., Correa, P. & Fraumeni, J.F., Jr (1988) Life-style risk factors for pancreatic cancer in Louisiana: a case–control study. *Am. J. Epidemiol.*, **128**, 324–336

Fan, W.Y., Ogusu, K., Kouda, K., Nakamura, H., Satoh, T., Ochi, H. & Takeuchi, H. (2000) Reduced oxidative DNA damage by vegetable juice intake: a controlled trial. *J. Physiol. Anthropol. Appl. Human Sci.*, **19,** 287–289

FAO Nutrition Country Profiles available at http://www.fao.org/es/esn/nutrition/profiles_by_country_en.stm

FAOSTAT (2000) Available at http://apps.fao.org/page/collections?subset=agriculture, under "Food Balance Sheets"

Farchi, S., Saba, A., Turrini, A., Forlani, F., Pettinelli, A. & D'Amicis, A. (1996) An ecological study of the correlation between diet and tumour mortality rates in Italy. *Eur. J. Cancer Prev.*, **5,** 113–120

Farquhar, J.W., Fortmann, S.P., Flora, J.A., Taylor, C.B., Haskell, W.L., Williams, P.T., Maccoby, N. & Wood, P.D. (1990) Effects of communitywide education on cardiovascular disease risk factors. The Stanford Five-City Project. *JAMA,* **264,** 359–365

Farrell, M., Catford, J., Aarum, A.O., Proctor, J., Bredenkamp, R., Matthews, D. & Tucker, N. (2000) 5 a day-type programmes throughout the world: lessons from Australia, Norway, Canada, Germany and Great Britain In: Stables, G. & Farrell, M., eds, *5 A Day International Symposium Proceedings*, Wallingford, CAB International, pp. 37–53

Farrow, D.C. & Davis, S. (1990) Diet and the risk of pancreatic cancer in men. *Am. J. Epidemiol.*, **132**, 423–431

Fehily, A.M., Yarnell, J.W., Sweetnam, P.M. & Elwood, P.C. (1993) Diet and incident ischaemic heart disease: the Caerphilly Study. *Br. J. Nutr.*, **69,** 303–314

Fenwick, G.R., Heaney, R.K. & Mawson, R. (1989) Glucosinolates. In: Cheeke, P.R., ed., *Toxicants of Plant Origin*, Volume II, Boca Raton, FL, CRC Press, pp. 1–41

Ferguson, L.R. & Harris, P.J. (1996) Studies on the role of specific dietary fibres in protection against colorectal cancer. *Mutat. Res.*, **350,** 173–184

Fergusson, D., Aaron, S.D., Guyatt, G. & Hébert, P. (2002) Post-randomisation exclusions: the intention to treat principle and excluding patients from analysis. *BMJ*, **325**, 652–654

Feskanich, D., Rimm, E.B., Giovannucci, E.L., Colditz, G.A., Stampfer, M.J., Litin, L.B. & Willett, W.C. (1993) Repro-ducibility and validity of food intake measurements from a semiquantitative food frequency questionnaire. *J. Am. Diet. Assoc.*, **93**, 790–796

References

Feskanich, D., Ziegler, R.G., Michaud, D.S., Giovannucci, E.L., Speizer, F.E., Willett, W.C. & Colditz, G.A. (2000) Prospective study of fruit and vegetable consumption and risk of lung cancer among men and women. *J. Natl Cancer Inst.*, **92**, 1812–1823

Field, A.E., Colditz, G.A., Fox, M.K., Byers, T., Serdula, M., Bosch, R.J. & Peterson, K.E. (1998) Comparison of 4 questionnaires for assessment of fruit and vegetable intake. *Am. J. Public Health*, **88**, 1216–1218

Fioretti, F., Bosetti, C., Tavani, A., Franceschi, S. & La Vecchia, C. (1999) Risk factors for oral and pharyngeal cancer in never smokers. *Oral Oncol.*, **35**, 375–378

Flegal, K.M. & Larkin, F.A. (1990) Partitioning macronutrient intake estimates from a food frequency questionnaire. *Am. J. Epidemiol.*, **131**, 1046–1058

Flood, A., Velie, E.M., Chaterjee, N., Subar, A.F., Thompson, F.E., Lacey, J.V., Jr, Schairer, C., Troisi, R. & Schatzkin, A. (2002) Fruit and vegetable intakes and the risk of colorectal cancer in the Breast Cancer Detection Demonstration Project follow-up cohort. *Am. J. Clin. Nutr.*, **75**, 936–943

Flynn, M.A. & Kearney, J.M. (1999) An approach to the development of food-based dietary guidelines for Ireland *Br J. Nutr.*, **81 Suppl. 2,** S77–S82

Foerster, S.B., Kizer, K.W., Disogra, L.K., Bal, D.G., Krieg, B.F. & Bunch, K.L. (1995) California's "5 a day—for better health!" campaign: an innovative population-based effort to effect large-scale dietary change. *Am. J. Prev. Med.*, **11**, 124–131

Fong, C.H., Hasegawa, S., Herman, Z. & Ou, P. (1989) Liminoid glucosides in commercial citrus juices. *J. Food Sci.*, **54**, 1505–1506

Fontham, E.T., Pickle, L.W., Haenszel, W., Correa, P., Lin, Y.P. & Falk, R.T. (1988) Dietary vitamins A and C and lung cancer risk in Louisiana. *Cancer*, **62**, 2267–2273

Food and Nutrition Research Institute (2001) *Philippine Nutrition: Facts & Figures*, Department of Science & Technology, Taguig, Metro Manila. Available at http://www.fnri.dost.gov.ph/facts/mainpn.html

Forman, M.R., Yao, S.X., Graubard, B.I., Qiao, Y.L., McAdams, M., Mao, B.L. & Taylor, P.R. (1992) The effect of dietary intake of fruits and vegetables on the odds ratio of lung cancer among Yunnan tin miners. *Int. J. Epidemiol.*, **21**, 437–441

Fowke, J.H., Longcope, C. & Hebert, J.R. (2000) Brassica vegetable consumption shifts estrogen metabolism in healthy postmenopausal women. *Cancer Epidemiol. Biomarkers Prev.*, **9**, 773–779

Franceschi, S., Bidoli, E., Baron, A.E. & La Vecchia, C. (1990) Maize and risk of cancers of the oral cavity, pharynx, and esophagus in northeastern Italy. *J. Natl Cancer Inst.*, **82**, 1407–1411

Franceschi, S., Bidoli, E., Baron, A.E., Barra, S., Talamini, R., Serraino, D. & La Vecchia, C. (1991a) Nutrition and cancer of the oral cavity and pharynx in northeast Italy. *Int. J. Cancer*, **47**, 20–25

Franceschi, S., Levi, F., Negri, E., Fassina, A. & La Vecchia, C. (1991b) Diet and thyroid cancer: a pooled analysis of four European case–control studies. *Int. J. Cancer*, **48**, 395–398

Franceschi, S., Favero, A., La Vecchia, C., Negri, E., Dal Maso, L., Salvini, S., Decarli, A. & Giacosa, A. (1995) Influence of food groups and food diversity on breast cancer risk in Italy. *Int. J. Cancer*, **63**, 785–789

Franceschi, S., Favero, A., La Vecchia, C., Negri, E., Conti, E., Montella, M., Giacosa, A., Nanni, O. & Decarli, A. (1997) Food groups and risk of colorectal cancer in Italy. *Int. J. Cancer*, **72**, 56–61

Franceschi, S., Favero, A., Conti, E., Talamini, R., Volpe, R., Negri, E., Barzan, L. & La Vecchia, C. (1999) Food groups, oils and butter, and cancer of the oral cavity and pharynx. *Br. J. Cancer*, **80**, 614–620

Franco, E.L., Kowalski, L.P., Oliveira, B.V., Curado, M.P., Pereira, R.N., Silva, M.E., Fava, A.S. & Torloni, H. (1989) Risk factors for oral cancer in Brazil: a case–control study. *Int. J. Cancer*, **43**, 992–1000

Fraser, G.E., Phillips, R.L. & Beeson, W.L. (1990) Hypertension, antihypertensive medication and risk of renal carcinoma in California Seventh-Day Adventists. *Int. J. Epidemiol.*, **19**, 832–838

Fraser, G.E., Beeson, W.L. & Phillips, R.L. (1991) Diet and lung cancer in California Seventh-day Adventists. *Am. J. Epidemiol.*, **133**, 683–693

Fraser, G.E., Sabaté, J., Beeson, W.L. & Strahan, T.M. (1992) A possible protective effect of nut consumption on risk of coronary heart disease. The Adventist Health Study. *Arch. Intern. Med.*, **152**, 1416–1424

Freudenheim, J.L., Marshall, J.R., Vena, J.E., Laughlin, R., Brasure, J.R., Swanson, M.K., Nemoto, T. & Graham, S. (1996) Premenopausal breast cancer risk and intake of vegetables, fruits, and related nutrients. *J. Natl Cancer Inst.*, **88**, 340–348

Friedenreich, C.M. (1993) Methods for pooled analyses of epidemiologic studies. *Epidemiology*, **4,** 295–302

Friedenreich, C.M. (1994) Methodologic issues for pooling dietary data. *Am. J. Clin. Nutr.*, **59,** 251S–252S

Friedenreich, C.M., Howe, G.R. & Miller, A.B. (1991) An investigation of recall bias in the reporting of past food intake among breast cancer cases and controls. *Ann. Epidemiol.*, **1,** 439–453

Fuhrman, B., Volkova, N., Rosenblat, M. & Aviram, M. (2000) Lycopene synergistically inhibits LDL oxidation in combination with vitamin E, glabridin, rosmarinic acid, carnosic acid, or garlic. *Antioxid. Redox. Signal.*, **2,** 491–506

Fukuda, K., Shibata, A., Hirohata, I., Tanikawa, K., Yamaguchi, G. & Ishii, M. (1993) A hospital-based case–control study on hepatocellular carcinoma in Fukuoka and Saga Prefectures, Northern Kyushu, Japan. *Jpn. J. Cancer Res.*, **84**, 708–714

Galanis, D.J., Kolonel, L.N., Lee, J. & Nomura, A. (1998) Intakes of selected foods and beverages and the incidence of gastric cancer among the Japanese residents of Hawaii: a prospective study. *Int. J. Epidemiol.*, **27**, 173–180

Galanti, M.R., Hansson, L., Bergström, R., Wolk, A., Hjartaker, A., Lund, E., Grimelius, L. & Ekbom, A. (1997) Diet and the risk of papillary and follicular thyroid carcinoma: a population-based case–control study in Sweden and Norway. *Cancer Causes Control*, **8**, 205–214

Gale, C.R., Martyn, C.N., Winter, P.D. & Cooper, C. (1995) Vitamin C and risk of death from stroke and coronary heart disease in cohort of elderly people. *BMJ*, **310,** 1563–1566

Gandini, S., Merzenich, H., Robertson, C. & Boyle, P. (2000) Meta-analysis of studies on breast cancer risk and diet: the role of fruit and vegetable consumption and the intake of associated micronutrients. *Eur. J. Cancer*, **36**, 636–646

Ganguly, C., De, S. & Das, S. (2000) Prevention of carcinogen-induced mouse skin papilloma by whole fruit aqueous extract of *Momordica charantia*. *Eur. J. Cancer Prev.*, **9,** 283–288

Gao, C.M., Tajima, K., Kuroishi, T., Hirose, K. & Inoue, M. (1993) Protective effects of raw vegetables and fruit against lung cancer among smokers and ex-smokers: a case–control study in the Tokai area of Japan. *Jpn J. Cancer Res.*, **84,** 594–600

Gao, Y.T., McLaughlin, J.K., Gridley, G., Blot, W.J., Ji, B.T., Dai, Q. & Fraumeni, J.F., Jr (1994) Risk factors for esophageal cancer in Shanghai, China. II. Role of diet and nutrients. *Int. J. Cancer*, **58**, 197–202

Gao, C.M., Takezaki, T., Ding, J.H., Li, M.S. & Tajima, K. (1999) Protective effect of allium vegetables against both esophageal and stomach cancer: a simultaneous case–referent study of a high-epidemic area in Jiangsu Province, China. *Jpn J. Cancer Res.*, **90**, 614–621

Garrote, L.F., Herrero, R., Reyes, R.M., Vaccarella, S., Anta, J.L., Ferbeye, L., Muñoz, N. & Franceschi, S. (2001) Risk factors for cancer of the oral cavity and oropharynx in Cuba. *Br. J. Cancer*, **85**, 46–54

Gaziano, J.M., Manson, J.E., Branch, L.G., Colditz, G.A., Willett, W.C. & Buring, J.E. (1995) A prospective study of consumption of carotenoids in fruits and vegetables and decreased cardiovascular mortality in the elderly. *Ann. Epidemiol.*, **5,** 255–260

Gillman, M.W., Cupples, L.A., Gagnon, D., Posner, B.M., Ellison, R.C., Castelli, W.P. & Wolf, P.A. (1995) Protective effect of fruits and vegetables on development of stroke in men. *JAMA*, **273,** 1113–1117

Giovanelli, L., Saieva, C., Masala, G., Testa, G., Salvini, S., Pitozzi, V., Riboli, E., Dolara, P. & Palli, D. (2002) Nutritional and lifestyle determinants of DNA oxidative damage: a study in a Mediterranean population. *Carcinogenesis*, **23,** 1483–1489

Giovannucci, E., Stampfer, M.J., Colditz, G.A., Manson, J.E., Rosner, B.A., Longnecker, M., Speizer, F.E. & Willett, W.C. (1993) A comparison of prospective and retrospective assessments of diet in the study of breast cancer. *Am. J. Epidemiol.*, **137,** 502–511

Giovannucci, E., Ascherio, A., Rimm, E.B., Stampfer, M.J., Colditz, G.A. & Willett, W.C. (1995) Intake of carotenoids and retinol in relation to risk of prostate cancer. *J. Natl Cancer Inst.*, **87**, 1767–1776

Gnarra, J.R., Tory, K., Weng, Y., Schmidt, L., Wei, M.H., Li, H., Tatif, F., Liu, S., Chen, F., Duh, F.M., Lubensky, I., Duan, D.R., Forence, C., Pozzati, R., Walther, M.M., Bander. N.H., Grossman, H.B., Brauch, H., Pomer, S., Brooks, J.D., Isaacs, W.B., Lerman, M.I., Zbar, B. & Linehan, W.M. (1994) Mutations of the VHL tumour suppressor gene in renal carcinoma. *Nat. Genet.*, **7**, 85–90

Gold, E.B., Gordis, L., Diener, M.D., Seltser, R., Boitnott, J.K., Bynum, T.E. & Hutcheon, D.F. (1985) Diet and other risk factors for cancer of the pancreas. *Cancer*, **55**, 460–467

Goldbohm, R.A., van den Brandt, P.A., Brants, H.A., van't Veer, P., Al, M., Sturmans, F. & Hermus, R.J. (1994) Validation of a dietary questionnaire used in a large-scale prospective cohort study on diet and cancer. *Eur. J. Clin. Nutr.*, **48**, 253–265

Goldbohm, R.A., van't Veer, P., van den Brandt, P.A., van't Hof, M.A., Brants, H.A., Sturmans, F. & Hermus, R.J. (1995) Reproducibility of a food frequency questionnaire and stability of dietary habits determined from five annually repeated measurements. *Eur. J. Clin. Nutr.*, **49,** 420–429

Gonzalez, C.A., Sanz, J.M., Marcos, G., Pita, S., Brullet, E., Saigi, E., Badia, A. & Riboli, E. (1991) Dietary factors and stomach cancer in Spain: a multi-centre case–control study. *Int. J. Cancer*, **49**, 513–519

Goodman, M.T., Hankin, J.H., Wilkens, L.R., Lyu, L.C., McDuffie, K., Liu, L.Q. & Kolonel, L.N. (1997) Diet, body size, physical activity, and the risk of endometrial cancer. *Cancer Res.*, **57**, 5077–5085

Graham, S., Dayal, H., Rohrer, T., Swanson, M., Sultz, H., Shedd, D. & Fischman, S. (1977) Dentition, diet, tobacco, and alcohol in the epidemiology of oral cancer. *J. Natl. Cancer Inst.*, **59**, 1611–1618

Graham, S., Dayal, H., Swanson, M., Mittelman, A. & Wilkinson, G. (1978) Diet in the epidemiology of cancer of the colon and rectum. *J. Natl Cancer Inst.*, **61**, 709–714

Graham, S., Haughey, B., Marshall, J., Brasure, J., Zielezny, M., Freudenheim, J., West, D., Nolan, J. & Wilkinson, G. (1990) Diet in the epidemiology of gastric cancer. *Nutr. Cancer*, **13**, 19–34

Graham, D.Y., Anderson, S.Y. & Lang, T. (1999) Garlic or jalapeño peppers for treatment of *Helicobacter pylori* infection. *Am. J. Gastroenterol.*, **94,** 1200–1202

Gramenzi, A., Gentile, A., Fasoli, M., Negri, E., Parazzini, F. & La Vecchia, C. (1990) Association between certain foods and risk of acute myocardial infarction in women. *BMJ*, **300,** 771–773

References

Grant, W.B. (1999) An ecologic study of dietary links to prostate cancer. *Altern. Med. Rev.*, **4**, 162–169

Greenland, S. (2001) Ecologic versus individual-level sources of bias in ecologic estimates of contextual health effects. *Int. J. Epidemiol.*, **30**, 1343–1350

Greenland, S. & Finkle, W.D. (1995) A critical look at methods for handling missing covariates in epidemiologic regression analyses. *Am. J. Epidemiol.*, **142**, 1255–1264

Gregory, J., Foster, K., Tyler, H. & Wiseman, M. (1990) *The Dietary and Nutritional Survey of British Adults: A Survey of the Dietary Behaviour, Nutritional Status and Blood Pressure of Adults Aged 16 to 64 Living in Great Britain,* London, Office of the Population Census and Surveys. Available at http://www.data-archive.ac.uk/findingData/snDescription.asp?sn=2836

Gridley, G., McLaughlin, J.K., Block, G., Blot, W.J., Winn, D.M., Greenberg, R.S., Schoenberg, J.B., Preston-Martin, S., Austin, D.F. & Fraumeni, J.F., Jr (1990) Diet and oral and pharyngeal cancer among blacks. *Nutr. Cancer*, **14**, 219–225

Gridley, G., McLaughlin, J.K., Block, G., Blot, W.J., Gluch, M. & Fraumeni, J.F., Jr (1992) Vitamin supplement use and reduced risk of oral and pharyngeal cancer. *Am. J. Epidemiol.*, **135**, 1083–1092

Guengerich, F.P. (2001) Forging the links between metabolism and carcinogenesis. *Mutat. Res.*, **488**, 195–209

Guo, W., Blot, W.J., Li, J.Y., Taylor, P.R., Liu, B.Q., Wang, W., Wu, Y.P., Zheng, W., Dawsey, S.M., Li, B. & Fraumeni, J.F., Jr (1994) A nested case–control study of oesophageal and stomach cancers in the Linxian nutrition intervention trial. *Int. J. Epidemiol.*, **23**, 444–450

Guo, X., Cheng, M. & Fei, S. (1995) A case–control study of the etiology of laryngeal cancer in Liaoning Province. *Chin. Med. J. (Engl.)*, **108**, 347–350

Gupta, P.C., Hebert, J.R., Bhonsle, R.B., Sinor, P.N., Mehta, H. & Mehta, F.S. (1998) Dietary factors in oral leukoplakia and submucous fibrosis in a population-based case control study in Gujarat, India. *Oral Dis.*, **4**, 200–206

Gupta, P.C., Hebert, J.R., Bhonsle, R.B., Murti, P.R., Mehta, H. & Mehta, F.S. (1999) Influence of dietary factors on oral precancerous lesions in a population-based case–control study in Kerala, India. *Cancer*, **85**, 1885–1893

Gwilt, P.R., Lear, C.L., Tempero, M.A., Birt, D.D., Grandjean, A.C., Ruddon, R.W. & Nagel, D.L. (1994) The effect of garlic extract on human metabolism of acetaminophen. *Cancer Epidemiol. Biomarkers Prev.*, **3**, 155–160

Hadziyannis, S., Tabor, E., Kaklamani, E., Tzonou, A., Stuver, S., Tassopoulos, N., Mueller, N. & Trichopoulos, D. (1995) A case–control study of hepatitis B and C virus infections in the etiology of hepatocellular carcinoma. *Int. J. Cancer*, **60**, 627–631

Hageman, G., Krul, C., van Herwijnen, M., Schilderman, P. & Kleinjans, J. (1997) Assessment of the anticarcinogenic potential of raw garlic in humans. *Cancer Lett.*, **114**, 161–162

Hagenlocher, T., Nair, J., Becker, N., Korfmann, A. & Bartsch, H. (2001) Influence of dietary fatty acid, vegetable, and vitamin intake on etheno-DNA adducts in white blood cells of healthy female volunteers: A pilot study. *Cancer Epidemiol. Biomarkers Prev.*, **10**, 1187–1191

Hagmar, L., Bonassi, S., Stromberg, U., Brogger, A., Knudsen, L.E., Norppa, H. & Reuterwall, C. (1998) Chromosomal aberrations in lymphocytes predict human cancer: a report from the European Study Group on Cytogenetic Biomarkers and Health (ESCH). *Cancer Res.*, **58**, 4117–4121

Häkkinen, S.H., Kärenlampi, S.O., Heinonen, I.M., Mykkänen, H.M. & Törrönen, A.R. (1999) Content of the flavonols quercetin, myricetin, and kaempferol in 25 edible berries. *J. Agric. Food Chem.*, **47**, 2274–2279

Halliwell, B. (2002) Effect of diet on cancer development: is oxidative DNA damage a biomarker? *Free Radic. Biol. Med.*, **32**, 968–974

Hallquist, A., Hardell, L., Degerman, A. & Boquist, L. (1994) Thyroid cancer: reproductive factors, previous diseases, drug intake, family history and diet. A case–control study. *Eur. J. Cancer Prev.*, **3**, 481–488

Hamada, G.S., Kowalski, L.P., Nishimoto, I.N., Rodrigues, J.J., Iriya, K., Sasazuki, S., Hanaoka, T. & Tsugane, S. (2002) Risk factors for stomach cancer in Brazil (II): a case–control study among Japanese Brazilians in Sao Paulo. *Jpn J. Clin. Oncol.*, **32**, 284–290

Hammar, N. & Norell, S.E. (1991) Retrospective versus original information on diet among cases of colorectal cancer and controls. *Int. J. Epidemiol.*, **20**, 621–627

Hanaoka, T., Tsugane, S., Ando, N., Ishida, K., Kakegawa, T., Isono, K., Takiyama, W., Takagi, I., Ide, H., Watanabe, H. & Iizuka T. (1994) Alcohol consumption and risk of esophageal cancer in Japan: a case–control study in seven hospitals. *Jpn J. Clin. Oncol.*, **24**, 241–246

Hankin, J.H. & Wilkens, L.R. (1994) Development and validation of dietary assessment methods for culturally diverse populations. *Am. J. Clin. Nutr.*, **59**, 198S–200S

Hankin, J.H., Stram, D.O., Arakawa, K., Park, S., Low, S.H., Lee, H.P. & Yu, M.C. (2001) Singapore Chinese Health Study: development, validation, and calibration of the quantitative food frequency questionnaire. *Nutr. Cancer*, **39**, 187–195

Hankinson, S.E., Stampfer, M.J., Seddon, J.M., Colditz, G.A., Rosner, B., Speizer, F.E. & Willett, W.C. (1992) Nutrient intake and cataract extraction in women: a prospective study. *BMJ*, **305**, 335–339

Hansson, L.E., Nyren, O., Bergström, R., Wolk, A., Lindgren, A., Baron, J. & Adami, H.O. (1993) Diet and risk of gastric cancer. A population-based case–control study in Sweden. *Int. J. Cancer*, **55**, 181–189

Haraldsdottir, J. (1999) Dietary guidelines and patterns of intake in Denmark. *Br. J. Nutr.*, **81 Suppl. 2**, S43–S48

Harats, D., Chevion, S., Nahir, M., Norman, Y., Sagee, O. & Berry, E.M. (1998) Citrus fruit supplementation reduces lipoprotein oxidation in young men ingesting a diet high in saturated fat: presumptive evidence for an interaction between vitamins C and E in vivo. *Am. J. Clin. Nutr.*, **67**, 240–245

Harris, T., Woteki, C., Briefel, R.R. & Kleinman, J.C. (1989) NHANES III for older persons: nutrition content and methodological considerations. *Am. J. Clin. Nutr.*, **50**, 1145–1149

Harris, P.J., Triggs, C.M., Roberton, A.M., Watson, M.E. & Ferguson, L.R. (1996) The adsorption of heterocyclic aromatic amines by model dietary fibres with contrasting compositions. *Chem. Biol. Interact.*, **100**, 13–25

Harris, G.K., Gupta, A., Nines, R.G., Kresty, L.A., Habib, S.G., Frankel, W.L., LaPerle, K., Gallaher, D.D., Schwartz, S.J. & Stoner, G.D. (2001) Effects of lyophilized black raspberries on azoxymethane-induced colon cancer and 8-hydroxy-2'-deoxyguanosine levels in the Fischer 344 rat. *Nutr. Cancer*, **40**, 125–133

Harrison, L.E., Zhang, Z.F., Karpeh, M.S., Sun, M. & Kurtz, R.C. (1997) The role of dietary factors in the intestinal and diffuse histologic subtypes of gastric adenocarcinoma: a case–control study in the U.S. *Cancer*, **80**, 1021–1028

Hartman, P.E. & Shankel, D.M. (1990) Antimutagens and anticarcinogens: a survey of putative interceptor molecules. *Environ. Mol. Mutagen.*, **15**, 145–182

Hayashi, T., Schimerlik, M. & Bailey, G. (1999) Mechanisms of chlorophyllin anticarcinogenesis: dose-responsive inhibition of aflatoxin uptake and biodistribution following oral co-administration in rainbow trout. *Toxicol. Appl. Pharmacol.*, **158**, 132–140

Hayes, R.B., Ziegler, R.G., Gridley, G., Swanson, C., Greenberg, R.S., Swanson, G.M., Schoenberg, J.B., Silverman, D.T., Brown, L.M., Pottern, L.M., Liff, J., Schwartz, A.G., Fraumeni, J.F., Jr & Hoover, R.N. (1999) Dietary factors and risks for prostate cancer among blacks and whites in the United States. *Cancer Epidemiol. Biomarkers Prev.*, **8**, 25–34

He, Y., Root, M.M., Parker, R.S. & Campbell, T.C. (1997) Effects of carotenoid-rich food extracts on the development of preneoplastic lesions in rat liver and on in vivo and in vitro antioxidant status. *Nutr. Cancer*, **27**, 238–244

Health Canada (2002) *Canada's Food Guide to Healthy Eating*. Office of Nutrition Policy and Promotion. Available at http://www.hc-sc.gc.ca/hpfb-dgpsa/onpp-bppn/food_guide_rainbow_e.html

Health Department of Western Australia (1990) *Fruit 'n' Veg with Every Meal Campaign Background Information Document*, Perth, Health Promotion Services Branch

Heber, D. & Bowerman, S. (2001) Applying science to changing dietary patterns. *J. Nutr.*, **131**, 3078S–3081S

Hebert, J.R. & Miller, D.R. (1994) A cross-national investigation of diet and bladder cancer. *Eur. J. Cancer*, **30A**, 778–784

Hebert, J.R. & Rosen, A. (1996) Nutritional, socioeconomic, and reproductive factors in relation to female breast cancer mortality: findings from a cross-national study. *Cancer Detect. Prev.*, **20**, 234–244

Hebert, J.R., Landon, J. & Miller, D.R. (1993) Consumption of meat and fruit in relation to oral and esophageal cancer: a cross-national study. *Nutr. Cancer*, **19**, 169–179

Hecht, S.S. (1995) Chemoprevention by isothiocyanates. *J. Cell Biochem.*, **22 Suppl.**, 195–209

Hecht, S.S., Chung, F.L., Richie, J.P., Jr, Akerkar, S.A., Borukhova, A., Skowronski, L. & Carmella, S.G. (1995) Effects of watercress consumption on metabolism of a tobacco-specific lung carcinogen in smokers. *Cancer Epidemiol. Biomarkers Prev.*, **4**, 877–884

Hecht, S.S., Carmella, S.G. & Murphy, S.E. (1999) Effects of watercress consumption on urinary metabolites of nicotine in smokers. *Cancer Epidemiol. Biomarkers Prev.*, **8**, 907–913

Helen, A., Krishnakumar, K., Vijayammal, P.L. & Augusti, K.T. (2000) Antioxidant effect of onion oil (Allium cepa. Linn) on the damages induced by nicotine in rats as compared to alpha-tocopherol. *Toxicol. Lett.*, **116**, 61–68

Helser, M.A., Hotchkiss, J.H. & Roe, D.A. (1992) Influence of fruit and vegetable juices on the endogenous formation of N-nitrosoproline and N-nitrosothiazolidine-4-carboxylic acid in humans on controlled diets. *Carcinogenesis*, **13**, 2277–2280

Hemminki, K., Jiang, Y., Ma, X., Yang, K., Egevad, L. & Lindblad P. (2002) Molecular epidemiology of VHL gene mutations in renal cell carcinoma patients: relation to dietary and other factors. *Carcinogenesis*, **23**, 809–815

Hermann-Kunz, E. & Thamm, M. (1999) Dietary recommendations and prevailing food and nutrient intakes in Germany. *Br. J. Nutr.*, **81 Suppl. 2**, S61–S69

Herrero, R., Potischman, N., Brinton, L.A., Reeves, W.C., Brenes, M.M., Tenorio, F., de Britton, R.C. & Gaitan, E. (1991) A case–control study of nutrient status and invasive cervical cancer. I. Dietary indicators. *Am. J. Epidemiol.*, **134**, 1335–1346

Herrmann, N. (1985) Retrospective information from questionnaires. I. Comparability of primary respondents and their next-of-kin. *Am. J. Epidemiol.*, **121**, 937–947

Hertog, M.G., Hollman, P.C. & Katan, M.B. (1992) Content of potentially anticarcinogenic flavonoids of 28 vegetables and 9 fruits commonly consumed in the Netherlands. *J. Agric. Food Chem.*, **40**, 2379–2383

Hertog, M.G., Feskens, E.J., Hollman, P.C., Katan, M.B. & Kromhout, D. (1993a) Dietary antioxidant flavonoids and risk of coronary heart disease: the Zutphen Elderly Study. *Lancet*, **342**, 1007–1011

Hertog, M.G., Hollman, P.C. & van de Putte, B. (1993b) Content of potentially anticarcinogenic flavonoids of tea infusions, wines, and fruit juices. *J. Agric. Food Chem.*, **41**, 1242–1246

References

Hininger, I., Chopra, M., Thurnham, D.I., Laporte, F., Richard, M.J., Favier, A. & Roussel, A.M. (1997) Effect of increased fruit and vegetable intake on the susceptibility of lipoprotein to oxidation in smokers. *Eur. J. Clin. Nutr.*, **51,** 601–606

Hirayama, T., ed (1990) *Life-style and Mortality. A Large-scale Census-based Cohort Study in Japan*, Vol. 6 (Contributions to Epidemiology and Biostatistics), Basel, Karger

Hirose, K., Tajima, K., Hamajima, N., Inoue, M., Takezaki, T., Kuroishi, T., Yoshida, M. & Tokudome, S. (1995) A large-scale, hospital-based case–control study of risk factors of breast cancer according to menopausal status. *Jpn J. Cancer Res.*, **86**, 146–154

Hirose, K., Tajima, K., Hamajima, N., Takezaki, T., Inoue, M., Kuroishi, T., Kuzuya, K., Nakamura, S. & Tokudome, S. (1996) Subsite (cervix/endometrium)-specific risk and protective factors in uterus cancer. *Jpn J. Cancer Res.*, **87**, 1001–1009

Ho, J. C.-M., Zheng, S., Comhair, S.A., Farver, C. & Erzurum, S.C. (2001) Differential expression of manganese superoxide dismutase and catalase in lung cancer. *Cancer Res.*, **61,** 8578–8585

Holden, J.M., Elridge, A.L., Beecher, G.R., Buzzard, I.M., Bhagwat, S., Davis, C.S., Douglass, L.W., Gebhardt, S., Haytowitz, D. & Schakel, S. (1999) Carotenoid content of US foods: An update of the database. *J. Food Comp. Anal.*, **12**, 169–196

Holick, C.N., Michaud, D.S., Stolzenberg-Solomon, R., Mayne, S.T., Pietinen, P., Taylor, P.R., Virtamo, J. & Albanes, D. (2002) Dietary carotenoids, serum β-carotene, and retinol and risk of lung cancer in the alpha-tocopherol, beta-carotene cohort study. *Am. J. Epidemiol.*, **156**, 536–547

Holmberg, L., Ohlander, E.M., Byers, T., Zack, M., Wolk, A., Bergström, R., Bergkvist, L., Thurfjell, E., Bruce, A. & Adami, H.O. (1994) Diet and breast cancer risk. Results from a population-based, case–control study in Sweden. *Arch. Intern. Med.*, **154**, 1805–1811

Holmberg, L., Ohlander, E.M., Byers, T., Zack, M., Wolk, A., Bruce, A., Bergström, R., Bergkvist, L. & Adami, H.O. (1996) A search for recall bias in a case-control study of diet and breast cancer. *Int. J. Epidemiol.*, **25,** 235–244

Holmqvist, O.H. (1997) Diet and colorectal cancer mortality: secular trends over 30 years in 15 European countries. *Cancer Lett.*, **114**, 247–250

Horner, N.K., Patterson, R.E., Neuhouser, M.L., Lampe, J.W., Beresford, S.A. & Prentice, R.L. (2002) Participant characteristics associated with errors in self-reported energy intake from the Women's Health Initiative food-frequency questionnaire. *Am. J. Clin. Nutr.*, **76,** 766–773

Hoshiyama, Y. & Sasaba, T. (1992) A case–control study of single and multiple stomach cancers in Saitama Prefecture, Japan. *Jpn J. Cancer Res.*, **83**, 937–943

Howard, D.J., Ota, R.B., Briggs, L.A., Hampton, M. & Pritsos, C.A. (1998) Environmental tobacco smoke in the workplace induces oxidative stress in employees, including increased production of 8-hydroxy-2'-deoxyguanosine. *Cancer Epidemiol. Biomarkers Prev.*, **7,** 141–146

Howe, G.R., Jain, M. & Miller, A.B. (1990) Dietary factors and risk of pancreatic cancer: results of a Canadian population-based case–control study. *Int. J. Cancer*, **45**, 604–608

Howe, G.R., Ghadirian, P., Bueno de Mesquita, H.B., Zatonski, W.A., Baghurst, P.A., Miller, A.B., Simard, A., Baillargeon, J., de Waard, F., Przewozniak, K., McMichael, A.J., Jain, M., Hsieh, C.C., Maisonneuve, P., Boyle, P. & Walker, A.M. (1992) A collaborative case–control study of nutrient intake and pancreatic cancer within the SEARCH programme. *Int. J. Cancer*, **51**, 365–372

Hsieh, C.C., Maisonneuve, P., Boyle, P., Macfarlane, G.J. & Roberston, C. (1991) Analysis of quantitative data by quantiles in epidemiologic studies: classification according to cases, noncases, or all subjects? *Epidemiology,* **2,** 137–140

Hsing, A.W., McLaughlin, J.K., Chow, W.H., Schuman, L.M., Co Chien, H.T., Gridley, G., Bjelke, E., Wacholder, S. & Blot, W.J. (1998a) Risk factors for colorectal cancer in a prospective study among U.S. white men. *Int. J. Cancer*, **77**, 549–553

Hsing, A.W., McLaughlin, J.K., Cocco, P., Co Chien, H.T. & Fraumeni, J.F., Jr (1998b) Risk factors for male breast cancer (United States). *Cancer Causes Control*, **9**, 269–275

Hsing, A.W., McLaughlin, J.K., Schuman, L.M., Bjelke, E., Gridley, G., Wacholder, S., Chien, H.T. & Blot, W.J. (1990) Diet, tobacco use, and fatal prostate cancer: results from the Lutheran Brotherhood Cohort Study. *Cancer Res.*, **50**, 6836–6840

Hu, J., Nyren, O., Wolk, A., Bergström, R., Yuen, J., Adami, H.O., Guo, L., Li, H., Huang, G. & Xu, X. (1994) Risk factors for oesophageal cancer in northeast China. *Int. J. Cancer*, **57**, 38–46

Hu, J., Johnson, K.C., Mao, Y., Xu, T., Lin, Q., Wang, C., Zhao, F., Wang, G., Chen, Y. & Yang, Y. (1997) A case–control study of diet and lung cancer in northeast China. *Int. J. Cancer*, **71**, 924–931

Hu, J., Johnson, K.C., Mao, Y., Guo, L., Zha, X., Jia, X., Bi, D., Huang, G. & Liu, R. (1998) Risk factors for glioma in adults: a case–control study in northeast China. *Cancer Detect. Prev.*, **22**, 100–108

Hu, J., La Vecchia, C., Negri, E., Chatenoud, L., Bosetti, C., Jia, X., Liu, R., Huang, G., Bi, D. & Wang, C. (1999) Diet and brain cancer in adults: a case–control study in northeast China. *Int. J. Cancer*, **81**, 20–23

Hu, J.F., Liu, Y.Y., Yu, Y.K., Zhao, T.Z., Liu, S.D. & Wang, Q.Q. (1991) Diet and cancer of the colon and rectum: a case–control study in China. *Int. J. Epidemiol.*, **20**, 362–367

Huang, A.S., Tanudjaja, L. & Lum, D. (1999) Content of alpha, beta-carotene, and dietary fiber in 18 sweetpotato varieties grown in Hawaii. *J. Food Comp. Anal.*, **12,** 147–151

Huang, X.E., Tajima, K., Hamajima, N., Xiang, J., Inoue, M., Hirose, K., Tominaga, S., Takezaki, T., Kuroishi, T. & Tokudome, S. (2000) Comparison of lifestyle and risk factors among Japanese with and without gastric cancer family history. *Int. J. Cancer*, **86**, 421–424

Hughes, R., Pollock, J.R. & Bingham, S. (2002) Effect of vegetables, tea, and soy on endogenous *N*-nitrosation, fecal ammonia, and fecal water genotoxicity during a high red meat diet in humans. *Nutr. Cancer*, **42**, 70–77

Humble, C.G., Samet, J.M. & Skipper, B.E. (1987) Use of quantified and frequency indices of vitamin A intake in a case–control study of lung cancer. *Int. J. Epidemiol.*, **16**, 341–346

Hunter, D. (1998) Biochemical indicators of dietary intake. In: Willett, W., ed., *Nutritional Epidemiology*, New York, Oxford, Oxford University Press, pp. 174–243

Hunter, D.J., Sampson, L., Stampfer, M.J., Colditz, G.A., Rosner, B. & Willett, W.C. (1988) Variability in portion sizes of commonly consumed foods among a population of women in the United States. *Am. J. Epidemiol.*, **127**, 1240–1249

Hussain, S.P., Jannu, L.N. & Rao, A.R. (1990) Chemopreventive action of garlic on methylcholanthrene-induced carcinogenesis in the uterine cervix of mice. *Cancer Lett.*, **49**, 175–180

IARC (1986) *Some Naturally Occurring and Synthetic Food Components, Furocoumarins and Ultraviolet Radiation* (IARC Monographs on the Evaluation of Carcinogenic Risk of Chemicals to Humans, Vol. 40), Lyon, IARCPress

IARC (1993) *Some Naturally Occurring Substances: Food Items and Constituents, Heterocyclic Aromatic Amines and Mycotoxins* (IARC Monographs on the Evaluation of Carcinogenic Risks to Humans, Vol. 56), Lyon, IARCPress

IARC (1998) *Carotenoids* (IARC Handbook of Cancer Prevention, Volume 2), Lyon, IARCPress

Ihaka, R. & Gentleman, R (1996) A language for data analysis and graphics. *J. Comput. Graph. Stat.*, **5**, 299–314

Imai, K., Matsuyama, S., Miyake, S., Suga, K. & Nakachi, K. (2000) Natural cytotoxic activity of peripheral-blood lymphocytes and cancer incidence: an 11-year follow-up study of a general population. *Lancet*, **356**, 1795–1799

INCAP/OPS (2000) *Guías Alimentarias para Guatemala. Los siete pasos para una alimentación sana*, Instituto de Nutrición de Centro América y Panamá. http://www.incap.org.gt/gu%C3%ADas_alimentarias_para_guate.htm

Ingram, D.M., Nottage, E. & Roberts, T. (1991) The role of diet in the development of breast cancer: a case–control study of patients with breast cancer, benign epithelial hyperplasia and fibrocystic disease of the breast. *Br. J. Cancer*, **64**, 187–191

Inoue, M., Tajima, K., Hirose, K., Kuroishi, T., Gao, C.M. & Kitoh, T. (1994) Life-style and subsite of gastric cancer – joint effect of smoking and drinking habits. *Int. J. Cancer*, **56**, 494–499

Inoue, M., Tajima, K., Kobayashi, S., Suzuki, T., Matsuura, A., Nakamura, T., Shirai, M., Nakamura, S., Inuzuka, K. & Tominaga, S. (1996) Protective factor against progression from atrophic gastritis to gastric cancer—data from a cohort study in Japan. *Int. J. Cancer*, **66**, 309–314

Institute of Nutrition and Food Hygiene (2002) *The Dietary and Nutritional Status of Chinese Population – 1992 National Nutrition Survey*, Volume 1, People's Medical Publishing House, pp. 43–113

Instituto Nacional de Estadística (1991) *Household budget survey – Spain 1990–1991. National Study on Nutrition and Food Consumption*, Volume 1, Madrid, Instituto Nacional de Estadística

Ioannidis, J.P.A., Haidich, A.B. & Lau, J. (2001) Any casualties in the clash of randomised and observational evidence? *BMJ*, **322**, 879–880

Ioannidis, J.P., Rosenberg, P.S., Goedert, J.J. & O'Brien, T.R. (2002) Commentary: meta-analysis of individual participants' data in genetic epidemiology. *Am. J. Epidemiol.*, **156**, 204–210

Ip, C. & Lisk, D.J. (1995) Efficacy of cancer prevention by high-selenium garlic is primarily dependent on the action of selenium. *Carcinogenesis*, **16**, 2649–2652

Ip, C. & Lisk, D.J. (1997) Modulation of phase I and phase II xenobiotic-metabolizing enzymes by selenium-enriched garlic in rats. *Nutr. Cancer*, **28**, 184–188

Ip, C., Lisk, D.J. & Stoewsand, G.S. (1992) Mammary cancer prevention by regular garlic and selenium-enriched garlic. *Nutr. Cancer*, **17**, 279–286

Irish Nutrition & Dietetic Institute (1990) *Irish National Nutrition Survey 1990*, Dublin, Fineprint, pp. 81–93

Iscovich, J.M., Iscovich, R.B., Howe, G., Shiboski, S. & Kaldor, J.M. (1989) A case–control study of diet and breast cancer in Argentina. *Int. J. Cancer*, **44**, 770–776

Iscovich, J.M., L'Abbé, K.A., Castelleto, R., Calzona, A., Bernedo, A., Chopita, N.A., Jmelnitzsky, A.C. & Kaldor, J. (1992) Colon cancer in Argentina. I: Risk from intake of dietary items. *Int. J. Cancer*, **51**, 851–857

Ishimoto, H., Nakamura, H. & Miyoshi, T. (1994) Epidemiological study on relationship between breast cancer mortality and dietary factors. *Tokushima J. Exp. Med.*, **41**, 103–114

Ito, Y., Maeda, S. & Sugiyama, T. (1986) Suppression of 7,12-dimethylbenz[a]anthracene-induced chromosome aberrations in rat bone marrow cells by vegetable juices. *Mutat. Res.*, **172**, 55–60

Ito, H., Hamajima, N., Takezaki, T., Matsuo, K., Tajima, K., Hatooka, S., Mitsudomi, T., Suyama, M., Sato, S. & Ueda, R. (2002) A limited association of OGG1 Ser326Cys polymorphism for adenocarcinoma of the lung. *J. Epidemiol.*, **12**, 258–265

Ito, L.S., Inoue, M., Tajima, K., Yamamura, Y., Kodera, Y., Horose, K., Takezaki, T., Hamajima, N., Kuroishi T., Tominaga, S. (2003) Dietary factors and the risk of gastric cancer among

References

Japanese women: a comparison between the differentiated and non-differentiated subtypes. *Ann. Epidemiol.*, **13**, 24–31

Jacobs, L.R. (1986) Relationship between dietary fiber and cancer: metabolic, physiologic, and cellular mechanisms. *Proc. Soc. Exp. Biol. Med.*, **183**, 299–310

Jafarey, N.A., Mahmood, Z. & Zaidi, S.H. (1977) Habits and dietary pattern of cases of carcinoma of the oral cavity and oropharynx. *J. Pak. Med. Assoc.*, **27**, 340–343

Jain, M., Burch, J.D., Howe, G.R., Risch, H.A. & Miller, A.B. (1990) Dietary factors and risk of lung cancer: results from a case–control study, Toronto, 1981–1985. *Int. J. Cancer*, **45**, 287–293

Jain, M.G., Hislop, G.T., Howe, G.R. & Ghadirian, P. (1999) Plant foods, antioxidants, and prostate cancer risk: findings from case–control studies in Canada. *Nutr. Cancer*, **34**, 173–184

Jain, M.G., Howe, G.R. & Rohan, T.E. (2000) Nutritional factors and endometrial cancer in Ontario, Canada. *Cancer Control*, **7**, 288–296

James, E.P., ed. (1988) *Healthy Nutrition: Preventing Nutrition-related Disease in Europe* (European Series), Copenhagen, WHO Regional Office for Europe

Jansen, M.C., Bueno de Mesquita, H.B., Rasanen, L., Fidanza, F., Nissinen, A.M., Menotti, A., Kok, F.J. & Kromhout, D. (2001) Cohort analysis of fruit and vegetable consumption and lung cancer mortality in European men. *Int. J. Cancer*, **92**, 913–918

Järvinen, R., Knekt, P., Seppanen, R. & Teppo, L. (1997) Diet and breast cancer risk in a cohort of Finnish women. *Cancer Lett.*, **114**, 251–253

Jedrychowski, W.A. & Popiela, T. (1986) Gastric cancer in Poland – a decreased malignancy due to changing nutritional habits of the population. *Neoplasma*, **33**, 97–106

Jedrychowski, W., Wahrendorf, J., Popiela, T. & Rachtan, J. (1986) A case–control study of dietary factors and stomach cancer risk in Poland. *Int. J. Cancer*, **37**, 837–842

Jedrychowski, W., Boeing, H., Popiela, T., Wahrendorf, J., Tobiasz-Adamczyk, B. & Kulig, J. (1992) Dietary practices in households as risk factors for stomach cancer: a familial study in Poland. *Eur. J. Cancer Prev.*, **1**, 297–304

Jenkins, D.J., Kendall, C.W., Popovich, D.G., Vidgen, E., Mehling, C.C., Vuksan, V., Ransom, T.P., Rao, A.V., Rosenberg-Zand, R., Tariq, N., Corey, P., Jones, P.J., Raeini, M., Story, J.A., Furumoto, E.J., Illingworth, D.R., Pappu, A.S. & Connelly, P.W. (2001) Effect of a very-high-fiber vegetable, fruit, and nut diet on serum lipids and colonic function. *Metabolism*, **50**, 494–503

Ji, B.T., Chow, W.H., Gridley, G., McLaughlin, J.K., Dai, Q., Wacholder, S., Hatch, M.C., Gao, Y.T. & Fraumeni, J.F., Jr (1995) Dietary factors and the risk of pancreatic cancer: A case–control study in Shanghai China. *Cancer Epidemiol. Biomarkers Prev.*, **4**, 885–893

Ji, B.T., Chow, W.H., Yang, G., McLaughlin, J.K., Zheng, W., Shu, X.O., Jin, F., Gao, R.N., Gao, Y.T. & Fraumeni, J.F., Jr (1998) Dietary habits and stomach cancer in Shanghai, China. *Int. J. Cancer*, **76**, 659–664

Jiao, H. & Wang, S.Y. (2000) Correlation of antioxidant capacities to oxygen radical scavenging enzyme activities in blackberry. *J. Agric. Food Chem.*, **48**, 5672–5676

Johansson, L. & Sovoll, K. (1999) *Norkost 1997 – Landsomfattende Kostholdsundersøkelse blant menn og kvinner i alderen 16–79 ar*, Oslo, Statens råd for ernaering og fysisk aktivitet

John, J.H., Ziebland, S., Yudkin, P., Roe, L.S. & Neil, H.A. (2002) Effects of fruit and vegetable consumption on plasma antioxidant concentrations and blood pressure: a randomised controlled trial. *Lancet*, **359**, 1969–1974

Johnson, K.C., Pan, S., Mao, Y. & Canadian Cancer Registries Epidemiology Research Group (2002) Risk factors for male breast cancer in Canada, 1994-1998. *Eur J Cancer Prev.*, **11**, 253–263

Joseph, J.A., Nadeau, D.A. & Underwood, A., eds (2002) *The Color Code. A Revolutionary Eating Plan for Optimum Health,* New York, Hyperion

Joshipura, K.J., Ascherio, A., Manson, J.E., Stampfer, M.J., Rimm, E.B., Speizer, F.E., Hennekens, C.H., Spiegelman, D. & Willett, W.C. (1999) Fruit and vegetable intake in relation to risk of ischemic stroke. *JAMA*, **282**, 1233–1239

Joshipura, K.J., Hu, F.B., Manson, J.E., Stampfer, M.J., Rimm, E.B., Speizer, F.E., Colditz, G., Ascherio, A., Rosner, B., Spiegelman, D. & Willett, W.C. (2001) The effect of fruit and vegetable intake on risk for coronary heart disease. *Ann. Intern. Med.*, **134**, 1106–1114

Kaaks, R., Riboli, E., Estève, J., van Kappel, A.L. & van Staveren, W.A. (1994a) Estimating the accuracy of dietary questionnaire assessments: validation in terms of structural equation models. *Stat. Med.*, **13**, 127–142

Kaaks, R., Plummer, M., Riboli, E., Estève, J. & van Staveren, W. (1994b) Adjustment for bias due to errors in exposure assessments in multicenter cohort studies on diet and cancer: a calibration approach. *Am. J. Clin. Nutr.*, **59**, 245S–250S

Kaaks, R., Riboli, E. & van Staveren, W. (1995) Calibration of dietary intake measurements in prospective cohort studies. *Am. J. Epidemiol.*, **142**, 548–556

Kaaks, R., Riboli, E. & Sinha, R. (1997a) Biochemical markers of dietary intake. In: Toniolo, P., Boffetta, P., Shuker, D.E.G., Rothman, N., Hulka, B. & Pearce, N., eds, *Application of Biomarkers in Cancer Epidemiology* (IARC Scientific Publications No. 142), Lyon, IARCPress, pp. 103–126

Kaaks, R., Slimani, N. & Riboli, E. (1997b) Pilot phase studies on the accuracy of dietary intake measurements in the EPIC project: overall evaluation of results. European Prospective Investigation into Cancer and Nutrition. *Int. J. Epidemiol.*, **26 Suppl. 1**, S26-S36

Kaaks, R., Ferrari, P., Ciampi, A., Plummer, M. & Riboli, E. (2002) Uses and limitations of statistical accounting for random error correlations, in the validation of dietary questionnaire assessments. *Public Health Nutr.*, **5**, 969–976

Kafatos, A.G. & Codrington, C.A. (2003) Eurodiet Reports and Proceedings (Special issue). *Public Health Nutr.*, **4**, 265–436

Kalandidi, A., Katsouyanni, K., Voropoulou, N., Bastas, G., Saracci, R. & Trichopoulos, D. (1990) Passive smoking and diet in the etiology of lung cancer among non-smokers. *Cancer Causes Control*, **1**, 15–21

Kall, M.A., Vang, O. & Clausen, J. (1996) Effects of dietary broccoli on human *in vivo* drug metabolizing enzymes: evaluation of caffeine, oestrone and chlorzoxazone metabolism. *Carcinogenesis*, **17**, 793–799

Kampman, E., Verhoeven, D., Sloots, L. & van't Veer, P. (1995) Vegetable and animal products as determinants of colon cancer risk in Dutch men and women. *Cancer Causes Control*, **6**, 225–234

Kandil, O., Abdullah, T., Tabuni, A.M. & Elkadi, A. (1988) Potential role of *Allium sativum* in natural cytotoxicity. *Arch. AIDS Res.*, **1**, 230–231

Karamanos, B., Thanopoulou, A., Angelico, F., Assaad-Khalil, S., Barbato, A., Del Ben, M., Dimitrijevic-Sreckovic, V., Djordjevic, P., Gallotti, C., Katsilambros, N., Migdalis, I., Mrabet, M., Petkova, M., Roussi, D. & Tenconi, M.T. (2002) Nutritional habits in the Mediterranean basin. The macronutrient composition of diet and its relation with the traditional Mediterranean diet. Multicentre study of the Mediterranean Group for the Study of Diabetes (MGSD). *Eur. J. Clin. Nutr.*, **56**, 983–991

Kasai, H., Crain, P.F., Kuchino, Y., Nishimura, S., Ootsuyama, A. & Tanooka, H. (1986) Formation of 8-hydroxyguanine moiety in cellular DNA by agents producing oxygen radicals and evidence for its repair. *Carcinogenesis*, **7**, 1849–1851

Kassie, F., Rabot, S., Uhl, M., Huber, W., Qin, H.M., Helma, C., Schulte-Hermann, R. & Knasmuller, S. (2002) Chemoprotective effects of garden cress (Lepidium sativum) and its constituents towards 2-amino-3-methyl-imidazo[4,5-f]quinoline (IQ)-induced genotoxic effects and colonic preneoplastic lesions. *Carcinogenesis*, **23**, 1155–1161

Kasum, C.M., Jacobs, D.R., Jr, Nicodemus, K. & Folsom, A.R. (2002) Dietary risk factors for upper aerodigestive tract cancers. *Int. J. Cancer*, **99**, 267–272

Kato, K., Akai, S., Tominaga, S. & Kato, I. (1989) A case–control study of biliary tract cancer in Niigata Prefecture, Japan. *Jpn J. Cancer Res.*, **80**, 932–938

Kato, I., Tominaga, S., Ito, Y., Kobayashi, S., Yoshii, Y., Matsuura, A., Kameya, A. & Kano, T. (1990) A comparative case–control analysis of stomach cancer and atrophic gastritis. *Cancer Res.*, **50**, 6559–6564

Kato, I., Tominaga, S. & Matsumoto, K. (1992) A prospective study of stomach cancer among a rural Japanese population: a 6-year survey. *Jpn J. Cancer Res.*, **83**, 568–575

Kato, I., Akhmedkhanov, A., Koenig, K., Toniolo, P.G., Shore, R.E. & Riboli, E. (1997) Prospective study of diet and female colorectal cancer: the New York University Women's Health Study. *Nutr. Cancer*, **28**, 276–281

Katsouyanni, K., Trichopoulos, D., Boyle, P., Xirouchaki, E., Trichopoulou, A., Lisseos, B., Vasilaros, S. & MacMahon, B. (1986) Diet and breast cancer: a case–control study in Greece. *Int. J. Cancer*, **38**, 815–820

Kay, C.D. & Holub, B.J. (2002) The effect of wild blueberry (*Vaccinium angustifolium*) consumption on postprandial serum antioxidant status in human subjects. *Br. J. Nutr.*, **88**, 389–398

Kelloff, G.J., Sigman, C.C., Johnson, K.M., Boone, C.W., Greenwald, P., Crowell, J.A., Hawk, E.T. & Doody, L.A. (2000) Perspectives on surrogate end points in the development of drugs that reduce the risk of cancer. *Cancer Epidemiol. Biomarkers Prev.*, **9**, 127–137

Key, T.J., Thorogood, M., Appleby, P.N. & Burr, M.L. (1996) Dietary habits and mortality in 11,000 vegetarians and health conscious people: results of a 17 year follow up. *BMJ*, **313**, 775–779

Key, T.J., Silcocks, P.B., Davey, G.K., Appleby, P.N. & Bishop, D.T. (1997) A case–control study of diet and prostate cancer. *Br. J. Cancer*, **76**, 678–687

Key, T., Allen, N., Appleby, P., Overvad, K., Tjønneland, A., Miller, A., Boeing, H., Karalis, D., Psaltopoulou, T., Berrino, F., Palli, D., Panico, S., Tumino, R., Vineis, P., Bueno de Mesquita, B., Kiemeney, L., Peeters, P., Martinez, C., Dorronsoro, M., González, C.A., Chirlaque, M.D., Ramon Quiros, J., Ardanaz, E., Berglund, G., Egevad, L., Hallmans, G., Stattin, P., Day, N., Gann, P., Kaaks, R., Ferrari, P. & Riboli, E. (2003) Fruit and vegetables and prostate cancer: no association among 1,104 cases in a prospective study of 130,544 men in the European Prospective Investigation into Cancer and Nutrition (EPIC). *Int. J. Cancer* (in press)

Keys, A., ed. (1980) *Seven Countries. A Multivariate Analysis of Death and Coronary Heart Disease*, London, Harvard University Press

Keys, A. (1983) From Naples to seven countries – a sentimental journey. *Prog. Biochem. Pharmacol.*, **19**, 1–30

Khoury, M.J., James, L.M. & Erickson, J.D. (1994) On the use of affected controls to address recall bias in case-control studies of birth defects. *Teratology*, **49**, 273–281

Kim, H.J., Chang, W.K., Kim, M.K., Lee, S.S. & Choi, B.Y. (2002) Dietary factors and gastric cancer in Korea: a case–control study. *Int. J. Cancer*, **97**, 531–535

Kipnis, V., Freedman, L.S., Brown, C.C., Hartman, A.M., Schatzkin, A. & Wacholder, S. (1997) Effect of measurement error on energy-adjustment models in nutritional epidemiology. *Am. J. Epidemiol.*, **146**, 842–855

Kipnis, V., Carroll, R.J., Freedman, L.S. & Li, L. (1999) Implications of a new dietary measurement error model for estimation of relative risk: application to four calibration studies. *Am. J. Epidemiol.*, **150**, 642–651

Kipnis, V., Midthune, D., Freedman, L.S., Bingham, S., Schatzkin, A., Subar, A. & Carroll, R.J. (2001) Empirical evidence of correlated biases in dietary assessment instruments and its implications. *Am. J. Epidemiol.*, **153**, 394–403

Kipnis, V., Subar, A.F., Midthune, D., Freedman, L.S., Ballard-Barbash, R., Troiano, R., Bingham, S., Schoeller, D.A., Schatzkin, A. & Carroll, R.J. (2003) The structure of dietary measurement error: Results of the OPEN biomarker study. *Am.J.Epidemiol.* **158**, 14–21

Kjaerheim, K., Gaard, M. & Andersen, A. (1998) The role of alcohol, tobacco, and dietary factors in upper aerogastric tract cancers: a prospective study of 10,900 Norwegian men. *Cancer Causes Control*, **9**, 99–108

Knekt, P., Reunanen, A., Järvinen, R., Seppänen, R., Heliövaara, M. & Aromaa, A. (1994) Antioxidant vitamin intake and coronary mortality in a longitudinal population study. *Am. J. Epidemiol.*, **139**, 1180–1189

Knekt, P., Järvinen, R., Reunanen, A. & Maatela, J. (1996) Flavonoid intake and coronary mortality in Finland: a cohort study. *BMJ*, **312**, 478–481

Kneller, R.W., McLaughlin, J.K., Bjelke, E., Schuman, L.M., Blot, W.J., Wacholder, S., Gridley, G., CoChien, H.T. & Fraumeni, J.F., Jr (1991) A cohort study of stomach cancer in a high-risk American population. *Cancer*, **68**, 672–678

Knight, T.M. & Forman, D. (1987) The availability of dietary nitrate for the endogenous nitrosation of L-proline. In: Bartsch, H., O'Neill, I. & Sculte-Hermann, R., eds, *The Relevance of N-Nitroso Compounds to Human Cancer: Exposure and Mechanisms* (IARC Scientific Publications No. 84), Lyon, IARC, pp. 518–523

Knize, M., Kulp, K., Salmon, C., Keating, G. & Felton, J. (2002) Factors affecting human heterocyclic amine intake and the metabolism of PhIP. *Mutat. Res.*, **506–507**, 153–162

Ko, Y.C., Lee, C.H., Chen, M.J., Huang, C.C., Chang, W.Y., Lin, H.J., Wang, H.Z. & Chang, P.Y. (1997) Risk factors for primary lung cancer among non-smoking women in Taiwan. *Int. J. Epidemiol.*, **26**, 24–31

Kobayashi, M., Tsubono, Y., Sasazuki, S., Sasaki, S. & Tsugane, S. (2002) Vegetables, fruit and risk of gastric cancer in Japan: A 10-year follow-up of the JPHC study Cohort I. *Int. J. Cancer*, **102**, 39–44

Kohno, H., Taima, M., Sumida, T., Azuma, Y., Ogawa, H. & Tanaka, T. (2001) Inhibitory effect of mandarin juice rich in beta-cryptoxanthin and hesperidin on 4-(methylnitrosamino)-1-(3-pyridyl)-1-butanone-induced pulmonary tumorigenesis in mice. *Cancer Lett.*, **174**, 141–150

Kolonel, L.N., Hankin, J.H., Whittemore, A.S., Wu, A.H., Gallagher, R.P., Wilkens, L.R., John, E.M., Howe, G.R., Dreon, D.M., West, D.W. & Paffenbarger, R.S., Jr (2000) Vegetables, fruits, legumes and prostate cancer: a multiethnic case–control study. *Cancer Epidemiol. Biomarkers Prev.*, **9**, 795–804

Kong, A.N., Owuor, E., Yu, R., Hebbar, V., Chen, C., Hu, R. & Mandlekar, S. (2001) Induction of xenobiotic enzymes by the MAP kinase pathway and the antioxidant or electrophile response element (ARE/EpRE). *Drug Metab. Rev.*, **33**, 255–271

Kono, S., Ikeda, M., Tokudome, S. & Kuratsune, M. (1988) A case–control study of gastric cancer and diet in northern Kyushu, Japan. *Jpn J. Cancer Res.*, **79**, 1067–1074

Koo, L.C. (1988) Dietary habits and lung cancer risk among Chinese females in Hong Kong who never smoked. *Nutr. Cancer*, **11**, 155–172

Kornitzer, M. & Bara, L. for the B.I.R.N.H. Study Group (1989) Clinical and anthropometric data, blood chemistry and nutritional patterns in the Belgian population according to age and sex. *Acta Cardiol.*, **44**, 101–144

Kossoy, G., Ben Hur, H., Stark, A., Zusman, I. & Madar, Z. (2001) Effects of a 15% orange-pulp diet on tumorigenesis and immune response in rats with colon tumors. *Oncol. Rep.*, **8**, 1387–1391

Kotake, K., Koyama, Y., Nasu, J., Fukutomi, T. & Yamaguchi, N. (1995) Relation of family history of cancer and environmental factors to the risk of colorectal cancer: a case–control study. *Jpn J. Clin. Oncol.*, **25**, 195–202

Krebs-Smith, S.M. & Kantor, L.S. (2001) Choose a variety of fruits and vegetables daily: understanding the complexities. *J. Nutr.*, **131**, 487S–501S

Krebs-Smith, S.M., Cook, A., Subar, A.F., Cleveland, L. & Friday, J. (1995) US adults' fruit and vegetable intakes, 1989 to 1991: a revised baseline for the Healthy People 2000 objective. *Am. J. Public Health*, **85**, 1623–1629

Kresty, L.A., Morse, M.A., Morgan, C., Carlton, P.S., Lu, J., Gupta, A., Blackwood, M. & Stoner, G.D. (2001) Chemoprevention of esophageal tumorigenesis by dietary administration of lyophilized black raspberries. *Cancer Res.*, **61**, 6112–6119

Kreuzer, M., Heinrich, J., Kreienbrock, L., Rosario, A.S., Gerken, M. & Wichmann, H.E. (2002) Risk factors for lung cancer among nonsmoking women. *Int. J. Cancer*, **100**, 706–713

Kristal, A.R., Vizenor, N.C., Patterson, R.E., Neuhouser, M.L., Shattuck, A.L. & McLerran, D. (2000) Precision and bias of food frequency-based measures of fruit and vegetable intakes. *Cancer Epidemiol. Biomarkers Prev.*, **9**, 939–944

Kubena, K.S. & McMurray, D.N. (1996) Nutrition and the immune system: a review of nutrient-nutrient interactions. *J. Am. Diet. Assoc.*, **96**, 1156–1164

Kubik, A., Zatloukal, P., Tomasek, L., Kriz, J., Petruzelka, L. & Plesko, I. (2001) Diet and the risk of lung cancer among women. A hospital-based case–control study. *Neoplasma*, **48**, 262–266

Kune, S., Kune, G.A. & Watson, L.F. (1987) Case–control study of dietary etiological factors: the Melbourne Colorectal Cancer Study. *Nutr. Cancer*, **9**, 21–42

Kune, G.A., Kune, S., Field, B., Watson, L.F., Cleland, H., Merenstein, D. & Vitetta, L. (1993) Oral and pharyngeal cancer, diet, smoking, alcohol, and serum vitamin A and beta-carotene levels: a case–control study in men. *Nutr. Cancer*, **20**, 61–70

Kuper, H., Tzonou, A., Lagiou, P., Mucci, L.A., Trichopoulos, D., Stuver, S.O. & Trichopoulou, A. (2000) Diet and hepatocellular carcinoma: a case–control study in Greece. *Nutr. Cancer*, **38**, 6–12

Kusamran, W.R., Tepsuwan, A. & Kupradinun, P. (1998a) Antimutagenic and anticarcinogenic potentials of some Thai vegetables. *Mutat. Res.*, **402**, 247–258

Kusamran, W.R., Ratanavila, A. & Tepsuwan, A. (1998b) Effects of neem flowers, Thai and Chinese bitter gourd fruits and sweet basil leaves on hepatic monooxygenases and glutathione S-transferase activities, and in vitro metabolic activation of chemical carcinogens in rats. *Food Chem. Toxicol.*, **36**, 475–484

Kushi, L.H., Sellers, T.A., Potter, J.D., Nelson, C.L., Munger, R.G., Kaye, S.A. & Folsom, A.R. (1992) Dietary fat and postmenopausal breast cancer. *J. Natl. Cancer Inst.*, **84,** 1092–1099

Kushi, L.H., Folsom, A.R., Prineas, R.J., Mink, P.J., Wu, Y. & Bostick, R.M. (1996) Dietary antioxidant vitamins and death from coronary heart disease in postmenopausal women. *New Engl. J. Med.*, **334,** 1156–1162

Kushi, L.H., Mink, P.J., Folsom, A.R., Anderson, K.E., Zheng, W., Lazovich, D. & Sellers, T.A. (1999) Prospective study of diet and ovarian cancer. *Am. J. Epidemiol.*, **149**, 21–31

Kuskowska-Wolk, A., Holte, S., Ohlander, E.M., Bruce, A., Holmberg, L., Adami, H.O. & Bergström, R. (1992) Effects of different designs and extension of a food frequency questionnaire on response rate, completeness of data and food frequency responses. *Int. J. Epidemiol.*, **21**, 1144–1150

Kvale, G., Bjelke, E. & Gart, J.J. (1983) Dietary habits and lung cancer risk. *Int. J. Cancer*, **31**, 397–405

Kwak, M.K., Kim, S.G. & Kim, N.D. (1995) Effects of garlic oil on rat hepatic P4502E1 expression. *Xenobiotica*, **25,** 1021–1029

La Vecchia, C., Decarli, A., Fasoli, M. & Gentile, A. (1986) Nutrition and diet in the etiology of endometrial cancer. *Cancer*, **57**, 1248–1253

La Vecchia, C., Decarli, A., Negri, E., Parazzini, F., Gentile, A., Cecchetti, G., Fasoli, M. & Franceschi, S. (1987a) Dietary factors and the risk of epithelial ovarian cancer. *J. Natl Cancer Inst.*, **79**, 663–669

La Vecchia, C., Negri, E., Decarli, A., D'Avanzo, B. & Franceschi, S. (1987b) A case–control study of diet and gastric cancer in northern Italy. *Int. J. Cancer*, **40**, 484–489

La Vecchia, C., Decarli, A., Fasoli, M., Parazzini, F., Franceschi, S., Gentile, A. & Negri, E. (1988a) Dietary vitamin A and the risk of intraepithelial and invasive cervical neoplasia. *Gynecol. Oncol.*, **30**, 187–195

La Vecchia, C., Negri, E., Decarli, A., D'Avanzo, B. & Franceschi, S. (1988b) Risk factors for hepatocellular carcinoma in northern Italy. *Int. J. Cancer*, **42**, 872–876

La Vecchia, C., Negri, E., Decarli, A., D'Avanzo, B., Gallotti, L., Gentile, A. & Franceschi, S. (1988c) A case–control study of diet and colorectal cancer in northern Italy. *Int. J. Cancer*, **41**, 492–498

La Vecchia, C., Negri, E., D'Avanzo, B., Ferraroni, M., Gramenzi, A., Savoldelli, R., Boyle, P. & Franceschi, S. (1990a) Medical history, diet and pancreatic cancer. *Oncology*, **47**, 463–466

La Vecchia, C., Negri, E., D'Avanzo, B., Franceschi, S., Decarli, A. & Boyle, P. (1990b) Dietary indicators of laryngeal cancer risk. *Cancer Res.*, **50**, 4497–4500

La Vecchia, C., Negri, E., D'Avanzo, B., Boyle, P. & Franceschi, S. (1991) Dietary indicators of oral and pharyngeal cancer. *Int. J. Epidemiol.*, **20**, 39–44

La Vecchia, C., Munoz, S.E., Braga, C., Fernandez, E. & Decarli, A. (1997) Diet diversity and gastric cancer. *Int. J. Cancer*, **72**, 255–257

La Vecchia, C., Braga, C., Franceschi, S., Dal Maso, L. & Negri E. (1999) Population-attributable risk for colon cancer in Italy. *Nutr. Cancer,* **33**, 196–200

Lampe, J.W. (1999) Health effects of vegetables and fruit: assessing mechanisms of action in human experimental studies. *Am. J. Clin. Nutr.*, **70,** 475S–490S

Lam, K.C., Yu, M.C., Leung, J.W. & Henderson, B.E. (1982) Hepatitis B virus and cigarette smoking: risk factors for hepatocellular carcinoma in Hong Kong. *Cancer Res.*, **42**, 5246–5248

Lampe, J.W., Slavin, J.L., Melcher, E.A. & Potter, J.D. (1992) Effects of cereal and vegetable fiber feeding on potential risk factors for colon cancer. *Cancer Epidemiol. Biomarkers Prev.*, **1**, 207–211

Lampe, J.W., Chen, C., Li, S., Prunty, J., Grate, M.T., Meehan, D.E., Barale, K.V., Dightman, D.A., Feng, Z. & Potter, J.D. (2000a) Modulation of human glutathione S-transferases by botanically defined vegetable diets. *Cancer Epidemiol. Biomarkers Prev.*, **9,** 787–793

Lampe, J.W., King, I.B., Li, S., Grate, M.T., Barale, K.V., Chen, C., Feng, Z. & Potter, J.D. (2000b) Brassica vegetables increase and apiaceous vegetables decrease cytochrome P450 1A2 activity in humans: changes in caffeine metabolite ratios in response to controlled vegetable diets. *Carcinogenesis*, **21**, 1157–1162

Landa, M.C., Frago, N. & Tres, A. (1994) Diet and the risk of breast cancer in Spain. *Eur. J. Cancer Prev.*, **3**, 313–320

Landi, M.T., Sinha, R., Lang, N.P. & Kadlubar, F.F. (1999) Human cytochrome P4501A2. In: Vineis, P., Malats, N., Lang, M., d'Errico,A., Caporaso, N., Cuzick, J. & Boffetta, P., eds, *Metabolic Polymorphisms and Susceptibility to Cancer,* (IARC Scientific Publications No. 148), Lyon, IARCPress, pp. 173–195

Lapidus, L., Andersson, H., Bengtsson, C. & Bosaeus, I. (1986) Dietary habits in relation to incidence of cardiovascular disease and death in women: a 12-year follow-up of participants in the population study of women in Gothenburg, Sweden. *Am. J. Clin. Nutr.,* **44,** 444–448

Lau, B.H. (2001) Suppression of LDL oxidation by garlic. *J. Nutr.,* **131,** 985S–988S

Launoy, G., Milan, C., Day, N.E., Pienkowski, M.P., Gignoux, M. & Faivre, J. (1998) Diet and squamous-cell cancer of the oesophagus: a French multicentre case–control study. *Int. J. Cancer,* **76,** 7–12

Le Marchand, L., Yoshizawa, C.N., Kolonel, L.N., Hankin, J.H. & Goodman, M.T. (1989) Vegetable consumption and lung cancer risk: a population-based case–control study in Hawaii. *J. Natl Cancer Inst.,* **81,** 1158–1164

Le Marchand, L., Kolonel, L.N., Wilkens, L.R., Myers, B.C. & Hirohata, T. (1994) Animal fat consumption and prostate cancer: a prospective study in Hawaii. *Epidemiology,* **5,** 276–282

Le Marchand, L., Hankin, J.H., Bach, F., Kolonel, L.N., Wilkens, L.R., Stacewicz-Sapuntzakis, M., Bowen, P.E., Beecher, G.R., Laudon, F., Baqué, P., Daniel, R., Seruvatu, L. & Henderson, B.E. (1995) An ecological study of diet and lung cancer in the South Pacific. *Int. J. Cancer,* **63,** 18–23

Lean, M.E., Noroozi, M., Kelly, I., Burns, J., Talwar, D., Sattar, N. & Crozier, A. (1999) Dietary flavonols protect diabetic human lymphocytes against oxidative damage to DNA. *Diabetes,* **48,** 176–181

Leclercq, I., Desager, J.P. & Horsmans, Y. (1998) Inhibition of chlorzoxazone metabolism, a clinical probe for CYP2E1, by a single ingestion of watercress. *Clin. Pharmacol. Ther.,* **64,** 144–149

Lee, H.P., Gourley, L., Duffy, S.W., Estève, J., Lee, J. & Day, N.E. (1989) Colorectal cancer and diet in an Asian population—a case–control study among Singapore Chinese. *Int. J. Cancer,* **43,** 1007–1016

Lee, H.H., Wu, H.Y., Chuang, Y.C., Chang, A.S., Chao, H.H., Chen, K.Y., Chen, H.K., Lai, G.M., Huang, H.H. & Chen, C.J. (1990) Epidemiologic characteristics and multiple risk factors of stomach cancer in Taiwan. *Anticancer Res.,* **10,** 875–881

Lee, S.W., Jang, I.J., Shin, S.G., Lee, K.H., Yim, D.S., Kim, S.W., Oh, S.J. & Lee, S.H. (1994) CYP1A2 activity as a risk factor for bladder cancer. *J. Korean Med. Sci.,* **9,** 482–489

Lee, J.-K., Park, B.-J., Yoo, K.-Y. & Ahn, Y.-O. (1995) Dietary factors and stomach cancer: a case–control study in Korea. *Int. J. Epidemiol.,* **24,** 33–41

Lee, S.K., Sobal, J. & Frongillo, E.A., Jr (1999) Acculturation and dietary practices among Korean Americans. *J. Am. Diet. Assoc.,* **99,** 1084–1089

Lee, A., Thurnham, D.I. & Chopra, M. (2000) Consumption of tomato products with olive oil but not sunflower oil increases the antioxidant activity of plasma. *Free Radic. Biol. Med.,* **29,** 1051–1055

Lei, Y.X., Cai, W.C., Chen, Y.Z. & Du, Y.X. (1996) Some lifestyle factors in human lung cancer: a case–control study of 792 lung cancer cases. *Lung Cancer,* **14,** S121–S136

Leighton, F., Cuevas, A., Guasch, V., Perez, D.D., Strobel, P., San Martin, A., Urzua, U., Diez, M.S., Foncea, R., Castillo, O., Mizon, C., Espinoza, M.A., Urquiaga, I., Rozowski, J., Maiz, A. & Germain, A. (1999) Plasma polyphenols and antioxidants, oxidative DNA damage and endothelial function in a diet and wine intervention study in humans. *Drugs Exp. Clin. Res.,* **25,** 133–141

Leuratti, C., Watson, M.A., Deag, E.J., Welch, A., Singh, R., Gottschalg, E., Marnett, L.J., Atkin, W., Day, N.E., Shuker, D.E. & Bingham, S.A. (2002) Detection of malondialdehyde DNA adducts in human colorectal mucosa: relationship with diet and the presence of adenomas. *Cancer Epidemiol. Biomarkers Prev.,* **11,** 267–273

Levi, F., Franceschi, S., Negri, E. & La Vecchia, C. (1993a) Dietary factors and the risk of endometrial cancer. *Cancer,* **71,** 3575–3581

Levi, F., La Vecchia, C., Gulie, C. & Negri, E. (1993b) Dietary factors and breast cancer risk in Vaud, Switzerland. *Nutr. Cancer,* **19,** 327–335

Levi, F., Pasche, C., La Vecchia, C., Lucchini, F., Franceschi, S. & Monnier, P. (1998) Food groups and risk of oral and pharyngeal cancer. *Int. J. Cancer,* **77,** 705–709

Levi, F., Pasche, C., La Vecchia, C., Lucchini, F. & Franceschi, S. (1999) Food groups and colorectal cancer risk. *Br. J. Cancer,* **79,** 1283–1287

Levi, F., Pasche, C., Lucchini, F., Bosetti, C., Franceschi, S., Monnier, P. & La Vecchia, C. (2000) Food groups and oesophageal cancer risk in Vaud, Switzerland. *Eur. J. Cancer Prev.,* **9,** 257–263

Li, J.Y., Ershow, A.G., Chen, Z.J., Wacholder, S., Li, G.Y., Guo, W., Li, B. & Blot, W.J. (1989) A case–control study of cancer of the esophagus and gastric cardia in Linxian. *Int. J. Cancer,* **43,** 755–761

Li, D., Wang, M., Cheng, L., Spitz, M.R., Hittelman, W.N. & Wei, Q. (1996) In vitro induction of benzo(a)pyrene diol epoxide-DNA adducts in peripheral lymphocytes as a susceptibility marker for human lung cancer. *Cancer Res.,* **56,** 3638–3641

Li, D., Walcott, F.L., Chang, P., Zhang, W., Zhu, J., Petrulis, E., Singletary, S.E., Sahin, A.A. & Bondy, M.L. (2002) Genetic and environmental determinants on tissue response to *in vitro* carcinogen exposure and risk of breast cancer. *Cancer Res.,* **62,** 4566–4570

Lin, X.Y., Liu, J.Z. & Milner, J.A. (1994) Dietary garlic suppresses DNA adducts caused by N-nitroso compounds. *Carcinogenesis,* **15,** 349–352

Lindblad, P., Wolk, A., Bergström, R. & Adami, H.O. (1997) Diet and risk of renal cell cancer: a population-based case–control study. *Cancer Epidemiol. Biomarkers Prev.*, **6**, 215–223

Lindqvist, R., Lendahls, L., Tollbom, O., Aberg, H. & Hakansson, A. (2002) Smoking during pregnancy: comparison of self-reports and cotinine levels in 496 women. *Acta Obstet. Gynecol. Scand.*, **81**, 240–244

Lindsted, K.D. & Kuzma, J.W. (1990) Reliability of eight-year diet recall in cancer cases and controls. *Epidemiology*, **1**, 392–401

Lindsted, K.D. & Kuzma, J.W. (1989) Long-term (24-year) recall reliability in cancer cases and controls using a 21-item food frequency questionnaire. *Nutr. Cancer*, **12**, 135–149

Lindström, J., Eriksson, J.G., Valle, T.T., Aunola, S., Cepaitis, Z., Hakumaki, M., Hamalainen, H., Ilanne-Parikka, P., Keinanen-Kiukaanniemi, S., Laakso, M., Louheranta, A., Mannelin, M., Martikkala, V., Moltchanov, V., Rastas, M., Salminen, V., Sundvall, J., Uusitupa, M. & Tuomilehto, J. (2003) Prevention of diabetes mellitus in subjects with impaired glucose tolerance in the Finnish diabetes prevention study: results from a randomized clinical trial. *J. Am. Soc. Nephrol.*, **14 Suppl. 2**, S108–S113

Lissowska, J., Pilarska, A., Pilarski, P., Samolczyk-Wanyura, D., Piekarczyk, J., Bardin-Mikollajczak, A., Zatonski, W., Herrero, R., Muñoz, N. & Franceschi, S. (2003) Smoking, alcohol, diet, dentition and sexual practices in the epidemiology of oral cancer in Poland. *Eur. J. Cancer Prev.*, **12**, 25–33

Littman, A.J., Beresford, S.A. & White, E. (2001) The association of dietary fat and plant foods with endometrial cancer (United States). *Cancer Causes Control*, **12**, 691–702

Liu, J., Lin, R.I. & Milner, J.A. (1992) Inhibition of 7,12-dimethylbenz[a]anthracene-induced mammary tumors and DNA adducts by garlic powder. *Carcinogenesis*, **13**, 1847–1851

Liu, S., Manson, J.E., Lee, I.M., Cole, S.R., Hennekens,C.H., Willett, W.C. & Buring, J.E. (2000) Fruit and vegetable intake and risk of cardiovascular disease: The Women's Health Study. *Am. J. Clin. Nutr.*, **72**, 922–928

Liu, S., Lee, I.M., Ajani, U., Cole, S.R., Buring, J.E. & Manson, J.E. (2001) Intake of vegetables rich in carotenoids and risk of coronary heart disease in men: the Physicians' Health Study. *Int. J. Epidemiol.*, **30**, 130–135

Livingstone, M.B. & Black, A.E. (2003) Markers of the validity of reported energy intake. *J. Nutr.*, **133**, 895S–920S

Livingstone, M.B., Prentice, A.M., Strain, J.J., Coward, W.A., Black, A.E., Barker, M.E., McKenna, P.G. & Whitehead, R.G. (1990) Accuracy of weighed dietary records in studies of diet and health. *BMJ*, **300**, 708–712

Loft, S., Vistisen, K., Ewertz, M., Tjonneland, A., Overvad, K. & Poulsen, H.E. (1992) Oxidative DNA damage estimated by 8-hydroxydeoxyguanosine excretion in humans: influence of smoking, gender and body mass index. *Carcinogenesis*, **13**, 2241–2247

Longnecker, M.P., Berlin, J.A., Orza, M.J. & Chalmers, T.C. (1988) A meta-analysis of alcohol consumption in relation to risk of breast cancer. *JAMA*, **260**, 652–656

Longnecker, M.P., Orza, M.J., Adams, M.E., Vioque, J. & Chalmers, T.C. (1990) A meta-analysis of alcoholic beverage consumption in relation to risk of colorectal cancer. *Cancer Causes Control*, **1**, 59–68

Lowenfels, A.B., Tuyns, A.J., Walker, E.A. & Roussel, A. (1978) Nitrite studies in oesophageal cancer. *Gut*, **19**, 199–201

Löwik, M.R., Hulshof, K.F. & Brussaard, J.H. (1999) Food-based dietary guidelines: some assumptions tested for The Netherlands. *Br. J. Nutr.*, **81 Suppl. 2**, S143–S149

Lu, Y.P., Lou, Y.R., Yen, P., Newmark, H.L., Mirochnitchenko, O.I., Inouye, M. & Huang, M.T. (1997) Enhanced skin carcinogenesis in transgenic mice with high expression of glutathione peroxidase or both glutathione peroxidase and superoxide dismutase. *Cancer Res.*, **57**, 1468–1474

Lubin, F., Rozen, P., Arieli, B., Farbstein, M., Knaani, Y., Bat, L. & Farbstein, H. (1997) Nutritional and lifestyle habits and water–fiber interaction in colorectal adenoma etiology. *Cancer Epidemiol. Biomarkers Prev.*, **6**, 79–85

Lubin, F., Farbstein, H., Chetrit, A., Farbstein, M., Freedman, L., Alfandary, E. & Modan, B. (2000) The role of nutritional habits during gestation and child life in pediatric brain tumour etiology. *Int. J. Cancer*, **86**, 139–143

Luepker, R.V., Murray, D.M., Jacobs, D.R., Jr, Mittelmark, M.B., Bracht, N., Carlaw, R., Crow, R., Elmer, P., Finnegan, J., Folsom, A.R., Grimm, R., Hannan, P.J., Jeffrey, R., Lando, H., McGovern, P., Mullis, R., Perry, C.L., Pechacek, T., Pirie, P., Sprafka, J.M., Weisbrod, R. & Blackburn, H. (1994) Community education for cardiovascular disease prevention: risk factor changes in the Minnesota Heart Health Program. *Am. J. Public Health*, **84**, 1383–1393

Lyles, R.H. & Allen, A.S. (2003) Missing data in the 2 x 2 table: patterns and likelihood-based analysis for cross-sectional studies with supplemental sampling. *Stat. Med.*, **22**, 517–534

Lyon, J.L., Egger, M.J., Robison, L.M., French, T.K. & Gao, R. (1992) Misclassification of exposure in a case-control study: the effects of different types of exposure and different proxy respondents in a study of pancreatic cancer. *Epidemiology*, **3**, 223–231

Lyon, J.L., Slattery, M.L., Mahoney, A.W. & Robison, L.M. (1993) Dietary intake as a risk factor for cancer of the exocrine pancreas. *Cancer Epidemiol. Biomarkers Prev.*, **2**, 513–518

Mack, T.M., Yu, M.C., Hanisch, R. & Henderson, B.E. (1986) Pancreas cancer and smoking, beverage consumption, and past medical history. *J. Natl. Cancer Inst.*, **76**, 49–60

MacLehose, R.R., Reeves, B.C., Harvey, I.M., Sheldon, T.A., Russell, I.T. & Black, A.M. (2000) A systematic review

References

of comparisons of effect sizes derived from randomised and non-randomised studies. *Health Technology Assessment*, **4,** 1–154

MacLennan, R., Da Costa, J., Day, N.E., Law, C.H., Ng, Y.K. & Shanmugaratnam, K. (1977) Risk factors for lung cancer in Singapore Chinese, a population with high female incidence rates. *Int. J. Cancer*, **20**, 854–860

Macquart-Moulin, G., Riboli, E., Cornée, J., Charnay, B., Berthezène, P. & Day, N. (1986) Case–control study on colorectal cancer and diet in Marseilles. *Int. J. Cancer*, **38**, 183–191

Macquart-Moulin, G., Riboli, E., Cornée, J., Kaaks, R. & Berthezène, P. (1987) Colorectal polyps and diet: a case–control study in Marseilles. *Int. J. Cancer*, **40**, 179–188

Madigan, M.P., Troisi, R., Potischman, N., Brogan, D., Gammon, M.D., Malone, K.E. & Brinton, L.A. (2000) Characteristics of respondents and non-respondents from a case-control study of breast cancer in younger women. *Int. J. Epidemiol.*, **29,** 793–798

Mahady, G.B. & Pendland, S. (2000) Garlic and *Helicobacter pylori*. *Am. J. Gastroenterol.*, **95,** 309

Maier, H. & Tisch, M. (1997) Epidemiology of laryngeal cancer: results of the Heidelberg case–control study. *Acta Otolaryngol*, **527**, 160–164

Mangels, A.R., Holden, J.M., Beecher, G.R., Forman, M.R. & Lanza, E. (1993) Carotenoid content of fruits and vegetables: an evaluation of analytic data. *J. Am. Diet. Assoc.*, **93**, 284–296

Männistö, S., Pietinen, P., Virtanen, M., Kataja, V. & Uusitupa, M. (1999) Diet and the risk of breast cancer in a case-control study: does the threat of disease have an influence on recall bias? *J. Clin. Epidemiol.*, **52,** 429–439

Manousos, O., Day, N.E., Trichopoulos, D., Gerovassilis, F., Tzonou, A. & Polychronopoulou, A. (1983) Diet and colorectal cancer: a case–control study in Greece. *Int. J. Cancer*, **32**, 1–5

Manson, J.E., Stampfer, M.J., Willett, W.C., Colditz, G.A., Rosner, B., Speizer, F.E. & Hennekens, C.H. (1992) A prospective study of vitamin C and incidence of coronary heart disease in women. *Circulation*, **85,** 865

Manson, J.E., Willett, W.C., Stampfer, M.J., Colditz, G.A., Speizer, F.E. & Hennekens, C.H. (1994) Vegetable and fruit consumption and incidence of stroke in women. *Circulation,* **89,** 932

Marchand, J.L., Luce, D., Goldberg, P., Bugel, I., Salomon, C. & Goldberg, M. (2002) Dietary factors and the risk of lung cancer in New Caledonia (South Pacific). *Nutr. Cancer*, **42**, 18–24

Margetts, B.M. & Nelson, M. (1991) Assessment of food consumption and nutrient intake. In: *Design Concepts in Nutritional Epidemiology,* New York, Oxford University Press, pp. 153–191

Margetts, B.M. & Pietinen, P. (1997) European Prospective Investigation into Cancer and Nutrition: validity studies on dietary assessment methods. *Int. J. Epidemiol.*, **26 Suppl. 1**, S1–S5

Marikovsky, M., Nevo, N., Vadai, E. & Harris-Cerruti, C. (2002) Cu/Zn superoxide dismutase plays a role in angiogenesis. *Int. J. Cancer*, **97**, 34–41

Marniemi, J., Hakala, P., Maki, J. & Ahotupa, M. (2000) Partial resistance of low density lipoprotein to oxidation in vivo after increased intake of berries. *Nutr. Metab. Cardiovasc. Dis.*, **10,** 331–337

Marshall, J.R. & Hastrup, J.L. (1996) Mismeasurement and the resonance of strong confounders: uncorrelated errors. *Am. J. Epidemiol.*, **143**, 1069–1078

Marshall, J., Priore, R., Haughey, B., Rzepka, T. & Graham, S. (1980) Spouse-subject interviews and the reliability of diet studies. *Am. J. Epidemiol.*, **112,** 675–683

Maruyama, C., Imamura, K., Oshima, S., Suzukawa, M., Egami, S., Tonomoto, M., Baba, N., Harada, M., Ayaori, M., Inakuma, T. & Ishikawa, T. (2001) Effects of tomato juice consumption on plasma and lipoprotein carotenoid concentrations and the susceptibility of low density lipoprotein to oxidative modification. *J. Nutr. Sci. Vitaminol. (Tokyo)*, **47,** 213–221

Masefield, G.B., Wallis, M., Harrison, S.G. & Nicholson, B.E., eds (1969) *The Oxford Book of Food Plants,* London, Oxford University Press

Maskarinec, G., Chan, C.L., Meng, L., Franke, A.A. & Cooney, R.V. (1999) Exploring the feasibility and effects of a high-fruit and -vegetable diet in healthy women. *Cancer Epidemiol. Biomarkers Prev.*, **8,** 919–924

Mathew, A., Gangadharan, P., Varghese, C. & Nair, M.K. (2000) Diet and stomach cancer: a case–control study in South India. *Eur. J. Cancer Prev.*, **9**, 89–97

Matullo, G., Guarrera, S., Carturan, S., Peluso, M., Malaveille, C., Davico, L., Piazza, A. & Vineis, P. (2001) DNA repair gene polymorphisms, bulky DNA adducts in white blood cells and bladder cancer in a case-control study. *Int. J. Cancer,* **92,** 562–567

Maynard, M., Gunnell, D., Emmett, P., Frankel, S. & Davey Smith, G. (2002) Fruits, vegetables, and antioxidants in childhood and risk of adult cancer: the Boyd Orr cohort. *J. Epidemiol. Community Health*, **57**, 218–225

Mayne, S.T. (2003) Antioxidant nutrients and chronic disease: use of biomarkers of exposure and oxidative stress status in epidemiologic research. *J. Nutr.*, **133**, 933S–940S

Mayne, S.T., Janerich, D.T., Greenwald, P., Chorost, S., Tucci, C., Zaman, M.B., Melamed, M.R., Kiely, M. & McKneally, M.F. (1994) Dietary beta carotene and lung cancer risk in U.S. nonsmokers. *J. Natl Cancer Inst.*, **86**, 33–38

Mayo Clinic, University of California Los Angeles & Dole Food Company Inc., eds (2002) *Encyclopedia of Foods. A Guide to Healthy Nutrition,* San Diego, CA, Academic Press

McCann, S.E., Freudenheim, J.L., Marshall, J.R., Brasure, J.R., Swanson, M.K. & Graham, S. (2000) Diet in the epidemiology of endometrial cancer in western New York (United States). *Cancer Causes Control*, **11**, 965–974

McCann, S.E., Moysich, K.B. & Mettlin, C. (2001) Intakes of selected nutrients and food groups and risk of ovarian cancer. *Nutr. Cancer*, **39**, 19–28

McCann, S.E., Moysich, K.B., Freudenheim, J.L., Ambrosone, C.B. & Shields, P.G. (2002) The risk of breast cancer associated with dietary lignans differs by *CYP17* genotype in women. *J. Nutr.*, **132**, 3036–3041

McCredie, M. & Stewart, J.H. (1992) Risk factors for kidney cancer in New South Wales – I. Cigarette smoking. *Eur. J. Cancer*, **28A**, 2050–2054

McCredie, M., Maisonneuve, P. & Boyle, P. (1994a). Antenatal risk factors for malignant brain tumours in New South Wales children. *Int. J. Cancer*, **56**, 6–10

McCredie, M., Maisonneuve, P. & Boyle, P. (1994b) Perinatal and early postnatal risk factors for malignant brain tumours in New South Wales children. *Int. J. Cancer*, **56**, 11–15

McCullough, M.L., Robertson, A.S., Jacobs, E.J., Chao, A., Calle, E.E. & Thun, M.J. (2001) A prospective study of diet and stomach cancer mortality in United States men and women. *Cancer Epidemiol. Biomarkers Prev.*, **10**, 1201–1205

McCullough, M.L., Robertson, A.S., Chao, A., Jacobs, E.J., Stampfer, M.J., Jacobs, D.R., Diver, W.R., Calle, E.E. & Thun, M.J. (2003) A prospective study of whole grains, fruits, vegetables and colon cancer risk. *Cancer Causes Control* (in press)

McDanell, R., McLean, A.E., Hanley, A.B., Heaney, R.K. & Fenwick, G.R. (1989) The effect of feeding brassica vegetables and intact glucosinolates on mixed-function-oxidase activity in the livers and intestines of rats. *Food Chem. Toxicol.*, **27**, 289–293

McDanell, R.E., Henderson, L.A., Russell, K. & McLean, A.E. (1992) The effect of brassica vegetable consumption on caffeine metabolism in humans. *Hum. Exp. Toxicol.*, **11**, 167–172

McDonald, A., Van Horn, L., Slattery, M., Hilner, J., Bragg, C., Caan, B., Jacobs, D., Jr., Liu, K., Hubert, H., Gernhofer, N., Betz, E. & Havlik, D. (1991) The CARDIA dietary history: development, implementation, and evaluation. *J. Am. Diet. Assoc.*, **91**, 1104–1112

McEligot, A.J., Rock, C.L., Flatt, S.W., Newman, V., Faerber, S. & Pierce, J.P. (1999) Plasma carotenoids are biomarkers of long-term high vegetable intake in women with breast cancer. *J. Nutr.*, **129**, 2258–2263

McLaughlin, J.K., Mandel, J.S., Blot, W.J., Schuman, L.M., Mehl, E.S. & Fraumeni, J.F., Jr (1984) A population-based case–control study of renal cell carcinoma. *J. Natl Cancer Inst.*, **72**, 275–284

McLaughlin, J.K., Gridley, G., Block, G., Winn, D.M., Preston-Martin, S., Schoenberg, J.B., Greenberg, R.S., Stemhagen, A., Austin, D.F. & Ershow, A.G. (1988) Dietary factors in oral and pharyngeal cancer. *J. Natl Cancer Inst.*, **80**, 1237–1243

McLaughlin, J.K., Gao, Y.T., Gao, R.N., Zheng, W., Ji, B.T., Blot, W.J. & Fraumeni, J.F., Jr (1992) Risk factors for renal-cell cancer in Shanghai, China. *Int. J. Cancer*, **52**, 562–565

McLennan, W. & Podger, A. (1999) *National Nutrition Survey: Foods eaten, Australia, 1995*, Canberra, Australian Bureau of Statistics

McMichael, A.J., Potter, J.D. & Hetzel, B.S. (1979) Time trends in colo-rectal cancer mortality in relation to food and alcohol consumption: United States, United Kingdom, Australia and New Zealand. *Int. J. Epidemiol.*, **8**, 295–303

McNulty, C.A., Wilson, M.P., Havinga, W., Johnston, B., O'Gara, E.A. & Maslin, D.J. (2001) A pilot study to determine the effectiveness of garlic oil capsules in the treatment of dyspeptic patients with Helicobacter pylori. *Helicobacter*, **6**, 249–253

McPhillips, J.B., Eaton, C.B., Gans, K.M., Derby, C.A., Lasater, T.M., McKenney, J.L. & Carleton, R.A. (1994) Dietary differences in smokers and non-smokers from two southeastern New England communities. *J. Am. Diet. Assoc.*, **94**, 287–292

Mellemgaard, A., McLaughlin, J.K., Overvad, K. & Olsen, J.H. (1996) Dietary risk factors for renal cell carcinoma in Denmark. *Eur. J. Cancer*, **32A**, 673–682

Memik, F., Gulten, M. & Nak, S.G. (1992a) The etiological role of diet, smoking, and drinking habits of patients with esophageal carcinoma in Turkey. *J. Environ. Pathol. Toxicol. Oncol.*, **11**, 197–200

Memik, F., Nak, S.G., Gulten, M. & Ozturk, M. (1992b) Gastric carcinoma in northwestern Turkey: epidemiologic characteristics. *J. Environ. Pathol. Toxicol. Oncol.*, **11**, 335–338

Meng, C.-L. & Shyu, K.-W. (1990) Inhibition of experimental carcinogenesis by painting with garlic extract. *Nutr. Cancer*, **14**, 207–217

Mertz, W. (1992) Food intake measurements: is there a "gold standard"? *J. Am. Med. Assoc.*, **92**, 1463–1465

Mettlin, C., Graham, S., Priore, R., Marshall, J. & Swanson, M. (1981) Diet and cancer of the esophagus. *Nutr. Cancer*, **2**, 143–147

Michaud, D.S., Spiegelman, D., Clinton, S.K., Rimm, E.B., Willett, W.C. & Giovannucci, E.L. (1999) Fruit and vegetable intake and incidence of bladder cancer in a male prospective cohort. *J. Natl Cancer Inst.*, **91**, 605–613

Michaud, D.S., Pietinen, P., Taylor, P.R., Virtanen, M., Virtamo, J. & Albanes, D. (2002) Intakes of fruits and vegetables, carotenoids and vitamins A, E, C in relation to the risk of bladder cancer in the ATBC cohort study. *Br. J. Cancer*, **87**, 960–965

Michels, K.B. & Wolk, A. (2002) A prospective study of variety of healthy foods and mortality in women. *Int. J. Epidemiol.*, **31**, 847–854

Michels, K.B., Giovannucci, E., Joshipura, K.J., Rosner, B.A., Stampfer, M.J., Fuchs, C.S., Colditz, G.A., Speizer, F.E. & Willett, W.C. (2000) Prospective study of fruit and vegetable consumption and incidence of colon and rectal cancers. *J. Natl Cancer Inst.*, **92**, 1740–1752

Miller, E.C. & Miller, J.A. (1981) Searches for ultimate chemical carcinogens and their reactions with cellular macromolecules. *Cancer,* **47**, 2327–2345

Miller, A.B., Howe, G.R., Jain, M., Craib, K.J. & Harrison, L. (1983) Food items and food groups as risk factors in a case–control study of diet and colo-rectal cancer. *Int. J. Cancer*, **32**, 155–161

Miller, M., Pollard, C.M. & Paterson, D. (1996) A public health nutrition campaign to promote fruit and vegetables in Australia In: Worsley, A., ed., *Multi-disciplinary Approaches to Food Choice. Proceedings of Food Choice Conference,* Adelaide, South Australia, University of Adelaide, pp. 152–158

Miller, M.R., Pollard, C.M. & Coli, T. (1997) Western Australian Health Department recommendations for fruit and vegetable consumption—how much is enough? *Aust. N.Z. J. Public Health,* **21,** 638–642

Miller, E.R., III, Appel, L.J. & Risby, T.H. (1998) Effect of dietary patterns on measures of lipid peroxidation: results from a randomized clinical trial. *Circulation,* **98**, 2390–2395

Miller, A.B., Bartsch, H., Boffetta, P., Dragsted, L.O. & Vainio, H., eds (2001) *Biomarkers in Cancer Chemoprevention* (IARC Scientific Publications No. 154), Lyon, International Agency for Research on Cancer

Miller, A. B., Altenburg, H. P., Bueno-de-Mesquita, H. B., Boshuizen, H., Agudo, A., Berrino, F., Gram, I. T., Janson, L., Linseisen, J., Overvad, K., Rasmuson, T., Vineis, P., Lukanova, A., Allen, N., Berglund, G., Boeing, H., Clavel-Chapelon, F., Day, N. E., Gonzalez, C. A., Hallmans, G., Lund, E., Martinez, C., Palli, D., Panico, S., Peeters, P. H., Tjonneland, A., Tumino, R., Trichopoulou, A., Trichopoulos, A., Slimani, N. & Riboli, E. (2003) Fruits and vegetables and lung cancer: Findings from the European Prospective Investigation into Cancer and Nutrition. *Int. J. Cancer* (in press)

Mills, P.K., Beeson, W.L., Abbey, D.E., Fraser, G.E. & Phillips, R.L. (1988) Dietary habits and past medical history as related to fatal pancreas cancer risk among Adventists. *Cancer*, **61**, 2578–2585

Mills, P.K., Beeson, W.L., Phillips, R.L. & Fraser, G.E. (1989) Cohort study of diet, lifestyle, and prostate cancer in Adventist men. *Cancer*, **64**, 598–604

Mirvish, S.S., Wallcave, L., Eagen, M. & Shubik, P. (1972) Ascorbate-nitrite reaction: possible means of blocking the formation of carcinogenic *N*-nitroso compounds. *Science,* **177,** 65–68

Mishina, T., Watanabe, H., Araki, H. & Nakao, M. (1985) Epidemiological study of prostatic cancer by matched-pair analysis. *Prostate*, **6**, 423–436

Miyagi, Y., Om, A.S., Chee, K.M. & Bennink, M.R. (2000) Inhibition of azoxymethane-induced colon cancer by orange juice. *Nutr. Cancer,* **36,** 224–229

Miyata, M., Takano, H., Takahashi, K., Sasaki, Y.F. & Yamazoe, Y. (2002) Suppression of 2-amino-1-methyl-6-phenylimidazo[4,5-*b*]pyridine-induced DNA damage in rat colon after grapefruit juice intake. *Cancer Lett.*, **183,** 17–22

Mollerup, S., Ryberg, D., Hewer, A., Phillips, D.H. & Haugen, A. (1999) Sex differences in lung CYP1A1 expression and DNA adduct levels among lung cancer patients. *Cancer Res.*, **59,** 3317–3320

Mongeau, R., Brassard, R., Cerkauskas, R., Chiba, M., Lok, E., Nera, E.A., Jee, P., McMullen, E. & Clayson, D.B. (1994) Effect of addition of dried healthy or diseased parsnip root tissue to a modified AIN-76A diet on cell proliferation and histopathology in the liver, oesophagus and forestomach of male Swiss Webster mice. *Food Chem. Toxicol.,* **32,** 265–271

Morgenstern, H. (1995) Ecologic studies in epidemiology: concepts, principles, and methods. *Annu. Rev. Public Health*, **16**, 61–81

Mori, M., Hariharan, M., Anandakumar, M., Tsutsumi, M., Ishikawa, O., Konishi, Y., Chellam, V.G., John, M., Praseeda, I., Priya, R. & Narendranathan, M. (1999) A case–control study on risk factors for pancreatic diseases in Kerala, India. *Hepatogastroenterology*, **46**, 25–30

Morris, J.N., Marr, J.W. & Clayton, D.G. (1977) Diet and heart: a postscript. *Br. Med. J.,* **2,** 1307–1314

Morse, D.E., Pendrys, D.G., Katz, R.V., Holford, T.R., Krutchkoff, D.J., Eisenberg, E., Kosis, D.L., Kerpel, S., Freedman, P., Freedman, P. & Mayne, S.T. (2000) Food group intake and the risk of oral epithelial dysplasia in a United States population. *Cancer Causes Control*, **11,** 713–720

Muñoz, S.E., Ferraroni, M., La Vecchia, C. & Decarli, A. (1997) Gastric cancer risk factors in subjects with family history. *Cancer Epidemiol. Biomarkers Prev.*, **6**, 137–140

Murata, M., Tagawa, M., Watanabe, S., Kimura, H., Takeshita, T. & Morimoto, K. (1999) Genotype difference of aldehyde dehydrogenase 2 gene in alcohol drinkers influences the incidence of Japanese colorectal cancer patients. *Jpn J. Cancer Res.*, **90**, 711–719

Murphy, S.P., Rose, D., Hudes, M. & Viteri, F.E. (1992) Demographic and economic factors associated with dietary quality for adults in the 1987-88 Nationwide Food Consumption Survey. *J. Am. Diet. Assoc.,* **92,** 1352–1357

Murphy, S.E., Johnson, L.M., Losey, L.M., Carmella, S.G. & Hecht, S.S. (2001) Consumption of watercress fails to alter coumarin metabolism in humans. *Drug Metab. Dispos.*, **29,** 786–788

Murray, S., Lake, B.G., Gray, S., Edwards, A.J., Springall, C., Bowey, E.A., Williamson, G., Boobis, A.R. & Gooderham, N.J. (2001) Effect of cruciferous vegetable consumption on heterocyclic aromatic amine metabolism in man. *Carcinogenesis,* **22,** 1413–1420

Nagano, J., Kono, S., Preston, D.L., Moriwaki, H., Sharp, G.B., Koyama, K. & Mabuchi, K. (2000) Bladder-cancer incidence in relation to vegetable and fruit consumption: a prospective study of atomic-bomb survivors. *Int. J. Cancer*, **86**, 132–138

Narisawa, T., Fukaura, Y., Hasebe, M., Nomura, S., Oshima, S., Sakamoto, H., Inakuma, T., Ishiguro, Y., Takayasu, J. & Nishino, H. (1998) Prevention of N-methylnitrosourea-induced colon carcinogenesis in F344 rats by lycopene and tomato juice rich in lycopene. *Jpn J. Cancer Res.*, **89**, 1003–1008

Naska, A., Vasdekis, V.G.S., Trichopoulou, A., Friel, S., Leonhäuser, I.U., Moreiras, O., Nelson, M., Remaut, A.M., Schmitt, A., Sekula, W., Trygg, K.U. & Zajkas, G. (2000) Fruit and vegetable availability among ten European countries: how does it compare with the 'five-a-day' recommendation? DAFNE I and II projects of the European Commission. *Br. J. Nutr.*, **84**, 549–556

National Cancer Institute (1986) *Cancer Control Objectives for the Nation, 1985–2000,* Washington, DC, US Government Printing Office

National Cancer Institute (1994) *DIETSYS version 3.0 User's Guide,* Bethesda, National Cancer Institute, Information Management Services I, Block Dietary Data Systems

National Cancer Institute (2002a) *5 A Day For Better Health Program Evaluation Report,* NIH/NCI, Publication No. 01–4904, Washington, DC, US Government Printing Office

National Cancer Institute (2002b) Savor the spectrum. Color Your daily diet with fruits and vegetables. 5 A Day Program for Better Health Press Kit Package. Available from: URL: http://www.5aday.gov

National Food Agency of Denmark (1990) *Food Monitoring in Denmark. Nutrients and Contaminants 1983–1987,* Soborg, National Food Agency of Denmark

National Health and Medical Research Council (1991) *Dietary Guidelines for Australians,* Canberra, Australian Government Publishing Service

National Institutes of Health and National Cancer Institute (2001) *5 A Day for Better Health Program* (NIH/NCI Publication 01–5019), Bethesda, MD, National Institutes of Health

National Public Health Institute of Finland (1998) *The 1997 Dietary Survey of Finnish Adults,* Helsinki, KTL, pp. 1–97

National Research Council (1989) *Diet and Health: Implications for Reducing Chronic Disease Risk,* Washington, DC, National Academy Press

Negri, E., La Vecchia, C., Franceschi, S., D'Avanzo, B. & Parazzini, F. (1991) Vegetable and fruit consumption and cancer risk. *Int. J. Cancer*, **48**, 350–354

Nelson, L.M., Longstreth, W.T., Jr., Koepsell, T.D. & van Belle, G. (1990) Proxy respondents in epidemiologic research. *Epidemiol. Rev.*, **12**, 71–86

Ness, A.R. & Powles, J.W. (1997) Fruit and vegetables, and cardiovascular disease: a review. *Int. J. Epidemiol.*, **26**, 1–13

Netherlands Nutrition Centre (1998) *Zo eet Nederland 1998. Resultaten van de Voedselconsumptiepeiling 1997–1998,* Den Haag, Voedingscentrum

Neuhouser, M.L., Patterson, R.E., Thornquist, M.D., Omenn, G.S., King, I.B. & Goodman, G.E. (2003) Fruits and vegetables are associated with lower lung cancer risk only in the placebo arm of the β-carotene and retinol efficacy trial (CARET). *Cancer Epidemiol. Biomarkers Prev.*, **12**, 350–358

NHMRC (National Health and Medical Research Council), eds (1999) *A Guide to the Development, Implementation and Evaluation of Clinical Practice Guidelines,* Canberra, NHMRC

Nho, C.W. & Jeffery, E. (2001) The synergistic upregulation of phase II detoxification enzymes by glucosinolate breakdown products in cruciferous vegetables. *Toxicol. Appl. Pharmacol.*, **174**, 146–152

Nielsen, S.E., Young, J.F., Daneshvar, B., Lauridsen, S.T., Knuthsen, P., Sandström, B. & Dragsted, L.O. (1999) Effect of parsley (*Petroselinum crispum*) intake on urinary apigenin excretion, blood antioxidant enzymes and biomarkers for oxidative stress in human subjects. *Br. J. Nutr.*, **81**, 447–455

Nijhoff, W.A., Mulder, T.P., Verhagen, H., van Poppel, G. & Peters, W.H. (1995a) Effects of consumption of brussels sprouts on plasma and urinary glutathione S-transferase class-α and -π in humans. *Carcinogenesis*, **16**, 955–957

Nijhoff, W.A., Grubben, M.J., Nagengast, F.M., Jansen, J.B., Verhagen, H., van Poppel, G. & Peters, W.H. (1995b) Effects of consumption of Brussels sprouts on intestinal and lymphocytic glutathione S-transferases in humans. *Carcinogenesis*, **16**, 2125–2128

Nishimoto, I.N., Hamada, G.S., Kowalski, L.P., Rodrigues, J.G., Iriya, K., Sasazuki, S., Hanaoka, T. & Tsugane, S. (2002) Risk factors for stomach cancer in Brazil (I): a case–control study among non-Japanese Brazilians in Sao Paulo. *Jpn J. Clin. Oncol.*, **32**, 277–283

Noethlings, U., Hoffmann, K., Bergmann, M.M. & Boeing, H. (2003) Portion size adds limited information on variance in food intake of participants in the EPIC-Potsdam study. *J. Nutr.*, **133**, 510–515

Nomura, A., Grove, J.S., Stemmermann, G.N. & Severson, R.K. (1990) A prospective study of stomach cancer and its relation to diet, cigarettes, and alcohol consumption. *Cancer Res.*, **50**, 627–631

Norell, S.E., Ahlbom, A., Erwald, R., Jacobson, G., Lindberg-Navier, I., Olin, R., Tornberg, B. & Wiechel, K.L. (1986) Diet and pancreatic cancer: a case–control study. *Am. J. Epidemiol.*, **124**, 894–902

Notani, P.N. & Jayant, K. (1987) Role of diet in upper aerodigestive tract cancers. *Nutr. Cancer*, **10**, 103–113

Nuttens, M.C., Romon, M., Ruidavets, J.B., Arveiler, D., Ducimetière, P., Lecerf, J.M., Richard, J.L., Cambou, J.P., Simon, C. & Salomez, J.L. (1992) Relationship between smoking and diet: the MONICA-France project. *J. Intern. Med.*, **231**, 349–356

References

Nyberg, F., Agrenius, V., Svartengren, K., Svensson, C. & Pershagen, G. (1998) Dietary factors and risk of lung cancer in never-smokers. *Int. J. Cancer*, **78**, 430–436

Obermeier, M.T., White, R.E. & Yang, C.S. (1995) Effects of bioflavonoids on hepatic P450 activities. *Xenobiotica*, **25**, 575–584

Ocké, M.C., Bueno de Mesquita, H.B., Feskens, E.J., van Staveren, W.A. & Kromhout, D. (1997a) Repeated measurements of vegetables, fruits, beta-carotene, and vitamins C and E in relation to lung cancer. The Zutphen Study. *Am. J. Epidemiol.*, **145**, 358–365

Ocké, M.C., Bueno de Mesquita, H.B., Goddijn, H.E., Jansen, A., Pols, M.A., van Staveren, W.A. & Kromhout, D. (1997b) The Dutch EPIC food frequency questionnaire. I. Description of the questionnaire, and relative validity and reproducibility for food groups. *Int. J. Epidemiol.*, **26 Suppl. 1**, S37–S48

Office for Life-Style Related Diseases Control (2002) *The National Nutrition Survey in Japan, 2000*, Tokyo, Ministry of Health, Labour and Welfare, pp. 1–185

Ohshima, H. & Bartsch, H. (1981) Quantitative estimation of endogenous nitrosation in humans by monitoring *N*-nitrosoproline excreted in the urine. *Cancer Res.*, **41**, 3658–3662

Ohyama, S., Inamasu, T., Ishizawa, M., Ishinishi, N. & Matsuura, K. (1987a) Mutagenicity of human urine after the consumption of fried salted salmon. *Food Chem. Toxicol.*, **25**, 147–153

Ohyama, S., Kitamori, S., Kawano, H., Yamada, T., Inamasu, T., Ishizawa, M. & Ishinishi, N. (1987b) Ingestion of parsley inhibits the mutagenicity of male human urine following consumption of fried salmon. *Mutat. Res.*, **192**, 7–10

Okajima, E., Tsutsumi, M., Ozono, S., Akai, H., Denda, A., Nishino, H., Oshima, S., Sakamoto, H. & Konishi, Y. (1998) Inhibitory effect of tomato juice on rat urinary bladder carcinogenesis after *N*-butyl-*N*-(4-hydroxybutyl)nitrosamine initiation. *Jpn J. Cancer Res.*, **89**, 22–26

Oishi, K., Okada, K., Yoshida, O., Yamabe, H., Ohno, Y., Hayes, R.B. & Schroeder, F.H. (1988) A case–control study of prostatic cancer with reference to dietary habits. *Prostate*, **12**, 179–190

Olsen, G.W., Mandel, J.S., Gibson, R.W., Wattenberg, L.W. & Schuman, L.M. (1989) A case–control study of pancreatic cancer and cigarettes, alcohol, coffee and diet. *Am. J. Public Health*, **79**, 1016–1019

Olson, S.H. (2001) Reported participation in case-control studies: changes over time. *Am. J. Epidemiol.*, **154**, 574–581

O'Neill, I.K., Loktionov, A., Manson, M.M., Ball, H., Bandaletova, T. & Bingham, S.A. (1997) Comparison of metabolic effects of vegetables and teas with colorectal proliferation and with tumour development in DMH-treated F344 rats. *Cancer Lett.*, **114**, 287–291

Onuk, M.D., Oztopuz, A. & Memik, F. (2002) Risk factors for esophageal cancer in eastern Anatolia. *Hepatogastroenterology*, **49**, 1290–1292

Oreggia, F., De Stefani, E., Correa, P. & Fierro, L. (1991) Risk factors for cancer of the tongue in Uruguay. *Cancer*, **67**, 180–183

O'Reilly, J.D., Mallet, A.I., McAnlis, G.T., Young, I.S., Halliwell, B., Sanders, T.A. & Wiseman, H. (2001) Consumption of flavonoids in onions and black tea: lack of effect on F_2-isoprostanes and autoantibodies to oxidized LDL in healthy humans. *Am. J. Clin. Nutr.*, **73**, 1040–1044

Osterholm, M.T. (1997) Cyclosporiasis and raspberries—lessons for the future. *New Engl. J. Med.*, **336**, 1597–1599

Ozasa, K., Watanabe, Y., Ito, Y., Suzuki, K., Tamakoshi, A., Seki, N., Nishino, Y., Kondo, T., Wakai, K., Ando, M. & Ohno, Y. (2001) Dietary habits and risk of lung cancer death in a large-scale cohort study (JACC Study) in Japan by sex and smoking habit. *Jpn J. Cancer Res.*, **92**, 1259–1269

Painter, J., Rah, J.H. & Lee, Y.K. (2002) Comparison of international food guide pictorial representations. *J. Am. Diet. Assoc.*, **102**, 483–489

Palli, D., Bianchi, S., Decarli, A., Cipriani, F., Avellini, C., Cocco, P., Falcini, F., Puntoni, R., Russo, A. & Vindigni, C. (1992) A case–control study of cancers of the gastric cardia in Italy. *Br. J. Cancer*, **65**, 263–266

Palli, D., Vineis, P., Russo, A., Berrino, F., Krogh, V., Masala, G., Munnia, A., Panico, S., Taioli, E., Tumino, R., Garte, S. & Peluso, M. (2000) Diet, metabolic polymorphisms and DNA adducts: The EPIC-Italy cross-sectional study. *Int. J. Cancer*, **87**, 444–451

Pandey, D.K., Shekelle, R., Selwyn, B.J., Tangney, C. & Stamler, J. (1995) Dietary vitamin C and β-carotene and risk of death in middle-aged men. The Western Electric Study. *Am. J. Epidemiol.*, **142**, 1269–1278

Pantuck, E.J., Pantuck, C.B., Garland, W.A., Min, B.H., Wattenberg, L.W., Anderson, K.E., Kappas, A. & Conney, A.H. (1979) Stimulatory effect of brussels sprouts and cabbage on human drug metabolism. *Clin. Pharmacol. Ther.*, **25**, 88–95

Pantuck, E.J., Pantuck, C.B., Anderson, K.E., Wattenberg, L.W., Conney, A.H. & Kappas, A. (1984) Effect of brussels sprouts and cabbage on drug conjugation. *Clin. Pharmacol. Ther.*, **35**, 161–169

Parkin, D.M., Srivatanakul, P., Khlat, M., Chenvidhya, D., Chotiwan, P., Insiripong, S., L'Abbé, K.A. & Wild, C.P. (1991) Liver cancer in Thailand. I. A case–control study of cholangiocarcinoma. *Int. J. Cancer*, **48**, 323–328

Passmore, R. & Eastwood, M.A., eds (1986) *Davidson and Passmore Human Nutrition and Dietetics*, Edinburgh, Churchill Livingstone

Pastor, S., Creus, A., Xamena, N., Siffel, C. & Marcos, R. (2002) Occupational exposure to pesticides and cytogenetic damage: results of a Hungarian population study using the micronucleus assay in lymphocytes and buccal cells. *Environ. Mol. Mutagen.*, **40**, 101–109

Pawlega, J. (1992) Breast cancer and smoking, vodka drinking and dietary habits. A case–control study. *Acta Oncol.*, **31**, 387–392

Pawlega, J., Rachtan, J. & Dyba, T. (1997) Evaluation of certain risk factors for lung cancer in Cracow (Poland) – a case–control study. *Acta Oncol.*, **36**, 471–476

Pedersen, C.B., Kyle, J., Jenkinson, A.M., Gardner, P.T., McPhail, D.B. & Duthie, G.G. (2000) Effects of blueberry and cranberry juice consumption on the plasma antioxidant capacity of healthy female volunteers. *Eur. J. Clin. Nutr.,* **54**, 405–408

Pedraza-Chaverri, J., Maldonado, P.D., Medina-Campos, O.N., Olivares-Corichi, I.M., Granados-Silvestre, M.A., Hernandez-Pando, R. & Ibarra-Rubio, M.E. (2000) Garlic ameliorates gentamicin nephrotoxicity: relation to antioxidant enzymes. *Free Radic. Biol. Med.*, **29**, 602–611

Pedraza-Chaverri, J., Granados-Silvestre, M.D., Medina-Campos, O.N., Maldonado, P.D., Olivares-Corichi, I.M. & Ibarra-Rubio, M.E. (2001) Post-transcriptional control of catalase expression in garlic-treated rats. *Mol. Cell Biochem.*, **216**, 9–19

Pedraza-Chaverri, J., Maldonado, P.D., Medina-Campos, O.N., Olivares-Corichi, I.M., Granados-Silvestre, M.A., Hernandez-Pando, R. & Ibarra-Rubio, M.E. (2000) Garlic ameliorates gentamicin nephrotoxicity: relation to antioxidant enzymes. *Free Radic. Biol. Med.*, **29**, 602–611

Pellegrini, N., Riso, P. & Porrini, M. (2000) Tomato consumption does not affect the total antioxidant capacity of plasma. *Nutrition*, **16**, 268–271

Peluso, M., Airoldi, L., Armelle, M., Martone, T., Coda, R., Malaveille, C., Giacomelli, G., Terrone, C., Casetta, G. & Vineis, P. (1998) White blood cell DNA adducts, smoking, and NAT2 and GSTM1 genotypes in bladder cancer: a case–control study. *Cancer Epidemiol. Biomarkers Prev.*, **7**, 341–346

Peluso, M., Airoldi, L., Magagnotti, C., Fiorini, L., Munnia, A., Hautefeuille, A.,
Malaveille, C. & Vineis, P. (2000) White blood cell DNA adducts and fruit and vegetable consumption in bladder cancer. *Carcinogenesis*, **21**, 183–187

Pennington, J.A. (2002) Food composition databases for bioactive food components. *J. Food Comp. Anal.*, **15**, 419–434

Perry, C.A., Dwyer, J., Gelfand, J.A., Couris, R.R. & McCloskey, W.W. (1996) Health effects of salicylates in foods and drugs. *Nutr. Rev.*, **54**, 225–240

Persson, I., He, L., Fang, C., Normén, L. & Rylander, R. (2000) Influence of vegetables on the expression of GSTP1 in humans – a pilot intervention study (Sweden). *Cancer Causes Control*, **11**, 359–361

Peters, R.K., Garabrant, D.H., Yu, M.C. & Mack, T.M. (1989) A case–control study of occupational and dietary factors in colorectal cancer in young men by subsite. *Cancer Res.*, **49**, 5459–5468

Peters, R.K., Pike, M.C., Garabrant, D. & Mack, T.M. (1992) Diet and colon cancer in Los Angeles County, California. *Cancer Causes Control*, **3**, 457–473

Peterson, J. & Dwyer, J. (1998) Taxonomic classification helps identify flavonoid-containing foods on a semi-quantitative food frequency questionnaire. *J. Am. Diet. Assoc.*, **98**, 677–685

Peterson, J. & Dwyer, J. (2000) An informatics approach to flavonoid database development. *J. Food Comp. Anal.*, **13**, 441–454

Peto, R., Pike, M.C., Armitage, P., Breslow, N.E., Cox, D.R., Howard, S.V., Mantel, N., McPherson, K., Peto, J. & Smith, P.G. (1976) Design and analysis of randomized clinical trials requiring prolonged observation of each patient. I. Introduction and design. *Br. J. Cancer*, **34**, 585–612

Phelps, S. & Harris, W.S. (1993) Garlic supplementation and lipoprotein oxidation susceptibility. *Lipids*, **28**, 475–477

Phukan, R.K., Chetia, C.K., Ali, M.S. & Mahanta, J. (2001) Role of dietary habits in the development of esophageal cancer in Assam, the north-eastern region of India. *Nutr. Cancer*, **39**, 204–209

Pickle, L.W., Greene, M.H., Ziegler, R.G., Toledo, A., Hoover, R., Lynch, H.T. & Fraumeni, J.F., Jr (1984) Colorectal cancer in rural Nebraska. *Cancer Res.*, **44**, 363–369

Pietinen, P., Hartman, A.M., Haapa, E., Rasanen, L., Haapakoski, J., Palmgren, J., Albanes, D., Virtamo, J. & Huttunen, J.K. (1988) Reproducibility and validity of dietary assessment instruments. I. A self-administered food use questionnaire with a portion size picture booklet. *Am. J. Epidemiol.*, **128**, 655–666

Pietinen, P., Malila, N., Virtanen, M., Hartman, T.J., Tangrea, J.A., Albanes, D. & Virtamo, J. (1999) Diet and risk of colorectal cancer in a cohort of Finnish men. *Cancer Causes Control*, **10**, 387–396

Pillow, P.C., Hursting, S.D., Duphorne, C.M., Jiang, H., Honn, S.E., Chang, S. & Spitz, M.R. (1997) Case–control assessment of diet and lung cancer risk in African Americans and Mexican Americans. *Nutr. Cancer*, **29**, 169–173

Pillow, P.C., Duphorne, C.M., Chang, S., Contois, J.H., Strom, S.S., Spitz, M.R. & Hursting, S.D. (1999) Development of a database for assessing dietary phytoestrogen intake. *Nutr. Cancer*, **33**, 3–19

Pisani, P., Faggiano, F., Krogh, V., Palli, D., Vineis, P. & Berrino, F. (1997) Relative validity and reproducibility of a food frequency dietary questionnaire for use in the Italian EPIC centres. *Int. J. Epidemiol.*, **26 Suppl.1**, S152–S160

Platz, E.A., Giovannucci, E., Rimm, E.B., Rockett, H.R., Stampfer, M.J., Colditz, G.A. & Willett, W.C. (1997) Dietary fiber and distal colorectal adenoma in men. *Cancer Epidemiol. Biomarkers Prev.*, **6**, 661–670

Plummer, M. & Clayton, D. (1993a) Measurement error in dietary assessment: an investigation using covariance structure models. Part I. *Stat. Med.*, **12**, 925–935

Plummer, M. & Clayton, D. (1993b) Measurement error in dietary assessment: an investigation using covariance structure models. Part II. *Stat. Med.*, **12**, 937–948

Poirier, M.C. (1997) DNA adducts as exposure biomarkers and indicators of cancer risk. *Environ. Health Perspect.*, **105**, 907–912

Polasa, K. & Krishnaswamy, K. (1997) Reduction of urinary mutagen excretion in rats fed garlic. *Cancer Lett.*, **114**, 185–186

Polsinelli, M.L., Rock, C.L., Henderson, S.A. & Drewnowski, A. (1998) Plasma carotenoids as biomarkers of fruit and vegetable servings in women. *J. Am. Diet. Assoc.*, **98**, 194–196

Pomerleau, J., McKee, M., Robertson, A., Kadziauskiene, K., Abaravicius, A., Vaask, S., Pudule, I. & Grinberga, D. (2001) Macronutrient and food intake in the Baltic republics. *Eur. J. Clin. Nutr.*, **55**, 200–207

Pool-Zobel, B.L., Bub, A., Muller, H., Wollowski, I. & Rechkemmer, G. (1997) Consumption of vegetables reduces genetic damage in humans: first results of a human intervention trial with carotenoid-rich foods. *Carcinogenesis*, **18**, 1847–1850

Pool-Zobel, B.L., Bub, A., Liegibel, U.M., Treptow-van Lishaut, S. & Rechkemmer, G. (1998) Mechanisms by which vegetable consumption reduces genetic damage in humans. *Cancer Epidemiol. Biomarkers Prev.*, **7**, 891–899

Porrini, M. & Riso, P. (2000) Lymphocyte lycopene concentration and DNA protection from oxidative damage is increased in women after a short period of tomato consumption. *J. Nutr.*, **130**, 189–192

Porrini, M., Riso, P. & Oriani, G. (2002) Spinach and tomato consumption increases lymphocyte DNA resistance to oxidative stress but this is not related to cell carotenoid concentrations. *Eur. J. Nutr.*, **41**, 95–100

Posner, B.M., Smigelski, C., Duggal, A., Morgan, J.L., Cobb, J. & Cupples, L.A. (1992) Validation of two-dimensional models for estimation of portion size in nutrition research. *J. Am. Diet. Assoc.*, **92**, 738–741

Potischman, N., Swanson, C.A., Brinton, L.A., McAdams, M., Barrett, R.J., Berman, M.L., Mortel, R., Twiggs, L.B., Wilbanks, G.D. & Hoover, R.N. (1993) Dietary associations in a case–control study of endometrial cancer. *Cancer Causes Control*, **4**, 239–250

Potischman, N., Weiss, H.A., Swanson, C.A., Coates, R.J., Gammon, M.D., Malone, K.E., Brogan, D., Stanford, J.L., Hoover, R.N. & Brinton, L.A. (1998) Diet during adolescence and risk of breast cancer among young women. *J. Natl Cancer Inst.*, **90**, 226–233

Potischman, N., Swanson, C.A., Coates, R.J., Gammon, M.D., Brogan, D.R., Curtin, J. & Brinton, L.A. (1999) Intake of food groups and associated micronutrients in relation to risk of early-stage breast cancer. *Int. J. Cancer*, **82**, 315–321

Potter, J.D. (1997) Diet and cancer: possible explanations for the higher risk of cancer in the poor. In: Kogevinas, M., Pearce, N., Susser, M. & Boffetta, P., eds, *Social Inequalities and Cancer* (IARC Scientific Publications No. 138), Lyon, IARCPress, pp. 265–283

Potter, J.D. & Steinmetz, K. (1996) Vegetables, fruit and phytoestrogens as preventive agents In: Stewart, B.W., McGregor, D. & Kleihues, P., eds, *Principles of Chemoprevention* (IARC Scientific Publications No. 139), Lyon, IARCPress, pp. 61–90

Pottern, L.M., Morris, L.E., Blot, W.J., Ziegler, R.G. & Fraumeni, J.F., Jr (1981) Esophageal cancer among black men in Washington, D.C. I. Alcohol, tobacco, and other risk factors. *J. Natl. Cancer Inst.*, **67**, 777–783

Prasad, M.P., Krishna, T.P., Pasricha, S., Krishnaswamy, K. & Quereshi, M.A. (1992) Esophageal cancer and diet – a case–control study. *Nutr. Cancer*, **18**, 85–93

Prentice, R.L. (1996) Measurement error and results from analytic epidemiology: dietary fat and breast cancer. *J. Natl. Cancer Inst.*, **88**, 1738–1747

Prieto-Ramos, F., Serra-Majem, L., La Vecchia, C., Ramon, J.M., Tresserras, R. & Salleras, L. (1996) Mortality trends and past and current dietary factors of breast cancer in Spain. *Eur. J. Epidemiol.*, **12**, 141–148

Prineas, R.J., Folsom, A.R., Zhang, Z.M., Sellers, T.A. & Potter, J. (1997) Nutrition and other risk factors for renal cell carcinoma in postmenopausal women. *Epidemiology*, **8**, 31–36

Prochaska, H.J. & Talalay, P. (1988) Regulatory mechanisms of monofunctional and bifunctional anticarcinogenic enzyme inducers in murine liver. *Cancer Res.*, **48**, 4776–4782

Produce for Better Health Foundation and National Cancer Institute (1999) *5-a-Day for Better Health Program Guidebook*, Bethesda, MD, National Cancer Institute

Prowse, A.H., Webster, A.R., Richards, F.M., Richard, S., Olschwang, S., Resche, F., Affara, N.A. & Maher, E.R. (1997) Somatic inactivation of the VHL gene in Von Hippel–Lindau disease tumors. *Am. J. Hum. Genet.*, **60**, 765–771

Puska, P., Nissinen, A., Salonen, J.T. & Toumilehto, J. (1983) Ten years of the North Karelia Project: results with community-based prevention of coronary heart disease. *Scand. J. Soc. Med.*, **11**, 65–68

Qi, X.Y., Zhang, A.Y., Wu, G.L. & Pang, W.Z. (1994) The association between breast cancer and diet and other factors. *Asia Pac. J. Public Health*, **7**, 98–104

Rachtan, J. (2002a) A case–control study of lung cancer in Polish women. *Neoplasma*, **49**, 75–80

Rachtan, J. (2002b) Dietary habits and lung cancer risk among Polish women. *Acta Oncologica*, **41**, 389–394

Rajkumar, T., Franceschi, S., Vaccarella, S., Gajalakshmi, V., Sharmila, A., Snijders, P.J.F., Muñoz, N., Meijer, C.J.L.M. & Herrero, R. (2003a) Role of paan chewing and dietary habits in cervical carcinoma in Chennai, India. *Br. J. Cancer*, **88**, 1388–1393

Rajkumar, T., Sridhar, H., Balaram, P., Vaccarella, S., Gajalakshmi, V.,

Nandakumar, A., Ramdas, K., Jayshree, R., Muñoz, N., Herrero, R., Franceschi, S. & Weiderpass, E. (2003b) Oral cancer in Southern India: the influence of body size, diet, infections and sexual practices. *Eur. J. Cancer Prev.*, **12**, 135–143

Ramon, J.M., Serra, L., Cerdo, C. & Oromi, J. (1993) Dietary factors and gastric cancer risk. A case–control study in Spain. *Cancer*, **71**, 1731–1735

Ranganna, S., Govindarajan, V.S. & Ramana, K.V. (1983) Citrus fruits—varieties, chemistry, technology, and quality evaluation. Part II. Chemistry, technology, and quality evaluation. A. Chemistry. *Crit. Rev. Food Sci. Nutr.*, **18**, 313–386

Rao, A.V. & Agarwal, S. (1998) Bioavailability and *in vivo* antioxidant properties of lycopene from tomato products and their possible role in the prevention of cancer. *Nutr. Cancer*, **31**, 199–203

Ravanat, J.L., Douki, T., Duez, P., Gremaud, E., Herbert, K., Hofer, T., Lasserre, L., Saint-Pierre, C., Favier, A. & Cadet, J. (2002) Cellular background level of 8-oxo-7,8-dihydro-2'-deoxyguanosine: an isotope based method to evaluate artefactual oxidation of DNA during its extraction and subsequent work-up. *Carcinogenesis*, **23**,1911–1918

Record, I.R., Dreosti, I.E. & McInerney, J.K. (2001) Changes in plasma antioxidant status following consumption of diets high or low in fruit and vegetables or following dietary supplementation with an antioxidant mixture. *Br. J. Nutr.*, **85**, 459–464

Reeve, L., (2000) Implementation and evaluation of the Coles 7-a-day program: a DAA partnership promoting fruit and vegetable intake in Australia. In: *Proceedings of the Dietitians Association of Australia 19th National Conference, 2000, May 18–21; Canberra*, Canberra, Dietitians Association of Australia, p. 14

Rehman, A., Bourne, L.C., Halliwell, B. & Rice-Evans, C.A. (1999) Tomato consumption modulates oxidative DNA damage in humans. *Biochem. Biophys. Res. Commun.*, **262**, 828–831

Reinli, K. & Block, G. (1996) Phytoestrogen content of foods – a compendium of literature values. *Nutr. Cancer*, **26**, 123–148

Renaud, S.C. & Lanzmann-Petithory, D. (2002) The beneficial effect of alpha-linolenic acid in coronary artery disease is not questionable. *Am. J. Clin. Nutr.*, **76**, 903–904

Renaud, S., de Lorgeril, M., Delaye, J., Guidollet, J., Jacquard, F., Mamelle, N., Martin, J.L., Monjaud, I., Salen, P. & Toubol, P. (1995) Cretan Mediterranean diet for prevention of coronary heart disease. *Am. J. Clin. Nutr.*, **61**, 1360S–1367S

Reuter, H.D., Koch, H.P. & Lawson, L.D. (1996) Therapeutic effects and applications of garlic and its preparation. In: Koch, H.P. & Lawson, L. D., eds, *Garlic: The Science and Therapeutic Application of Allium sativum L. and Related Species*, Baltimore, Williams and Wilkins, pp. 135–212

Riboli, E. (1992) Nutrition and cancer: background and rationale of the European Prospective Investigation into Cancer and Nutrition (EPIC). *Ann. Oncol.*, **3**, 783–791

Riboli, E. & Kaaks, R. (1997) The EPIC project: rationale and study design. European Prospective Investigation into Cancer and Nutrition. *Int. J. Epidemiol.*, **26 Suppl 1**, S6–14

Riboli, E. & Norat T. (2003) Epidemiological evidence of the protective effect of fruits and vegetables on cancer risk. *Am. J. Clin. Nutr.*, **78**, 559S–569S

Riboli, E., Gonzalez, C.A., Lopez-Abente, G., Errezola, M., Izarzugaza, I., Escolar, A., Nebot, M., Hémon, B. & Agudo, A. (1991) Diet and bladder cancer in Spain: a multi-centre case–control study. *Int. J. Cancer*, **49**, 214–219

Riboli, E., Hunt, K.J., Slimani, N., Ferrari, P., Norat, T., Fahey, M., Charrondière, R.U., Hémon, B., Casagrande, C., Vignat, J., Overvad, K., Tjonneland, A., Clavel-Chapelon, F., Thiébaut, A., Wahrendorf, J., Boeing, H., Trichopoulos, D., Trichopoulou, A., Vineis, P., Palli, D., Bueno de Mesquita, H.B., Peeters, P.H., Lund, E., Engeset, D., Gonzalez, C.A., Barricarte, A., Berglung, G., Hallmans, G., Day, N.E., Key, T.J., Kaaks, R. & Saracci, R. (2002) European Prospective Investigation into Cancer and Nutrition (EPIC): Study populations and data collection. *Public Health Nutr.*, **5**, 1113–1124

Richardson, S., Gerber, M. & Cenee, S. (1991) The role of fat, animal protein and some vitamin consumption in breast cancer: a case control study in southern France. *Int. J. Cancer*, **48**, 1–9

Richter, E., Rosler, S. & Becker, A. (2000) Effect of diet on haemoglobin adducts from 4-aminobiphenyl in rats. *Arch. Toxicol.*, **74**, 203–206

Rieder, A., Adamek, M. & Wrba, H. (1983) Delay of diethylnitrosamine-induced hepatoma in rats by carrot feeding. *Oncology*, **40**, 120–123

Riggs, D.R., DeHaven, J.I. & Lamm, D.L. (1997) *Allium sativum* (garlic) treatment for murine transitional cell carcinoma. *Cancer*, **79**, 1987–1994

Rijnkels, J.M. & Alink, G.M. (1998) Effects of a vegetables–fruit mixture on liver and colonic 1,2-dimethylhydrazine-metabolizing enzyme activities in rats fed low- or high-fat diets. *Cancer Lett.*, **128**, 171–175

Rijnkels, J.M., Hollanders, V.M.H., Woutersen, R.A., Koeman, J.H. & Alink, G.M. (1997a) Interaction of dietary fat and of a vegetables/fruit mixture on 1,2-dimethylhydrazine- or *N*-methyl-*N'*-nitro-*N*-nitrosoguanidine-induced colorectal cancer in rats. *Cancer Lett.*, **114**, 297–298

Rijnkels, J.M., Hollanders, V.M.H., Woutersen, R.A., Koeman, J.H. & Alink, G.M. (1997b) Interaction of dietary fat with a vegetables–fruit mixture on 1,2-dimethylhydrazine-induced colorectal cancer in rats. *Nutr. Cancer*, **27**, 261–266

Rijnkels, J.M., Hollanders, V.M.H., Woutersen, R.A., Koeman, J.H. & Alink, G.M. (1997c) Modulation of dietary fat-enhanced colorectal carcinogenesis in *N*-methyl-*N'*-nitro-*N*-nitrosoguanidine-treated rats by a vegetables-fruit mixture. *Nutr. Cancer*, **29**, 90–95

Rijnkels, J.M., Hollanders, V.M.H., Woutersen, R.A., Koeman, J.H. & Alink, G.M. (1998) Absence of an inhibitory effect of a vegetables–fruit mixture on the initiation and promotion phases of azoxymethane-induced colorectal carcinogenesis in rats fed low- or high-fat diets. *Nutr. Cancer,* **30,** 124–129

Rimm, E.B., Stampfer, M.J., Ascherio, A., Giovannucci, E., Colditz, G.A. & Willett, W.C. (1993) Vitamin E consumption and the risk of coronary heart disease in men. *New Engl. J. Med.,* **328,** 1450–1456

Risch, H.A., Jain, M., Choi, N.W., Fodor, J.G., Pfeiffer, C.J., Howe, G.R., Harrison, L.W., Craib, K.J. & Miller, A.B. (1985) Dietary factors and the incidence of cancer of the stomach. *Am. J. Epidemiol.,* **122,** 947–959

Riso, P., Pinder, A., Santangelo, A. & Porrini, M. (1999) Does tomato consumption effectively increase the resistance of lymphocyte DNA to oxidative damage? *Am. J. Clin. Nutr.,* **69,** 712–718

Rissanen, T.H., Voutilainen, S., Virtanen, J.K., Venho, B., Vanharanta, M., Mursu, J. & Salonen, J.T. (2003) Low intake of fruits, berries and vegetables is associated with excess mortality in men: the Kuopio Ischaemic Heart Disease Risk Factor (KIHD) Study. *J. Nutr.,* **133,** 199–204

Rock, C.L., Jacob, R.A. & Bowen, P.E. (1996) Update on the biological characteristics of the antioxidant micronutrients: vitamin C, vitamin E, and the carotenoids. *J. Am. Diet. Assoc.,* **96,** 693–702

Rohan, T.E., Howe, G.R., Friedenreich, C.M., Jain, M. & Miller, A.B. (1993) Dietary fiber, vitamins A, C, and E, and risk of breast cancer: a cohort study. *Cancer Causes Control,* **4,** 29–37

Rolon, P.A., Castellsague, X., Benz, M. & Muñoz, N. (1995) Hot and cold mate drinking and esophageal cancer in Paraguay. *Cancer Epidemiol. Biomarkers Prev.,* **4,** 595–605

Ronco, A., De Stefani, E., Boffetta, P., Deneo-Pellegrini, H., Mendilaharsu, M. & Leborgne, F. (1999) Vegetables, fruits, and related nutrients and risk of breast cancer: a case–control study in Uruguay. *Nutr. Cancer,* **35,** 111–119

Rose, D.P., Boyar, A.P. & Wynder, E.L. (1986) International comparisons of mortality rates for cancer of the breast, ovary, prostate, and colon, and *per capita* food consumption. *Cancer,* **58,** 2363–2371

Rosenberger, G. (1939) Anaemie und Haemoglobinurie beim Rind nach Markstammkohl-Fütterung. *Deutsche tierärztliche Wochenschrift,* **47,** 244–246

Rosenblatt, K.A., Thomas, D.B., Jimenez, L.M., Fish, B., McTiernan, A., Stalsberg, H., Stemhagen, A., Thompson, W.D., Curnen, M.G., Satariano, W., Austin, D.F., Greenberg, R.S., Key, C., Kolonel, L.N. & West, D.W. (1999) The relationship between diet and breast cancer in men (United States). *Cancer Causes Control,* **10,** 107–113

Rosner, B. & Gore, R. (2001) Measurement error correction in nutritional epidemiology based on individual foods, with application to the relation of diet to breast cancer. *Am. J. Epidemiol.,* **154,** 827–835

Rosner, B. & Willett, W.C. (1988) Interval estimates for correlation coefficients corrected for within-person variation: implications for study design and hypothesis testing. *Am. J. Epidemiol.,* **127,** 377–386

Rosner, B., Willett, W.C. & Spiegelman, D. (1989) Correction of logistic regression relative risk estimates and confidence intervals for systematic within-person measurement error. *Stat. Med.,* **8,** 1051–1069

Ross, J.A., Davies, S.M., Wentzlaff, K.A., Campbell, D.R., Martini, M.C., Slavin, J.L. & Potter, J.D. (1995) Dietary modulation of serum platelet-derived growth factor-AB levels. *Cancer Epidemiol. Biomarkers Prev.,* **4,** 485–489

Russell, C., Palmer, J.R., Adams-Campbell, L.L. & Rosenberg, L. (2001) Follow-up of a large cohort of Black women. *Am. J. Epidemiol.,* **154,** 845–853

Sadek, I., Abdel-Salam, F. & Al-Qattan, K. (1995) Chemopreventive effects of cabbage on 7,12-dimethylbenz(a)-anthracene-induced hepatocarcinogenesis in toads (*Bufo viridis*). *J. Nutr. Sci. Vitaminol. (Tokyo),* **41,** 163–168

Safe, S. (2001) Molecular biology of the Ah receptor and its role in carcinogenesis. *Toxicol. Lett.,* **120,** 1–7

Salazar-Martinez, E., Lazcano-Ponce, E.C., Gonzalez Lira-Lira, G., Escudero-De los, R.P. & Hernandez-Avila, M. (2002) Nutritional determinants of epithelial ovarian cancer risk: a case–control study in Mexico. *Oncology,* **63,** 151–157

Samet, J.M., Humble, C.G. & Skipper, B.E. (1984) Alternatives in the collection and analysis of food frequency interview data. *Am. J. Epidemiol.,* **120,** 572–581

Sampson, L., Rimm, E., Hollman, P.C., de Vries, J.H. & Katan, M.B. (2002) Flavonol and flavone intakes in US health professionals. *J. Am. Diet. Assoc.,* **102,** 1414–1420

Sánchez, M.J., Martínez, C., Nieto, A., Castellsagué, X., Quintana, M.J., Bosch, F.X., Muñoz, N., Herrero, R. & Franceschi, S. (2003) Oral and oropharyngeal cancer in Spain: influence of dietary patterns. *Eur. J. Cancer Prev.,* **12,** 49–56

Sanchez-Diez, A., Hernandez-Mejia, R. & Cueto-Espinar, A. (1992) Study of the relation between diet and gastric cancer in a rural area of the Province of Leon, Spain. *Eur. J. Epidemiol.,* **8,** 233–237

Sandler, R.S., Lyles, C.M., Peipins, L.A., McAuliffe, C.A., Woosley, J.T. & Kupper, L.L. (1993) Diet and risk of colorectal adenomas: macronutrients, cholesterol, and fiber. *J. Natl Cancer Inst.,* **85,** 884–891

Sankaranarayanan, R., Varghese, C., Duffy, S.W., Padmakumary, G., Day, N.E. & Nair, M.K. (1994) A case–control study of diet and lung cancer in Kerala, south India. *Int. J. Cancer,* **58,** 644–649

Sauvaget, C., Nagano, H.J., Hayashi, M., Spencer, E., Shimizu, Y. & Allen, N. (2003) Vegetables and fruit intake and cancer mortality in the Hiroshima/Nagasaki Life span Study. *Br. J. Cancer,* **88,** 689–694

Schaffer, E.M., Liu, J.Z., Green, J., Dangler, C.A. & Milner, J.A. (1996) Garlic and associated allyl sulfur components inhibit N-methyl-N-nitrosourea induced rat mammary carcinogenesis. *Cancer Lett.*, **102**, 199–204

Schaffer, E.M., Liu, J.Z. & Milner, J.A. (1997) Garlic powder and allyl sulfur compounds enhance the ability of dietary selenite to inhibit 7,12-dimethylbenz[a]anthracene-induced mammary DNA adducts. *Nutr. Cancer*, **27**, 162–168

Schatzkin, A., Freedman, L.S., Dawsey, S.M. & Lanza, E. (1994) Interpreting precursor studies: what polyp trials tell us about large-bowel cancer. *J. Natl Cancer Inst.*, **86**, 1053–1057

Schatzkin, A., Lanza, E., Corle, D., Lance, P., Iber, F., Caan, B., Shike, M., Weissfeld, J., Burt, R., Cooper, M.R., Kikendall, J.W. & Cahill, J. (2000) Lack of effect of a low-fat, high-fiber diet on the recurrence of colorectal adenomas. Polyp Prevention Trial Study Group. *New Engl. J. Med.*, **342**, 1149–1155

Schroll, K., Carbajal, A., Decarli, B., Martins, I., Grunenberger, F., Blauw, Y.H., de Groot, C.P.G.M. for the SENECA Investigators (1996) Food patterns of elderly Europeans. *Eur. J. Clin. Nutr.*, **50 Suppl. 2**, S86–S100

Schroll, K., Moreiras-Varela, O., Schlettwein-Gsell, D., Decarli, B., de Groot, L. & van Staveren, W. (1997) Cross-cultural variations and changes in food-group intake among elderly women in Europe: results from the Survey in Europe on Nutrition and the Elderly a Concerted Action (SENECA). *Am. J. Clin. Nutr.*, **65 Suppl.**, 1282S–1289S

Schuurman, A.G., Goldbohm, R.A., Dorant, E. & van den Brandt, P.A. (1998) Vegetable and fruit consumption and prostate cancer risk: a cohort study in The Netherlands. *Cancer Epidemiol. Biomarkers Prev.*, **7**, 673–680

Seow, A., Poh, W.T., Teh, M., Eng, P., Wang, Y.T., Tan, W.C., Chia, K.S., Yu, M.C. & Lee, H.P. (2002) Diet, reproductive factors and lung cancer risk among Chinese women in Singapore: evidence for a protective effect of soy in nonsmokers. *Int. J. Cancer*, **97**, 365–371

Serafini, M., Maiani, G. & Ferro-Luzzi, A. (1998) Alcohol-free red wine enhances plasma antioxidant capacity in humans. *J. Nutr.*, **128**, 1003–1007

Serafini, M., Bellocco, R., Wolk, A. & Ekström, A.M. (2002) Total antioxidant potential of fruit and vegetables and risk of gastric cancer. *Gastroenterology*, **123**, 985–991

Serdula, M., Coates, R., Byers, T., Mokdad, A., Jewell, S., Chavez, N., Mares-Perlman, J., Newcomb, P., Ritenbaugh, C. & Treiber, F. (1993) Evaluation of a brief telephone questionnaire to estimate fruit and vegetable consumption in diverse study populations. *Epidemiology*, **4**, 455–463

Serdula, M.K., Byers, T., Mokdad, A.H., Simoes, E., Mendlein, J.M. & Coates, R.J. (1996) The association between fruit and vegetable intake and chronic disease risk factors. *Epidemiology*, **7**, 161–165

Severson, R.K., Nomura, A.M., Grove, J.S. & Stemmermann, G.N. (1989) A prospective study of demographics, diet, and prostate cancer among men of Japanese ancestry in Hawaii. *Cancer Res.*, **49**, 1857–1860

Shannon, J., White, E., Shattuck, A.L. & Potter, J.D. (1996) Relationship of food groups and water intake to colon cancer risk. *Cancer Epidemiol. Biomarkers Prev.*, **5**, 495–502

Sharif, S.I. & Ali, B.H. (1994) Effect of grapefruit juice on drug metabolism in rats. *Food Chem. Toxicol.*, **32**, 1169–1171

Sharp, L., Chilvers, C.E., Cheng, K.K., McKinney, P.A., Logan, R.F., Cook-Mozaffari, P., Ahmed, A. & Day, N.E. (2001) Risk factors for squamous cell carcinoma of the oesophagus in women: a case–control study. *Br. J. Cancer*, **85**, 1667–1670

Sheen, L.Y., Chen, H.W., Kung, Y.L., Liu, C.T. & Lii, C.K. (1999) Effects of garlic oil and its organosulfur compounds on the activities of hepatic drug-metabolizing and antioxidant enzymes in rats fed high- and low-fat diets. *Nutr. Cancer*, **35**, 160–166

Shibata, A., Paganini-Hill, A., Ross, R.K. & Henderson, B.E. (1992) Intake of vegetables, fruits, β-carotene, vitamin C and vitamin supplements and cancer incidence among the elderly: a prospective study. *Br. J. Cancer*, **66**, 673–679

Shibata, A., Mack, T.M., Paganini-Hill, A., Ross, R.K. & Henderson, B.E. (1994) A prospective study of pancreatic cancer in the elderly. *Int. J. Cancer*, **58**, 46–49

Shimada, A. (1986) Regional differences in gastric cancer mortality and eating habits of people [in Japanese]. *Gan No Rinsho*, **32**, 692–698

Shoichet, S.A., Baumer, A.T., Stamenkovic, D., Sauer, H., Pfeiffer, A.F., Kahn, C.R., Muller-Wieland, D., Richter, C. & Ristow, M. (2002) Frataxin promotes antioxidant defense in a thiol-dependent manner resulting in diminished malignant transformation in vitro. *Hum. Mol. Genet.*, **11**, 815–821

Shu, X.O., Gao, Y.T., Yuan, J.M., Ziegler, R.G. & Brinton, L.A. (1989) Dietary factors and epithelial ovarian cancer. *Br. J. Cancer*, **59**, 92–96

Shu, X.O., Zheng, W., Potischman, N., Brinton, L.A., Hatch, M.C., Gao, Y.T. & Fraumeni, J.F., Jr (1993) A population-based case–control study of dietary factors and endometrial cancer in Shanghai, People's Republic of China. *Am. J. Epidemiol.*, **137**, 155–165

Shyu, K.W. & Meng, C.L. (1987) The inhibitory effect of oral administration of garlic on experimental carcinogenesis in hamster buccal pouches by DMBA painting. *Proc. Natl Sci. Counc. Repub. China B*, **11**, 137–147

Sichieri, R., Everhart, J.E. & Mendonça, G.A. (1996) Diet and mortality from common cancers in Brazil: an ecological study. *Cad. Saude Publica*, **12**, 53–59

Sidenvall, B., Fjellström, C., Andersson, J., Gustafsson, K., Nygren, U. & Nydahl, M. (2002) Reasons among older Swedish women of not participating in a food survey. *Eur. J. Clin. Nutr.*, **56**, 561–567

References

SIGN, eds (2001) http://www.sign.ac.uk/guidelines/fulltext/50/index.html, Edinburgh, Scottish Intercollegiate Guidelines Network

Sigurdson, A.J., Chang, S., Annegers, J.F., Duphorne, C.M., Pillow, P.C., Amato, R.J., Hutchinson, L.P., Sweeney, A.M. & Strom, S.S. (1999) A case–control study of diet and testicular carcinoma. *Nutr. Cancer*, **34**, 20–26

Silverman, D.T., Swanson, C.A., Gridley, G., Wacholder, S., Greenberg, R.S., Brown, L.M., Hayes, R.B., Swanson, G.M., Schoenberg, J.B., Pottern, L.M., Schwartz, A.G., Fraumeni, J.F., Jr & Hoover, R.N. (1998) Dietary and nutritional factors and pancreatic cancer: A case–control study based on direct interviews. *J. Natl Cancer Inst.*, **90**, 1710–1719

Slattery, M.L. (2001) Does an apple a day keep breast cancer away? *JAMA*, **285,** 799–801

Slattery, M.L., Sorenson, A.W., Mahoney, A.W., French, T.K., Kritchevsky, D. & Street, J.C. (1988) Diet and colon cancer: assessment of risk by fiber type and food source. *J. Natl Cancer Inst.*, **80**, 1474–1480

Slimani, N., Ferrari, P., Ocke, M., Welch, A., Boeing, H., Liere, M., Pala, V., Amiano, P., Lagiou, A., Mattisson, I., Stripp, C., Engeset, D., Charrondière, R., Buzzard, M., Staveren, W. & Riboli, E. (2000) Standardization of the 24-hour diet recall calibration method used in the European Prospective Investigation into Cancer and Nutrition (EPIC): general concepts and preliminary results. *Eur. J. Clin. Nutr.*, **54**, 900–917

Slimani, N., Kaaks, R., Ferrari, P., Casagrande, C., Clavel-Chapelon, F., Lotze, G., Kroke, A., Trichopoulos, D., Trichopoulou, A., Lauria, C., Bellegotti, M., Ocké, M.C., Peeters, P.H., Engeset, D., Lund, E., Agudo, A., Larranaga, N., Mattisson, I., Andren, C., Johansson, I., Davey, G., Welch, A., Overvad, K., Tjonneland, A., van Staveren, W.A., Saracci, R. & Riboli, E. (2002) European Prospective Investigation into Cancer and Nutrition (EPIC) calibration study: rationale, design and population characteristics. *Public Health Nutr.*, **5**, 1125–1145

Smith, R.H. (1978) S-Methyl cysteine sulphoxide, the *Brassica* anaemia factor: a valuable dietary factor for man? *Vet. Sci. Commun.*, **2,** 47–62

Smith, A.F., Jobe, J.B. & Mingay, D.J. (1991) Question-induced cognitive biases in reports of dietary intake by college men and women. *Health Psychol.*, **10**, 244–251

Smith, S.A., Campbell, D.R., Elmer, P.J., Martini, M.C., Slavin, J.L. & Potter, J.D. (1995) The University of Minnesota Cancer Prevention Research Unit vegetable and fruit classification scheme (United States). *Cancer Causes Control*, **6,** 292–302

Smith-Warner, S.A., Elmer, P.J., Fosdick, L., Tharp, T.M. & Randall, B. (1997) Reliability and comparability of three dietary assessment methods for estimating fruit and vegetable intakes. *Epidemiology*, **8**, 196–201

Smith-Warner, S.A., Elmer, P.J., Tharp, T.M., Fosdick, L., Randall, B., Gross, M., Wood, J. & Potter, J.D. (2000) Increasing vegetable and fruit intake: randomized intervention and monitoring in an at-risk population. *Cancer Epidemiol. Biomarkers Prev.*, **9**, 307–317

Smith-Warner, S.A., Spiegelman, D., Yaun, S.S., Adami, H.O., Beeson, W.L., van den Brandt, P.A., Folsom, A.R., Fraser, G.E., Freudenheim, J.L., Goldbohm, R.A., Graham, S., Miller, A.B., Potter, J.D., Rohan, T.E., Speizer, F.E., Toniolo, P., Willett, W.C., Wolk, A., Zeleniuch-Jacquotte, A. & Hunter, D.J. (2001a) Intake of fruits and vegetables and risk of breast cancer: a pooled analysis of cohort studies. *JAMA*, **285**, 769–776

Smith-Warner, S.A., Spiegelman, D., Yaun, S.S., Adami, H.O., Beeson, W.L., van den Brandt, P.A., Folsom, A.R., Fraser, G.E., Freudenheim, J.L., Goldbohm, R.A., Graham, S., Miller, A.B., Potter, J.D., Rohan, T.E., Speizer, F.E., Toniolo, P., Willett, W.C., Wolk, A., Zeleniuch-Jacquotte, A. & Hunter, D.J. (2001) Intake of fruits and vegetables and risk of breast cancer: a pooled analysis of cohort studies. *JAMA*, **285**, 769–776

Smith-Warner, S.A., Spiegelman, D. & Hunter, D. (2002a) Fruits and vegetables and colorectal cancer: A pooled analysis of cohort studies. *Am. J. Epidemiol.*, **155**, S106 (SER Abstract)

Smith-Warner, S.A., Elmer, P.J., Fosdick, L., Randall, B., Bostick, R.M., Grandits, G., Grambsch, P., Louis, T.A., Wood, J.R. & Potter, J.D. (2002b) Fruits, vegetables, and adenomatous polyps: the Minnesota Cancer Prevention Research Unit case–control study. *Am. J. Epidemiol.*, **155**, 1104–1113

Smith-Warner, S.A., Spiegelman, D., Yaun, S.S., Albanes, D., Beeson, W.L., van den Brandt, P.A., Feskanich, D., Folsom, A.R., Fraser, G.E., Freudenheim, J.L., Giovannucci, E., Goldbohm, R.A., Graham, S., Kushi, L.H., Miller, A.B., Pietinen, P., Rohan, T.E., Speizer, F.E., Willett, W.C. & Hunter, D.J. (2003) Fruits and vegetables and lung cancer: A pooled analysis of cohort studies. *Int. J. Cancer* (in press)

Song, K. & Milner, J.A. (1999) Heating garlic inhibits its ability to suppress 7,12-dimethylbenz(a)anthracene-induced DNA adduct formation in rat mammary tissue. *J. Nutr.*, **129,** 657–661

Sørensen, M., Jensen, B.R., Poulsen, H.E., Deng, X., Tygstrup, N., Dalhoff, K. & Loft, S. (2001) Effects of a Brussels sprouts extract on oxidative DNA damage and metabolising enzymes in rat liver. *Food Chem. Toxicol.*, **39**, 533–540

Sousa, J., Nath, J. & Ong, T. (1985) Dietary factors affecting the urinary mutagenicity assay system. II. The absence of mutagenic activity in human urine following consumption of red wine or grape juice. *Mutat. Res.*, **156,** 171–176

Spanos, G.A. & Wrolstad, R.E. (1992) Phenolics of apple, pear, and white grape juices and their changes with processing and storage – a review. *J. Agric. Food Chem.*, **40**, 1478–1487

Sparnins, V.L., Venegas, P.L. & Wattenberg, L.W. (1982) Glutathione S-transferase activity: enhancement by compounds inhibiting chemical carcinogenesis and by dietary constituents. *J. Natl Cancer Inst.*, **68**, 493–496

Sreerama, L., Hedge, M.W. & Sladek, N.E. (1995) Identification of a class 3 aldehyde dehydrogenase in human saliva and increased levels of this enzyme, glutathione S-transferases, and DT-diaphorase in the saliva of subjects who continually ingest large quantities of coffee or broccoli. *Clin. Cancer Res.*, **1**, 1153–1163

Srivatanakul, P., Parkin, D.M., Khlat, M., Chenvidhya, D., Chotiwan, P., Insiripong, S., L'Abbé, K.A. & Wild, C.P. (1991) Liver cancer in Thailand. II. A case–control study of hepatocellular carcinoma. *Int. J. Cancer*, **48**, 329–332

Stables, G.J., Subar, A.F., Patterson, B.H., Dodd, K., Heimendinger, J., Van Duyn, M.A. & Nebeling, L. (2002) Changes in vegetable and fruit consumption and awareness among US adults: results of the 1991 and 1997 5 A Day for Better Health Program surveys. *J. Am. Diet. Assoc.*, **102**, 809–817

Steineck, G., Norell, S.E. & Feychting, M. (1988) Diet, tobacco and urothelial cancer. A 14-year follow-up of 16,477 subjects. *Acta Oncol.*, **27**, 323–327

Steiner, M. & Lin, R.S. (1998) Changes in platelet function and susceptibility of lipoproteins to oxidation associated with administration of aged garlic extract. *J. Cardiovasc. Pharmacol.*, **31**, 904–908

Steinmaus, C.M., Nuñez, S. & Smith, A.H. (2000) Diet and bladder cancer: a meta-analysis of six dietary variables. *Am. J. Epidemiol.*, **151**, 693–702

Steinmetz, K.A. & Potter, J.D. (1991) Vegetables, fruit, and cancer. II. Mechanisms. *Cancer Causes Control*, **2**, 427–442

Steinmetz, K.A. & Potter, J.D. (1993) Food-group consumption and colon cancer in the Adelaide Case–Control Study. I. Vegetables and fruit. *Int. J. Cancer*, **53**, 711–719

Steinmetz, K.A., Potter, J.D. & Folsom, A.R. (1993) Vegetables, fruit, and lung cancer in the Iowa Women's Health Study. *Cancer Res.*, **53**, 536–543

Steinmetz, K.A., Kushi, L.H., Bostick, R.M., Folsom, A.R. & Potter, J.D. (1994) Vegetables, fruit, and colon cancer in the Iowa Women's Health Study. *Am. J. Epidemiol.*, **139**, 1–15

Stern, K.R., ed. (1988) *Introductory Plant Biology*, Dubuque, IA, W.C. Brown

Stoewsand, G.S. (1995) Bioactive organosulfur phytochemicals in Brassica oleracea vegetables – a review. *Food Chem. Toxicol.*, **33**, 537–543

Stoewsand, G.S., Anderson, J.L. & Munson, L. (1988) Protective effect of dietary brussels sprouts against mammary carcinogenesis in Sprague-Dawley rats. *Cancer Lett.*, **39**, 199–207

Stoewsand, G.S., Anderson, J.L., Munson, L. & Lisk, D.J. (1989) Effect of dietary Brussels sprouts with increased selenium content on mammary carcinogenesis in the rat. *Cancer Lett.*, **45**, 43–48

Stolzenberg-Solomon, R.Z., Pietinen, P., Taylor, P.R., Virtamo, J. & Albanes, D. (2002) Prospective study of diet and pancreatic cancer in male smokers. *Am. J. Epidemiol.*, **155**, 783–792

Stoner, G.D., Kresty, L.A., Carlton, P.S., Siglin, J.C. & Morse, M.A. (1999) Isothiocyanates and freeze-dried strawberries as inhibitors of esophageal cancer. *Toxicol. Sci.*, **52 (Suppl.)**, 95–100

Story, M. & Harris, L.J. (1989) Food habits and dietary change of Southeast Asian refugee families living in the United States. *J. Am. Diet. Assoc.*, **89**, 800–803

Stram, D.O., Hankin, J.H., Wilkens, L.R., Pike, M.C., Monroe, K.R., Park, S., Henderson, B.E., Nomura, A.M., Earle, M.E., Nagamine, F.S. & Kolonel, L.N. (2000) Calibration of the dietary questionnaire for a multiethnic cohort in Hawaii and Los Angeles. *Am. J. Epidemiol.*, **151**, 358–370

Stram, D.O., Huberman, M. & Wu, A.H. (2002) Is residual confounding a reasonable explanation for the apparent protective effects of beta-carotene found in epidemiologic studies of lung cancer in smokers? *Am. J. Epidemiol.*, **155**, 622–628

Strandhagen, E., Hansson, P.O., Bosaeus, I., Isaksson, B. & Eriksson, H. (2000) High fruit intake may reduce mortality among middle-aged and elderly men. The Study of Men Born in 1913. *Eur. J. Clin. Nutr.*, **54**, 337–341

Stroup, D.F. & Thacker, S.B. (2000) Meta-analysis in epidemiology. In: Gail, M.H. & Bénichou, J., eds, *Encyclopedia of Epidemiologic Methods*, Chichester, New York, Wiley, pp. 557–570

Stucker, I., Jacquet, M., de, W., I, Cenee, S., Beaune, P., Kremers, P. & Hemon, D. (2000) Relation between inducibility of CYP1A1, GSTM1 and lung cancer in a French population. *Pharmacogenetics*, **10**, 617–627

Subar, A.F., Harlan, L.C. & Mattson, M.E. (1990) Food and nutrient intake differences between smokers and non-smokers in the US. *Am. J. Public Health*, **80**, 1323–1329

Subar, A.F., Thompson, F.E., Smith, A.F., Jobe, J.B., Ziegler, R.G., Potischman, N., Schatzkin, A., Hartman, A., Swanson, C., Kruse, L., Hayes, R.B., Riedel Lewis, D. & Harlan, L.C. (1995) Improving food frequency questionnaires: a qualitative approach using cognitive interviewing. *J. Am. Diet. Assoc.*, **95**, 781–788

Subar, A.F., Midthune, D., Kulldorff, M., Brown, C.C., Thompson, F.E., Kipnis, V. & Schatzkin, A. (2000) Evaluation of alternative approaches to assign nutrient values to food groups in food frequency questionnaires. *Am. J. Epidemiol.*, **152**, 279–286

Sung, J.F., Lin, R.S., Pu, Y.S., Chen, Y.C., Chang, H.C. & Lai, M.K. (1999) Risk factors for prostate carcinoma in Taiwan: a case–control study in a Chinese population. *Cancer*, **86**, 484–491

References

Suzuki, I., Hamada, G.S., Zamboni, M.M., Cordeiro, P.B., Watanabe, S. & Tsugane, S. (1994) Risk factors for lung cancer in Rio de Janeiro, Brazil: a case–control study. *Lung Cancer*, **11**, 179–190

Swan, S.H., Shaw, G.M. & Schulman, J. (1992) Reporting and selection bias in case-control studies of congenital malformations. *Epidemiology*, **3**, 356–363

Swanson, C.A., Mao, B.L., Li, J.Y., Lubin, J.H., Yao, S.X., Wang, J.Z., Cai, S.K., Hou, Y., Luo, Q.S. & Blot, W.J. (1992) Dietary determinants of lung-cancer risk: results from a case–control study in Yunnan Province, China. *Int. J. Cancer*, **50**, 876–880

Swerdlow, A.J., De Stavola, B.L., Swanwick, M.A., Mangtani, P. & Maconochie, N.E. (1999) Risk factors for testicular cancer: a case–control study in twins. *Br. J. Cancer*, **80**, 1098–1102

Swistak, E., Sawicka, B., Rejman, K. & Berger, S. (1996) Nutrition and mortality from some diet-related diseases [in Polish]. *Rocz. Panstw. Zakl. Hig.*, **47**, 303–312

Szeto, Y.T., Tomlinson, B. & Benzie, I.F. (2002) Total antioxidant and ascorbic acid content of fresh fruits and vegetables: implications for dietary planning and food preservation. *Br. J. Nutr.*, **87**, 55–59

Tagesson, C., Kallberg, M., Klintenberg, C. & Starkhammar, H. (1995) Determination of urinary 8-hydroxydeoxyguanosine by automated coupled-column high performance liquid chromatography: a powerful technique for assaying in vivo oxidative DNA damage in cancer patients. *Eur. J. Cancer*, **31A**, 934–940

Takezaki, T., Gao, C.M., Ding, J.H., Liu, T.K., Li, M.S. & Tajima, K. (1999) Comparative study of lifestyles of residents in high and low risk areas for gastric cancer in Jiangsu Province, China; with special reference to allium vegetables. *J. Epidemiol.*, **9**, 297–305

Takezaki, T., Hirose, K., Inoue, M., Hamajima, N., Kuroishi, T., Nakamura, S., Koshikawa, T., Matsuura, H. & Tajima, K. (1996) Tobacco, alcohol and dietary factors associated with the risk of oral cancer among Japanese. *Jpn J. Cancer Res.*, **87**, 555–562

Takezaki, T., Hirose, K., Inoue, M., Hamajima, N., Yatabe, Y., Mitsudomi, T., Sugiura, T., Kuroishi, T. & Tajima, K. (2001) Dietary factors and lung cancer risk in Japanese: with special reference to fish consumption and adenocarcinomas. *Br. J. Cancer*, **84**, 1199–1206

Talalay, P., De Long, M.J. & Prochaska, H.J. (1988) Identification of a common chemical signal regulating the induction of enzymes that protect against chemical carcinogenesis. *Proc. Natl Acad. Sci. USA*, **85**, 8261–8265

Talalay, P. & Fahey, J.W. (2001) Phytochemicals from cruciferous plants protect against cancer by modulating carcinogen metabolism. *J. Nutr.*, **131**, 3027S–3033S

Talamini, R., Baron, A.E., Barra, S., Bidoli, E., La Vecchia, C., Negri, E., Serraino, D. & Franceschi, S. (1990) A case–control study of risk factor for renal cell cancer in northern Italy. *Cancer Causes Control*, **1**, 125–131

Talamini, R., Franceschi, S., La Vecchia, C., Serraino, D., Barra, S. & Negri, E. (1992) Diet and prostatic cancer: a case–control study in northern Italy. *Nutr. Cancer*, **18**, 277–286

Tanaka, T., Kohno, H., Murakami, M., Shimada, R., Kagami, S., Sumida, T., Azuma, Y. & Ogawa, H. (2000) Suppression of azoxymethane-induced colon carcinogenesis in male F344 rats by mandarin juices rich in β-cryptoxanthin and hesperidin. *Int. J. Cancer*, **88**, 146–150

Tang, D., Cho, S., Rundle, A., Chen, S., Phillips, D., Zhou, J., Hsu, Y., Schnabel, F., Estabrook, A. & Perera, F.P. (2002) Polymorphisms in the DNA repair enzyme XPD are associated with increased levels of PAH-DNA adducts in a case–control study of breast cancer. *Breast Cancer Res. Treat.*, **75**, 159–166

Tavani, A., Negri, E., Franceschi, S. & La Vecchia, C. (1993) Risk factors for esophageal cancer in women in northern Italy. *Cancer*, **72**, 2531–2536

Tavani, A., Negri, E., Franceschi, S. & La Vecchia, C. (1994) Risk factors for esophageal cancer in lifelong nonsmokers. *Cancer Epidemiol. Biomarkers Prev.*, **3**, 387–392

Tavani, A., Negri, E., Franceschi, S. & La Vecchia, C. (1996) Tobacco and other risk factors for oesophageal cancer in alcohol non-drinkers. *Eur. J. Cancer Prev.*, **5**, 313–318

Tavani, A., Pregnolato, A., Negri, E., Franceschi, S., Serraino, D., Carbone, A. & La Vecchia, C. (1997) Diet and risk of lymphoid neoplasms and soft tissue sarcomas. *Nutr. Cancer*, **27**, 256–260

Tavani, A., Gallus, S., La Vecchia, C., Negri, E., Montella, M., Dal Maso, L. & Franceschi, S. (1999) Risk factors for breast cancer in women under 40 years. *Eur. J. Cancer*, **35**, 1361–1367

Tavani, A., Gallus, S., La Vecchia, C., Talamini, R., Barbone, F., Herrero, R. & Franceschi, S. (2001) Diet and risk of oral and pharyngeal cancer. An Italian case–control study. *Eur. J. Cancer Prev.*, **10**, 191–195

Teel, R.W. (1986) Ellagic acid binding to DNA as a possible mechanism for its antimutagenic and anticarcinogenic action. *Cancer Lett.*, **30**, 329–336

Temple, N.J. & Basu, T.K. (1987) Selenium and cabbage and colon carcinogenesis in mice. *J. Natl Cancer Inst.*, **79**, 1131–1134

Temple, N.J. & el Khatib, S.M. (1987) Cabbage and vitamin E: their effect on colon tumor formation in mice. *Cancer Lett.* **35**, 71–77

Terry, P., Nyren, O. & Yuen, J. (1998) Protective effect of fruits and vegetables on stomach cancer in a cohort of Swedish twins. *Int. J. Cancer*, **76**, 35–37

Terry, P., Baron, J.A., Weiderpass, E., Yuen, J., Lichtenstein, P. & Nyren, O. (1999) Lifestyle and endometrial cancer risk: a cohort study from the Swedish Twin Registry. *Int. J. Cancer*, **82**, 38–42

Terry, P., Giovannucci, E., Michels, K.B., Bergkvist, L., Hansen, H., Holmberg, L. & Wolk, A. (2001a) Fruit, vegetables, dietary fiber, and risk of colorectal cancer. *J. Natl Cancer Inst.*, **93**, 525–533

Terry, P., Lagergren, J., Hansen, H., Wolk, A. & Nyren, O. (2001b) Fruit and vegetable consumption in the prevention of oesophageal and cardia cancers. *Eur. J. Cancer Prev.*, **10**, 365–369

Terry, P., Wolk, A., Persson, I. & Magnusson, C. (2001c) Brassica vegetables and breast cancer risk. *JAMA*, **285**, 2975–2977

Terry, P., Vainio, H., Wolk, A. & Weiderpass, E. (2002) Dietary factors in relation to endometrial cancer: a nationwide case–control study in Sweden. *Nutr. Cancer*, **42**, 25–32

Thompson, F.E. & Byers, T. (1994) Dietary assessment resource manual. *J. Nutr.*, **124**, 2245S–2317S

Thompson, C.H., Head, M.K. & Rodman, S.M. (1987) Factors influencing accuracy in estimating plate waste. *J. Am. Diet. Assoc.*, **87**, 1219–1220

Thompson, H.J., Heimendinger, J., Haegele, A., Sedlacek, S.M., Gillette, C., O'Neill, C., Wolfe, P. & Conry, C. (1999a) Effect of increased vegetable and fruit consumption on markers of oxidative cellular damage. *Carcinogenesis*, **20**, 2261–2266

Thompson, P.A., Seyedi, F., Lang, N.P., MacLeod, S.L., Wogan, G.N., Anderson, K.E., Tang, Y.M., Coles, B. & Kadlubar, F.F. (1999b) Comparison of DNA adduct levels associated with exogenous and endogenous exposures in human pancreas in relation to metabolic genotype. *Mutat. Res.*, **424**, 263–274

Thompson, F.E., Kipnis, V., Subar, A.F., Krebs-Smith, S.M., Kahle, L.L., Midthune, D., Potischman, N. & Schatzkin, A. (2000) Evaluation of 2 brief instruments and a food-frequency questionnaire to estimate daily number of servings of fruit and vegetables. *Am. J. Clin. Nutr.*, **71**, 1503–1510

Thompson, F.E., Subar, A.F., Brown, C.C., Smith, A.F., Sharbaugh, C.O., Jobe, J.B., Mittl, B., Gibson, J.T. & Ziegler, R.G. (2002) Cognitive research enhances accuracy of food frequency questionnaire reports: results of an experimental validation study. *J. Am. Diet. Assoc.*, **102**, 212–225

Thorand, B., Kohlmeier, L., Simonsen, N., Croghan, C. & Thamm, M. (1998) Intake of fruits, vegetables, folic acid and related nutrients and risk of breast cancer in postmenopausal women. *Public Health Nutr*, **1**, 147–156

Thouez, J.P., Ghadirian, P., Petitclerc, C. & Hamelin, P. (1990) International comparisons of nutrition and mortality from cancers of the oesophagus, stomach and pancreas. *Geogr. Med.*, **20**, 39–50

Thun, M.J., Calle, E.E., Namboodiri, M.M., Flanders, W.D., Coates, R.J., Byers, T., Boffetta, P., Garfinkel, L. & Heath, C.W., Jr (1992) Risk factors for fatal colon cancer in a large prospective study. *J. Natl Cancer Inst.*, **84**, 1491–1500

Tjonneland, A., Haraldsdottir, J., Overvad, K., Stripp, C., Ewertz, M. & Jensen, O.M. (1992) Influence of individually estimated portion size data on the validity of a semiquantitative food frequency questionnaire. *Int. J. Epidemiol.*, **21**, 770–777

Todd, K.S., Hudes, M. & Calloway, D.H. (1983) Food intake measurement: problems and approaches. *Am. J. Clin. Nutr.*, **37**, 139–146

Tominaga, S. & Kuroishi, T. (1997) An ecological study on diet/nutrition and cancer in Japan. *Int. J. Cancer*, **71 Suppl. 10**, 2–6

Toniolo, P., Riboli, E., Protta, F., Charrel, M. & Cappa, A.P. (1989) Calorie-providing nutrients and risk of breast cancer. *J. Natl Cancer Inst.*, **81**, 278–286

Trichopoulou, A., Katsouyanni, K., Stuver, S., Tzala, L., Gnardellis, C., Rimm, E. & Trichopoulos, D. (1995a) Consumption of olive oil and specific food groups in relation to breast cancer risk in Greece. *J. Natl Cancer Inst.*, **87**, 110–116

Trichopoulou, A., Kouris-Blazos, A., Vassilakou, T., Gnardellis, C., Polychronopoulos, E., Venizelos, M., Lagiou, P., Wahlqvist, M.L. & Trichopoulos, D. (1995b) Diet and survival of elderly Greeks: a link to the past. *Am. J. Clin. Nutr.*, **61 Suppl**, 1346S–1350S

Trichopoulou, A., Lagiou, P., Nelson, M., Remaut-De Winter, A.M., Kelleher, C., Leonhauser, I.U., Moreiras, O., Schmitt, A., Sekula, W., Trygg, K. & Zaykas, G. (1999) Food disparities in 10 European countries: Their detection using household budget survey data – The DAta Food NEtworking (DAFNE) initiative. *Nutr. Today*, **34**, 129–139

Tsubono, Y., Kobayashi, M. & Tsugane, S. (1997) Food consumption and gastric cancer mortality in five regions of Japan. *Nutr. Cancer*, **27**, 60–64

Tuomilehto, J., Lindström, J., Eriksson, J.G., Valle, T.T., Hämäläinen, H., Ilanne-Parikka, P., Keinänen-Kiukaanniemi, S., Laakso, M., Louheranta, A., Rastas, M., Salminen, V. & Uusitupa, M. (2001) Prevention of type 2 diabetes mellitus by changes in lifestyle among subjects with impaired glucose tolerance. *New Engl. J. Med.*, **344**, 1343–1350

Turrell, G., Hewitt, B., Patterson, C., Oldenburg, B. & Gould T. (2002) Socioeconomic differences in food purchasing behaviour and suggested implications for diet-related health promotion. *J. Hum. Nutr. Dietet.*, **15**, 355–364

Turrini, A., Saba, A., Perrone, D., Cialfa, E. & D'Amicis, A. (2001) Food consumption patterns in Italy: the INN-CA Study 1994–1996. *Eur. J. Clin. Nutr.*, **55**, 571–588

Tuyns, A.J., Riboli, E., Doornbos, G. & Péquignot, G. (1987) Diet and esophageal cancer in Calvados (France). *Nutr. Cancer*, **9**, 81–92

Tuyns, A.J., Kaaks, R. & Haelterman, M. (1988) Colorectal cancer and the consumption of foods: a case–control study in Belgium. *Nutr. Cancer*, **11**, 189–204

Tuyns, A.J., Kaaks, R., Haelterman, M. & Riboli, E. (1992) Diet and gastric cancer. A case–control study in Belgium. *Int. J. Cancer*, **51**, 1–6

Tylavsky, F.A. & Sharp, G.B. (1995) Misclassification of nutrient and energy

References

intake from use of closed-ended questions in epidemiologic research. *Am. J. Epidemiol.*, **142**, 342–352

Tzonou, A., Kalandidi, A., Trichopoulou, A., Hsieh, C.C., Toupadaki, N., Willett, W. & Trichopoulos, D. (1993) Diet and coronary heart disease: a case–control study in Athens, Greece. *Epidemiology*, **4**, 511–516

Tzonou, A., Lipworth, L., Garidou, A., Signorello, L.B., Lagiou, P., Hsieh, C. & Trichopoulos, D. (1996a) Diet and risk of esophageal cancer by histologic type in a low-risk population. *Int. J. Cancer*, **68**, 300–304

Tzonou, A., Lipworth, L., Kalandidi, A., Trichopoulou, A., Gamatsi, I., Hsieh, C.C., Notara, V. & Trichopoulos, D. (1996b) Dietary factors and the risk of endometrial cancer: a case–control study in Greece. *Br. J. Cancer*, **73**, 1284–1290

Tzonou, A., Signorello, L.B., Lagiou, P., Wuu, J., Trichopoulos, D. & Trichopoulou, A. (1999) Diet and cancer of the prostate: a case–control study in Greece. *Int. J. Cancer*, **80**, 704–708

Ubukata, T., Oshima, A. & Fujimoto, I. (1986) Mortality among Koreans living in Osaka, Japan, 1973–1982. *Int. J. Epidemiol.*, **15**, 218–225

Uchino, H. & Itokawa, Y. (1972) Studies on the nutritional value of S-methylcysteine sulfoxide. II. Splenic hypertrophy of rats on an increased S-methyl cysteine sulfoxide diet and effect of *S*-methylcysteine sulfoxide administration on splenectomized rats. *Nippon Eiseigaku Zasshi*, **27**, 253–256

Uchino, H. & Otokami, Y. (1972) Studies on the nutritional value of S-methylcysteine sulfoxide. I. Effect of increased dietary S-methylcysteine sulfoxide on growth and tissues in rats. *Nippon Eiseigaku Zasshi*, **27**, 248–252

United States General Accounting Office (2002) *Fruits and Vegetables. Enhanced Federal Efforts to Increase Consumption could Yield Health Benefits for America.* Available at: URL: http://www.gao.gov (Report to Congressional Requesters), Washington, DC

US Department of Agriculture Food Surveys Research Group (2003a) http://www.barc.usda.gov/bhnrc/foodsurvey/Questionnaires.html and http://www.barc.usda.gov/bhnrc/foodsurvey/pdf/FIB.pdf

(2003b) http://www.barc.usda.gov/bhnrc/foodsurvey/pdf/Portion.pdf

(2003c) http://www.barc.usda.gov/bhnrc/foodsurvey/pdf/Region.pdf

(2003d) http://www.barc.usda.gov/bhnrc/foodsurvey/pdf/Income.pdf

(2003e) http://www.barc.usda.gov/bhnrc/foodsurvey/pdf/Origin94.pdf

US Department of Health and Human Services (1990) *Healthy People 2000: National Health Promotion and Disease Prevention Objectives* (DHHS Publication No. (PHS) 91-50212), Washington, DC, US Government Printing Office

US Department of Health and Human Services (2000) *Nutrition and your Health: Dietary Guidelines for Americans*, 5th edition (Home and Garden Bulletin No. 232)

US Public Health Service, Office of the Surgeon General (1988) *The Surgeon General's Report on Nutrition and Health* (DHHS Publication No. PHS 88–50210), Washington, DC, US Government Printing Office

USDA (1998) *Carotenoid Database*, Available from: URL: http://www.nal.usda.gov/fnic.foodcomp/Data/car98/caro98.html Washington, DC, United States Department of Agriculture

USDA (1999a) *Database on the Isoflavone Content of Food.* Available from: URL: http://www.nal.usda.gov/fnic/foodcomp/Data/isoflav/isoflav/html

USDA (1999b) *America's Eating Habits: Changes and Consequences, No. 750* (Agriculture Information Bulletin), Washington, DC, US Department of Agriculture, Economic Research Service, Food and Rural Economic Division

USDA (2002) *National Nutrient Database for Standard.* Available from: URL: http://www.nal.usda.gov/fnic/foodcomp/ Washington, DC, United States Department of Agriculture

Vach, W. & Blettner, M. (1991) Biased estimation of the odds ratio in case-control studies due to the use of ad hoc methods of correcting for missing values for confounding variables. *Am. J. Epidemiol.*, **134**, 895–907

Valsta, L.M. (1999) Food-based dietary guidelines for Finland—a staged approach. *Br. J. Nutr.*, **81 Suppl. 2**, S49–S55

Van Beijsterveldt, C.E., van Boxtel, M.P., Bosma, H., Houx, P.J., Buntinx, F. & Jolles, J. (2002) Predictors of attrition in a longitudinal cognitive aging study: the Maastricht Aging Study (MAAS). *J. Clin. Epidemiol.*, **55**, 216–223

van den Berg, R., van Vliet, T., Broekmans, W.M., Cnubben, N.H. & Vaes, W.H. (2001) A vegetable/fruit concentrate with high antioxidant capacity has no effect on biomarkers of antioxidant status in male smokers. *J. Nutr.*, **131**, 1714–1722

Van Kranen, H.J., Van Iersel, P.W.C., Rijnkels, J.M., Beems, D.B., Alink, G.M. & Van Kreijl, C.F. (1998) Effects of dietary fat and a vegetable–fruit mixture on the development of intestinal neoplasia in the Apc^{Min} mouse. *Carcinogenesis*, **19**, 1597–1601

van Liere, M.J., Lucas, F., Clavel, F., Slimani, N. & Villeminot, S. (1997) Relative validity and reproducibility of a French dietary history questionnaire. *Int. J. Epidemiol.*, **26 Suppl.1**, S128–S136

van Poppel, G., Verhoeven, D.T., Verhagen, H. & Goldbohm, R.A. (1999) Brassica vegetables and cancer prevention. Epidemiology and mechanisms. *Adv. Exp. Med. Biol.*, **472**, 159–168

Vang, O., Jensen, H. & Autrup, H. (1991) Induction of cytochrome P-450IA1, IA2, IIB1, IIB2 and IIE1 by broccoli in rat liver and colon. *Chem. Biol. Interact.*, **78**, 85–96

Vang, O., Rasmussen, B.F. & Andersen, O. (1997) Combined effects of complex mixtures of potentially anti-carcinogenic compounds on antioxidant enzymes and carcinogen metabolizing enzymes in the rat. *Cancer Lett*, **114**, 283–286

Vang, O., Mehrota, K., Georgellis, A. & Andersen, O. (1999) Effects of dietary broccoli on rat testicular xenobiotic metabolizing enzymes. *Eur. J. Drug Metab. Pharmacokin.*, **24**, 353–359

Vang, O., Frandsen, H., Hansen, K.T., Sorensen, J.N., Sorensen, H. & Andersen, O. (2001) Biochemical effects of dietary intakes of different broccoli samples. I. Differential modulation of cytochrome P-450 activities in rat liver, kidney, and colon. *Metabolism*, **50**, 1123–1129

van't Hof, M.A. & Burema, J. (1996) Assessment of bias in the SENECA study. *Eur. J. Clin. Nutr.*, **50 Suppl. 2**, 4–8

van't Veer, P., Kolb, C.M., Verhoef, P., Kok, F.J., Schouten, E.G., Hermus, R.J. & Sturmans, F. (1990) Dietary fiber, beta-carotene and breast cancer: results from a case–control study. *Int. J. Cancer*, **45**, 825–828

Venti, C.A. & Johnston, C.S. (2002) Modified food guide pyramid for lactovegetarians and vegans. *J. Nutr.*, **132**, 1050–1054

Verhagen, H., Poulsen, H.E., Loft, S., van Poppel, G., Willems, M.I. & van Bladeren, P.J. (1995) Reduction of oxidative DNA-damage in humans by brussels sprouts. *Carcinogenesis*, **16**, 969–970

Verhagen, H., de Vries, A., Nijhoff, W.A., Schouten, A., van Poppel, G., Peters, W.H. & van den Berg, H. (1997) Effect of Brussels sprouts on oxidative DNA-damage in man. *Cancer Lett.*, **114**, 127–130

Verhoeven, D.T., Assen, N., Goldbohm, R.A., Dorant, E., van't Veer, P., Sturmans, F., Hermus, R.J. & van den Brandt, P.A. (1997a) Vitamins C and E, retinol, beta-carotene and dietary fibre in relation to breast cancer risk: a prospective cohort study. *Br. J. Cancer*, **75**, 149–155

Verhoeven, D.T., Verhagen, H., Goldbohm, R.A., van den Brandt, P.A. & van Poppel, G. (1997b) A review of mechanisms underlying anticarcinogenicity by brassica vegetables. *Chem.*

Biol. Interact., **103**, 79–129

Vernon, S.W., Roberts, R.E. & Lee, E.S. (1984) Ethnic status and participation in longitudinal health surveys. *Am. J. Epidemiol.*, **119**, 99–113

Verreault, R., Chu, J., Mandelson, M. & Shy, K. (1989) A case–control study of diet and invasive cervical cancer. *Int. J. Cancer*, **43**, 1050–1054

Victora, C.G., Muñoz, N., Day, N.E., Barcelos, L.B., Peccin, D.A. & Braga, N.M. (1987) Hot beverages and oesophageal cancer in southern Brazil: a case–control study. *Int. J. Cancer*, **39**, 710–716

Villeneuve, P.J., Johnson, K.C., Kreiger, N. & Mao, Y. (1999) Risk factors for prostate cancer: results from the Canadian National Enhanced Cancer Surveillance System. The Canadian Cancer Registries Epidemiology Research Group. *Cancer Causes Control*, **10**, 355–367

Vinson, J.A., Hao, Y., Su, X. & Zubik, L.S. (1998) Phenol antioxidant quantity and quality in foods: vegetables. *J. Agric. Food Chem.*, **46**, 3630–3634

Vinson, J.A., Su, X., Zubik, L.S. & Bose, P. (2001) Phenol antioxidant quantity and quality in foods: Fruits. *J. Agric. Food Chem.*, **49**, 5315–5321

Vioque, J., Gonzalez, S.L. & Cayuela, D.A. (1990) Cancer of the pancreas: an ecologic study [in Spanish]. *Med. Clin. (Barc.)*, **95**, 121–125

Vistisen, K., Poulsen, H.E. & Loft, S. (1992) Foreign compound metabolism capacity in man measured from metabolites of dietary caffeine. *Carcinogenesis*, **13**, 1561–1568

Vogel, U., Møller, P., Dragsted, L., Loft, S., Pedersen, A. & Sandström, B. (2002) Inter-individual variation, seasonal variation and close correlation of *OGG1* and *ERCC1* mRNA levels in full blood from healthy volunteers. *Carcinogenesis*, **23**, 1505–1509

Voirol, M., Infante, F., Raymond, L., Hollenweger, V., Zurkirch, M.C., Tuyns, A. & Loizeau, E. (1987) Profil alimentaire des malades atteints de cancer du pan-

creas. *Schweiz. Med. Wochenschr.*, **117**, 1101–1104

Volatier, J.L. & Verger, P. (1999) Recent national French food and nutrient intake data. *Br. J. Nutr.*, **81 Suppl. 2**, S57–S59

Vollset, S.E. & Bjelke, E. (1983) Does consumption of fruit and vegetables protect against stroke? *Lancet*, **2**, 742

Voorrips, L.E., Goldbohm, R.A., van Poppel, G., Sturmans, F., Hermus, R.J. & van den Brandt, P.A. (2000a) Vegetable and fruit consumption and risks of colon and rectal cancer in a prospective cohort study: The Netherlands Cohort Study on Diet and Cancer. *Am. J. Epidemiol.*, **152**, 1081–1092

Voorrips, L.E., Goldbohm, R.A., Verhoeven, D.T., van Poppel, G.A., Sturmans, F., Hermus, R.J. & van den Brandt, P.A. (2000b) Vegetable and fruit consumption and lung cancer risk in the Netherlands Cohort Study on diet and cancer. *Cancer Causes Control*, **11**, 101–115

Wacholder, S., Silverman, D.T., McLaughlin, J.K. & Mandel, J.S. (1992) Selection of controls in case-control studies. II. Types of controls. *Am. J. Epidemiol.*, **135**, 1029–1041

Wacholder, S., Chatterjee, N. & Hartge, P. (2002) Joint effect of genes and environment distorted by selection biases: implications for hospital-based case-control studies. *Cancer Epidemiol. Biomarkers Prev.*, **11**, 885–889

Wagner, S. & Breiteneder, H. (2002) The latex-fruit syndrome. *Biochem. Soc. Trans.*, **30**, 935–940

Wakai, K., Takashi, M., Okamura, K., Yuba, H., Suzuki, K., Murase, T., Obata, K., Itoh, H., Kato, T., Kobayashi, M., Sakata, T., Otani, T., Ohshima, S. & Ohno, Y. (2000) Foods and nutrients in relation to bladder cancer risk: a case–control study in Aichi Prefecture, Central Japan. *Nutr. Cancer*, **38**, 13–22

Wallstrom, P., Wirfalt, E., Janzon, L., Mattisson, I., Elmstahl, S., Johansson, U. & Berglund, G. (2000) Fruit and vegetable consumption in relation to risk factors for cancer: a report from the

Malmö Diet and Cancer Study. *Public Health Nutr.*, **3**, 263–271

Wang, L.D. & Hammond, E.C. (1985) Lung cancer, fruit, green salad and vitamin pills. *Chin. Med. J. (Engl.)*, **98**, 206–210

Wang, H. & Murphy, P.A. (1994) Isoflavone content in commercial soybean foods. *J. Agric. Food Chem.*, **42**, 1666–1673

Wang, Z.Y., Cheng, S.J., Zhou, Z.C., Athar, M., Khan, W.A., Bickers, D.R. & Mukhtar, H. (1989) Antimutagenic activity of green tea polyphenols. *Mutat. Res.*, **223**, 273–285

Wang, M., Dhingra, K., Hittelman, W.N., Liehr, J.G., de Andrade, M. & Li, D. (1996) Lipid peroxidation-induced putative malondialdehyde–DNA adducts in human breast tissues. *Cancer Epidemiol. Biomarkers Prev.*, **5**, 705–710

Wang, Y., Ichiba, M., Oishi, H., Iyadomi, M., Shono, N. & Tomokuni, K. (1997) Relationship between plasma concentrations of beta-carotene and alpha-tocopherol and life-style factors and levels of DNA adducts in lymphocytes. *Nutr. Cancer*, **27**, 69–73

Ward, M.H. & Lopez-Carrillo, L. (1999) Dietary factors and the risk of gastric cancer in Mexico City. *Am. J. Epidemiol.*, **149**, 925–932

Ward, M.H., Zahm, S.H., Weisenburger, D.D., Gridley, G., Cantor, K.P., Saal, R.C. & Blair, A. (1994) Dietary factors and non-Hodgkin's lymphoma in Nebraska (United States). *Cancer Causes Control*, **5**, 422–432

Wattenberg, L.W. (1975) Effects of dietary constituents on the metabolism of chemical carcinogens. *Cancer Res.*, **35**, 3326–3331

Wattenberg, L.W., Loub, W.D., Lam, L.K. & Speier, J.L. (1976) Dietary constituents altering the responses to chemical carcinogens. *Fed. Proc.*, **35**, 1327–1331

Watzl, B., Bub, A., Brandstetter, B.R. & Rechkemmer, G. (1999) Modulation of human T-lymphocyte functions by the consumption of carotenoid-rich vegetables. *Br. J. Nutr.*, **82**, 383–389

Watzl, B., Bub, A., Blockhaus, M., Herbert, B.M., Luhrmann, P.M., Neuhauser-Berthold, M. & Rechkemmer, G. (2000) Prolonged tomato juice consumption has no effect on cell-mediated immunity of well-nourished elderly men and women. *J. Nutr.*, **130**, 1719–1723

WCRF/AICR (World Cancer Research Fund and American Institute for Cancer Research) (1997) *Food, Nutrition and the Prevention of Cancer: A Global Perspective*, Washington, DC

Weisburger, J.H., Reddy, B.S., Rose, D.P., Cohen, L.A., Kendall, M.E. & Wynder, E.L. (1993) Protective mechanisms of dietary fibers in nutritional carcinogenesis. *Basic Life Sci.*, **61**, 45–63

WHO (1990) *Diet, Nutrition, and the Prevention of Chronic Diseases* (WHO Technical Report No. 797), Geneva, World Health Organization

WHO (1998) *Preparation and Use of Food-based Dietary Guidelines: Report of a Joint FAO/WHO Consultation* (WHO Technical Report Series), Geneva, World Health Organization

WHO (2002) *National Cancer Control Programmes. Policies and Managerial Guidelines*, 2nd edition, Geneva, World Health Organization

WHO (2003) *Diet, Nutrition and the Prevention of Chronic Diseases. Report of a Joint FAO/WHO Expert Consultation* (WHO Technical Report Series 916), Geneva, World Health Organization

WHO/EURO (2000) *CINDI Dietary Guide*, Copenhagen, WHO Regional Office for Europe

Wilkens, L.R., Hankin, J.H., Yoshizawa, C.N., Kolonel, L.N. & Lee, J. (1992) Comparison of long-term dietary recall between cancer cases and noncases. *Am. J. Epidemiol.*, **136**, 825–835

Willett, W.C. (1990) Total energy intake and nutrient composition: dietary recommendations for epidemiologists. *Int. J. Cancer*, **46**, 770–771

Willett, W. (1998a) Food frequency methods. In: Willett, W., ed., *Nutritional Epidemiology*, 2nd edition, New York, Oxford, Oxford University Press, pp. 74–94

Willett, W. (1998b) Recall of remote diet. In: Willett, W., ed., *Nutritional Epidemiology*, 2nd edition, New York, Oxford, Oxford University Press, pp. 148–156

Willett, W. (1998c) Correction for the effects of measurement error. In: Willett, W., ed., *Nutritional Epidemiology*, 2nd edition, New York, Oxford, Oxford University Press, pp. 302–320

Willett, W. (1998d) 24-hour dietary recall and food record methods In: Willett, W., ed., *Nutritional Epidemiology*, 2nd edition, New York, Oxford University Press, pp. 50–73

Willett, W. (1998e) Issues in analysis and presentation of dietary data. In: Willett, W., ed., *Nutritional Epidemiology*, 2nd edition, New York, Oxford University Press, pp. 321–345

Willett, W. (2001a) Commentary: Dietary diaries versus food frequency questionnaires – a case of undigestible data. *Int. J. Epidemiol.*, **30**, 317–319

Willett, W. (2001b) Invited commentary: a further look at dietary questionnaire validation. *Am. J. Epidemiol.*, **154**, 1100–1102

Willett, W. (2001c) Commentator's response. *Int. J. Epidemiol.*, **30**, 694–695

Willett, W.C. (2001d) Diet and cancer: one view at the start of the millennium. *Cancer Epidemiol. Biomarkers Prev.*, **10**, 3–8

Willett, W. & Lenart, E. (1998) Reproducibility and validity of food frequency questionnaires. In: Willett, W., ed., *Nutritional Epidemiology*, New York, Oxford, Oxford University Press, pp. 101–147

Willett, W.C., Sampson, L., Stampfer, M.J., Rosner, B., Bain, C., Witschi, J., Hennekens, C.H. & Speizer, F.E. (1985) Reproducibility and validity of a semiquantitative food frequency questionnaire. *Am. J. Epidemiol.*, 122, 51–65

Williams, D.E., Prevost, A.T., Whichelow, M.J., Cox, B.D., Day, N.E. & Wareham, N.J. (2000) A cross-sectional study of dietary patterns with glucose intolerance and other features of the metabolic syndrome. *Br. J. Nutr.*, **83**, 257–266

Winn, D.M., Ziegler, R.G., Pickle, L.W., Gridley, G., Blot, W.J. & Hoover, R.N. (1984) Diet in the etiology of oral and pharyngeal cancer among women from the southern United States. *Cancer Res.*, **44**, 1216–1222

Witte, J.S., Longnecker, M.P., Bird, C.L., Lee, E.R., Frankl, H.D. & Haile, R.W. (1996) Relation of vegetable, fruit, and grain consumption to colorectal adenomatous polyps. *Am. J. Epidemiol.*, **144**, 1015–1025

Wolf, C.R. (2001) Chemoprevention: increased potential to bear fruit. *Proc. Natl Acad. Sci. USA*, **98**, 2941–2943

Wolfgarten, E., Rosendahl, U., Nowroth, T., Leers, J., Metzger, R., Hölscher, A.H. & Bollschweiler, E. (2001) Coincidence of nutritional habits and esophageal cancer in Germany. *Onkologie*, **24**, 546–551

Wolk, A., Gridley, G., Niwa, S., Lindblad, P., McCredie, M., Mellemgaard, A., Mandel, J.S., Wahrendorf, J., McLaughlin, J.K. & Adami, H.O. (1996) International renal cell cancer study. VII. Role of diet. *Int. J. Cancer*, **65**, 67–73

World Health Organization & Tufts University School of Nutrition and Policy (2002) *Keep Fit for Life. Meeting the Nutritional Needs of Older Persons*, Geneva, WHO

Wortelboer, H.M., de Kruif, C.A., van Iersel, A.A., Noordhoek, J., Blaauboer, B.J., van Bladeren, P.J. & Falke, H.E. (1992) Effects of cooked brussels sprouts on cytochrome P-450 profile and phase II enzymes in liver and small intestinal mucosa of the rat. *Food Chem. Toxicol.*, **30**, 17–27

Wu, A.H. & Bernstein, L. (1998) Breast cancer among Asian Americans and Pacific Islanders. *Asian Am. Pac. Isl. J. Health*, **6**, 327–343

Wu-Williams, A.H., Yu, M.C. & Mack, T.M. (1990) Life-style, workplace, and stomach cancer by subsite in young men of Los Angeles County. *Cancer Res.*, **50**, 2569–2576

Wynder, E.L. (1985) Large bowel cancer: prospects for control. *Cancer Detect. Prev.*, **8**, 413–420

Wynder, E.L. & Bross, I.J. (1961) A study of etiological factors in cancer of the esophagus. *Cancer*, **14**, 389–413

Wynder, E.L., Bross, I.J. & Feldman, R.M. (1957) A study of the etiological factors in cancer of the mouth. *Cancer*, **10**, 1301–1323

Xie, B., Gilliland, F.D., Li, Y.F. & Rockett, H.R.H. (2003) Effects of ethnicity, family income, and education on dietary intake among adolescents. *Prev. Med.*, **36**, 30–40

Xu, G.P., Song, P.J. & Reed, P.I. (1993) Effects of fruit juices, processed vegetable juice, orange peel and green tea on endogenous formation of *N*-nitrosoproline in subjects from a high-risk area for gastric cancer in Moping County, China. *Eur. J. Cancer Prev.*, **2**, 327–335

Xu, Z., Brown, L.M., Pan, G.W., Liu, T.F., Gao, G.S., Stone, B.J., Cao, R.M., Guan, D.X., Sheng, J.H., Yan, Z.S., Dosemeci, M., Fraumeni, J.F., Jr & Blot, W.J. (1996) Cancer risks among iron and steel workers in Anshan, China, Part II: Case–control studies of lung and stomach cancer. *Am. J. Ind. Med.*, **30**, 7–15

Yamaguchi, M., ed. (1983) *World Vegetables. Principles, Production and Nutritive Values*, Westport, CT, AVI Publishing Co.

Yang, C.S., Smith, T.J. & Hong, J.Y. (1994) Cytochrome P-450 enzymes as targets for chemoprevention against chemical carcinogenesis and toxicity: opportunities and limitations. *Cancer Res.*, **54**, 1982s–1986s

Yang, K., Lindblad, P., Egevad, L. & Hemminki, K. (1999) Novel somatic mutations in the VHL gene in Swedish archived sporadic renal cell carcinomas. *Cancer Lett.*, **141**, 1–8

Yokoyama, A., Kato, H., Yokoyama, T., Tsujinaka, T., Muto, M., Omori, T., Haneda, T., Kumagai, Y., Igaki, H., Yokoyama, M., Watanabe, H., Fukuda, H. & Yoshimizu, H. (2002) Genetic polymorphisms of alcohol and aldehyde dehydrogenases and glutathione *S*-transferase M1 and drinking, smoking, and diet in Japanese men with esophageal squamous cell carcinoma. *Carcinogenesis*, **23**, 1851–1859

You, W.C., Blot, W.J., Chang, Y.S., Ershow, A.G., Yang, Z.T., An, Q., Henderson, B., Xu, G.W., Fraumeni, J.F., Jr & Wang, T.G. (1988) Diet and high risk of stomach cancer in Shandong, China. *Cancer Res.*, **48**, 3518–3523

Young, T.B. & Wolf, D.A. (1988) Case–control study of proximal and distal colon cancer and diet in Wisconsin. *Int. J. Cancer*, **42**, 167–175

Young, J.F., Nielsen, S.E., Haraldsdottir, J., Daneshvar, B., Lauridsen, S.T., Knuthsen, P., Crozier, A., Sandstrom, B. & Dragsted, L.O. (1999) Effect of fruit juice intake on urinary quercetin excretion and biomarkers of antioxidative status. *Am. J. Clin. Nutr.*, **69**, 87–94

Young, J.F., Dragsted, L.O., Daneshvar, B., Lauridsen, S.T., Hansen, M. & Sandstrom, B. (2000) The effect of grape-skin extract on oxidative status. *Br. J. Nutr.*, **84**, 505–513

Yu, M.W. & Chen, C.J. (1993) Elevated serum testosterone levels and risk of hepatocellular carcinoma. *Cancer Res.*, **53**, 790–794

Yu, G.P. & Hsieh, C.C. (1991) Risk factors for stomach cancer: a population-based case–control study in Shanghai. *Cancer Causes Control*, **2**, 169–174

Yu, M.C., Mack, T.M., Hanisch, R., Cicioni, C. & Henderson, B.E. (1986) Cigarette smoking, obesity, diuretic use, and coffee consumption as risk factors for renal cell carcinoma. *J. Natl Cancer Inst.*, **77**, 351–356

Yu, M.C., Garabrant, D.H., Peters, J.M. & Mack, T.M. (1988) Tobacco, alcohol, diet, occupation, and carcinoma of the esophagus. *Cancer Res.*, **48**, 3843–3848

References

Yu, M.C., Huang, T.B. & Henderson, B.E. (1989) Diet and nasopharyngeal carcinoma: a case–control study in Guangzhou, China. *Int. J. Cancer*, **43**, 1077–1082

Yu, Y., Taylor, P.R., Li, J.Y., Dawsey, S.M., Wang, G.Q., Guo, W.D., Wang, W., Liu, B.Q., Blot, W.J. & Shen, Q. (1993) Retrospective cohort study of risk factors for esophageal cancer in Linxian, People's Republic of China. *Cancer Causes Control*, **4**, 195–202

Yu, M.W., Hsieh, H.H., Pan, W.H., Yang, C.S. & Chen, C.J. (1995) Vegetable consumption, serum retinol level, and risk of hepatocellular carcinoma. *Cancer Res.*, **55**, 1301–1305

Yuan, J.M., Gago-Dominguez, M., Castelao, J.E., Hankin, J.H., Ross, R.K. & Yu, M.C. (1998) Cruciferous vegetables in relation to renal cell carcinoma. *Int. J. Cancer*, **77**, 211–216

Zaridze, D., Lifanova, Y., Maximovitch, D., Day, N.E. & Duffy, S.W. (1991) Diet, alcohol consumption and reproductive factors in a case–control study of breast cancer in Moscow. *Int. J. Cancer*, **48**, 493–501

Zatonski, W., Becher, H., Lissowska, J. & Wahrendorf, J. (1991) Tobacco, alcohol, and diet in the etiology of laryngeal cancer: a population-based case–control study. *Cancer Causes Control*, **2**, 3–10

Zeegers, M.P., Goldbohm, R.A. & van den Brandt, P.A. (2001) Consumption of vegetables and fruits and urothelial cancer incidence: a prospective study. *Cancer Epidemiol. Biomarkers Prev.*, **10**, 1121–1128

Zemla, B. (1984) The role of selected dietary elements in breast cancer risk among native and migrant populations in Poland. *Nutr. Cancer*, **6**, 187–195

Zemla, B., Guminski, S. & Banasik, R. (1986) Study of risk factors in invasive cancer of the corpus uteri. *Neoplasma*, **33**, 621–629

Zhang, X.H., Maxwell, S.R., Thorpe, G.H., Thomason, H., Rea, C.A., Connock, M.J. & Maslin, D.J. (1997) The action of garlic upon plasma total antioxidant capacity. *Biochem. Soc Trans.*, **25,** 523S

Zhang, S., Hunter, D.J., Forman, M.R., Rosner, B.A., Speizer, F.E., Colditz, G.A., Manson, J.E., Hankinson, S.E. & Willett, W.C. (1999) Dietary carotenoids and vitamins A, C, and E and risk of breast cancer. *J. Natl Cancer Inst.*, **91**, 547–556

Zhang, S.M., Hunter, D.J., Rosner, B.A., Giovannucci, E.L., Colditz, G.A., Speizer, F.E. & Willett, W.C. (2000) Intakes of fruits, vegetables, and related nutrients and the risk of non-Hodgkin's lymphoma among women. *Cancer Epidemiol. Biomarkers Prev.*, **9**, 477–485

Zhang, Y., Chen, S.Y., Hsu, T. & Santella, R.M. (2002a) Immunohisto-chemical detection of malondialdehyde–DNA adducts in human oral mucosa cells. *Carcinogenesis,* **23,** 207–211

Zhang, M., Yang, Z.Y., Binns, C.W. & Lee, A.H. (2002b) Diet and ovarian cancer risk: a case–control study in China. *Br. J. Cancer*, **86**, 712–717

Zhao, Y., Xue, Y., Oberley, T.D., Kiningham, K.K., Lin, S.M., Yen, H.C., Majima, H., Hines, J. & St Clair, D. (2001) Overexpression of manganese superoxide dismutase suppresses tumor formation by modulation of activator protein-1 signaling in a multistage skin carcinogenesis model. *Cancer Res.*, **61,** 6082–6088

Zheng, W., Blot, W.J., Shu, X.O., Diamond, E.L., Gao, Y.T., Ji, B.T. & Fraumeni, J.F., Jr (1992a) Risk factors for oral and pharyngeal cancer in Shanghai, with emphasis on diet. *Cancer Epidemiol. Biomarkers Prev.*, **1**, 441–448

Zheng, W., Blot, W.J., Shu, X.O., Gao, Y.T., Ji, B.T., Ziegler, R.G. & Fraumeni, J.F., Jr (1992b) Diet and other risk factors for laryngeal cancer in Shanghai, China. *Am. J. Epidemiol.*, **136**, 178–191

Zheng, W., McLaughlin, J.K., Gridley, G., Bjelke, E., Schuman, L.M., Silverman, D.T., Wacholder, S., Co-Chien, H.T., Blot, W.J. & Fraumeni, J.F., Jr (1993) A cohort study of smoking, alcohol consumption, and dietary factors for pancreatic cancer (United States). *Cancer Causes Control*, **4**, 477–482

Zheng, W., Shu, X.O., Ji, B.T. & Gao, Y.T. (1996) Diet and other risk factors for cancer of the salivary glands: a population-based case–control study. *Int. J. Cancer*, **67**, 194–198

Zhuo, X.G. & Watanabe, S. (1999) Factor analysis of digestive cancer mortality and food consumption in 65 Chinese counties. *J. Epidemiol.*, **9**, 275–284

Ziegler, R.G., Morris, L.E., Blot, W.J., Pottern, L.M., Hoover, R. & Fraumeni, J.F., Jr (1981) Esophageal cancer among black men in Washington, D.C. II. Role of nutrition. *J. Natl Cancer Inst.*, **67**, 1199–1206

Ziegler, R.G., Mason, T.J., Stemhagen, A., Hoover, R., Schoenberg, J.B., Gridley, G., Virgo, P.W. & Fraumeni, J.F., Jr (1986) Carotenoid intake, vegetables, and the risk of lung cancer among white men in New Jersey. *Am. J. Epidemiol.*, **123**, 1080–1093

Ziegler, R.G., Brinton, L.A., Hamman, R.F., Lehman, H.F., Levine, R.S., Mallin, K., Norman, S.A., Rosenthal, J.F., Trumble, A.C. & Hoover, R.N. (1990) Diet and the risk of invasive cervical cancer among white women in the United States. *Am. J. Epidemiol.*, **132**, 432–445

Ziegler, R.G., Jones, C.J., Brinton, L.A., Norman, S.A., Mallin, K., Levine, R.S., Lehman, H.F., Hamman, R.F., Trumble, A.C., Rosenthal, J.F. & Hoover, R.N. (1991) Diet and the risk of *in situ* cervical cancer among white women in the United States. *Cancer Causes Control*, **2**, 17–29

Ziegler, R.G., Hoover, R.N., Pike, M.C., Hildesheim, A., Nomura, A.M., West, D.W., Wu-Williams, A.H., Kolonel, L.N., Horn-Ross, P.L., Rosenthal, J.F. & Hyer, M.B. (1993) Migration patterns and breast cancer risk in Asian-American women. *J. Natl. Cancer Inst.*, **85**, 1819–1827

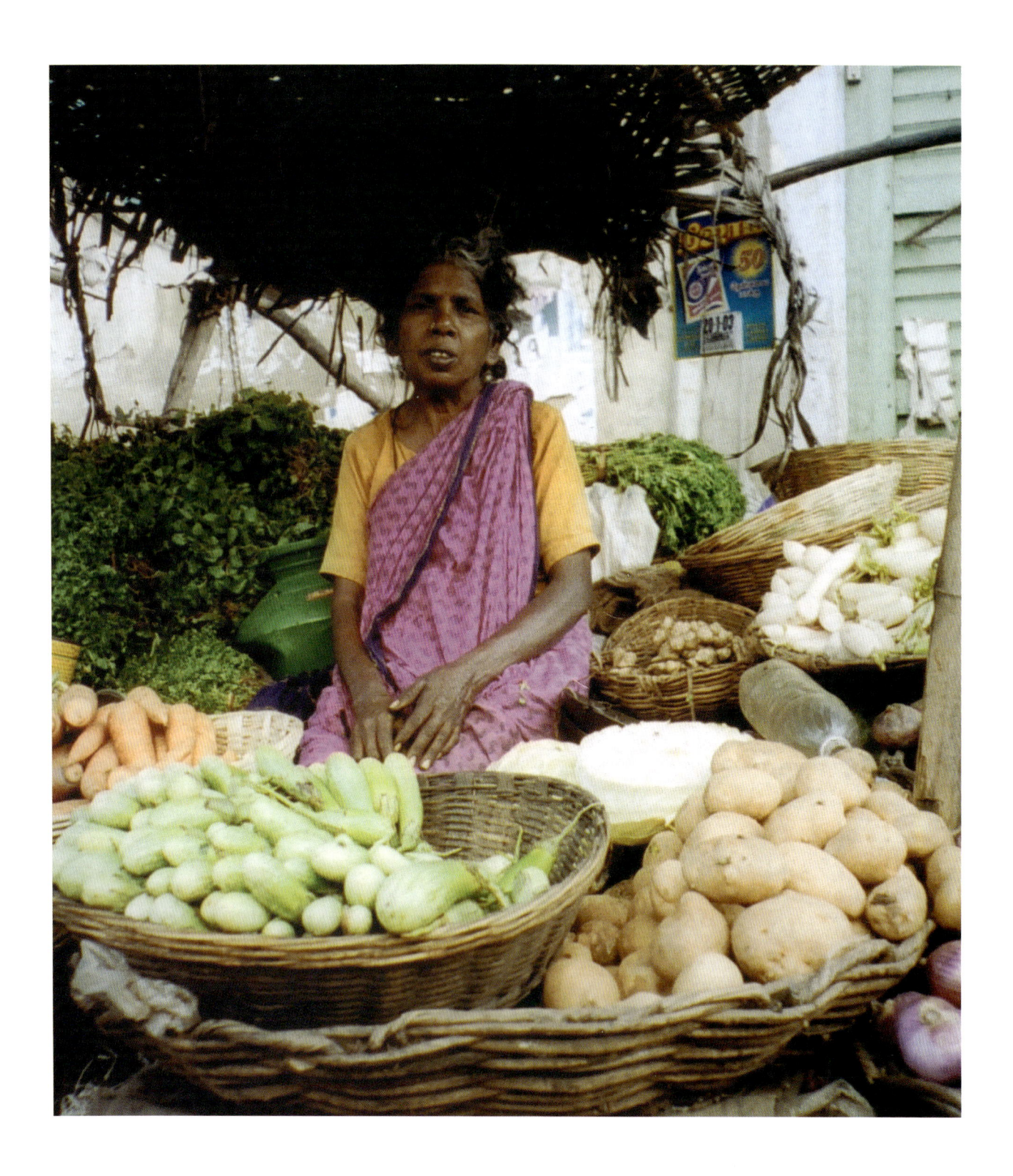

Working Procedures for the *IARC Handbooks of Cancer Prevention*

The prevention of cancer is one of the key objectives of the International Agency for Research on Cancer (IARC). This may be achieved by avoiding exposures to known cancer-causing agents, by increasing host defences through immunization or chemoprevention or by modifying lifestyle. The aim of the series of *IARC Handbooks of Cancer Prevention* is to evaluate scientific information on agents and interventions that may reduce the incidence of or mortality from cancer.

Scope

Cancer-preventive strategies embrace chemical, immunological, dietary and behavioural interventions that may retard, block or reverse carcinogenic processes or reduce underlying risk factors. The term 'chemoprevention' is used to refer to interventions with pharmaceuticals, vitamins, minerals and other chemicals to reduce cancer incidence. The *IARC Handbooks* address the efficacy, safety and mechanisms of cancer-preventive strategies and the adequacy of the available data, including those on timing, dose, duration and indications for use.

Preventive strategies can be applied across a continuum of: (1) the general population; (2) subgroups with particular predisposing host or environmental risk factors, including genetic susceptibility to cancer; (3) persons with precancerous lesions; and (4) cancer patients at risk for second primary tumours. Use of the same strategies or agents in the treatment of cancer patients to control the growth, metastasis and recurrence of tumours is considered to be patient management, not prevention, although data from clinical trials may be relevant when making a *Handbooks* evaluation.

Objective

The objective of the *Handbooks* programme is the preparation of critical reviews and evaluations of evidence for cancer-prevention and other relevant properties of a wide range of potential cancer-preventive agents and strategies by international working groups of experts. The resulting *Handbooks* may also indicate when additional research is needed.

The Handbooks may assist national and international authorities in devising programmes of health promotion and cancer prevention and in making benefit–risk assessments. The evaluations of IARC working groups are scientific judgements about the available evidence for cancer-preventive efficacy and safety. No recommendation is given with regard to national and international regulation or legislation, which are the responsibility of individual governments and/or other international authorities.

Working Groups

Reviews and evaluations are formulated by international working groups of experts convened by the IARC. The tasks of each group are: (1) to ascertain that all appropriate data have been collected; (2) to select the data relevant for the evaluation on the basis of scientific merit; (3) to prepare accurate summaries of the data to enable the reader to follow the reasoning of the Working Group; (4) to evaluate the significance of the available data from human studies and experimental models on cancer-preventive activity, and other beneficial effects and also on adverse effects; and (5) to evaluate data relevant to the understanding of the mechanisms of preventive activity.

Approximately 13 months before a working group meets, the topics of the *Handbook* are announced, and participants are selected by IARC staff in consultation with other experts. Subsequently, relevant clinical, experimental and human data are collected by the IARC from all available sources of published information. Representatives of producer or consumer associations may assist in the preparation of sections on production and use, as appropriate.

Working Group participants who contributed to the considerations and evaluations within a particular *Handbook* are listed, with their addresses, at the beginning of each publication. Each participant serves as an individual scientist and not as a representative of any organization, government or industry. In addition, scientists nominated by national and international agencies, industrial associations and consumer and/or environmental organizations may be invited as observers. IARC staff involved in the preparation of the *Handbooks* are listed.

About eight months before the meeting, the material collected is sent to meeting participants to prepare sections for the first drafts of the *Handbooks*. These are then compiled by IARC staff and sent, before the meeting, to all participants of the Working Group for review. There is an opportunity to return the compiled specialized sections of the draft to the experts, inviting preliminary comments, before the complete first-draft document is distributed to all members of the Working Group.

Data for Handbooks

The *Handbooks* do not necessarily cite all of the literature on the agent or strategy being evaluated. Only those data considered by the Working Group to be relevant to making the evaluation are included. In principle, meeting abstracts and other reports that do not provide sufficient detail upon which to base an assessment of their quality are not considered.

With regard to data from toxicological, epidemiological and experimental studies and from clinical trials, only reports that have been published or accepted for publication in the openly available scientific literature are reviewed by the Working Group. In certain instances, government agency reports that have undergone peer review and are widely available are considered. Exceptions may be made on an ad-hoc basis to include unpublished reports that are in their final form and publicly available, if their inclusion is considered pertinent to making a final evaluation. In the sections on chemical and physical properties, on production, on use, on analysis and on human exposure, unpublished sources of information may be used.

The available studies are summarized by the Working Group. In general, numerical findings are indicated as they appear in the original report; units are converted when necessary for easier comparison. The Working Group may conduct additional analyses of the published data and use them in their assessment of the evidence. Important aspects of a study, directly impinging on its interpretation, are brought to the attention of the reader.

Criteria for selection of topics for evaluation

Agents, classes of agents and interventions to be evaluated in the *Handbooks* are selected on the basis of one or more of the following criteria.
- The available evidence suggests potential for significantly reducing the incidence of cancers.
- There is a substantial body of human, experimental, clinical and/or mechanistic data suitable for evaluation.
- The agent is in widespread use and of putative protective value, but of uncertain efficacy and safety.
- The agent shows exceptional promise in experimental studies but has not been used in humans.
- The agent is available for furthe studies of human use.

Evaluation of cancer-preventive agents

A wide range of findings must be taken into account before a particular agent can be recognized as preventing cancer and a systematized approach to data presentation has been adopted for *Handbooks* evaluations.

Characteristics of the agent or intervention

Chemical identity and other definitive information (such as genus and species of plants) are given as appropriate. Data relevant to identification, occurrence and biological activity are included. Technical products of chemicals, including trade names, relevant specifications and information on composition and impurities are mentioned.

Preventive interventions can be broad, community-based interventions, or interventions targeted to individuals (counselling, behavioural, chemopreventive).

Occurrence, trends, analysis
Occurrence

Information on the occurrence of an agent in the environment is obtained from monitoring and surveillance in occupational environments, air, water, soil, foods and animal and human tissues. When available, data on the generation, persistence and bioaccumulation of the agent are included. For interventions, data on prevalence are supplied. The data on the prevalence of a factor (e.g., overweight) in different populations are collected as widely as possible.

Production and use

The dates of first synthesis and of first commercial production of a chemical or mixture are provided, the dates of first reported occurrence. In addition, methods of synthesis used in past and present commercial production and methods of production that may give rise to various impurities are described. For interventions, the dates of first mention of their use are given.

Data on the production, international trade and uses and applications of agents are obtained for representative regions. In the case of drugs, mention of their therapeutic applications does not necessarily represent current practice, nor does it imply judgement as to their therapeutic efficacy.

If an agent is used as a prescribed or over-the-counter pharmaceutical product, then the type of person receiving the product in terms of health status, age, sex and medical condition being treated are described. For non-pharmaceutical agents, particularly those taken because of cultural traditions, the characteristics of use or exposure and the relevant populations are described. In all cases, quantitative data, such as dose–response relationships, are considered to be of special importance.

Metabolism of and metabolic responses to the agent or metabolic consequences of an intervention

In evaluating the potential utility of a suspected cancer-preventive agent or strategy, a number of different properties, in addition to direct effects upon cancer incidence, are described and weighed. Furthermore, as many of the data leading to an evaluation are expected to come from studies in experimental animals, information that facilitates interspecies extrapolation is particularly important; this includes metabolic, kinetic and genetic data. Whenever possible, quantitative data, including information on dose, duration and potency, are considered.

Information is given on absorption, distribution (including placental transfer), metabolism and excretion in humans and experimental animals. Kinetic properties within the target species may affect the interpretation and extrapolation of dose–response relationships, such as blood concentrations, protein binding, tissue concentrations, plasma half-lives and elimination rates. Comparative information on the relationship between use or exposure and the dose that reaches the target site may be of particular importance for extrapolation between species. Studies that indicate the metabolic pathways and fate of an agent in humans and experimental animals are summarized, and data on humans and experimental animals are compared when possible. Observations are made on inter-individual variations and relevant metabolic polymorphisms. Data indicating long-term accumulation in human tissues are included. Physiologically based pharmacokinetic models and their parameter values are relevant and are included whenever they are available. Information on the fate of the compound within tissues and cells (transport, role of cellular receptors, compartmentalization, binding to macromolecules) is given.

The metabolic consequences of interventions are described.

Genotyping will be used increasingly, not only to identify subpopulations at increased or decreased risk for cancers but also to characterize variation in the biotransformation of and responses to cancer-preventive agents. This subsection can include effects of the compound on gene expression, enzyme induction or inhibition, or pro-oxidant status, when such data are not described elsewhere. It covers data obtained in humans and experimental animals, with particular attention to effects of long-term use and exposure.

Cancer-preventive effects
Human studies
Types of study considered

Human data are derived from experimental and non-experimental study designs and are focused on cancer, precancer or intermediate biological end-points. The experimental designs include randomized controlled trials and short-term experimental studies; non-experimental designs include cohort, case–control and cross-sectional studies.

Cohort and case–control studies relate individual use of, or exposure to, the agent or invervention under study to the occurrence of cancer in individuals and provide an estimate of relative risk (ratio of incidence or mortality in those exposed to incidence or mortality in those not exposed) as the main measure of association. Cohort and case–control studies follow an observational approach, in which the use of, or exposure to, the agent is not controlled by the investigator.

Intervention studies are experimental in design — that is, the use of, or exposure to, the agent or intervention is assigned by the investigator. The intervention study or clinical trial is the design that can provide the strongest and most direct evidence of a protective or preventive effect; however, for practical and ethical reasons, such studies are limited to observation of the effects among specifically defined study subjects of interventions of 10 years or fewer, which is relatively short when compared with the overall lifespan.

Intervention studies may be undertaken in individuals or communities and may or may not involve randomization to use or exposure. The differences between these designs is important in relation to analytical methods and interpretation of findings.

In addition, information can be obtained from reports of correlation (ecological) studies and case series; however, limitations inherent in these approaches usually mean that such studies carry limited weight in the evaluation of a preventive effect.

Quality of studies considered

The *Handbooks* are not intended to summarize all published studies. The Working Group considers the following aspects: (1) the relevance of the study; (2) the appropriateness of the design and analysis to the question being asked; (3) the adequacy and completeness of the presentation of the data; and (4) the degree to which chance, bias and confounding may have affected the results.

Studies that are judged to be inadequate or irrelevant to the evaluation are generally omitted. They may be mentioned briefly, particularly when the information is considered to be a useful supplement to that in other reports or when it provides the only data available. Their inclusion does not imply acceptance of the adequacy of the study design, nor of the analysis and interpretation of the results, and their limitations are outlined.

Assessment of the cancer-preventive effect at different doses and durations

The Working Group gives special attention to quantitative assessment of the preventive effect of the agent under study, by assessing data from studies at different doses. The Working Group also addresses issues of timing and duration of use or exposure. Such quantitative assessment is important to clarify the circumstances under which a preventive effect can be achieved, as well as the dose at which a toxic effect has been shown.

Criteria for a cancer-preventive effect
After summarizing and assessing the individual studies, the Working Group makes a judgement concerning the evidence that the agent or intervention in question prevents cancer in humans. In making the judgement, the Working Group considers several criteria for each relevant cancer site.

Evidence of protection derived from intervention studies of good quality is particularly informative. Evidence of a substantial and significant reduction in risk, including a 'dose'–response relationship, is more likely to indicate a real effect. Nevertheless, a small effect, or an effect without a dose–response relationship, does not imply lack of real benefit and may be important for public health if the cancer is common.

Evidence is frequently available from different types of study and is evaluated as a whole. Findings that are replicated in several studies of the same design or using different approaches are more likely to provide evidence of a true protective effect than isolated observations from single studies.

The Working Group evaluates possible explanations for inconsistencies across studies, including differences in use of, or exposure to, the agent, differences in the underlying risk of cancer and metabolism and genetic differences in the population.

The results of studies judged to be of high quality are given more weight. Note is taken of both the applicability of preventive action to several cancers and of possible differences in activity, including contradictory findings, across cancer sites.

Data from human studies (as well as from experimental models) that suggest plausible mechanisms for a cancer-preventive effect are important in assessing the overall evidence.

The Working Group may also determine whether, on aggregate, the evidence from human studies is consistent with a lack of preventive effect.

Experimental models
Experimental animals
Animal models are an important component of research into cancer prevention. They provide a means of identifying effective compounds, of carrying out fundamental investigations into their mechanisms of action, of determining how they can be used optimally, of evaluating toxicity and, ultimately, of providing an information base for developing intervention trials in humans. Models that permit evaluation of the effects of cancer-preventive agents on the occurrence of cancer in most major organ sites are available. Major groups of animal models include: those in which cancer is produced by the administration of chemical or physical carcinogens; those involving genetically engineered animals; and those in which tumours develop spontaneously. Most cancer-preventive agents investigated in such studies can be placed into one of three categories: compounds that prevent molecules from reaching or reacting with critical target sites (blocking agents); compounds that decrease the sensitivity of target tissues to carcinogenic stimuli; and compounds that prevent evolution of the neoplastic process (suppressing agents). There is increasing interest in the use of combinations of agents as a means of improving efficacy and minimizing toxicity. Animal models are useful in evaluating such combinations. The development of optimal strategies for human intervention trials can be facilitated by the use of animal models that mimic the neoplastic process in humans.

Specific factors to be considered in such experiments are: (1) the temporal requirements of administration of the cancer-preventive agents; (2) dose–response effects; (3) the site-specificity of cancer-preventive activity; and (4) the number and structural diversity of carcinogens whose activity can be reduced by the agent being evaluated.

An important variable in the evaluation of the cancer-preventive response is the time and the duration of administration of the agent or intervention in relation to any carcinogenic treatment, or in transgenic or other experimental models in which no carcinogen is administered. Furthermore, concurrent administration of a cancer-preventive agent may result in a decreased incidence of tumours in a given organ and an increase in another organ of the same animal. Thus, in these experiments it is important that multiple organs be examined.

For all these studies, the nature and extent of impurities or contaminants present in the cancer-preventive agent or agents being evaluated are given when available. For experimental studies of mixtures, consideration is given to the possibility of changes in the physico-chemical properties of the test substance during collection, storage, extraction, concentration and delivery. Chemical and toxicological interactions of the components of mixtures may result in nonlinear dose–response relationships.

As certain components of commonly used diets of experimental animals are themselves known to have cancer-preventive activity, particular consideration should be given to the interaction between the diet and the apparent effect of the agent or intervention being studied. Likewise, restriction of diet may be important. The appropriateness of the diet given relative to the composition of human diets may be commented on by the Working Group.

Qualitative aspects. An assessment of the experimental prevention of cancer involves several considerations of qualitative importance, including: (1) the experimental conditions under which the test was performed (route and schedule of exposure, species, strain, sex and age of animals studied, duration of the exposure, and duration of the study); (2) the consistency of the results, for example across species and target organ(s); (3) the stage or stages of the neoplastic process, from preneoplastic lesions and benign tumours to malignant neoplasms, studied and (4) the possible role of modifying factors.

Considerations of importance to the Working Group in the interpretation and evaluation of a particular study include: (1) how clearly the agent was defined and, in the case of mixtures, how adequately the sample composition was reported; (2) the composition of the diet and the stability of the agent in the diet; (3) whether the source, strain and quality of the animals was reported; (4) whether the dose and schedule of treatment with the known carcinogen were appropriate in assays of combined treatment; (5) whether the doses of the cancer-preventive agent were adequately monitored; (6) whether the agent(s) was absorbed, as shown by blood concentrations; (7) whether the survival of treated animals was similar to that of controls; (8) whether the body and organ weights of treated animals were similar to those of controls; (9) whether there were adequate numbers of animals, of appropriate age, per group; (10) whether animals of each sex were used, if appropriate; (11) whether animals were allocated randomly to groups; (12) whether appropriate respective controls were used; (13) whether the duration of the experiment was adequate; (14) whether there was adequate statistical analysis; and (15) whether the data were adequately reported. If available, recent data on the incidence of specific tumours in historical controls, as well as in concurrent controls, are taken into account in the evaluation of tumour response.

Quantitative aspects. The probability that tumours will occur may depend on the species, sex, strain and age of the animals, the dose of carcinogen (if any), the dose of the agent and the route and duration of exposure. A decreased incidence and/or decreased multiplicity of neoplasms in adequately designed studies provides evidence of a cancer-preventive effect. A dose-related decrease in incidence and/or multiplicity further strengthens this association.

Statistical analysis. Major factors considered in the statistical analysis by the Working Group include the adequacy of the data for each treatment group: (1) the initial and final effective numbers of animals studied and the survival rate; (2) body weights; and (3) tumour incidence and multiplicity. The statistical methods used should be clearly stated and should be the generally accepted techniques refined for this purpose. In particular, the statistical methods should be appropriate for the characteristics of the expected data distribution and should account for interactions in multifactorial studies. Consideration is given as to whether appropriate adjustment was made for differences in survival.

In-vitro models

Cell systems *in vitro* contribute to the early identification of potential cancer-preventive agents and to elucidation of mechanisms of cancer prevention. A number of assays in prokaryotic and eukaryotic systems are used for this purpose. Evaluation of the results of such assays includes consideration of: (1) the nature of the cell type used; (2) whether primary cell cultures or cell lines (tumorigenic or nontumorigenic) were studied; (3) the appropriateness of controls; (4) whether toxic effects were considered in the outcome; (5) whether the data were appropriately summated and analysed; (6) whether appropriate controls were used; (7) whether appropriate concentration ranges were used; (8) whether adequate numbers of independent measurements were made per group; and (9) the relevance of the end-points, including inhibition of mutagenesis, morphological transformation, anchorage-independent growth, cell–cell communication, calcium tolerance and differentiation.

Intermediate biomarkers

Other types of study include experiments in which the end-point is not cancer but a defined preneoplastic lesion or tumour-related intermediate biomarker.

The observation of effects on the occurrence of lesions presumed to be preneoplastic or the emergence of benign or malignant tumours may aid in assessing the mode of action of the presumed cancer-preventive agent or intervention. Particular attention is given to assessing the reversibility of these lesions and their predictive value in relation to cancer development.

Mechanisms of cancer prevention

Data on mechanisms can be derived from both human studies and experimental models. For a rational implementation of cancer preventive measures, it is essential not only to assess protective end-points but also to understand the mechanisms by which the agents or interventions exert their anticarcinogenic action. Information on the mechanisms of cancer-preventive activity can be inferred from relationships between chemical structure and biological activity, from analysis of interactions between agents and specific molecular targets, from studies of specific end-points *in vitro*, from studies of the inhibition of tumorigenesis *in vivo*, from the effects of modulating intermediate biomarkers, and from human studies. Therefore, the Working Group takes account of data on mechanisms in making the final evaluation of cancer prevention.

Several classifications of mechanisms have been proposed, as have several systems for evaluating them. Cancer-preventive agents may act at several distinct levels. Their action may be: (1) extracellular, for example, inhibiting the uptake or endogenous formation of carcinogens, or forming complexes with, diluting and/or deactivating carcinogens; (2) intracellular, for example, trapping carcinogens in non-target cells, modifying transmembrane transport, modulating metabolism, blocking reactive molecules, inhibiting cell replication or modulating gene expression or DNA metabolism; or (3) at the level of the cell, tissue or organism, for example, affecting cell differentiation, intercellular communication, proteases, signal transduction, growth factors, cell adhesion molecules, angiogenesis, interactions with the extracellular matrix, hormonal status and the immune system.

Many cancer-preventive agents are known or suspected to act by several mechanisms, which may operate in a coordinated manner and allow them a broader spectrum of anticarcinogenic activity. Therefore, multiple mechanisms of action are taken into account in the evaluation of cancer-prevention.

Beneficial interactions, generally resulting from exposure to inhibitors that work through complementary mechanisms, are exploited in combined cancer-prevention. Because organisms are naturally exposed not only to mixtures of carcinogenic agents but also to mixtures of protective agents, it is also important to understand the mechanisms of interactions between inhibitors.

Other beneficial effects

An expanded description is given, when appropriate, of the efficacy of the agent in the maintenance of a normal healthy state and the treatment of particular diseases. Information on the mechanisms involved in these activities is described. Reviews, rather than individual studies, may be cited as references.

The physiological functions of agents such as vitamins and micronutrients can be described briefly, with reference to reviews. Data on the therapeutic effects of drugs approved for clinical use are summarized.

Toxic effects

Toxic effects are of particular importance in the case of agents or interventions that may be used widely over long periods in healthy populations. Data are given on acute and chronic toxic effects, such as organ toxicity, increased cell proliferation, immunotoxicity and adverse endocrine effects. Some agents or interventions may have both carcinogenic and anticarcinogenic activities. If the agent has been evaluated within the *IARC Monographs on the Evaluation of Carcinogenic Risks to Humans*, that evaluation is accepted, unless significant new data have appeared that may lead the Working Group to reconsider the evidence. If the agent occurs naturally or has been in clinical use previously, the doses and durations used in cancer-prevention trials are compared with intakes from the diet, in the case of vitamins, and previous clinical exposure, in the case of drugs already approved for human use. When extensive data are available, only summaries are presented; if adequate reviews are available, reference may be made to these. If there are no relevant reviews, the evaluation is made on the basis of the same criteria as are applied to epidemiological studies of cancer. Differences in response as a consequence of species, sex, age and genetic variability are presented when the information is available.

Data demonstrating the presence or absence of adverse effects in humans are included; equally, lack of data on specific adverse effects is stated clearly.

Information is given on carcinogenicity, immunotoxicity, neurotoxicity, cardiotoxicity, haematological effects and toxicity to other target organs. Specific case reports in humans and any previous clinical data are noted. Other biochemical effects thought to be relevant to adverse effects are mentioned.

The results of studies of genetic and related effects in mammalian and non-mammalian systems *in vivo* and *in vitro* are summarized. Information on whether DNA damage occurs via direct interaction with the agent or via indirect mechanisms (e.g. generation of free radicals) is included, as is information on other genetic effects such as mutation, recombination, chromosomal damage, aneuploidy, cell immortalization and transformation, and effects on cell–cell communication. The presence and toxicological significance of cellular receptors for the cancer-preventive agent are described.

Structure–activity relationships that may be relevant to the evaluation of the toxicity of an agent are described.

Summary of data

In this section, the relevant human and experimental data are summarized. Inadequate studies are generally not included but are identified in the preceding text.

Evaluation

Evaluations of the strength of the evidence for cancer-preventive activity and carcinogenic effects from studies in humans and experimental models are made, using standard terms. These terms may also be applied to other beneficial and adverse effects, when indicated. When appropriate, reference is made to specific organs and populations.

It is recognized that the criteria for these evaluation categories, described below, cannot encompass all factors that may be relevant to an evaluation of cancer-preventive activity. In considering all the relevant scientific data, the Working Group may assign the agent or intervention to a higher or lower category than a strict interpretation of these criteria would indicate.

Cancer-preventive activity

The evaluation categories refer to the strength of the evidence that an agent or intervention prevents cancer. The evaluations may change as new information becomes available.

Evaluations are inevitably limited to the cancer sites, conditions and levels of exposure and length of observation covered by the available studies. An evaluation of degree of evidence, whether for an agent or intervention, is limited to the materials tested, as defined physically, chemically or biologically, or to the intensity or frequency of an intervention. When agents are considered by the Working Group to be sufficiently closely related, they may be grouped for the purpose of a single evaluation of degree of evidence.

Information on mechanisms of action is taken into account when evaluating the strength of evidence in humans and in experimental animals, as well as in assessing the consistency of results between studies in humans and experimental models.

Cancer-preventive activity in humans

The evidence relevant to cancer prevention in humans is classified into one of the following categories.

- *Sufficient evidence of cancer-preventive activity*

The Working Group considers that a causal relationship has been established between use of the agent or intervention and the prevention of human cancer in studies in which chance, bias and confounding could be ruled out with reasonable confidence.

- *Limited evidence of cancer-preventive activity*

The data suggest a reduced risk for cancer with use of the agent or intervention but are limited for making a definitive evaluation either because chance, bias or confounding could not be ruled out with reasonable confidence or because the data are restricted to intermediary biomarkers of uncertain validity in the putative pathway to cancer.

- *Inadequate evidence of cancer-preventive activity*

The available studies are of insufficient quality, consistency or statistical power to permit a conclusion regarding a cancer-preventive effect of the agent or intervention, or no data on the prevention of cancer in humans are available

- *Evidence suggesting lack of cancer-preventive activity*

Several adequate studies of use or exposure to the agent or intervention are mutually consistent in not showing a preventive effect.

The strength of the evidence for any carcinogenic effect is assessed in parallel.

Both cancer-preventive activity and carcinogenic effects are identified and, when appropriate, tabulated by organ site. The evaluation also cites the population subgroups concerned, specifying age, sex, genetic or environmental predisposing risk factors and the relevance of precancerous lesions.

Cancer-preventive activity in experimental animals

Evidence for cancer prevention in experimental animals is classified into one of the following categories.

- *Sufficient evidence of cancer-preventive activity*

The Working Group considers that a causal relationship has been established between the agent or intervention and a decreased incidence and/or multiplicity of neoplasms.

- *Limited evidence of cancer-preventive activity*

The data suggest a cancer-preventive effect but are limited for making a definitive evaluation because, for example, the evidence of cancer prevention is restricted to a single experiment, the agent or intervention decreases the incidence and/or multiplicity only of benign neoplasms or lesions of uncertain neoplastic potential or there is conflicting evidence.

- *Inadequate evidence of cancer-preventive activity*

The studies cannot be interpreted as showing either the presence or absence of a preventive effect because of major or quantitative limitations (unresolved questions regarding the adequacy of the design, conduct or interpretation of the study), or no data on cancer prevention in experimental animals are available.

- *Evidence suggesting lack of cancer-preventive activity*

Adequate evidence from conclusive studies in several models shows that, within the limits of the tests used, the agent or intervention does not prevent cancer.

Overall evaluation

Finally, the body of evidence is considered as a whole, and summary statements are made that emcompass the effects of the agent or intervention in humans with regard to cancer-preventive activity and other beneficial effects or adverse effects, as appropriate.

Recommendations

During the evaluation process, it is likely that opportunities for further research will be identified. These are clearly stated, with the understanding that the areas are recommended for future investigation. It is made clear that these research opportunities are identified in general terms on the basis of the data currently available.

Recommendations for public health action are listed, based on the analysis of the existing scientific data.

Available in the same series:

IARC Handbooks of Cancer Prevention:

Volume 1   Non-Steroidal Anti-inflammatory Drugs (NSAIDs)
Volume 2   Carotenoids
Volume 3   Vitamin A
Volume 4   Retinoids
Volume 5   Sunscreens
Volume 6   Weight Control and Physical Activity
Volume 7   Breast Cancer Screening

These books can be ordered from:

IARC*Press*	IARC*Press*	Oxford University Press
150 Cours Albert Thomas	WHO Office	Walton Street
69372 Lyon cedex 08	Suite 480	Oxford OX2 6DP
France	1775 K Street	UK
Fax.: + 33 4 72 73 83 02	Washington DC 20006	Fax.: + 44 1865 267782
	USA	
	Fax.: + 1 202 223 1782	